Principles and Practice of Regional Anaesthesia

Wildsmith & Armitage's
Principles and Practice of Regional Anaesthesia

FOURTH EDITION

Edited by

Graeme A. McLeod, MD MRCGP FRCA FFPMRCA
Consultant & Clinical Reader in Anaesthesia
Ninewells Hospital & Medical School, Dundee, UK

Colin J. L. McCartney, MBChB FCARCSI FRCA FRCPC
Staff Anesthesiologist & Associate Professor
Sunnybrook Health Sciences Centre & University of Toronto, Ontario, Canada

J. A. W. Wildsmith, MD FRCA FRCPEd FRCSEd FDSRCSEng
Emeritus Professor of Anaesthesia
University of Dundee, Dundee, UK

Illustrated by
Patrick Elliott
BSc(Hons) ATC MMAA RMIP

Photographs by
Ken Crowe

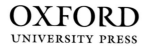

OXFORD
UNIVERSITY PRESS

OXFORD
UNIVERSITY PRESS

Great Clarendon Street, Oxford, OX2 6DP,
United Kingdom

Oxford University Press is a department of the University of Oxford.
It furthers the University's objective of excellence in research, scholarship,
and education by publishing worldwide. Oxford is a registered trade mark of
Oxford University Press in the UK and in certain other countries

First Edition published in 1987 © Longman Group
Second Edition published in 1993 © Churchill Livingstone
Third Edition published in 2003 © Elsevier Science Limited
Fourth Edition published in 2013 © Oxford University Press

Impression: 1

British Library Cataloguing in Publication Data

Data available

Library of Congress Cataloguing in Publication Data

Library of Congress Control Number: 2012937864

ISBN 978-0-19-958669-1

Printed in China
C&C Offset Printing Co., Ltd.

This book is dedicated to the memory of
Edward N Armitage: MBBS DObsRCOG FRCA 1935–2009

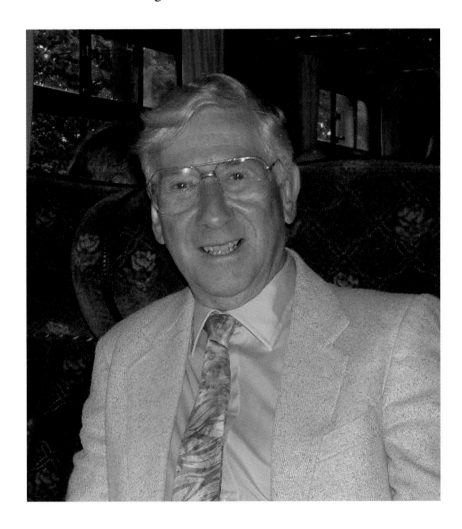

'No system of analgesia will yield its full potential unless it is targeted at prevention rather than relief. The continued use of the term 'pain relief' is probably doing more than anything else to retard progress in this field.'

Foreword

The modern concept of detailed anaesthesia monographs dedicated to various aspects of our speciality really began in the United Kingdom with the first edition of this book in 1987. Tony Wildsmith and Edward Armitage had the then unique concept of writing a clinical text purely about regional anaesthetic techniques, and what an original idea it was! At only 200 pages, and essentially with a practical bias, its spacious, attractive layout made it an instant success with all grades of anaesthetist. The popularity of subsequent editions never waned and now it has an international reputation as a reference textbook on regional block. What is more, its style became so popular that it set a trend for a multiplicity of monographs on other areas of anaesthetic practice.

The original editorial pairing of an academic interested in local anaesthetic pharmacology and central neuraxial blocks (Wildsmith), and an NHS consultant interested in paediatric anaesthesia and postoperative analgesia (Armitage) was an ideal combination. Well known and greatly respected by me in their different roles each had, in his own way and area of practice, the essential qualities of good authorship: clarity of thought; vision; and meticulous attention to detail. These characteristics, together with their considerable work ethic, were the sure foundations for the book's success. For the third, enlarged edition they were joined by a third editor, John McClure, a teaching hospital consultant with extensive experience of obstetric anaesthesia and local anaesthetic clinical research.

For this fourth edition, there has been significant editorial change as a consequence of the untimely death of Edward Armitage, the retirement from clinical practice of the other two editors, and the need for the book to continue to develop. Tony Wildsmith provides continuity, but he has been joined by two younger editors, Graeme McLeod and Colin McCartney, who bring other expertise, notably in major peripheral nerve block techniques and the use of ultrasound guidance. This latest edition has been updated and expanded to include these and all other new developments: it could not be more comprehensive. The original authorship was entirely British, but the addition of an editor and several authors based overseas will ensure that the text's international standing will only increase as it keeps pace with modern developments in our speciality.

However, the book still has a predominantly Scottish flavour (with a picture of Sir James Young Simpson on the first page). This is apposite as there have never been better human anatomists anywhere in the world than in Scotland, and this book gives all the relevant anatomical details required for good regional anaesthesia practice. This is well seen in the detailed diagrams and figures which I have always appreciated and which improve with every edition; what other book tells you in a figure legend which foot to maintain one's balance on during a regional technique (page 141)?

This, the fourth edition of *Principles and Practice of Regional Anaesthesia*, is the first to be published by Oxford University Press, so it joins the prestigious Oxford Medical Textbook stable. I am confident that it will continue to be the mainstay of regional anaesthetic practice for generations to come, serving as an excellent teaching aid for trainees and consultants alike.

Finally, I wish to congratulate Professor Wildsmith heartily on his massive contribution to regional anaesthesia over his professional lifetime. This text and will be a lasting legacy to his academic work. I wish his new editors every success and urge them, for the sake of our speciality, to continue this pivotal contribution to regional anaesthetic practice in the future.

Jennifer M Hunter, University of Liverpool, UK

Preface

To be introducing a fourth edition of *Principles and Practice of Regional Anaesthesia* is a matter of some quiet satisfaction, albeit tinged with the sadness that my original co-editor, Edward Armitage, is no longer with us to celebrate the event. We first met at the founding meeting of the European Society of Regional Anaesthesia in Edinburgh, exactly 30 years ago in 1982, and quickly found that we shared many views on regional anaesthesia, including the need for a British book to meet British conditions. Edward brought to our collaboration his dry Yorkshire humour, an erudition born of *not* having studied science in the sixth form at school, and particular expertise in the use of postoperative epidural analgesia and, above all, in paediatric anaesthesia. A fairly long-distance (Scotland–Sussex) collaboration turned into a long-lasting friendship, and I still find myself reaching for the telephone when searching for the right form of words.

One of the principles which Edward was adamant should apply to producing this book was that those no longer practising regional anaesthesia (through retirement or change of interest) should soon stop writing about it. Thus, he indicated, once the third edition was complete, that he would make no contribution in this one, but I am pleased that he did discuss with me (and approve) the proposed new editors: Graeme McLeod and Colin McCartney. They bring considerable clinical, academic, and literary experience to the project, and have particular interest in two areas of considerable development over the last decade: the wider use of major peripheral nerve blocks and the introduction of ultrasound guidance for nerve localization.

Ultrasound guidance is an exciting development, and it has driven a welcome increase in the interest in, and use of, regional anaesthesia. However, it does not, as some seem to believe, negate the need for anatomical knowledge and technical skills, although it does change the emphasis of both. Its use has been incorporated into all of the relevant chapters, but primarily as an *addition* to the armamentarium, not as an alternative to what went before. Apart from anything else, the development of ultrasound for regional anaesthesia is still very much work in progress, particularly because current equipment was designed for diagnostic use, not the performance of invasive procedures. Further, it will never change the need for thoughtful patient assessment and block selection, for understanding of the relevant physiology and pharmacology, and for skills in patient management before, during, and after block performance.

Thus the aim of the book remains as it ever was: to help the specialist anaesthetist learn about, and understand, the use of regional anaesthesia. The book is divided into two parts: the first outlines the general principles of safe, effective practice; and the second describes anatomy, techniques, and their application in some of the main clinical areas. Some topics are mentioned in both parts to allow each chapter to stand alone, but we have tried to avoid too much repetition by providing the necessary cross references. Recommendations for local anaesthetic doses for particular blocks should really be in milligrams, but long standing practice is to state a definitive volume of a specified percentage so we have followed that standard, although occasionally stated the milligram dose when it is really crucial. It is a pleasure to welcome adrenaline back to the fold for this edition, but it seems that lidocaine is here to stay!

No attempt has been made to describe every known block, but only those which our authors find useful in their, predominantly British, clinical practice. Few anaesthetists, if any, can expect to master the whole range of regional techniques to a level at which they can instruct others so the expertise of our many authors is vital. However, each chapter has been subject to detailed editorial review to try and produce a cohesive literary style, and all the illustrations were prepared by the same artist, photographer, or sonographer to ensure consistency of appearance as well.

However, regional anaesthesia is an intensely practical aspect of our specialty and any book has to be supplemented by clinical training and graded experience of the various techniques. Even knowledge of anatomy should be supplemented by visits to the dissecting room and by asking surgical colleagues to demonstrate relevant structures exposed during surgery. Now, theoretical and practical training in ultrasound is needed also, and *before* it is used clinically. It is only when all the knowledge and skills have been acquired, and are applied with much attention to detail, that regional anaesthesia can deliver its potential to make patient care better. As I follow Dr Armitage's example and retire from future involvement I trust that this will always be the aim.

Tony Wildsmith

Acknowledgements

Previous editions of this book were well received, and this new one is built firmly on their foundations, so we must acknowledge those who have contributed in the past. Particular thanks are due to John McClure, who was a co-editor for the third edition, and to Bill Macrae, Vaughan Martin, Tony Rubin, and the late Ed Charlton, who were not only long-term contributors, but also, from the beginning, great supporters of the aims of the project.

Producing a book with full colour illustrations is an expensive exercise, and some form of sponsorship is essential if the cover price is to be kept at a realistic level. Thus special thanks are due to Philips Healthcare for an educational grant, and also for lending an ultrasound scanner so that all the sonograms could be produced from the same source. This enabled us to maintain consistency of appearance, paralleling the excellent results achieved by having Ken Crowe and Patrick Elliott produce all the photographs and drawings over the four editions.

We would like to thank Oxford University Press for publishing this edition in the Oxford Textbooks in Anaesthesia series. We thank Christopher Reid for taking us on, Fiona Richardson for her support, and Tessa Eaton for seeing it through to production.

Illustrations set in the clinical setting must be obtained there, and we thank patients and staff in Ninewells Hospital, Dundee and Sunnybrook Health Sciences Centre, Toronto for their collaboration in obtaining these. We also thank Sherif Abbas MD for his assistance in formatting the sonograms ready for publication.

Last, but not least, we thank our families for their support during the editorial process.

Graeme McLeod
Colin McCartney
Tony Wildsmith

Contents

Abbreviations

AMPA	amino-3-hydroxy-5-methylisoxazole-4-propionic acid		LDCV	large dense-core vesicle
APTT	activated partial thromboplastin time		LIA	local infiltration analgesia
ATP	adenosine triphosphate		LMWH	low-molecular-weight heparin
BMI	body mass index		mcg	microgram/s
CAE	carotid endarterectomy		MEGX	monoethylglycinexylidide
CAT	computerized axial tomography		mGluR	metabotropic glutamate receptor
CES	cauda equina syndrome		mg	milligram/s
CIEA	continuous infusion epidural analgesia		ml	millilitre/s
CNS	central nervous system		MRI	magnetic resonance imaging
CRPS	complex regional pain syndrome		MS	multiple sclerosis
CSA	continuous spinal anaesthesia		NMDA	N-methyl-D-aspartate
CSE	combined spinal–epidural		NSAID	non-steroidal anti-inflammatory drug
CSEA	combined spinal–epidural analgesia		OP	occipitoposterior
CSF	cerebrospinal fluid		PAG	periaqueductal grey
CT	computed tomography		PCEA	patient-controlled epidural analgesia
ECG	electrocardiogram		PDPH	postdural puncture headache
EMLA	eutectic mixture of local anaesthetics		PNS	peripheral nerve stimulator *or* peripheral nervous system
GABA	γ-amino-butyric acid		PONV	postoperative nausea & vomiting
GX	glycinexylidide		PPX	pipecolylxylidide
h	hour/s		SG	specific gravity
IL	interleukin		STT	spinothalamic tract
INR	international normalized ratio		TAP	transversus abdominis plane
IVRA	intravenous regional anaesthesia		TNS	transient neurological symptoms
IVRSB	intravenous regional sympathetic block		VAS	visual analogue scale
l	litre/s			

Contributors

Nigel M Bedforth BMBS BMedSci FRCA
Consultant Anaesthetist & Honorary Special Lecturer
Queen's Medical Centre Campus, Nottingham, UK

W Alastair Chambers MD MEd FRCA FRCPEd
Consultant & Honorary Professor of Anaesthesia
Aberdeen Royal Infirmary, Aberdeen, UK

Matthew R Checketts MBChB FRCA
Consultant Anaesthetist
Ninewells Hospital & Medical School, Dundee, UK

Lesley A Colvin BSc MBChB PhD FRCA FFPMRCA
Consultant in Anaesthesia & Pain Medicine
Western General Hospital, Edinburgh, UK

Catriona Connolly MBChB FRCA
Consultant Anaesthetist
Ninewells Hospital & Medical School, Dundee, UK

George A Corner PhD
Professor & Head of Instrumentation
Department of Medical Physics
Ninewells Hospital & Medical School, Dundee, UK

David M Coventry MBChB FRCA
Consultant Anaesthetist
Ninewells Hospital & Medical School, Dundee, UK

Edward Doyle MD FRCA
Consultant Paediatric Anaesthetist
Royal Hospital for Sick Children, Edinburgh, UK

H Barrie J Fischer MBChB FRCA
Consultant Anaesthetist
The Alexandra Hospital, Redditch, UK

Andreas Goebel PhD MSc FRCA
Senior Lecturer in Pain Medicine
University of Liverpool, Liverpool UK

Calum Grant MBChB FRCA
Consultant Anaesthetist
Ninewells Hospital & Medical School, Dundee, UK

Stuart A Grant MBChB FRCA
Professor of Anesthesiology
Duke University Medical Center, Durham, NC, USA

Jonathan G Hardman BMedSci(Hons) BMBS DM FANZCA FRCA
Professor of Anaesthesia
University of Nottingham, Nottingham, UK

Dominic Harmon MD FCARCSI
Professor of Anaesthesia & Consultant in Pain Medicine
Mid-Western Regional Hospitals & University of Limerick, Ireland

Stephen Hickey MBChB FRCA
Consultant & Honorary Senior Lecturer in Anaesthesia
Glasgow Royal Infirmary, Glasgow, UK

Colin J L McCartney MBChB FCARCSI FRCA FRCPC
Staff Anesthesiologist & Associate Professor
Sunnybrook Health Sciences Centre & University of Toronto, Ontario, Canada

John H McClure BSc(Hons) MBChB FRCA
Retired Consultant Anaesthetist
The Royal Infirmary, Edinburgh, UK

Jonathan McCormack MBChB MRCP FRCA
Consultant in Paediatric Anaesthesia & Intensive Care Retrieval
Royal Hospital for Sick Children, Edinburgh, UK

John G McDonnell MBChB FCARCSI
Consultant Anaesthetist
Galway University Hospitals & National University of Ireland, Galway, Eire

Graeme A McLeod MD MRCGP FRCA FFPMRCA
Consultant & Clinical Reader in Anaesthesia
Ninewells Hospital & Medical School, Dundee, UK

Hamish McLure MBChB FRCA
Consultant Anaesthetist
St James's University Teaching Hospital, Leeds, UK

Alastair F Nimmo MBChB FRCA FFPMRCA
Consultant & Honorary Clinical Senior Lecturer in Anaesthesia
The Royal Infirmary, Edinburgh, UK

Susan M Nimmo BSc(Hons) MBChB(Hons) MRCP FRCA
Consultant & Honorary Clinical Senior Lecturer in Anaesthesia
Western General Hospital, Edinburgh, UK

Ian G Parkin MBChB
Professor of Applied Clinical Anatomy
Ninewells Hospital & Medical School, Dundee, UK

Jennifer M Porter MD FCARCSI
Consultant Anaesthetist
St James's Hospital, Dublin, Eire

Stephen Roberts MBChB FRCA(Hons)
Consultant Paediatric Anaesthetist
Alder Hey Children's NHS Foundation Trust, Liverpool, UK

Nicholas B Scott MBChB FFARCSI FRCSEd
Lead Clinician for Pain Services
Golden Jubilee National Hospital, Clydebank, UK

Michael G Serpell MBChB FRCA FFPMRCA
Consultant & Senior Lecturer in Anaesthesia
Gartnavel General Hospital, Glasgow, UK

Neil G Smart BSc(Hons) MBChB FFARCSI
Consultant & Honorary Senior Lecturer in Anaesthesia
Victoria Infirmary, Glasgow, UK

Gary R Strichartz BS AM(Hons) PhD
Professor of Anesthesia (Pharmacology)
Brigham & Women's Hospital, Boston, MA, USA

Geoffrey T Tucker BPharm PhD FRCPEd FRCA FFPM
Emeritus Professor of Clinical Pharmacology
University of Sheffield, Sheffield, UK

Bernadette Th Veering MD PhD
Staff Anaesthesiologist
Leiden University Medical Centre, Leiden, The Netherlands

Cameron J Weir BSc(Hons) MBChB FRCA PhD
Consultant Anaesthetist & Honorary Clinical Senior Lecturer
Ninewells Hospital & Medical School, Dundee, UK

Jonathan B Whiteside MBChB FRCA
Consultant Anaesthetist
Raigmore Hospital, Inverness, UK

J A W Wildsmith MD FRCA FRCPEd FRCSEd FDSRCSEng
Emeritus Professor of Anaesthesia
University of Dundee, Dundee, UK

PART 1

General principles

CHAPTER 1

History and development of local anaesthesia

Tony Wildsmith

The first steps

The possible production of local anaesthesia by this or by other means, is certainly an object well worthy of study and attainment. Surgeons everywhere seem more and more acknowledging the facility, certainty, and safety with which the state of general anaesthesia can be produced at will before operating, as well as the moral and professional necessity of saving their patients from all requisite pain. But if we could by any means induce a local anaesthesia, without that temporary absence of consciousness, which is found in the state of general anaesthesia, many would regard it as a still greater improvement in this branch of practice. If a man, for instance, could have his hand so obtunded that he could see, but not feel, the performance of amputation upon his own fingers, the practice of anaesthesia in surgery would, in all likelihood, advance and progress even still more rapidly than it has done.

This striking commentary was published by James Young Simpson (Figure 1.1) in 1848, decades before local anaesthesia became a practical possibility, and his paper describes his (unsuccessful) experiments with the topical application of various liquids and vapours (Simpson 1848). Because it was published less than 2 years after Oliver Wendell Holmes had suggested the word 'anaesthesia' to William Morton, it probably represents the first use of the term 'local anaesthesia'. However, Simpson was aware that his were far from being the first attempts to produce peripheral insensibility because the paper refers to some ancient methods (which he considered 'apocryphal') and to Moore's method of nerve compression (Figure 1.2) which had been used with some success towards the end of the 18th century.

In direct response to Simpson's paper James Arnott proposed that cold, produced by the application of ice and salt mixtures, would be effective, but his technique was rather cumbersome (Bird 1949). Another eminent Victorian interested in producing local anaesthesia was Benjamin Ward Richardson (Figure 1.3) who experimented with electricity before trying the effect of cold (Richardson 1866). As with nerve compression, reports of the numbing effect of cold go back to antiquity, the best known being by Napoleon's surgeon, Baron Larrey. Richardson's work culminated in the introduction of the ether spray (Figure 1.4), which worked by evaporation and was the only practical method of local anaesthesia until the local action of cocaine was fully appreciated. Ethyl chloride supplanted ether as the cooling agent after 1880.

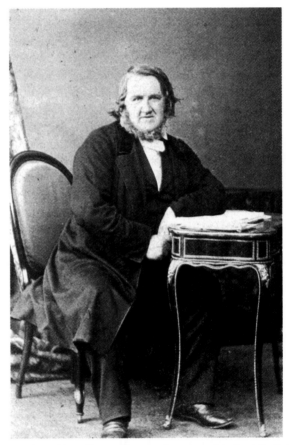

Figure 1.1 James Young Simpson. Photograph courtesy of the Royal Medical Society.

The development of the hypodermic syringe and needle was an important prerequisite for local anaesthesia by injection, but these items evolved over many years so their introduction cannot be ascribed to any one person. However, Alexander Wood (Figure 1.5), an Edinburgh contemporary of Simpson, was, in 1853, the first to combine them for hypodermic medication (Figure 1.6). Wood was

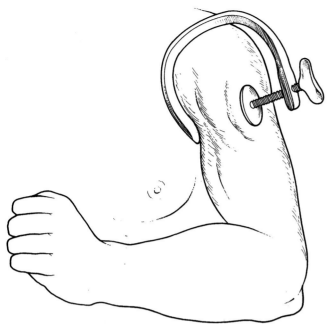

Figure 1.2 James Moore's method of nerve compression.

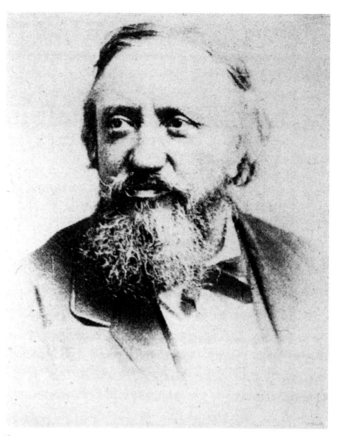

Figure 1.3 Benjamin Ward Richardson. Photograph from Disciples of Aesculapius.

interested in the treatment of neuralgia and he reasoned that morphine might be more effective if it were injected close to the nerve supplying the affected area (Wood 1855). Although morphine may have some peripheral actions, the effect of Wood's morphine was probably central, but he was nevertheless the first to think of the possibility of producing nerve block by drug injection and he has been called the 'father-in-lore' of local anaesthesia—all he lacked was an agent which worked locally.

The introduction of cocaine

The events leading to the introduction of cocaine, the alkaloid in the leaves of *Erythroxylon coca*, into clinical practice began shortly after Wood's experiments with local morphine injection. Sporadic reports of the systemic effects of chewing the leaves had reached Europe from the time of the Spanish conquest, but it was not until 1857 that Montegazza gave the first detailed description of these actions. Prior to that, Gaedke had extracted some reddish crystals, but it was Niemann in 1860 who produced pure white crystals

which he named cocaine. Niemann noted that these crystals produced numbness of the tongue, an observation subsequently confirmed by several other workers. Alexander Hughes Bennett was the first to demonstrate (in animals) that injection of cocaine produces sensory block, but, as with the work of others, the significance of his observation was not appreciated (Wildsmith 1983).

During this time cocaine came to be looked upon as a universal panacea and was even used to treat morphine addiction. This latter use attracted the attention of Sigmund Freud, who reviewed the literature and started a programme of research on the drug's systemic effects. In this he was assisted by his friend Carl Koller (Figure 1.7),

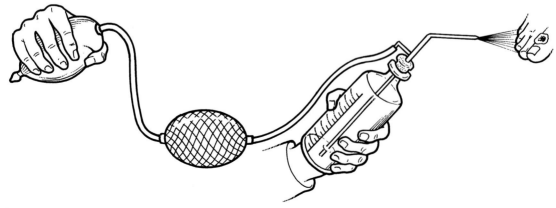

Figure 1.4 Richardson's ether spray.

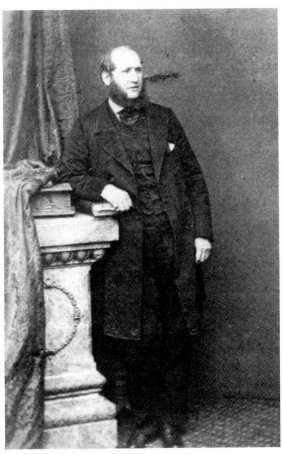

Figure 1.5 Alexander Wood. Photograph courtesy of the Royal Medical Society.

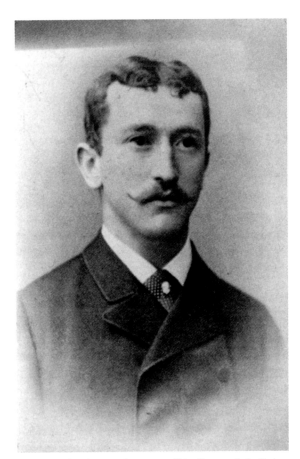

Figure 1.7 Carl Koller. Photograph courtesy of Mrs Hortense Koller Becker.

another young graduate of the Vienna medical school also working part-time in Stricker's research laboratories. Koller hoped to become an ophthalmologist and, having heard from his teacher—Ferdinand Arlt—of the disadvantages of general anaesthesia for eye surgery, he had applied a variety of agents to the conjunctiva without success (Wildsmith 1984). However, not even Koller appreciated the significance of the reports of local insensibility until a chance comment from a colleague made him realize that he had in his possession the local anaesthetic agent for which he had been searching (Becker 1963). Experiments, firstly with animals, then on himself and colleagues, led on to clinical trials during the summer of 1884. A preliminary communication was read (by a colleague—Joseph Brettaur—because Koller could not afford the trip) at the Heidelberg meeting of the German Ophthalmological Society on 15 September 1884, and from there the news spread with amazing speed.

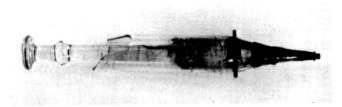

Figure 1.6 Syringe devised by Wood. Photograph courtesy of the Royal College of Surgeons of Edinburgh.

Immediate developments

The full account of his work (Koller 1884) appeared shortly after, and many others reported their experience before the end of the year. Although there is evidence (Faulconer & Keys 1965) that William Burke may have absolute priority for the first nerve block (performed before the end of November 1884), credit is usually given to William Halsted and Richard Hall of New York. Before the end of 1885 they had blocked virtually every peripheral somatic nerve, including the brachial plexus, and had demonstrated the effectiveness of such methods (Boulton 1984).

Central neural block may be considered to have been performed almost as early. We will never know for certain whether the New York neurologist, Leonard Corning, produced epidural or subarachnoid block in 1885, but there is no doubt that at that early stage he deliberately injected cocaine between the posterior spinous processes of both a dog and a patient and produced block of the lower half of the body. Although he suggested that it might be used in surgery, no further development took place until the end of the century. In 1891, Quincke in Kiel, Germany, showed that lumbar puncture was a practical procedure, and it was in the same centre that August Bier performed the first spinal blocks for surgery in 1898. However, Bier abandoned the technique before he had gained much experience with it, and it was Tuffier, working independently in Paris, who was responsible for popularizing the method in Europe. In the USA Tait, Caglieri, and Matas were the early pioneers.

Pharmacological advances

The major factor in Bier's decision to abandon spinal anaesthesia was the toxicity of cocaine. It was also difficult to sterilize, brief in duration, and had exacted a terrible price from pioneers like Halsted and Hall who became addicted to it as a result of self-experimentation. Because of these factors the early use of cocaine was largely limited to topical application. Later, Schleich in Germany and Reclus in France developed safe dose regimens for, and popularized, infiltration anaesthesia. Braun increased its duration and reduced its toxicity, first by the use of a tourniquet and later by adding adrenaline to the solution.

However, widespread use of local methods had to await the introduction of safer drugs. Niemann, in his pioneer work, had hydrolysed benzoic acid from cocaine and it was the search for other benzoic acid esters that produced new local anaesthetics. Amylocaine (Stovaine) was introduced in 1903 and was popular for spinal anaesthesia until it was shown to be irritant, but it was the development of procaine by Einhorn in 1904 that was the really significant advance. Its low toxicity, lack of addictive properties, and relative stability ensured its popularity for the techniques already in use, and made feasible the development of new ones for which larger doses of drug were required.

Procaine is still far from ideal because it hydrolyses when heated in solution, has a short duration of action, and may induce allergic reactions. Many agents were tried, but the only others to become well established were amethocaine and cinchocaine. Both are potent and toxic, but were well suited to spinal anaesthesia for which they became widely used. Chloroprocaine is the only ester-type drug to be developed successfully in more recent times, but even it is of relatively limited availability. The 1930s saw the start of the next major advance. Trying to synthetize the alkaloid gramine, Erdtman, a Swedish chemist believing in the importance of the senses in analysis, tasted one of the substances which had been produced. The significance of the ensuing numbness was appreciated and the search for a clinically useful derivative was pursued by Nils Lofgren, who synthesized lidocaine in 1943. Perhaps almost as important was Lofgren's systematic study of a whole range of compounds (Lofgren 1948), so laying the foundations for all subsequent studies of local anaesthetic drugs. From these studies have come derivatives of lidocaine such as mepivacaine, prilocaine, bupivacaine, and ropivacaine.

While the introduction of these agents has considerably widened the scope of local anaesthesia, they are essentially variations on a theme. Since the development of lidocaine the most important work has been in the field of membrane physiology. Many workers have contributed to this, the most notable being Hodgkin and Huxley. Use of apparatus such as the voltage clamp has produced major advances in our knowledge of the mechanism of nerve conduction and its block by drugs at the molecular level. This has yet to lead to the development of new drugs, but the research continues to examine ever more detailed aspects of the transmission of nerve impulses (see Chapter 6).

Concurrent studies of the pharmacokinetics of local anaesthetic drugs have made a more practical contribution to our knowledge because they have indicated the most appropriate doses and agents for the various techniques. They have thus played an important part in basing clinical local anaesthesia on sound scientific principles.

In more recent years, pharmaceutical research has led to the development of novel ways of delivering local anaesthetics. The first local anaesthetic preparation to be effective on application to intact skin (EMLA—the eutectic mixture of local anaesthetics) is a classic example, and depot preparations (such as liposomal local anaesthetics) continue to be evaluated.

Developments in technique

As has been mentioned, most local techniques had been described by 1900, even if they were not widely used. In 1906, Sellheim introduced paravertebral and intercostal block, and 2 years later Bier, taking advantage of the low toxicity of procaine, developed his technique of intravenous regional anaesthesia. Another important development at this time was Barker's description of the way in which the curves of the lumbar spine and gravity interact to affect the spread of intrathecally injected solutions. Epidural block is very much a product of the 20th century. The sacral approach, described independently by Sicard and Cathelin in 1901, was used by Stoeckel for analgesia during vaginal delivery in 1909. The lumbar approach was first described by Pages in Spain in 1921, but he died soon afterwards and the technique was 'rediscovered' and popularized by Dogliotti in Italy a decade later. The lumbar approach was first used in labour in 1938 by Graffagnino and Seyler, and Massey Dawkins performed the first epidural in Britain in 1942.

Most other subsequent advances in technique may be looked upon as being refinements or rediscoveries of techniques which had been described previously. This is not to deny the importance of these later authors because they did a great deal to improve and popularize the practice of local anaesthesia. One important technical development which does deserve specific mention is the introduction of catheter methods. Continuous spinal anaesthesia was introduced in the USA in 1940 by Lemmon who left the spinal needle *in situ* (projecting through a gap in the operating table) and connected it to a length of rubber tubing for the repeat injections. In 1945, Tuohy described his needle for the insertion of a catheter into the subarachnoid space, and in 1949 Curbelo adapted it for lumbar epidural block, although the first continuous epidural blocks are attributed to Hingson and Edwards who used the caudal route in 1942.

The popularity and use of local anaesthesia

Ever since Koller's original work, the popularity of local anaesthesia has waxed and waned, like that of many other medical developments. The announcement of his work produced a massive wave of enthusiasm, which was tempered as the problems of cocaine became appreciated. The first resurgence of interest came with the introduction of safer drugs at the beginning of the century, and the second as a result of the efforts of Labat, Lundy, Maxson, Odom, and Pitkin in the USA in the years between the two world wars.

In Britain at the same time, general anaesthesia was preferred, perhaps because it was usually administered by doctors who, though rarely specialists, were entirely responsible for its conduct and achieved acceptable standards. By contrast, local and regional techniques, if they were used at all, were performed by the surgeon, whose interest and attention were divided between anaesthetic and operation so that the methods were not seen to best advantage. Nevertheless, when the examination for the Diploma in Anaesthesia was instituted in 1935, the curriculum included local techniques. This, together with the establishment of anaesthesia as an independent speciality within the British National Health Service in 1948, did much to encourage use of the methods.

Unfortunately, the years between 1950 and 1955 saw a sharp decrease in the use of local, particularly spinal, anaesthesia in Britain. The many contemporary advances in general anaesthesia were partly responsible because they encouraged the belief that a local technique was unnecessary, but more important was the fear of severe neurological damage. The 1950 report 'The grave spinal cord paralyses caused by spinal anesthesia' by a British-trained New York neurologist, Foster Kennedy (Kennedy et al. 1950), was followed by the Woolley and Roe case (Cope 1954, Hutter 1990), and the use of local anaesthesia all but died out. That it did not do so entirely was due to anaesthetists such as Macintosh, Gillies, Dawkins, Doughty, Lee, and Scott who were prepared to advocate, use, and teach local techniques, and to encourage formal research into their features. Subsequently, many reports appeared describing very large numbers of cases without neurological sequelae, and local anaesthesia became re-established in British practice during the 1980s, although concerns about sequelae have persisted, particularly in patients receiving antithrombotic drugs.

There were more positive influences. The advantages of lidocaine and its derivatives—potent, predictable, heat-resistant, and virtually free of allergic side effects—should not be underestimated. The introduction of bupivacaine was particularly important because its long duration of action allows repeated injection with relatively little risk of cumulative toxicity. This was a major factor in the increased use of continuous epidural techniques in labour where local techniques are very appropriate because they are effective and exert minimal effects on the child. Anaesthetists observing these benefits were encouraged to try them in other areas, especially as they became aware that general anaesthesia cannot provide the ideal answer to every anaesthetic problem. The formation of the American (1975) and European (1982) Societies of Regional Anaesthesia were important in providing platforms where clinicians could hear the issues debated and obtain the necessary theoretical education.

Regional techniques are of value in blocking afferent stimuli after any type of surgery, reducing both the pain and stress suffered by the patient, with the approach even extending today to cardiac surgery, but the concept is far from new. As early as 1902, Harvey Cushing was advocating the combination of local with general anaesthesia to reduce surgical 'shock', a concept which was developed by Crile into 'anoci-association'. The term 'balanced anaesthesia' often implies the triad of sleep (using the inhalational or intravenous route), profound analgesia with opioid drugs, and muscle relaxation by neuromuscular block, but when Lundy first used the term in 1926 the second and third components were produced by a local block. This combination has now developed into the 'fast-track' approach where high-quality pain relief allows rapid mobilization and early discharge even after major surgery.

There have been other advances which, although more difficult to quantify, have directly or indirectly helped the cause of local anaesthesia in the last 50 years. For example, developments in the field of medical plastics have resulted in safe and reliable syringes, catheters, and filters; and the anaesthetist can select from a wide variety of sedative and anxiolytic drugs which, carefully used, can greatly improve the patient's acceptance of a nerve block. Of great importance has been the understanding of the effects, and treatment, of sympathetic block. Ephedrine became available in 1924 and was first used to treat hypotension during spinal anaesthesia in 1927, but readily available intravenous fluids and equipment for their administration came later.

Recent developments

Over the last 20 years, as regional techniques have been used more widely, there have been a number of attempts to 'prove' that they have a positive impact on the outcomes of surgery. These issues are considered in Chapter 2, but fundamental difficulties have been recruiting sufficiently large numbers of patients to produce a study of sufficient 'power' and, possibly more important, ensuring that those managing the patients have equal competence in managing the surgery with and without a block. Significant reductions in postoperative pain are easy to demonstrate, and no study has even suggested that the outcome may be worse when regional methods are used, but it is difficult to draw valid comparisons when the regional technique is less than fully effective in a large proportion of the patients who are supposed to receive it (Rigg et al. 2002).

As noted earlier, there have been concerns about the risks of major sequelae, especially after central nerve block, but an UK-wide audit of such problems suggested that the incidence is much lower than some had feared (Cook et al. 2009). These worries did encourage wider use of more peripheral blocks such as paravertebral for thoracotomy, interpleural, subcostal, rectus sheath, and transversus abdominis plane blocks for abdominal surgery, and femoral/sciatic block and intra-articular techniques for lower limb arthroplasty. The French led in the development of peripheral nerve stimulation techniques, but this method is being displaced by the other major, recent driver to the increased use of regional techniques, the availability of portable ultrasound devices for the identification of the precise position of target nerves prior to injection. There is much enthusiasm for their use, but their efficacy is not yet clearly proven, although technical advances and greater experience may soon confirm that they increase success rates and decrease the risk of complications.

Overview

Ever since the first recognition of the significance of the local effects of cocaine the popularity of local and regional methods of anaesthesia has varied considerably. New drugs, techniques, and equipment have all stimulated enthusiasm and usage, but the risk of complications, sometimes related to other aspects of patient care such as thromboprophylaxis, balance the equation. This is sometimes over-simplified and presented as a 'regional versus general' anaesthesia debate, but the real issues are to identify how a regional technique may contribute to a patient's care and then perform the block in such a way so as to *both* maximize efficacy and minimize complications. This is the underlying theme for all which follows.

Further reading

Ellis ES (1946). *Ancient anodynes: primitive anaesthesia and allied conditions*. London: Heinemann.

Liljestrand G (1971). The historical development of local anesthesia. In Lechat P (Ed) *International encyclopedia of pharmacology and therapeutics*, vol 1, pp. 1–38. New York: Pergamon.

On-line resource

http://www.histansoc.org.uk Proceedings of the History of Anaesthesia Society.

References

Becker HK (1963) Carl Koller and cocaine. *Psychoanalytic Quarterly* 32: 309–73.

Bird HM (1949) James Arnott, M.D. (Aberdeen) 1797–1883: A pioneer in refrigeration anaesthesia. *Anaesthesia* 4: 10–17.

Boulton TB (1984) Classical file. *Survey of Anesthesiology* 28: 150–2.

Cook TM, Counsell D, Wildsmith JAW (2009) Major complications of central neuraxial block: report on the Third National Audit Project of the Royal College of Anaesthetists. *British Journal of Anaesthesia* 102: 179–90.

Cope RW (1954) The Woolley and Roe case. *Anaesthesia* 9: 249–70.

Faulconer A, Keys TE (1965) *Foundations of Anesthesiology*, vol II, pp. 769–845. Springfield, IL: Charles C Thomas.

Hutter CDD (1990) The Woolley and Roe case: A reassessment. *Anaesthesia* 45: 859–64.

Kennedy FG, Effron AS, Perry G (1950) The grave spinal cord paralyses caused by spinal anesthesia. *Surgery, Gynecology and Obstetrics* 91: 385–98.

Koller C (1884) On the use of cocaine for producing anaesthesia of the eye. *Lancet* ii: 990–2.

Lee JA, Atkinson RS (1978) *Sir Robert Macintosh's Lumbar Puncture and Spinal Analgesia: Intradural and Extradural*, 4th edn pp. 179–81. Edinburgh: Churchill Livingstone.

Lofgren N (1948) *Studies on Local Anesthetics: Xylocaine, a New Synthetic Drug*. Worcester, MA: Morin Press [reprinted].

Richardson BW (1866) On a new and ready method of producing local anaesthesia. *Medical Times and Gazette* I: 115–17.

Rigg JR, Jamrozik K, Myles PS, et al. (2002) Epidural anaesthesia and analgesia and outcome of major surgery: a randomised trial. The MASTER Anaesthesia Trial Study Group. *Lancet* 359: 1276–82.

Simpson JY (1848) Local anaesthesia, notes on its production by chloroform etc in the lower animals, and in man. *Lancet* ii: 39–42.

Wildsmith JAW (1983) Three Edinburgh men. *Regional Anesthesia* 8: 1–5.

Wildsmith JAW (1984) Carl Koller (1857–1944) and the introduction of cocaine into anesthetic practice. *Regional Anesthesia* 9: 161–4.

Wood A (1855) New method of treating neuralgia by the direct application of opiates to the painful points. *Edinburgh Medical Journal* 82: 265–81.

CHAPTER 2

Anatomy and physiology of pain

Lesley Colvin

Pain is defined by the International Association for the Study of Pain (1986) as 'an unpleasant sensory and emotional experience associated with actual or potential tissue damage, or described in terms of such damage', and so it encompasses much more than the simple reflex response to a noxious stimulus. Sensory impulses arising from noxious stimuli undergo considerable processing at all levels in the central nervous system, the conscious perception of pain resulting from an integration of sensory, cognitive, and affective/emotional components modified in the context of social and cultural factors (the biopsychosocial model) (Gatchel et al. 2007). In the biological situation pain prevents further damage by leading to the removal of injured tissue from the stimulus, and promotes wound healing by discouraging movement. This type of pain has been termed physiological because it serves a purpose (Woolf 1989). However, in some situations pain may persist for much longer than would be expected from the severity of the original injury so that it actually interferes with recovery of function. Abnormal processes beginning at the time of injury may result in long-term alterations in central responses to peripheral stimuli, so that conventional treatment may no longer be effective. Chronic pain syndromes have been termed pathological pain (Woolf 1995), and any consideration of pain physiology must explain how such syndromes occur.

Traditionally, pain was thought to be a 'hard-wired' system with fixed neuronal connections conducting impulses directly from the periphery to the brain (Duncan 2000). Melzack and Wall's (1965) *gate control theory of pain* recognized that modulation of sensory input could occur in the spinal cord, by both local interneurones and descending connections from the brain. Current knowledge has developed from this concept, but it is clear that the actual situation is much more complex with functional, and even anatomical, changes occurring in neurones and other cells in response to pain. Modern brain imaging techniques, such as functional magnetic resonance imaging, reveal the dynamic nature of the system, with complex interactions modulating pain transmission at every level from the periphery to the cortex (Flor 2000, Tracey 2008). Prolonged stimulation, particularly, can induce alterations in neuronal phenotype, with 'up-' or 'down-' regulation of a variety of genes leading to changes in the type and pattern of neurotransmitter release, altered neuronal response characteristics, and recruitment of previously inactive neurones (Latremoliere & Woolf 2009).

Both peripheral and central nervous systems may respond to both noxious stimuli and pharmacological interventions with alterations in their connections and function—the phenomenon of *plasticity* (Besson & Chaouch 1987).

It is apparent that there is not a single, defined 'pain pathway', although it is possible to outline the basic components of the systems involved in the transmission and modulation of pain (Figure 2.1), and to recognize functional components within these:

1. The primary afferent neurones in the peripheral nerves.

2. Signal transduction by neurotransmitters in the spinal cord.

3. Modulation by supraspinal systems.

4. Peripheral and central sensitization mechanisms.

The peripheral nerves

A peripheral nerve may contain any combination of sensory (primary afferent), motor, and autonomic fibres, the exact anatomical arrangement depending on the particular nerve. For example, the femoral nerve contains fibres serving all three broad functions, but its most distal continuation, the saphenous nerve, contains mainly sensory fibres (Willis & Coggeshall 1991). If a mixed peripheral nerve is stimulated adequately, an electrode placed some distance away will record the resulting electrical activity (Figure 2.2). The latencies of the various peaks in this *compound action potential* indicate the conduction velocities of the different fibre types, and the amplitudes of those peaks relate to the number of fibres of that type. Several classifications of nerve fibres have been proposed, but the one most commonly used relates the function subserved by the fibre to its diameter and conduction velocity (Table 2.1).

The physical structure of peripheral nerves, the physiology of axonal conduction, and the pharmacology of its block are considered in Chapter 6.

Nerve distribution

Specific segmental nerves are formed in the vertebral canal by the joining of dorsal (sensory) and ventral (motor) roots after they emerge from the spinal cord (Figure 2.1). The course which these nerves take towards the periphery is determined during development and is regulated by growth factor substances (Stoeckli 1997). In general, distribution of both motor and sensory neurones

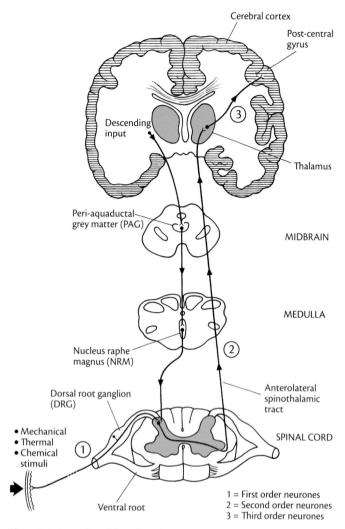

Figure 2.1 An outline of the pain pathway.

1 = First order neurones
2 = Second order neurones
3 = Third order neurones

the viscera can result in pain perception in areas distant from those that would be expected. Thus, block of cutaneous sensation does not necessarily imply block of either underlying visceral sensation or motor function.

Pain originating in the thoracic and abdominal viscera is transmitted by afferent sympathetic fibres through the sympathetic chain to segmental nerves (T_1–L_2) and by parasympathetic vagal (X) fibres. Other parasympathetic fibres transmit deep pain from structures in the pelvis (S_2–S_3) and the head and neck (cranial nerves III, VII, and IX). Referred pain, such as shoulder tip pain secondary to diaphragmatic irritation, indicates the common embryonic origin of the nerve supply to the two structures involved. Stimulation of sympathetic and parasympathetic afferent fibres which transmit nociceptive information to the spinal cord results in pain, which tends to be diffuse and poorly localized in nature (Janig 1995).

Primary afferent (sensory) neurone

A typical primary afferent neurone consists of:

1. Peripheral nerve ending(s) and any associated receptor(s);

2. The axon (nerve fibre) connecting centrally;

3. The cell body in the dorsal root ganglion; and

4. Its central termination(s) in the dorsal horn of the spinal cord.

Peripheral nerve endings

Many sensory nerve endings are associated with specialized receptors (e.g. Merkel discs, Pacinian corpuscles) for stimulus transduction, but nociceptors are not specialized, consisting of fine branches of the nerve fanning out through the dermis and, sometimes, the epidermis. Signal transduction is by the generation of action potentials, although the nerve endings contain neuroactive substances, the release of which may modify their own responsiveness, particularly after tissue damage has occurred. The type of stimulus to which each neurone responds tends to be highly specific, so that thermal receptors, for example, are not activated by mechanical or chemical stimuli. Additionally, the intensity of the stimulus required to activate a peripheral receptor varies: light touch will only activate low-threshold mechanoreceptors, whereas a much more severe stimulus is needed to activate nociceptors.

If these nociceptors are related to Aδ fibres, rapid impulse transmission occurs, with immediate perception of relatively well-localized pain. However, the majority of neurones concerned with nociceptive transmission are small, unmyelinated, slowly conducting C fibres, with receptors which respond to a variety of stimuli. There are different types of C fibres, characterized by the receptors and neurotransmitters which they produce. Some are purely nociceptive, whereas some are polymodal and also respond, in particular, to thermal stimuli via specific receptors (Eid & Cortright 2009). Their activation results in perception of a more diffuse and persistent pain which is poorly localized. The initial activation of the peripheral receptor is responsible for encoding the type of stimulus, but further information about its exact nature is transmitted proximally by alterations in the frequency and pattern of impulse generation (Julius & Basbaum 2001). For instance, a 'firing' rate of less than 5 Hz in a C fibre does not result in the perception of pain (Wiesenfeld & Lindblom 1980). A range of G-protein coupled receptors and ion channels (e.g. the transient receptor potential family) located on peripheral nerve endings may

follows a well-defined pattern, with the sensory component of each segmental nerve innervating a specific area of skin known as a dermatome (Figure 2.3). The distribution of these varies among individuals and there is some degree of overlap between adjacent dermatomes, possibly related to local connections within the spinal cord. In addition, contributions from afferent autonomic fibres to

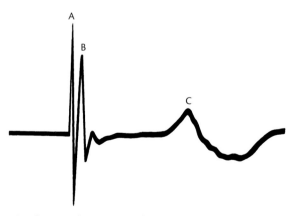

Figure 2.2 Compound action potential recorded from a peripheral nerve.

Table 2.1 Classification of nerve fibres. (Adapted from Erlanger & Gasser 1937.)

Fibre type	Function	Diameter (μm)	Conduction velocity (m s⁻¹)
Large myelinated			
Aα	Proprioception, motor	12–20	70–120
Aβ	Light touch, pressure	5–12	30–70
Aγ	Motor to muscle spindles	3–6	15–30
Small myelinated			
Aδ	Pain, cold, touch	2–5	12–30
B	Preganglionic autonomic	<3	3–15
Unmyelinated			
C	Pain, temperature, postganglionic sympathetics	0.4–1.3	0.5–2

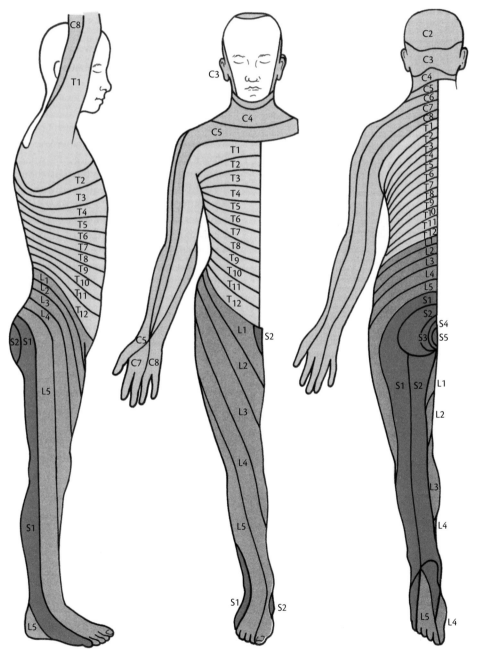

Figure 2.3 Cutaneous dermatomes.

modulate nociceptive transmission, and their modulation may have analgesic potential (Bevan & Andersson 2009, Wemmie et al. 2006).

Axonal functions

In the past, the only significant function of the axon was thought to be the electrical transmission of the nerve impulse (see Chapter 6), but axoplasmic transport (both peripheral and central) is also important. This provides a slower method of communication whereby structural components and transmitter substances produced in the cell body are transported distally to maintain the neuronal phenotype or (after release peripherally) to modulate impulse generation. There is also evidence that peripherally-derived growth factor substances (neurotrophins) are transported centrally to the dorsal root ganglia to regulate neurotransmitter synthesis (McMahon & Jones 2004, Merighi et al. 2004). More recently there has been increased interest in the role of supporting cells, such as Schwann cells, previously thought to be important only for their electrical 'insulating' properties. They appear to have a much more dynamic interaction with the neurone itself. They produce neurotrophic substances and cytokines, particularly in response to injury (Friedman et al. 1995). These substances may be transported retrogradely or anterogradely, and produce significant effects in both the periphery and the cell body of the neurone. It is thus apparent that the axons and the surrounding glial cells have a much more active role than was previously thought, and that there is the potential for longer-term modulation by neuroactive compounds, as well as control of the rate and direction of neuronal growth.

The cell body and its central terminations

The cell bodies of primary sensory neurones lie in the dorsal root ganglia, situated within the confines of the vertebral canal. The neurone dies if the cell body is damaged because it contains the nucleus of the cell, its DNA, and the systems which manufacture cell components, including the neurotransmitters which are essential for survival. In general, the diameter of the cell body correlates well with the diameter of its nerve fibre. Thus, small-diameter cells in the dorsal root ganglia are thought to be concerned mainly with the transmission of nociceptive information, whereas large-diameter cells are related to their fibres' discriminatory functions such as light touch or pressure. Transmission of information within neurones occurs by electrical conduction of action potentials (see Chapter 6), but at the 'synapse' in the dorsal horn of the spinal cord, chemicals (neurotransmitters) are released to activate the second order neurones.

One of the characteristic differences between the dorsal root ganglia cell bodies is in the neurotransmitters synthesized and 'packaged' in them (Bean et al. 1994). The small-diameter cells synthesize peptides which are stored in large dense-core vesicles (LDCVs), whereas the larger cells do not produce significant amounts of such peptides under normal conditions (Landry et al. 2000, Zhang et al. 1995). Other neurotransmitters, such as amino acids and purines, are also produced and, although common to many other neuronal subtypes, they are often stored in the same LDCVs. The transmitters are released at the first central synapse in the dorsal horn of the spinal cord, a point with great potential for manipulation of the pain signal because of the significant degree of impulse modulation which takes place there (Ji & Strichartz 2004).

Transmission in the spinal cord
Neural connections

The circuitry in the dorsal horn is complex, with many neurones converging and diverging at the synapse. There are many influences, both pre- and postsynaptic, on the pain signal at the termination of the primary afferent neurone before it is transmitted onwards in the spinothalamic tracts. The incoming afferent volley may be modulated by the actions of intrinsic dorsal horn neurones, as well as by fibres descending from supraspinal systems (Figure 2.4). Equally, that initial afferent input can spread to proximal and distal segments of the cord as well as acting where the primary neurone terminates.

The concept that there are specific areas and pathways in the spinal cord is an old one, there being obvious distinctions between motor and sensory systems, and between sensory information which is noxious and innocuous. Previous work has shown some correlation between neuronal type and area of termination in the spinal cord (Brown 1982), although this may be altered in certain abnormal situations, such as after nerve injury. Additionally, it is possible to correlate peripheral receptive fields within each area of the cord with central terminations (Handwerker et al. 1975). This has also been demonstrated at supraspinal levels.

The spinal cord, in cross-section, has been divided into various areas according to their characteristic histological appearances: Rexed's laminae (Figure 2.5). There is some slight species variation, but lamina II, also known as the substantia gelatinosa, is the area of the cord thought to be concerned with nociceptive transmission (Molander et al. 1984). This is where the majority of C and Aδ fibres terminate, although some Aδ fibres also terminate more deeply at lamina V. The larger, Aβ fibres terminate in laminae III/IV, and large proprioceptive fibres terminate deeper still, in laminae VI/VII (Willis & Coggeshall 1991).

Many neurotransmitters and their receptors can be located in the dorsal horn, with a particularly high density in the superficial layers. This reflects the major degree of modulation which can be

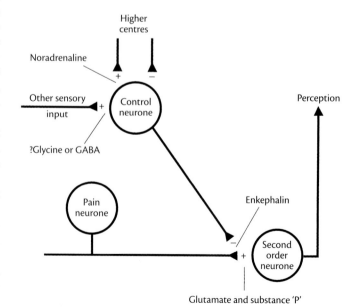

Figure 2.4 Gate control theory of pain. Release of enkephalin by the control neurone inhibits transmitter release. Exogenous opioids have the same effect.

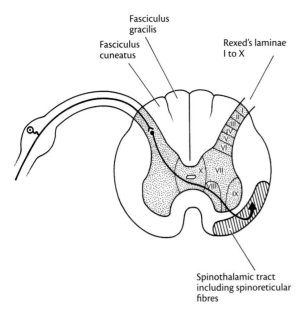

Figure 2.5 Transverse section of the spinal cord to show Rexed's laminae.

applied to the incoming signal in these areas. Neural transmission is also modulated by cells of the immune system, in particular, glial cells such as astrocytes and oligodendrocytes. These can not only alter neurotransmitter reuptake, but may themselves release neurotransmitters (Watkins & Maier 2003, Watkins et al. 2009). The complexity of the system is outside the scope of this book, but a brief summary of the major neurotransmitters considered important in the processing of nociception at spinal cord level is appropriate.

Neurotransmitters

Amino acids

The 'classical', fast-acting neurotransmitters include amino acids, which may be either excitatory (glutamate and aspartate) or inhibitory (γ-amino-butyric acid (GABA) and glycine) (Aanonsen et al. 1990). Characteristically, their release, reuptake, and metabolism are rapid, and the major site of action is very close to the site of release, usually within the synaptic cleft. Each of these transmitters acts on several subtypes of receptor, allowing a whole series of actions to be initiated. If, in the future, it is possible to develop highly specific agonists or antagonists, each able to target the actions of a specific receptor subtype, and so minimize side effects, some very useful analgesic drugs would be available (Yaksh 1999).

Glutamate is one of the main excitatory amino acids involved in pain transmission, and it acts at two different groups of receptors. The *ionotropic* receptors, which include N-methyl-D-aspartate (NMDA), amino-3-hydroxy-5-methylisoxazole-4-propionic acid (AMPA), and kainate receptors have rapid response times. They activate ligand-gated ion channels and thus produce changes in intracellular ionic concentrations (e.g. increased calcium with NMDA receptor stimulation) (Gogas 2006). The NMDA receptor, at which glutamate acts, is known to be important in the development of central sensitization (Davis & Lodge 1987, and see 'Sensitization mechanisms' section), as well as the rapid transmission of nociceptive information. In contrast to the receptors associated with ion channels, the *metabotropic* glutamate receptors

(mGluRs) are G-protein coupled, and have effects on a variety of intracellular second messenger systems. At least seven subtypes, some of which are involved in pain processing, have been identified. The role of mGluRs in nociception is not yet clear, with some evidence that certain subtypes may facilitate NMDA receptor function, while others may have an inhibitory role (Pin & Acher 2002).

Neuropeptides

Normally, neuropeptides are synthesized by the majority of primary afferent neurones involved in nociception, but many of the neurones intrinsic to the dorsal horn, and some of those in the descending systems, also contain neuropeptides. Unlike amino acids, the majority of the neuropeptides do not act at ligand-gated ion channels, but at G-protein coupled receptors. There is no evidence of rapid reuptake systems for neuropeptides, their termination of action being determined by their rate of metabolism. Thus, they may diffuse beyond the synaptic zone to act at distant sites, an effect which has been termed *volume transmission* (Fuxe & Agnati 1991) and which reflects the possible 'paracrine' action of these neurotransmitters.

Substance P, a member of the tachykinin family, is synthesized by primary afferent neurones and is thought to play a major role in pain transmission (Duggan et al. 1995, Honore et al. 2000a, Liu et al. 1997). Its predominantly excitatory action (at the neurokinin-1 receptor) is in contrast to the opioid peptides (e.g. enkephalins, endorphins, and dynorphin) which have predominantly inhibitory actions and normally act as endogenous analgesics. Opioid peptides are synthesized and released by intrinsic dorsal horn neurones and also by neurones which form part of descending modulatory systems (Mollereau et al. 2005, Schafer et al. 2000). There is a high density of opioid receptors in the superficial dorsal horn, approximately 70% of them being of the μ subtype, 20% δ, and 10% κ. Opioids acting in this area may have both pre- and postsynaptic effects. Dependent on their location and receptor subtype they may also have pro-nociceptive actions rather than being analgesic (Colvin & Fallon 2010, Davis et al. 2007).

The classification of opioid receptors has been revised following their genetic cloning, and now includes the 'orphan' opioid receptor (Table 2.2). When it was originally cloned it was found to have a high degree of sequence homology with the μ receptor, but it was named 'orphan' because none of the known opioid peptides activated it, and naloxone did not antagonize its activation. However, an endogenously produced peptide, nociceptin (or orphanin FQ), which acts on this receptor, has been identified (Calo et al. 2000). It is of interest that insults (traumatic or surgical), causing either inflammation or nerve injury, dramatically alter neuropeptide synthesis in primary afferent neurones (Calza et al. 2000, Hokfelt et al. 1994). Although the functional significance of these changes is not fully understood, it is likely that the neuropeptides play a major role in the response to such stimuli.

Table 2.2 Classification of opioid receptors.

Original classification	New classification
Mu (μ)	OP3
Delta (δ)	OP1
Kappa (κ)	OP2
Orphan	ORL1

It is relatively common for neurones to release more than one type of neurotransmitter in response to a specific stimulus. In some primary afferent neurones, amino acids, catecholamines, and neuropeptides may be stored and released together, there being some evidence that the type and quantity of neurotransmitter released may vary with the character of the incoming signal (De Potter et al. 1997).

Ascending pathways

Some of the neurones with which primary afferent neurones synapse project to adjacent segments. The remainder join the anterolateral spinothalamic tract (STT), from which some fibres separate at the brainstem (the spinoreticular tract) to terminate in the reticular formation. The STT neurones display certain characteristics which allow their identification in functional studies. They have small receptive fields, respond maximally to noxious or thermal stimulation at the periphery, receive convergent inputs from deep and visceral structures, and are able to code for threshold and intensity of stimulation. Although the majority of these fibres cross to the contralateral side before ascending, a small proportion ascend ventrally on the same side of the spinal cord.

The STT is the major ascending pathway involved in nociceptive processing. The monosynaptic connection of each of its fibres has allowed anatomical studies using antidromic activation and retrograde tracers to determine the termination of specific neurones (Bolton & Tracey 1992). Within the thalamus are groups of nuclei—ventral, posterior, medial, and lateral—each with further subdivisions. Their function varies between species and the relative contribution of each nucleus to nociceptive processing has been reviewed, with clinical brain imaging studies adding to our knowledge (Apkarian et al. 2005, Treede et al. 2000). From the thalamus the tertiary neurones of the pain pathway project widely throughout the brain, although brain imaging consistently shows activation of several areas, including the insula and anterior cingulate cortex (Bingel & Tracey 2008).

Descending modulation

Pathways descending from the brainstem play a significant role in modulating the level of tonic excitability of the spinal cord. This has previously been termed diffuse noxious inhibitory control because cord transection results in a marked increase in basal excitability at the spinal level (Morgan et al. 1994). Stimulation of certain areas of the brainstem, including the nucleus raphe magnus and the locus coeruleus, has been shown to result in release of neurotransmitters (including catecholamines, such as noradrenaline and serotonin) in the spinal cord and behavioural signs of decreased pain perception (Mokha et al. 1985). It may be that analgesics such as tramadol act through this system, as well as the more unconventional agents, such as antidepressants, used in the treatment of chronic pain. Neuropeptides, including endogenous opioids and substance P, also play a role in this descending control (Stamford 1995). More recently it has become apparent that descending modulation from the brain may also have facilitatory effects, particularly in chronic pain states (Bannister et al. 2009, Porreca et al. 2002).

Supraspinal systems

The conscious perception of pain has never been localized to any specific part of the brain, and it seems that many areas are involved. Several parts of the brainstem are thought to be of particular importance, including the periaqueductal grey (PAG) matter (where the locus coeruleus is situated), the nucleus raphe magnus, and the surrounding reticular formation. The hypothalamus, the amygdala, and the PAG are thought to make major contributions to nociceptive processing, and are involved in the integration of the responses to a noxious stimulus, including activation of the autonomic, endocrine, and motor elements of these responses (Giesler et al. 1994).

Modern imaging methods are providing much useful information on both the brain's acute response to a noxious stimulus and the modification of this response after tissue injury (Casey et al. 2003, Svensson et al. 1997). Thus, clinical and volunteer studies have confirmed the involvement of many areas of the brain, reflecting the multifaceted nature of pain perception. The acute response has been shown to involve the PAG, the hypothalamus, the prefrontal, insular, anterior cingulate, and posterior parietal areas of the cerebral cortex, the primary motor and sensory areas, the supplementary motor area, and the cerebellum. Interestingly, imaging studies in chronic pain patients have demonstrated activation of quite different areas of the brain in response to noxious stimuli. This may reflect altered spinal processing, but could also indicate plasticity at supraspinal levels (Geha et al. 2008).

Sensitization mechanisms

Peripheral sensitization

Normally, a high-intensity noxious stimulus is required to activate peripheral nociceptors. This results in the central transmission of action potentials which encode the site and character of the pain, but after tissue injury peripheral 'sensitization' may occur. This lowers the threshold for activation of nociceptors, so that previously innocuous stimuli generate action potentials in nociceptive neurones. This may result in *hyperalgesia*, which is an exaggerated response to a painful stimulus, or *allodynia*, which is perception of a previously innocuous stimulus as painful. An additional feature may be recruitment of larger myelinated Aβ fibres, normally concerned with light touch transmission, to become involved in pain transmission (Cervero & Laird 1996).

Peripheral sensitization involves mast cells, neutrophils, the surrounding vascular bed, the autonomic nervous system, and the primary afferent neurones themselves. A complex series of processes is activated, the exact mechanisms of which are not yet fully understood (Stein et al. 2009). One effect of the activation of these interlinked cascades is the development of what has been termed an *inflammatory soup*, an alteration in the milieu of the peripheral nerve endings that lowers their activation threshold (Figure 2.6).

Other peripheral changes may result in alterations in primary afferent 'drive', the final result of which is increased peripheral sensitivity. After peripheral nerve damage, the injured fibres start to generate action potentials spontaneously at sites other than the nociceptors. Increased 'mechanosensitivity' occurs at the site of injury, and impulses also arise *de novo* at the cell bodies in the dorsal root ganglia. These 'ectopic discharges' may correlate with the generation of spontaneous pain because clinical microneurography studies have demonstrated a correlation between its severity and the rate of ectopic discharge (Devor 1991). The factors causing these ectopic discharges are unclear, but they may be related to peripherally produced mediators, such as tumour necrosis factor,

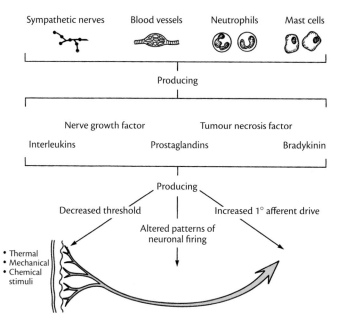

Sympathetic nerves   Blood vessels   Neutrophils   Mast cells

Producing

Nerve growth factor   Tumour necrosis factor
Interleukins   Prostaglandins   Bradykinin

Producing

Decreased threshold   Increased 1° afferent drive

Altered patterns of
neuronal firing

• Thermal
• Mechanical
• Chemical
  stimuli

Figure 2.6 Mechanisms involved in peripheral sensitization.

with involvement of glutaminergic and histaminergic systems (Sorkin et al. 1997, Suzuki et al. 2004).

The end result of peripheral sensitization is an amplification of peripheral sensory input so that there is an increase in the transmission of impulses to the spinal cord.

Central sensitization

The process of central sensitization begins in the spinal cord, initially as a response to increased excitatory input from the injured tissue, and may be associated with changes in the transport from the periphery of substances involved in maintenance of neuronal phenotype. There are several components to the central response:

1. The acute response to repeated noxious stimulation, the phenomenon known as *wind up*, is an increase in the responsiveness of the secondary neurone. The end result is amplification of the response to a defined peripheral stimulus, with an increase in neuronal firing rate and summation of action potentials. One of the principal excitatory amino acids in the spinal cord, glutamate, acting through both NMDA (Woolf & Thompson 1991) and mGlu receptor subtypes (Mutel 2002), appears to be important in the development of central sensitization.

2. In addition to the rapid change in firing pattern mediated by glutamate receptor activation, there are rapid alterations in the dorsal horn cell bodies. Increases in the activity of *immediate early genes* and in their protein products (e.g. c-fos and c-jun), can be detected within hours of intense noxious stimulation. Potentially, these can produce rapid alterations in neuronal phenotype and function (Csillik et al. 2003, Li et al. 2004).

3. There are major changes in neurotransmitter concentrations in both the dorsal root ganglia and the spinal cord, their specific nature being dependent on the type and severity of tissue damage. For example, synthesis of substance P is increased in primary afferent neurones in response to inflammation, but is reduced after peripheral nerve injury (Honore et al. 2000b). After nerve injury, there may also be preferential damage to

inhibitory neurones, with decreases in both glycine and GABA concentrations within the dorsal horn. A corresponding increase in spontaneous and evoked activity within the dorsal horn has been found (Baba et al. 2003, Moore et al. 2002).

4. In the longer term, functional anatomical connections within the dorsal horn may alter. For example, after peripheral nerve injury large myelinated Aβ fibres, which normally synapse in the deeper dorsal horn, make functional connections with the substantia gelatinosa. Previously these were thought to be due to sprouting of Aβ fibres, but it is now thought to be more likely due to unmasking of silent synapses (Cafferty et al. 2008, Jaken et al. 2010, Zhang & Strong 2008). Additionally, sprouting of sympathetic fibres has been found around dorsal root ganglia, with evidence of cross excitation between these fibres and primary afferent neurones (Hayashida et al. 2008, McLachlan et al. 1993).

Conduction block

The pain pathway may be interrupted at many points along its course. Opioids and other analgesic drugs affect pain receptors or the synaptic transmission of pain, while local anaesthetics have the advantage of producing a complete, yet reversible block of axonal transmission. In addition, local anaesthetics may be used at many points along the pain pathway (Figure 2.7), although the anaesthetist must consider carefully the deep and superficial innervation of the operative field when choosing the point of block. The standard methods of local anaesthetic administration are as follows:

Topical

Local anaesthetics may be applied directly to the mucous membranes of the nose, mouth, throat, and urethra, and also to the

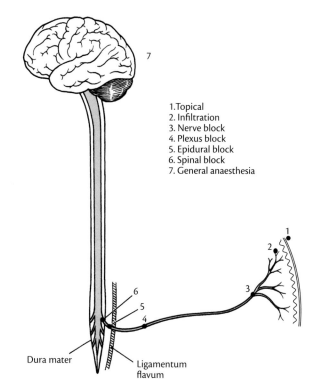

1. Topical
2. Infiltration
3. Nerve block
4. Plexus block
5. Epidural block
6. Spinal block
7. General anaesthesia

Dura mater   Ligamentum flavum

Figure 2.7 Possible sites (1–7) of local anaesthetic action. Other analgesic drugs act at some of these points: opioids at 1, 2, and 5–7; α₂-agonists and ketamine at 5–7; and NSAIDs at 1, 2, and 7.

external surfaces of the eye. Standard preparations will penetrate these surfaces, but intact skin requires special formulations because it presents a significant barrier to diffusion. The eutectic mixture (lidocaine and prilocaine) of local anaesthetics (EMLA) in a cream formulation and a 4% tetracaine gel both overcome this difficulty. Five per cent lidocaine plasters are also available for the topical treatment of neuropathic pain (Attal & Bouhassira 2004, Baron et al. 2009).

Infiltration

The extent of infiltration will depend on the area of anaesthesia required, and large volumes of dilute local anaesthetic solution are sometimes used. An alternative term for this, 'tumescent anaesthesia', has been applied in recent years. It involves injection of very large volumes of local anaesthetic, with associated safety concerns (Fettes & Wildsmith 2003), for liposuction for cosmetic purposes. A more elegant variant, using ultrasound to identify the relevant fascial planes, is employed for the laser ablation of varicose veins (Boezem et al. 2011).

Peripheral nerve block

Many small peripheral nerves are readily accessible and easily blocked, given a reasonable knowledge of the distribution and anatomical relations of the peripheral nerves.

Proximal nerve block

Accessibility is the essential prerequisite for a proximal nerve block. The brachial plexus may be located at a number of points by reference to anatomical landmarks, but the lumbosacral plexus is not so easily identified, and the sciatic nerve is deeply placed in the buttock and upper leg. Paravertebral somatic block involves injecting local anaesthetic close to the vertebral column where the segmental nerves emerge from the intervertebral foramina. (This technique had been virtually superseded by epidural block, which anaesthetizes several nerves with a single injection, but it has recently increased in popularity again.)

Epidural block

Ease of identification of the epidural space and unimpeded spread of the local anaesthetic solution make this a most useful technique. Continuous block can be produced with catheter techniques.

Spinal (subarachnoid) block

This is a simpler technique than the epidural approach because identification of cerebral spinal fluid is an unambiguous end-point. It is usually performed in the lumbar region to avoid needle damage to the spinal cord.

General anaesthesia

Local anaesthetic drugs stabilize all excitable membranes. Procaine infusion has been used to produce general anaesthesia, but the technique is rarely used now.

Summary

It is apparent that the 'pain pathway' is not a static, hard-wired component of the nervous system, but is a very dynamic one. Both the nature of the peripheral stimulus and the degree of tissue damage can influence the level of neuronal activity and even the actual phenotype of the primary sensory neurone. This in turn can have major effects on signal processing at spinal level, initiating long-term changes within the spinal cord which alter all subsequent processing of sensory information. Any attempt to produce analgesia with local anaesthetics or other agents which act at the various accessible points in the pathway (Figure 2.7) must therefore take account of the changes which may already have occurred, and also of the possibility of preventing the development of detrimental long-term changes.

Clinical implementation of the theory of 'pre-emptive analgesia', that is, inducing impulse block prior to injury to prevent the initiation and development of peripheral and central sensitization, remains controversial. Much of the work from animal studies supports the effectiveness of pre-treatment, but the results from clinical studies have been disappointing (Dahl & Moiniche 2004, Kissin 2000), perhaps because of the complexity and plasticity of the system. It is now clear that a multiplicity of neurotransmitters are involved at a variety of sites so that use of a single agent is almost bound to fail. It has become evident, therefore, that optimal analgesia can only be obtained by using a 'balanced' or 'multi-modal' approach (Kehlet & Dahl 1993), that is, systemic analgesics (e.g. opioids and non-steroidal anti-inflammatory drugs) combined with site-directed local anaesthetics (Wilmore & Kehlet 2001).

Key references

Bingel U, Tracey I (2008) Imaging CNS modulation of pain in humans. *Physiology* 23: 371–80.

Eid SR, Cortright DN (2009) Transient receptor potential channels on sensory nerves. *Handbook of Experimental Pharmacology* 194: 261–81.

Giesler GJ Jr, Katter JT, Dado RJ (1994) Direct spinal pathways to the limbic system for nociceptive information. *Trends in Neurological Sciences* 17: 244–50.

Julius D, Basbaum AI (2001) Molecular mechanisms of nociception. *Nature* 413: 203–10.

Kehlet H, Dahl JB (1993) The value of 'multi-modal' or 'balanced analgesia' in post-operative pain treatment. *Anesthesia & Analgesia* 77: 1048–66.

McMahon SB, Jones NG (2004) Plasticity of pain signaling: role of neurotrophic factors exemplified by acid-induced pain. *Journal of Neurobiology* 61: 72–87.

Mollereau C, Roumy M, Zajac JM (2005) Opioid-modulating peptides: mechanisms of action. *Current Topics in Medicinal Chemistry* 5: 341–55.

Porreca F, Ossipov MH, Gebhart GF (2002) Chronic pain and medullary descending facilitation. *Trends in Neurosciences* 25: 319–25.

Watkins LR, Hutchinson MR, Rice KC, Maier SF (2009) The 'toll' of opioid-induced glial activation: improving the clinical efficacy of opioids by targeting glia. *Trends in Pharmacological Sciences* 30: 581–91.

References

Aanonsen LM, Sizheng L, Wilcox GL (1990) Excitatory amino acid receptors and nociceptive neurotransmission in rat spinal cord. *Pain* 41: 309–21.

Apkarian AV, Bushnell MC, Treede RD, et al. (2005) Human brain mechanisms of pain perception and regulation in health and disease. *European Journal of Pain* 9: 463–84.

Attal N, Bouhassira D (2004) Neuropathic pain: experimental advances and clinical applications. *Revue Neurologique* 160: 199–203.

Baba H, Ji RR, Kohno T, Moore KA, et al. (2003) Removal of GABAergic inhibition facilitates polysynaptic A fiber-mediated excitatory transmission to the superficial spinal dorsal horn. *Molecular & Cellular Neurosciences* 24: 818–30.

Bannister K, Bee LA, Dickenson AH (2009) Preclinical and early clinical investigations related to monoaminergic pain modulation. *Neurotherapeutics* 6: 703–12.

Baron R, Mayoral V, Leijon G, et al. (2009) Efficacy and safety of 5% lidocaine (lignocaine) medicated plaster in comparison with pregabalin in patients with postherpetic neuralgia and diabetic polyneuropathy: interim analysis from an open-label, two-stage adaptive, randomized, controlled trial. *Clinical Drug Investigation* 29: 231–41.

Bean AJ, Zhang X, Hökfelt T (1994) Peptide secretion: What do we know? *FASEB Journal* 8: 630–8.

Besson J-M, Chaouch A (1987) Peripheral and spinal mechanisms of nociception. *Physiological Review* 67: 67–186.

Bevan S, Andersson DA (2009) TRP channel antagonists for pain—opportunities beyond TRPV1. *Current Opinion in Investigational Drugs* 10: 655–63.

Boezem PB van dem, Klem TMAL, Cocq d'Armandville E le, Wittens CH (2011) The management of superficial venous incompetence. *British Medical Journal* 343: d4489.

Bolton PS, Tracey DJ (1992) Spinothalamic and propriospinal neurons in the upper cervical cord of the rat—terminations of primary afferent-fibers on soma and primary dendrites. *Experimental Brain Research* 92: 59–68.

Brown AG (1982) The dorsal horn of the spinal-cord. *Quarterly Journal of Experimental Physiology and Cognate Medical Sciences* 67: 193–212.

Cafferty WB, McGee AW, Strittmatter SM (2008) Axonal growth therapeutics: regeneration or sprouting or plasticity? *Trends in Neurosciences* 31: 215–20.

Calo G, Guerrini R, Rizzi A, et al. (2000) Pharmacology of nociceptin and its receptor: a novel therapeutic target. *British Journal of Pharmacology* 129: 1261–83.

Calza L, Pozza M, Arletti R, et al. (2000) Long-lasting regulation of galanin, opioid, and other peptides in dorsal root ganglia and spinal cord during experimental polyarthritis. *Experimental Neurology* 164: 333–43.

Casey KL, Lorenz J, Minoshima S, et al. (2003) Insights into the pathophysiology of neuropathic pain through functional brain imaging. *Experimental Neurology* 184(Suppl 1): S80–8.

Cervero F, Laird JMA (1996) Mechanisms of touch-evoked pain (allodynia): a new model. *Pain* 68: 13–23.

Colvin LA, Fallon MT (2010) Opioid-induced hyperalgesia—a clinical challenge. *British Journal of Anaesthesia* 104: 125–7.

Csillik B, Janka Z, Boncz I, et al. (2003) Molecular plasticity of primary nociceptive neurons: relations of the NGF-c-jun system to neurotomy and chronic pain. *Annals of Anatomy* 185: 303–14.

Dahl JB, Moiniche S (2004) Pre-emptive analgesia. *British Medical Bulletin* 71: 13–27.

Davis MP, Shaiova LA, Angst MS (2007) When opioids cause pain. *Journal of Clinical Oncology* 25: 4497–8.

Davis SN, Lodge D (1987) Evidence for involvement of N-methyl-D-aspartatic acid receptors in 'wind up' of class 2 neurons in the dorsal horn of the rat. *Brain Research* 424: 402–6.

De Potter WP, Partoens P, Schoups A, et al. (1997) Noradrenergic neurons release both noradrenaline and neuropeptide Y from a single pool: the large dense cored vesicles. *Synapse* 25: 44–55.

Devor M (1991) Neuropathic pain and injured nerve: peripheral mechanisms. *British Medical Bulletin* 47: 619–30.

Duggan AW, Riley RC, Mark MA, et al. (1995) Afferent volley patterns and the spinal release of immunoreactive substance P in the dorsal horn of the anaesthetized spinal cat. *Neuroscience* 65: 849–58.

Duncan G (2000) Mind-body dualism and the biopsychosocial model of pain: what did Descartes really say? *Journal of Medicine & Philosophy* 25: 485–513.

Erlanger J, Gasser HS (1937) *Electrical Signs of Nervous Activity.* Philadelphia, PA: University of Pennsylvania Press.

Fettes PDF, Wildsmith JAW (2003) Tumescent anaesthesia. *Royal College of Anaesthetists Bulletin* 17: 826–9.

Flor H (2000) The functional organization of the brain in chronic pain. *Progress in Brain Research* 129: 313–22.

Friedman B, Wong V, Lindsay RM (1995) Axons, Schwann cells and neurotrophic factors. *The Neuroscientist* 1: 192–8.

Fuxe K, Agnati LF (1991) Two principal modes of electrochemical communication in the brain: volume versus wiring transmission. In Fuxe K (Ed) *Volume Transmission in the Brain*, pp. 1–9. New York: Raven Press.

Gatchel RJ, Peng YB, Peters ML, et al. (2007) The biopsychosocial approach to chronic pain: scientific advances and future directions. *Psychological Bulletin* 133: 581–624.

Geha PY, Baliki MN, Wang X, et al. (2008) Brain dynamics for perception of tactile allodynia (touch-induced pain) in postherpetic neuralgia. *Pain* 138: 641–56.

Gogas KR (2006) Glutamate-based therapeutic approaches: NR2B receptor antagonists. *Current Opinion in Pharmacology* 6: 68–74.

Handwerker HO, Iggo A, Zimmermann M (1975) Segmental and supraspinal actions on dorsal horn neurons responding to noxious and non-noxious skin stimuli. *Pain* 1: 147–65.

Hayashida K, Clayton BA, Johnson JE, Eisenach JC (2008) Brain derived nerve growth factor induces spinal noradrenergic fiber sprouting and enhances clonidine analgesia following nerve injury in rats. *Pain* 136: 348–55.

Hokfelt T, Zhang X, Wiesenfeld-Hallin Z (1994) Messenger plasticity in primary sensory neurons following axotomy and its functional implications. *Trends in Neurological Sciences* 17: 22–9.

Honore P, Menning PM, Rogers SD, et al. (2000a) Neurochemical plasticity in persistent inflammatory pain. *Progress in Brain Research* 129: 357–63.

Honore P, Rogers SD, Schwei MJ, et al. (2000b) Murine models of inflammatory, neuropathic and cancer pain each generates a unique set of neurochemical changes in the spinal cord and sensory neurons. *Neuroscience* 98: 585–98.

International Association for the Study of Pain (1986) http://www.iasp-pain.org/Content/NavigationMenu/GeneralResourceLinks/PainDefinitions/default.htm

Jaken RJ, Joosten EA, Knuwer M, et al. (2010) Synaptic plasticity in the substantia gelatinosa in a model of chronic neuropathic pain. *Neuroscience Letters* 469: 30–3.

Janig W (1995) The sympathetic nervous system in pain. *European Journal of Anaesthesiology* 12: 53–60.

Ji RR, Strichartz GR (2004) Cell signaling and the genesis of neuropathic pain. *Science's STKE* 2004(252): reE14 [DOI: 10.1126/stke.2522004re14].

Kissin I (2000) Preemptive analgesia. *Anesthesiology* 93: 1138–43.

Landry M, Holmberg K, Zhang X, Hokfelt T (2000) Effect of axotomy on expression of NPY, galanin, and NPVY1 and Y2. *Experimental Neurology* 162: 361–84.

Latremoliere A, Woolf CJ (2009) Central sensitization: a generator of pain hypersensitivity by central neural plasticity. *Journal of Pain* 10: 895–926.

Li X, Lighthall G, Liang DY, Clark JD (2004) Alterations in spinal cord gene expression after hindpaw formalin injection. *Journal of Neuroscience Research* 78: 533–41.

Liu H, Mantyh PW, Basbaum AI (1997) NMDA-receptor regulation of substance P release from primary afferent nociceptors. *Nature* 386: 721–4.

McLachlan EM, Janig W, Devor M, Michaelis M (1993) Peripheral nerve injury triggers noradrenergic sprouting within dorsal root ganglia. *Nature* 363: 543–5.

Melzack R, Wall PD (1965) Pain mechanisms: a new theory. *Science* 150: 971–9.

Merighi A, Carmignoto G, Gobbo S, et al. (2004) Neurotrophins in spinal cord nociceptive pathways. *Progress in Brain Research* 146: 291–321.

Meunier JC (2003) Utilizing functional genomics to identify new pain treatments: the example of nociceptin. *American Journal of PharmacoGenomics* 3: 117–30.

Mokha SS, McMillan JA, Iggo A (1985) Descending control of spinal nociceptive transmission. Actions produced on spinal multireceptive neurones from the nuclei locus coeruleus (LC) and raphe magnus (NRM). *Experimental Brain Research* 58: 213–26.

Molander C, Xu Q, Grant G (1984) The cytoarchitectonic organization of the spinal cord in the rat. i. the lower thoracic and lumbosacral cord. *Journal of Comparative Neurology* 230: 133–41.

Moore KA, Kohno T, Karchewski LA, et al. (2002) Partial peripheral nerve injury promotes a selective loss of GABAergic inhibition in the superficial dorsal horn of the spinal cord. *Journal of Neuroscience* 22: 6724–31.

Morgan NM, Gogas KR, Basbaum AI (1994) Diffuse noxious inhibitory controls reduce the expression of noxious stimulus-evoked fos-like immunoreactivity in the superficial and deep laminae of the rat spinal cord. *Pain* 56: 347–52.

Mutel V (2002) Therapeutic potential of non-competitive, subtype-selective metabotropic glutamate receptor ligands. *Expert Opinion on Therapeutic Patents* 12: 1845–52.

Pin JP, Acher F (2002) The metabotropic glutamate receptors: structure, activation mechanism and pharmacology. *Current Drug Targets – CNS & Neurological Disorders* 1: 297–317.

Schafer M, Brack A, Stein C (2000) Dynorphin a peptides—Potential role in pain transmission and therapy. *CNS Drugs* 13: 161–6.

Sorkin LS, Xiao WH, Wagner R, Myers RR (1997) Tumour necrosis factor-alpha induces ectopic activity in nociceptive primary afferent fibres. *Neuroscience* 81: 255–62.

Stamford JA (1995) Descending control of pain. *British Journal of Anaesthesia* 75: 217–27.

Stein C, Clark JD, Oh U, et al. (2009) Peripheral mechanisms of pain and analgesia. *Brain Research Reviews* 60: 90–113.

Stoeckli ET (1997) Molecular mechanisms of growth cone guidance: stop and go? *Cell and Tissue Research* 290: 441–9.

Suzuki R, Rahman W, Hunt SP, Dickenson AH (2004) Descending facilitatory control of mechanically evoked responses is enhanced in deep dorsal horn neurones following peripheral nerve injury. *Brain Research* 1019: 68–76.

Svensson P, Minoshima S, Beydoun A, et al. (1997) Cerebral processing of acute skin and muscle pain in humans. *Journal of Neurophysiology* 78: 450–60.

Tracey I (2008) Imaging pain. *British Journal of Anaesthesia* 101: 32–9.

Treede RD, Apkarian AV, Bromm B, et al. (2000) Cortical representation of pain: functional characterization of nociceptive areas near the lateral sulcus. *Pain* 87: 113–19.

Watkins LR, Maier SF (2003) Glia: a novel drug discovery target for clinical pain. *Nature Reviews Drug Discovery* 2: 973–85.

Wemmie JA, Price MP, Welsh MJ (2006) Acid-sensing ion channels: advances, questions and therapeutic opportunities. *Trends in Neurosciences* 29: 578–86.

Wiesenfeld Z, Lindblom U (1980) Behavioural and electrophysiological effects of various types of peripheral nerve lesions in the rat: a comparison of possible models for chronic pain. *Pain* 8: 285–98.

Willis WD, Coggeshall RE (1991) *Sensory Mechanisms of the Spinal Cord* (2nd edn). New York & London: Plenum Press.

Wilmore DW, Kehlet H (2001) Management of patients in fast track surgery. *British Medical Journal* 322: 473–6.

Woolf CJ (1989) Recent advances in the pathophysiology of acute pain. *British Journal of Anaesthesia* 63: 139–46.

Woolf CJ (1995) Somatic pain—pathogenesis and prevention. *British Journal of Anaesthesia* 75: 169–76.

Woolf CJ, Thompson SWN (1991) The induction and maintenance of central sensitization is dependent on N-methyl-D-aspartic acid receptor activation; Implications for the treatment of post-injury pain hypersensitivity states. *Pain* 44: 293–9.

Yaksh TL (1999) Spinal systems and pain processing: development of novel analgesic drugs with mechanistically defined models. *Trends in Pharmacological Sciences* 20: 329–37.

Zhang JM, Strong JA (2008) Recent evidence for activity-dependent initiation of sympathetic sprouting and neuropathic pain. *Sheng Li Hsueh Pao – Acta Physiologica Sinica* 60: 617–27.

Zhang X, Nicholas AP, Hokfelt T (1995) Ultrastructural studies on peptides in the dorsal horn of the rat spinal cord—II. Co-existence of galanin with other peptides in local neurons. *Neuroscience* 64: 875–91.

CHAPTER 3

The potential benefits

Nick Scott

As the preceding historical review has indicated, the popularity of local and regional techniques has waxed and waned over the years. The last great increase in interest started during the late 1960s with the recognition of the benefits (for both mother and fetus) of these methods in obstetric practice, and was followed by the recognition that some of its features are relevant to other areas, especially as developments in surgery of the aging population increased the anaesthetic challenge. This led to attempts to define the advantages in comparative 'outcome' studies, but these have produced less than definitive results, primarily because of the difficulties associated with such studies even when they are combined by meta-analysis (Wildsmith 2002). Thus there has been some questioning of the place of regional techniques, especially for the provision of analgesia after major surgery, driven also by concerns about major complications such as vertebral canal haematoma and epidural abscess. The more recent Royal College of Anaesthetists UK-wide audit of adverse outcome after central nerve block has defined such risks more clearly (Cook et al. 2009), but the doubts about the benefits remain (Low et al. 2008). The aim of this chapter is to review the potential for regional anaesthetic methods to improve patient care.

The fundamental consideration to achieving the benefits of regional methods after major surgery is the physiological ('stress') response to surgery, a process which is the same after any form of 'trauma'. The changes comprising the response evolved as mechanisms for the repair of relatively simple injuries, but the scale and range of the responses after major surgery are anything but beneficial, even increasing its adverse consequences. Conventional anaesthetic and analgesic techniques have minimal effect on these changes, yet managing (and minimizing) their impact is a major component of perioperative care, particularly those aspects delivered by anaesthetists. Regional techniques have much to offer in this area, but they must be delivered both safely and effectively if the patient is to benefit. This requires knowledge of the adverse physiological consequences of surgery, the moderating effects which regional methods can provide, and an understanding of the ways in which the features of different techniques may (or may not) contribute to patient safety and comfort. These issues are reviewed here.

The physiological stress response

The stress response to trauma, originally described by Cuthbertson in 1929 (Wilmore 2002) as a neuroendocrine response, occurs after all types of surgery, with the degree being proportional to the severity of that surgery (Kehlet 1998). Surgery to the extremities produces little effect, but open thoracic and abdominal procedures quickly produce major changes. Historically, the stress response was thought to be protective, but there is now a great deal of evidence to show that its reduction *decreases* morbidity and mortality (Wilmore 2002). It has five different components or 'cascades' (sequential changes in homeostatic mechanisms), all of which interact with each other and may be modified by pre-existing patient co-morbidities. These five cascades relate to the pain pathway, the sympathetic nervous system, inflammation & immunosuppression, hypercatabolism, and hypercoagulation (Figure 3.1).

Pain

The pain pathway was long thought to be a simple conduit to provide a warning of, and withdrawal from, harmful stimuli, but it is now recognized that it also has many complex components and functions (see Chapter 2). Importantly, pain and the other cascade mechanisms are all interconnected, and attempting to provide analgesia using a single drug is unlikely to succeed, hence the development of the concept of multimodal analgesia. General anaesthesia overcomes what would otherwise be the immediate 'behavioural'

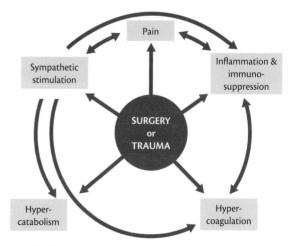

Figure 3.1 The five components of the stress response and their major interactions. See text for details.

response to surgery, and opioid analgesics provide some relief from the psychological effects of postoperative pain, but neither has any significant impact on the physiological processes which the pain pathway activates. Recently, pain and cytokine release have been shown to modulate one another, with neuropathic pain and hyperalgesia (both components of chronic pain) being increased by interleukin (IL)-1b and IL-6, while IL-6 and IL-8 induce peripheral and central sensitization, and are activated by sympathetic nervous system stimulation (Sommer & Kreiss 2004).

The most immediate of these responses is a reflex increase in muscle tone ('splinting') to decrease movement and minimize subsequent pain, but this limits mobilization after limb surgery and has significant respiratory impact after abdominal and thoracic procedures. Postoperative pain reduces both static and dynamic lung parameters, most notably functional residual capacity and peak flow rate (Craig 1981). Basal atelectasis occurs rapidly, and both deep breathing and effective coughing are impaired (Bromage 1978). Secretion retention, airway collapse, and venous admixture predispose to hypoxia, hypercapnia, and sepsis, each of which can amplify other aspects of the stress response.

Subsequent changes within the pain pathway itself can amplify and prolong the pain experienced by the patient, even resulting in chronic pain states developing. Stimulation of the pain pathway is also the key to the activation of all other components of the physiological stress response.

Sympathetic activation

The increased sympathetic activity which follows *peripheral* surgery is stimulated mainly by somatic afferent pathways, and is both minimal and localized, even after lengthy procedures. However, breaching of the thoracic or abdominal cavities (particularly with handling of the viscera) produces widespread stimulation of sympathetic afferent pathways, triggering a multitude of inhibitory reflexes which impair major organ function as well as releasing adrenal catecholamines and further interacting with the other cascades. Because the effects are widespread, block of one or two spinal cord segments is insufficient to prevent these effects which may persist for several days or even weeks.

Cardiovascular effects

The physiological effects of noradrenaline, adrenaline, and dopamine on the heart and circulation are well known, but, in summary, tachycardia and increased contractility both result in increased myocardial work and oxygen consumption. In the presence of increased systemic vascular resistance these may cause myocardial ischaemia and infarction, especially if there is pre-existing disease. Decreased organ blood flow, most notably to the heart, liver, and kidneys, may also result in ischaemia and cell necrosis. Adrenaline has been shown, in animal studies, to increase pulmonary arterio-venous admixture by producing non-uniform vasodilatation/constriction within the pulmonary vasculature. Both α- and β-block can reduce this (Berk et al. 1973, 1976). During cardiac catheterization there is a close correlation between pulmonary vascular resistance and pulmonary artery catecholamine concentrations in the presence of pulmonary arterial hypertension.

Respiratory effects

For many years it has been known that reflexes mediated through sympathetic nerves result in substantial inhibition of normal breathing patterns, particularly after abdominal and thoracic procedures (Ford & Guenter 1984), stimulation of bulbosplanchnic pathways inhibiting normal respiration (Albano & Garnier 1983). Furthermore, even in the virtual or complete absence of pain, pulmonary function remains depressed for many days after surgery (Benhamou et al. 1983), with multiple factors affecting this: diaphragmatic contractility, abdominal distension, secondary ileus, age, obesity, type of surgery and incision, personality, pre-existing lung disease, smoking habits, neuromuscular disease and muscle weakness, changes in thoracoabdominal blood volume, and, of considerable importance, the position of the patient (Hedenstierna 1988). Local neurogenic stimuli have also been shown to contribute to the pulmonary platelet trapping seen in shock (Thorne et al. 1980).

Gastrointestinal effects

Catecholamines have potentially harmful effects on gastrointestinal blood flow and function. In hypovolaemic states, splanchnic blood flow is greatly decreased so that healing may be compromised in patients with gastrointestinal anastomoses (Tagart 1981). Intestinal secretions and sphincter tone are increased, while motility is decreased. Gastric dilatation and paralytic ileus are known to be caused by local sympathetic inhibitory reflexes both within the gut wall and the spinal cord (Hedenstierna 1988). A similar state occurs within the genitourinary tract resulting in acute retention of urine.

Inflammation and immunosuppression

Current understanding of the mechanisms which initiate postoperative immunosuppression is poor, but the magnitude of the stress response correlates directly with both serum cortisol and the degree of immunosuppression (Carli & Shricker 2009). Triggers include transient episodes of ischaemia or malperfusion of vulnerable organs or surgical handling of major vessels and organs. Cardiac surgery with extracorporeal bypass induces the most severe inflammatory response, and concomitant complement activation has been associated with exacerbation of ischaemic brain, kidney, and myocardial injury through increased capillary permeability, neutrophil activation, and protease-activated receptor upregulation. The primary agent is probably the neutrophil, activated in the general circulation and coronary vasculature by myocytes.

Ischaemic cardiac myocytes produce *pro-inflammatory* IL-1b, IL-8, and IL-18 which allow neutrophils to adhere to the myocytes and release proteolytic enzymes (Suleiman 2008). Cardiac myocytes produce *anti-inflammatory* IL-6 and IL-10 which in turn lead to C-reactive protein production in the liver. IL-6 produces negative inotropic effects and myocardial stunning, its concentration correlating with left ventricular dysfunction and poor clinical outcome, while IL-8 exacerbates cardiac injury, correlating with cardiac troponin-I concentrations (Landis 2009). Thus elective major surgery may be regarded as inducing a 'pro-inflammatory, hypercoagulable, pseudo-septic state', with IL-1, IL-6, and IL-8 also promoting the discharge of A- and C-fibres, and leading to increased pain and hyperalgesia (Sommer & Kress 2004).

In addition, postoperative immunosuppression has been implicated in the formation of tumour metastases (Ben-Eliyahu et al. 1999). After tumour resection there is downregulation of the cellular immune system, and T-helper lymphocytes are decreased, causing an imbalance between these and the suppressor lymphocytes (Hole & Bakke 1984). After major surgery both helper and suppressor cells are suppressed, and the numbers of circulating natural killer cells, which have a wide range of cytotoxic activity particularly against tumour cells, are reduced also (Tonnesen et al. 1984). Thus, cellular immunity is disturbed for up to 7 days postoperatively (Lennard et al. 1985). There is a growing body of evidence from retrospective data to suggest these findings need further scientific evaluation (Biki et al. 2008, Tsui et al. 2010, Wada et al. 2007).

Hypercatabolism

It has long been appreciated that the metabolic consequences of surgery are generated by somatic and autonomic neuronal input, but humoral factors (e.g. tumour necrosis factor and the interleukins) are also involved. Reflex responses in several organs increase plasma concentrations of cortisol, glucose, catecholamines, and antidiuretic hormone soon after the start of surgery (Gordon et al. 1973), and the results include increased catabolism (especially of protein), negative nitrogen balance, hyperglycaemia, and salt & water retention. These effects may last for several weeks after surgery and are associated with weight loss of up to 5 kg in the first month, mainly secondary to protein breakdown. In clean, uncontaminated surgery the response is generated solely by neuronal reflexes, but acidosis, anxiety, haemorrhage, heat loss, hyperglycaemia, hypoxia, and infection will amplify the response (Kehlet 1998).

Catecholamines, particularly adrenaline, have a crucial role, promoting the catabolic state and increasing blood sugar, plasma lactate, and free fatty acid concentrations. In addition, adrenaline contributes to the retention of sodium and water, the excretion of potassium, and the displacement of fluid from the extracellular to vascular and intracellular compartments. By inhibiting pancreatic release of insulin and antagonizing its peripheral effects on glucose utilization, adrenaline inhibits anabolism and promotes a negative nitrogen balance (Frayn 1986, Little & Frayn 1985, Wilmore et al. 1988).

The combination of the cytokine, neuroendocrine, and catecholamine responses may have some beneficial effects, but they can be seriously detrimental as well. In the presence of severe trauma (such as major surgery) or sepsis their actions can lead to rapid depletion of lean body mass and organ failure (Carli & Shricker 2009), and while the changes are well documented, little is known about the specific trigger mechanisms. The gastrointestinal tract is known to have a central role in the protein catabolism which follows injury (Wilmore 1983), this being recognized as a major factor in delaying convalescence after surgery. Mucosal cell atrophy may occur secondary to ischaemia and hypoxia, resulting in breakdown of the gut barrier to micro-organisms and endotoxin, and further stimulating the glucocorticoid response and immunosuppression.

Hypercoagulation

Venous thromboembolism remains one of the most frequent and most serious complications of major trauma or surgery. Again the risk correlates with the degree of tissue damage and today only minor surgery in healthy patients is considered risk-free. The clotting cascade does not simply lead to clot formation, but is an inherent component of both the tissue repair process and the immune response to infection and tumour metastases (Bombeli & Spahn 2004). Many factors can trigger the hypercoagulable state, including autonomic afferent and efferent pathways (Kehlet 1998). Usually, any increase in coagulation during surgery is offset by an equivalent increase in fibrinolysis, but the latter decreases again postoperatively, so increasing the likelihood of clot formation (Murphy et al. 1993).

Ameliorating the stress response

A block technique will modify the response to surgery in two ways: first by preventing afferent input from producing the adverse changes outlined previously (analgesia at its simplest), but also through more subtle effects on autonomic efferent activity (sympatholysis) and the other components of the response.

Analgesia

The most outstanding feature of even a single-shot regional technique is the excellent analgesia (without central depression) which is produced. After more major surgery, recent meta-analyses provide definitive evidence that blocks are superior to opioid analgesia for any procedure at any time in the first 3 days (Richman et al. 2006, Wu et al. 2005). Thus the long-held and widespread belief that opioids are the 'gold standard' for postoperative pain is clearly no longer true, particularly with the recognition that their significant side effects limit the potential for the pain relief to promote rapid mobilization. 'Multimodal analgesia' is designed to substitute opioids with analgesics which have less troublesome side effects, but provide good quality pain relief (Kehlet & Dahl 1993). Pain will develop on block regression, but administration of supplementary oral or parenteral analgesics should be timed so that they become effective before the block wears off. This results in a gradual, rather than a sudden, awareness of pain and reduces the requirement for (and complications of) subsequent analgesic therapy. Where needed, catheter techniques allow the period of profound analgesia to be prolonged well into the postoperative period.

Sympatholysis

Regional techniques produce sympathetic block in the relevant area for the duration of the block, its influence depending not only on the site and level of the block, but also on the dose of local anaesthetic and any vasoconstrictor used, the presence of intercurrent disease, and the pre-existing state of the circulation. In *peripheral surgery* (i.e. of the head, neck, and limbs), afferent somatic and sympathetic block are usually complete, but with the effects on the circulation being minimal when peripheral blocks are used. The haemodynamic effects of central blocks used during peripheral surgery are usually easy to control, with the cause of any significant hypotension being readily apparent. In *body cavity surgery*, the consequences of central techniques are more variable, but there is now considerable evidence that sympathetic block is effective in reducing the duration and severity of postoperative systemic organ dysfunction, particularly after major procedures. However, full knowledge of these effects is needed so that the patient can be managed appropriately (Chapter 11) and the benefits gained (Chapter 5).

In the past decade, improved postoperative outcomes in patients receiving both α-2 agonists and β-adrenoceptor blocking agents have led to widespread adoption of their routine use for many types of surgery. However, the role of β-blockade in perioperative care has now been questioned by a large prospective randomized study of 8,351 patients. They all had established vascular disease and were undergoing thoracoabdominal surgery, and received sustained-release metoprolol. The results demonstrated that this was indeed associated with reduced cardiac morbidity, but surprisingly was also associated with an increased risk of infectious complications, stroke, and mortality (POISE Study Group 2008). A number of reasons might explain the findings, but perhaps the most likely is that the bradycardia and hypotension produced by β-adrenergic blocking agents led anaesthetists to 'lighten' the general anaesthetic, thereby actually increasing the stress response.

Cardiovascular system

In supine, healthy volunteers block up to, and including, the upper thoracic segments may have remarkably little effect on arterial pressure. Cardiac output and limb and organ blood flow are maintained, or even increased. Studies in normovolaemic patients without pain tend to confirm this except that hypotension is more likely to be seen as the block extends above T_5, when the sympathetic innervation to the heart is interrupted. Peripheral flow is usually increased in spite of the hypotension. When a block is performed in a patient in pain, cardiac output and arterial pressure decrease, but this is usually only to 'normal' levels because pain causes an increase in sympathetic activity. Sympathetic block may result in cardiovascular collapse in the sitting or hypovolaemic patient, because the circulation has been maintained by the increased sympathetic activity. The patient with severe valvular heart disease may be less able to compensate for peripheral vasodilatation because cardiac output may be relatively 'fixed'. Sympathetic block may also cause an unexpected degree of hypotension in the anxious patient, because the accompanying parasympathetic overactivity is then unopposed, and the patient simply faints.

The effects of an epidural block may be different from those of a spinal of similar extent. Very high systemic concentrations of local anaesthetic may be produced by the former and may contribute to circulatory depression, but it is usually considered that an epidural is less likely to cause hypotension. This may be because epidural block usually spreads more slowly than spinal so that there is more time for auto-compensation to occur. However, hypotension may be more marked when a local anaesthetic solution containing adrenaline is used for an epidural (Kennedy et al. 1966) because the dose absorbed is only sufficient to produce β-adrenergic effects. A comparison of the cardiovascular effects of epidurals and spinals was carried out by Ward and colleagues (1965).

Moderate hypotension improves the surgical field and decreases blood loss by a combination of arterial and venous hypotension (Modig 1988). Even in the cardiac patient, a moderate degree of hypotension will improve performance because it is accompanied by reductions in preload, afterload, and heart rate (Merin 1981). Sympathetic block produces an increase in lower limb blood (and arterial graft) flow and this may be partly responsible for the reduction in thromboembolic disease reported after regional anaesthesia (Thorburn et al. 1980). This antithrombotic effect may also be related to a direct pharmacological action of the local anaesthetic drug on blood coagulability and fibrinolysis (Modig et al. 1983a,b).

This analysis relates to central block techniques extending to the mid-thoracic level, but the tentative use of high thoracic epidural block for cardiac surgery has revealed some surprising features. Early work showed that thoracic epidural techniques improve endocardial blood flow (Klassen et al. 1980), and epidural block restricted to the upper thoracic dermatomes (T_{1-6}) has little impact on blood pressure and cardiac output (Berendes et al. 2003, Hejmanns 2007, Lagunilla 2006, Suttner et al. 2005). There are

positive effects on indices of myocardial function (Table 3.1), and even the patient with a 'fixed' cardiac output state may benefit (Chakravaty et al. 2005). However, the management of such a block requires experienced and skilled care, and the negative impact of co-morbid factors such as hypovolaemia and parasympathetic activity remains very relevant.

Respiratory system

The adverse effects of surgery on both breathing patterns and pulmonary function have been mentioned, and their prevention clearly explain the well-documented beneficial effect of high spinal or epidural block on postoperative respiratory function. However, these techniques also block the sympathetic supply to the lungs and airways, leaving parasympathetic activity unopposed. This can precipitate bronchospasm in the asthmatic patient; problems are rare, but the risk is always there. Bronchospasm may also develop during general anaesthesia, and regional anaesthesia may help prevent this complication by removing the need for airway instrumentation and by blocking afferent stimuli (both potent causes of reflex bronchospasm).

Gastrointestinal system

Because of unopposed parasympathetic activity, sympathetic block (in contrast to opioid analgesia) leads to preservation of oesophageal sphincter tone, an increase in gastrointestinal motility, and relaxation of many sphincters, promoting increased gastrointestinal transit (Thoren et al. 1988). Large bowel incontinence is a theoretical consequence, but occurs no more often than during general anaesthesia. Potentially, bowel rupture may be more likely if there is an obstruction, and this is a situation where spinal and epidural blocks should be used with great caution, if at all, and certainly not until the obstruction has been relieved. In elective bowel surgery the physiological consequences of sympathetic block may be more beneficial (Jorgensen et al. 2000), increasing hepatic (Meierhenrich et al. 2009) and colonic blood flow (Johansson et al. 1988), and reducing ileus (Basse et al. 2001). The accompanying muscle relaxation avoids the need to administer neostigmine, which may increase the incidence of anastomotic breakdown.

Neuroendocrine and metabolic effects

There are now many studies in the literature which demonstrate that reduction in the stress response hormones is associated with decreased mortality and morbidity (Wilmore 2002). Neither general

Table 3.1 Established benefits of T_{1-5} block on indices of myocardial function.

Decreases	Increases
Heart rate/blood pressure—clinically insignificant	Diseased artery diameter by up to 64%
Metabolism and O_2 consumption	Atrial and ventricular arrhythmia thresholds
Infarct size by up to 50%	Endo:epicardial blood flow ratio
Afterload	O_2 supply to ischaemic areas
Myocardial stunning and H^+ during ischaemia	Systolic and diastolic dysfunction
ST depression during stress test	

anaesthesia nor opioid analgesia has any significant impact, general anaesthesia doing little more than reducing the response transiently (Roizen et al. 1988). However, the metabolic and hormonal changes noted when surgery is performed under general anaesthesia are reduced considerably when regional techniques are employed. The effect extends to decreasing the incidence of postoperative insulin resistance, a risk factor for coronary artery disease and stroke in non-surgical individuals (Donatelli et al. 2007).

Epidural anaesthesia is known to have an anticatabolic effect which, by inhibiting protein breakdown, results in a positive nitrogen balance and retention of skeletal muscle and body mass. The reduction in response has been shown most convincingly during and after lower abdominal surgery and the effect is more marked if the regional block extends from T_4 to S_5 (Engquist et al. 1977). During upper abdominal surgery, epidural block, even when combined with vagal nerve block, may be insufficient to prevent some increase in the plasma concentrations of stress-related hormones (Traynor et al. 1982), but the catecholamine response to cardiac surgery is completely obtunded by continuous thoracic epidural analgesia (Fawcett et al. 1997).

The immune response

Changes in immunocompetence parallel the endocrine response after major surgery, and they have been implicated in the formation of tumour metastases and postoperative sepsis (Lennard et al. 1985). Non-specific humoral and cellular elements are involved, are proportional to the degree of 'trauma', are unaffected by general anaesthesia, and may be exacerbated by opioids (Scott 1991). More specifically, depression of lymphocyte transformation has been shown to be reduced by regional anaesthesia (Cullen & van Belle 1975), and the ratio of 'T' helper 1 to 'T' helper 2 cells was higher after transurethral resection of the prostate under spinal compared to general anaesthesia (LeCras et al. 1998). More recently, combined spinal and general anaesthesia was shown to attenuate liver metastasis formation by preserving Th1/Th2 cytokine balance (Wada 2007). These findings suggest that use of central blocks may

result in less immunosuppression, although there is still relatively little objective evidence to indicate whether such effects influence outcome.

Blood loss and thromboembolism

Although spinal anaesthesia was the earliest technique used for induced hypotension, the relationship between blood pressure and blood loss is far from clear. Notably, it has been shown that artificial maintenance of blood pressure during spinal anaesthesia does not increase blood loss (Thorburn 1985), and other studies have suggested that the main effect of the blocks is to diminish venous oozing (Modig 1988). Controlled studies show that a consistent decrease in bleeding with regional anaesthesia occurs, but that the effect is only statistically significant in surgery to the lower half of the body (Kehlet 1998).

A large number of studies have now shown that regional anaesthesia has a significant impact on the incidence of thromboembolic complications of surgery to the lower half of the body. Fewer studies have been performed on patients undergoing surgery to the upper half of the body and they have tended to show that regional anaesthesia makes little difference. However, one study did find that epidural block was as effective as low-dose heparin (Hjortso et al. 1985).

Early mobilization after surgery is now known to be a major contributing factor in reducing the incidence of postoperative thromboembolism, especially after orthopaedic procedures. This does not obviate the benefit of regional anaesthesia in minimizing these complications, although some of the benefit may simply be due to better analgesia improving mobilization.

Advantages and disadvantages, or features?

It is traditional to assess regional anaesthesia by considering its advantages and disadvantages, but this ignores the very real possibility that what is an advantage in one situation may be a disadvantage in another (Table 3.2). It is better to think in terms of the features of a particular block and then consider whether it will be

Table 3.2 Examples of positive and negative effects of the features of regional anaesthesia. The benefits are due to the combination of direct effects with reduced need for systemic opioids.

Feature	Benefits	Potential problems
Simplicity of administration	Minor surgery facilitated	Uninformed practice
Preservation of consciousness	Airway preserved	Heightened patient anxiety
	Improved childbirth 'experience'	
Profound analgesia	Improved patient comfort	Pressure sores from numbness
Sympathetic block	Stress response ameliorated	Unopposed vagal activity
Vasodilatation	Increased organ blood flow Reduced thromboembolism	Hypotension
Hypotension	Reduced surgical bleeding	Inadequate perfusion pressure
Muscle relaxation	Improved operating conditions	Hyperextension injuries Impaired mobilization
Gastrointestinal motility enhanced	Less nausea and vomiting	Increased intraluminal pressure
Side effects and sequelae	Traditional general anaesthetic sequelae reduced	Needle track discomfort Systemic local anaesthetic toxicity

advantageous (or not) in the individual patient. Hypotension is a good example of a feature of regional anaesthesia which is traditionally considered undesirable, but which can be an advantage during certain surgical procedures. Conversely, preservation of consciousness—commonly considered an advantage—may be unacceptable to the severely anxious patient undergoing anything more than the most minor procedure. When choosing an anaesthetic for a particular patient and operation, the anaesthetist should be able to assess the potential of all possible techniques, local and general, and decide which is the most appropriate. Some of these issues merit more detailed review.

Pain relief

Even simple peripheral nerve blocks may provide much greater comfort for the patient and simplify the administration of a general anaesthetic, notably for relatively minor, but extremely painful, operations such as nail-bed ablation, distal orthopaedic procedures (e.g. Mitchell's osteotomy, release of Dupuytren's contracture) and, in children, herniotomy and circumcision. Even if the block might, in itself, be insufficient for the surgery, a lighter plane of general anaesthesia can be used so that recovery is faster and the pain-free patient can mobilize sooner. However, even this, the most obvious benefit of regional anaesthesia, has its potentially negative side. Some patients find prolonged numbness distressing, and skin damage may result if the nursing staff are unaware of its implications for their care of the patient. Any associated muscle weakness may also cause problems (see 'Muscle relaxation' section).

Simplicity of administration

Local anaesthesia is a safe simple technique for the non-specialist anaesthetist undertaking relatively minor surgery. For the specialist involved with more major surgery, regional anaesthesia may also simplify the procedure. A single intrathecal injection of one drug will produce excellent conditions for many procedures—complete anaesthesia, muscle relaxation, and a reduction in blood loss. The patient's life is less dependent on the proper functioning and constant monitoring of complex general anaesthetic equipment. Moreover, simplicity of administration means that the practitioner with a good knowledge of anatomy can easily become proficient in these methods.

The ease of administration, particularly of infiltration and topical anaesthesia, can produce problems, and a meticulous technique is required for even minor procedures. Wound infiltration has enjoyed a renaissance in the past decade for a variety of procedures where central neuraxial block was performed previously (Kehlet & Kristensen 2009, Kehlet & Liu 2007). However, minimal training or complacency may result in a cavalier attitude to administration, with incorrect injection technique and thus failed analgesia. Lack of awareness of, or an inability to treat, complications may lead to disaster. Systemic toxicity due to drug overdosage, cardiorespiratory arrest due to poorly managed high spinal or epidural block, and pneumothorax after supraclavicular brachial plexus block are all potentially fatal complications. It is important to be aware that the combination of sympathetic block with even a minor degree of hypovolaemia (from whatever cause) will cause more hypotension than will general anaesthesia in the same circumstances. Thus, knowledge of the pharmacology of drugs, of the complications of the techniques to be used, and training in appropriate methods of resuscitation are essential. The availability of ultrasound to guide nerve identification and block performance does not obviate this requirement.

Preservation of consciousness

By its nature, uncomplicated regional anaesthesia will preserve consciousness, a desirable end in itself for the patient who wishes to remain awake. However, it is the avoidance of the secondary effects of unconsciousness that is important for the majority of patients. For example, the obstetric patient receiving regional analgesia is aware of her surroundings and the birth of her child, is able to maintain and protect her own airway and can co-operate with her attendant staff. There is also minimal fetal depression. These factors add up to a major argument for the use of local techniques.

The ability of the conscious patient to maintain and protect the airway and to co-operate is also of great value in dental practice, a field where airway obstruction during general anaesthesia is an ever present risk. Minor orthopaedic trauma is often dealt with under general anaesthesia, although it is recognized that gastric emptying is delayed in such patients. The majority of these injuries are peripheral and eminently suitable for local techniques.

In some circumstances general anaesthesia may be preferred even though the risk of pulmonary aspiration is high, as, for example, in emergency surgery for gastrointestinal obstruction. The general condition of these patients tends to be poor because of the effects of the obstruction, particularly dehydration leading to hypovolaemia, and the presence of intercurrent disease. If a spinal or an epidural is to be used, a block to the mid-thoracic region is required because the extent of surgery is unpredictable in this setting so blood loss may lead to severe hypotension. Nevertheless, an epidural sited at the time of surgery, but activated later when the patient's physiology has been stabilized and the risk of bowel rupture has passed (see 'Gastrointestinal system' section), can be invaluable. Equally, an elderly patient with limited respiratory reserve undergoing aortic valve surgery may benefit from this approach.

A conscious, co-operative patient is an advantage in other situations. Surgery for varicose veins on the back of the legs or for pilonidal sinus requires the patient to be prone. If a regional technique is used, patients can help to position themselves, indicate that the position is comfortable, and confirm that respiration is unimpeded. A spinal anaesthetic can be used very effectively, although a full understanding of the factors which influence block height is particularly important, so a solution which will not spread to the upper thoracic dermatomes is used. Treatment of a high block in a prone patient is difficult. Further, the conscious or lightly sedated patient may be able to warn of the subjective effects of complications at an early stage. The diabetic patient may recognize and report the initial symptoms of hypoglycaemia, and patient agitation or distress during transurethral surgery may arouse suspicion that bladder irrigation fluid has entered the circulation.

Most of the problems of regional anaesthesia due to preservation of consciousness relate to patients' anxiety about being aware during the performance of the block and the surgical procedure. The majority of British patients expect to be asleep, and it is at least arguable that many European and North American patients might prefer to be asleep, even though they expect to be awake during surgery. To undergo major surgery under regional anaesthesia alone is an unpleasant experience and patients subjected to this may faint, even in the supine position, and this may be mistaken for other causes of hypotension. Finally, because most operating tables are uncomfortable, the conscious patient may become restless and unable to remain still—one of the few situations where the surgeon may justifiably be upset by an anaesthetic technique.

Explanation and reassurance can help, but the more nervous the patient and the longer and more extensive the surgery, the greater is the need for some kind of sedation. Oral premedication is rarely contraindicated, and intravenous or inhalational sedation can both be used to produce amnesia while preserving the benefits of consciousness. However, some patients may be so frightened that they will not tolerate surgery with anything but complete loss of consciousness, and then of course some benefits may be lost.

Muscle relaxation

Local techniques produce motor as well as sensory block. This means that for the majority of patients undergoing even major surgery the need to use muscle relaxants is virtually abolished, thereby avoiding all their side effects and the risk of developing postoperative pulmonary complications (Berg et al. 1997). The muscle relaxation which results from regional anaesthesia has the specific advantage of being confined to the operative field (unlike that due to neuromuscular-blocking drugs), so the patient can continue to breathe spontaneously. Spinal and epidural block may result in impairment of the nerve supply to some respiratory muscles, but unless a very high block is produced this is of little clinical consequence. Blocks to the level normally required for abdominal surgery produce only a slight decrease in expiratory reserve volume and expulsive ability (Bowler et al. 1988). However, these latter effects may be more important in patients with respiratory disease, although the effect of the block in preventing pain and reducing the requirement for opioid drugs will more than compensate for any decrease in muscle power. The latter will, in any case, be minimized by careful choice of local anaesthetic and use of an appropriate concentration.

Weakness of the legs may be relatively prolonged after spinal anaesthesia, because the highest concentration of local anaesthetic in the cerebrospinal fluid will be around the lumbar and sacral nerve roots. Provided patients are warned in advance that motor block is likely, they should not become very concerned about it, although some patients may prefer an alternative, albeit less effective, analgesic technique which preserves more motor power and mobility than an epidural infusion of local anaesthetic. Complete analgesia accompanied by lower limb motor weakness is a real hazard for the patient being mobilized after a knee arthroplasty with femoral nerve block, and thus with paralysis of the quadriceps femoris muscle (Kandesami et al. 2009). This can lead to complications such as falling during mobilization (Sharma et al. 2010), although the use of less local anaesthetic than is 'traditional' (e.g. 20 ml ropivacaine 0.2%) can provide good quality analgesia *without* the risk of limb weakness (see Chapter 5). Similarly, a patient with an arm paralysed by a brachial plexus block must be moved slowly or a hyperextension injury may result because of the limb's 'inertia'.

Side effects and sequelae

In addition to its effect on postoperative pain, regional anaesthesia may also reduce the incidence of other less major sequelae of anaesthesia and surgery, although freedom from wound pain may make the patient more aware of other sources of discomfort such as a venepuncture site or a nasogastric tube. Few controlled studies have been performed of the relative incidence of these sequelae, but

Table 3.3 shows data from two reasonably comparable groups of patients having surgery with either spinal or general anaesthesia. All but one of the symptoms occurred less frequently after spinal anaesthesia, the exception being headache, although the proportion of patients who graded this as 'severe' was the same in each group.

Others (Lanz et al. 1982) have suggested that differences in minor sequelae are not quite so clearly in favour of regional anaesthesia, although in their study the patient was responsible for the choice of anaesthetic technique. Patients who have suffered severe nausea and vomiting after previous general anaesthetics are particularly appreciative of regional techniques, especially those which minimize the need for opioids. However, no method can prevent certain patients from reacting to the psychological stress of surgery by becoming nauseated or even vomiting, particularly if they are given little in the way of perioperative sedation. Untreated hypotension and bradycardia are, in turn, potent causes of nausea and vomiting during central blocks.

In addition, there are some disadvantages to the extension of the effects of these techniques into the postoperative period. As noted, some patients find prolonged lack of feeling, especially in the legs, unpleasant and urinary retention may occur, notably if large volumes of intravenous fluids have been used in an attempt to maintain blood pressure. A high standard of medical and nursing care will minimize these complications, and the staff/patient ratio in the obstetric unit is high enough for this to be provided. In the general ward even single-injection nerve block techniques may cause concern unless the nursing staff are properly educated in the care of such patients. The routine use of continuous techniques requires careful appraisal of the staff available to monitor the patient and ensure both effective delivery of analgesia and identification of complications at an early stage. These issues are considered further in Chapters 4, 11, and 14.

Finally, there will always be concern about the rare, but major sequelae of continuous blocks such as haematoma and abscess formation (see Chapter 4). In a review of 505,000 obstetric epidurals there were two cases of epidural haematoma and one abscess, with two of the patients suffering permanent sequelae (Scott & Hibbard 1990). Only constant vigilance and early diagnosis and treatment can minimize the effects on the patient. All of these points have been reinforced by the recent Royal College of Anaesthetists audit of complications (Cook et al. 2009).

Table 3.3 Total incidence (%) of minor postoperative complications after spinal and general anaesthesia (data from Dempster 1984). The incidence of complications graded 'severe' by the patient is also shown.

Complications	Spinal anaesthesia		General anaesthesia	
	Total	Severe	Total	Severe
Nausea	9	0	40	6
Vomiting	15	2	43	6
Headache	34	6	23	6
Sore throat	2	0	30	0
Muscle pains	4	0	9	0
Backache	28	2	32	6
Urinary difficulty	6	0	30	0

Benefits to the anaesthetist

A most important benefit to the specialty as a whole is the way in which local techniques have enabled anaesthetists to extend their practice beyond the operating theatre. The provision of epidural services in the labour wards and the staffing of chronic pain clinics are two good examples, and the wider use of these methods in the management of acute pain is an area of continuing interest. An additional benefit of these activities is that the anaesthetist maintains and improves both communication skills and, perhaps more importantly, professional identity with the patient.

The anaesthetist who is prepared to learn and practise regional anaesthesia has a larger armamentarium with which to deal with the many clinical problems which present in routine practice. Those who use these methods successfully obtain considerable satisfaction, not only from the technical skill required, but also from the benefits which accrue to their patients, particularly in the period immediately after surgery. If, by the use of a single technique, it is possible to offer complete neural block which results in control of pain, abolition of the stress response, efferent sympathetic block with increased regional blood flow, early ambulation, deep vein thrombosis prophylaxis, reduced susceptibility to infection, and reductions in nausea and vomiting, respiratory depression, and hypoxia, then such a technique should be more expertly taught and more widely advocated. At the same time significant efforts should be made to overcome its avoidable side effects. Today, neural block makes it possible to provide a quality of recovery and convalescence after major surgery that was undreamed of 20 or 30 year ago.

Conclusion

Local and regional techniques have much to offer patients and practitioners. The benefits over general anaesthesia are self-evident in minor surgery, but as the operation becomes more major a more complex judgement needs to be made although the *potential* for benefit, as outlined throughout this chapter, is quite clear. As the use of regional methods for very major surgery has increased over the last 20-plus years many attempts have been made to 'prove' that these benefits translate into reductions in perioperative morbidity and mortality. The issues surrounding this aspect are considered in Chapter 5.

Key reference

Carli F, Shricker T (2009) Modification of metabolic responses to surgery by neural blockade. In Cousins MJ, Carr DB, Horlocker TT, Bridenbaugh PO (Eds) *Neural blockade in clinical anesthesia and pain medicine*, 4th edn, pp. 133–43. Philadelphia, PA: Lippincott Williams & Wilkins.

On-line resource

www.neuralblockadepainmanagement.com This is the electronic version of the Cousins et al. (2009) text listed in the 'Key reference' section, but a subscription is required.

References

Albano JP, Garnier L (1983) Bulbo-spinal respiratory effects originating from splanchnic afferents. *Respiration Physiology* 51: 229–39.

Basse L, Madsen JL, Kehlet H (2001) Normal gastrointestinal transit after colonic resection using epidural analgesia, enforced oral nutrition and laxative. *British Journal of Surgery* 88: 1498–500.

Ben-Eliyahu S, Page GG, Yirmiya R, Shakhar G (1999) Evidence that stress and surgical interventions promote tumor development by suppressing natural killer cell activity. *International Journal of Cancer* 80: 880–8.

Benhamou D, Samii K, Noviant Y (1983) Effect of analgesia on respiratory muscle function after upper abdominal surgery. *Acta Anaesthesiologica Scandinavica* 27: 22–5.

Berendes E, Schmidt C, Van Aken H et al. (2003) Reversible cardiac sympathectomy by high thoracic epidural anesthesia improves regional left ventricular function in patients undergoing coronary artery bypass grafting: a randomized trial. *Archives of Surgery* 138: 1283–90.

Berk JL, Hagen JF, Koo R (1973) Pulmonary insufficiency caused by epinephrine. *Annals of Surgery* 178: 423–34.

Berk JL, Hagan JF, Koo R (1976) Effect of alpha and beta adrenergic blockade on epinephrine induced pulmonary insufficiency. *Annals of Surgery* 183: 369–76.

Berg H, Viby-Mogensen J, Roed J, et al. (1997) Residual neuromuscular block is a risk factor for postoperative pulmonary complications. A prospective, randomised, and blinded study of postoperative pulmonary complications after atracurium, vecuronium and pancuronium. *Acta Anaesthesiologica Scandinavica* 41: 1095–103.

Biki B, Mascha E, Moriarty DC, et al. (2008) Anesthetic technique for radical prostatectomy surgery affects cancer recurrence: a retrospective analysis. *Anesthesiology* 109: 180–7.

Bombeli T, Spahn DR (2004) Updates in perioperative coagulation home: physiology and management of thromboembolism and haemorrhage. *British Journal of Anaesthesia* 93: 275–87.

Bowler GMR, Wildsmith JAW, Scott DB (1988) Epidural administration of anesthetics. *Clinics in Critical Care Medicine: Acute Pain Management* 8: 187–235.

Bromage PR (1978) *Epidural analgesia*. Philadelphia, PA: WB Saunders.

Carli F, Shricker T (2009) Modification of metabolic responses to surgery by neural blockade. In Cousins MJ, Carr DB, Horlocker TT, Bridenbaugh PO (Eds) *Neural blockade in clinical anesthesia and pain medicine*, 4th edn, pp. 133–43. Philadelphia, PA: Lippincott Williams & Wilkins.

Chakravarthy M, Thimmangowda P, Krishnamurhy J, et al. (2005) Thoracic epidural anesthesia in cardiac surgical patients: a prospective audit of 2,113 cases. *Journal of Cardiothoracic & Vascular Anesthesia* 119: 44–8.

Cook TM, Counsel D, Wildsmith JAW (2009) Major complications of central neuraxial block: report on the 3rd National Audit Project of the Royal College of Anaesthetists. *British Journal of Anaesthesia* 102: 179–90.

Craig DB (1981) Postoperative recovery of pulmonary function. *Anesthesia and Analgesia* 60: 46–52.

Cullen BF, van Belle G (1975) Lymphocyte transformation and changes in leukocyte count: effects of anesthesia and operation. *Anesthesiology* 43: 563–9.

Dempster S (1984) The sequelae of spinal analgesia as opposed to general anaesthesia. Undergraduate prize essay: Association of Anaesthetists of Great Britain and Ireland.

Donatelli, F, Vavassori A, Bonfanti S, et al. (2007) Epidural anesthesia and analgesia decrease the postoperative incidence of insulin resistance in preoperative insulin-resistant subjects only. *Anesthesia & Analgesia* 104: 1587–93.

Engquist A, Brandt MR, Fernandes A, Kehlet H (1977) The blocking effect of epidural anaesthesia on the adrenocortical responses to surgery. *Acta Anaesthesiologica Scandinavica* 21: 330–5.

Fawcett WJ, Edwards RE, Quinn AC et al. (1997) Thoracic epidural analgesia started after cardiopulmonary bypass. Adrenergic, cardiovascular and respiratory sequelae. *Anaesthesia* 52: 294–9.

Ford GT, Guenter CA (1984) Toward prevention of postoperative pulmonary complications. *American Review of Respiratory Disease* 130(1): 4–5.

Frayn KN (1986) Hormonal control of metabolism in trauma and sepsis. *Clinical Endocrinology* 24: 577–99.

Gordon NH, Scott DB, Percy-Robb IW (1973) Modification of plasma corticosteroid concentrations during and after surgery by epidural blockade. *British Medical Journal* i: 581–3.

Hedenstierna G (1988) Mechanisms of postoperative pulmonary dysfunction. *Acta Chirurgica Scandinavica Supplement* 550: 152–8.

Heijmans J, Fransen E, Buurman W, et al. (2007) Comparison of the modulatory effects of four different fast-track anesthetic techniques on the inflammatory response to cardiac surgery with cardiopulmonary bypass. *Journal of Cardiothoracic & Vascular Anesthesia* 21: 512–18.

Hjortso NC, Andersen T, Frosig F (1985 A controlled study of the effect of epidural analgesia with local anaesthetics and morphine on morbidity after abdominal surgery. *Acta Anesthesiologica Scandinavica* 29: 790.

Hole A, Bakke O (1984) T-lymphocytes and the subpopulations of T-helper and T-suppressor cells measured by monoclonal antibodies (T11, T4 and T8) in relation to surgery under epidural and general anaesthesia. *Acta Anaesthesiologica Scandinavica* 28: 296–300.

Johansson K, Ahn H, Lindhagen J, Tryselius U (1988) Effect of epidural anaesthesia on intestinal blood flow. *British Journal of Surgery* 75: 73–6.

Jørgensen H, Wetterslev J, Møiniche S, Dahl JB (2000) Epidural LA versus opioid-based analgesic regimens on postoperative gastrointestinal paralysis, PONV and pain after abdominal surgery. *Cochrane Database of Systemic Reviews* 4: CD001893.

Kandasami M, Kinninmonth AW, Sarungi M, et al. (2009) Femoral nerve block for total knee replacement—a word of caution. *Knee* 16: 98–100.

Kehlet H, Dahl JB (1993) The value of 'multimodal' or 'balanced analgesia' in post-operative pain treatment. *Anesthesia & Analgesia* 77: 1048–56.

Kehlet H (1998) Modification of responses to surgery by neural blockade: clinical implications. In Cousins MJ, Bridenbaugh PO (Eds) *Neural blockade in clinical anesthesia and management of pain*, 3rd edn, pp. 129–78. Philadelphia, PA: Lippincott-Raven.

Kehlet H, Kristensen BB (2009) Local anesthetics in the surgical wound—is the pendulum swinging toward increased use? *Regional Anesthesia & Pain Medicine* 34: 389–90.

Kehlet H, Liu SS (2007) Continuous local anesthetic wound infusion to improve postoperative outcome: back to the periphery? *Anesthesiology* 107: 369–71.

Kennedy WF, Bonica JJ, Ward RJ, et al. (1966) Cardiorespiratory effects of epinephrine when used in regional anesthesia. *Acta Anaesthesiologica Scandinavica Supplement* 26: 320–33.

Klassen GA, Bramwell RS, Bromage PR, et al. (1980) Effect of acute sympathectomy by epidural anesthesia on the canine coronary circulation. *Anesthesiology* 52: 8–15.

Lagunilla J, Garcia-Bengochea JB, Fernandez AL, et al. (2006) High thoracic epidural blockade increases myocardial oxygen availability in coronary surgery patients. *Acta Anaesthesiologica Scandinavica* 50: 780–6.

Landis RC (2009) Redefining the systemic inflammatory response. *Seminars in Cardiothoracic & Vascular Anesthesia* 13: 87–94.

Lanz E, Theiss D, Emmerich EA, Emmerich M (1982) Regional versus general anaesthesia: attitudes and experiences of patients. *Regional Anaesthesia* 7: S163–71.

LeCras AE, Galley HF, Webster NR (1998) Spinal but not general anesthesia increases the ratio of T helper 1 to T helper 2 cell subsets in patients undergoing transurethral resection of the prostate. *Anesthesia and Analgesia* 87: 1421–5.

Lennard TW, Shenton BK, Bortotta A, et al. (1985) The influence of surgical operation on components of the immune system. *British Journal of Surgery* 72: 771–6.

Little RA, Frayn KN (Eds) (1985) *The scientific basis for the care of the critically ill*. Manchester: Manchester University Press.

Low J, Johnston N, Morris C (2008) Epidural analgesia: First do no harm. *Anaesthesia* 63: 1–3.

Meierhenrich R, Wagner F, Schutz W, et al. (2009) The effects of thoracic epidural anesthesia on hepatic blood flow in patients under general anesthesia. *Anesthesia & Analgesia* 108: 1331–7.

Merin RG (1981) Local and regional anesthetic techniques for the patient with ischaemic heart disease. *Cleveland Clinic Quarterly* 48: 72–4.

Modig J (1988) Beneficial effects on blood loss in total hip replacement when performed under lumbar epidural anaesthesia versus general anaesthesia: an exploratory study. *Acta Chirurgica Scandinavica Supplement* 550: 95–103.

Modig J, Borg T, Bagge L, Saldeen T (1983a) Role of extradural and of general anaesthesia in fibrinolysis and coagulation after total hip replacement. *British Journal of Anaesthesia* 55: 625–9.

Modig J, Borg T, Karlstrom G, et al. (1983b) Thromboembolism after total hip replacement: role of epidural and general anesthesia. *Anesthesia & Analgesia* 62: 174–80.

Murphy WG, Davies MJ, Eduardo A (1993) The haemostatic response to surgery and trauma. *British Journal of Anaesthesia* 70: 205–13.

POISE Study Group (2008) Effects of extended release metoprolol succinate in patients undergoing non-cardiac surgery (POISE trial): a randomised controlled trial. *Lancet* 371: 1839–47.

Richman JM, Liu SS, Courpas G, et al. (2006) Does continuous peripheral nerve block provide superior pain control to opioids? A meta-analysis. *Anesthesia & Analgesia* 102: 248–57.

Roizen MF (1988) Should we all have a sympathectomy at birth? Or at least preoperatively? *Anesthesiology* 68: 482–4.

Scott NB (1991) The effects of pain and its treatment. In McClure JH, Wildsmith JAW (eds) *Mechanisms and management of conduction blockade for postoperative analgesia*, pp. 78–110. London: Arnold.

Scott DB, Hibbard BM (1990) Serious non-fatal complications associated with extradural block in obstetric practice. *British Journal of Anaesthesia* 64: 547–1.

Sharma S, Iorio R, Specht LM, et al. (2010) Complications of femoral nerve block for total knee arthroplasty. *Clinical Orthopaedics & Related Research* 468: 135–40.

Sommer C, Kress M (2004) Recent findings on how proinflammatory cytokines cause pain: peripheral mechanisms in inflammatory and neuropathic hyperalgesia. *Neuroscience Letters* 361: 184–7.

Suleiman MS, Zacharowski K, Angelini GD (2008) Inflammatory response and cardioprotection during open-heart surgery: the importance of anaesthetics. *British Journal of Pharmacology* 153: 21–33.

Suttner S, Lang K, Piper SN, et al. (2005) Continuous intra- and postoperative thoracic epidural analgesia attenuates brain natriuretic peptide release after major abdominal surgery. *Anesthesia & Analgesia* 101: 896–903.

Tagart REB (1981) Colorectal anastomosis: factors influencing success. *Journal of the Royal Society of Medicine* 74: 111–18.

Thorburn J (1985) Subarachnoid blockade and total hip replacement: effect of ephedrine on intraoperative blood loss. *British Journal of Anaesthesia* 57: 290–3.

Thorburn J, Louden JR, Vallance R (1980) Spinal and general anaesthesia in total hip replacement: frequency of deep vein thrombosis. *British Journal of Anaesthesia* 52: 1117–21.

Thoren T, Carlsson E, Sandmark S, Watwil M (1988) Effects of thoracic epidural analgesia with morphine or bupivacaine on lower oesophageal sphincter pressure: an experimental study in man. *Acta Anaesthesiologica Scandinavica* 32: 391–4.

Thorne LJ, Kuenzig M, McDonald HM, Schwartz SI (1980) Effect of denervation of a lung on pulmonary platelet trapping associated with traumatic shock. *Surgery* 88: 208–14.

Tonnesen E, Huttel MS, Christensen NJ, Schmitz O (1984) Natural killer cell activity in patients undergoing upper abdominal surgery: relationship to the endocrine stress response. *Acta Anaesthesiologica Scandinavica* 28: 654–60.

Traynor C, Paterson JL, Ward ID, et al. (1982) Effects of extradural analgesia and vagal blockade on the metabolic and endocrine response to upper abdominal surgery. *British Journal of Anaesthesia* 54: 319–23.

Tsui BC, Rashiq S, Schopflocher D, et al. (2010) Epidural anesthesia and cancer recurrence rates after radical prostatectomy. *Canadian Journal of Anaesthesia* 57: 107–12.

Wada H, Seki S, Takahashi T, et al. (2007) Combined spinal and general anaesthesia attenuates liver metastasis by preserving Th1/Th2 cytokine balance. *Anesthesiology* 106: 499–506.

Ward RJ, Bonica JJ, Freund FG, et al. (1965) Epidural and subarachnoid anesthesia: cardiovascular and respiratory effects. *Journal of the American Medical Association* 191: 275–8.

Wildsmith JAW (2002) No sceptic me, but the long day's task is not yet done: The 2002 Gaston Labat Lecture. *Regional Anesthesia & Pain Management* 27: 503–8.

Wilmore DW (1983) Alterations in protein, carbohydrate and fat metabolism in injured and septic patients. *Journal of the American College of Nutrition* 2: 3–13.

Wilmore DW (2002) From Cuthbertson to fast-track surgery: 70 years of progress in reducing stress in surgical patients. *Annals of Surgery* 236: 643–8.

Wilmore DW, Smith RJ, O'Dwyer ST, et al. (1988) The gut: a central organ after surgical stress. *Surgery* 104: 917–23.

Wu CL, Cohen SR, Richman JM, et al. (2005) Efficacy of postoperative patient-controlled and continuous infusion epidural analgesia versus patient-controlled analgesia with opioids: a meta-analysis. *Anesthesiology* 103: 1079–88.

CHAPTER 4

Neurological complications

Colin McCartney

Gentleness is the first requisite of the anesthetist.
Gaston Labat 1922

Regional techniques have the potential to provide many benefits for patients (Chapter 3), but a major barrier to their wider use is the fear of neurological injury even though this is very rare. Adverse events can occur after any medical intervention, but nerve injury after regional anaesthesia is so rare that it is very difficult to study, even the true incidence being difficult to ascertain although estimates have been made (Table 4.1). However, when these complications occur they can be devastating: devastating for the patient, for the anaesthetist, and for the practice of regional anaesthesia. Some 60 years ago, reports of severe spinal cord damage after spinal anaesthesia (Cope 1954, Kennedy et al. 1950) resulted in regional methods being almost abandoned in the UK. Although others soon showed that spinal anaesthesia can be used safely with proper attention to detail (Dripps & Vandam 1954), the reports of injury are required reading because they show what can happen if that detail is ignored.

Because of their severity, and in spite of their rarity, the problems require close scrutiny to determine aetiology, establish principles of management to minimize disability, and indicate how they may be avoided altogether. Even the brain may be injured by complications of regional anaesthesia: ischaemia after cardiovascular collapse and the consequences of cerebrospinal fluid (CSF) leak from an uncontrolled dural puncture are two examples, but they are dealt with elsewhere (Chapters 9 and 13). The focus of this chapter is to identify how the spinal cord and peripheral nerves may be damaged

during regional anaesthesia, although the investigation of an individual patient should recognize that other factors are more frequent causes of postoperative nerve injury (see later in chapter). In the last decade knowledge of these issues has advanced significantly, and the aetiology, incidence, diagnosis, management, and prevention of neurological complications of both central and peripheral block will be discussed. However, prevention has to be the guiding principle because of the nervous system's very limited capacity for either repair or recovery.

Injury after central neuraxial block

The spinal cord and the nerve roots within the vertebral canal are provided with very considerable protection from harm, but the insertion of a needle or catheter bypasses all of that protection, particularly when the dura mater is punctured. A wide range of mechanisms can then lead to harm, and the spinal cord and nerve roots may be injured *directly* by infection, physical trauma, compression (by both haematoma and abscess) or chemical insult, or *indirectly* by ischaemia, with study often showing that several factors may be involved.

Direct trauma

The spinal cord

The spinal cord terminates at the L_{1-2} level in most adults so spinal anaesthesia is usually performed at the mid/low lumbar level to avoid the conus medullaris. The site of needle insertion is traditionally identified by reference to Tuffier's line, the level of the iliac crests (typically the fourth lumbar vertebra), but determination of level using this landmark can be inaccurate (Furness et al. 2002). Further, the cord may actually terminate anywhere between T_{12} and L_4 (Kim et al. 2003) so direct trauma may be associated with inaccurate determination of vertebral level, an abnormally caudad conus, or a combination of the two.

In reporting a series of seven patients with needle damage to spinal cord, Reynolds (2001) placed much emphasis on errors in identification of vertebral level. However, spinal anaesthesia must, on occasion, be performed (apparently uneventfully) in patients with longer than usual spinal cords. Further, it is quite possible, with an appropriately gentle and careful technique, to deliberately perform spinal anaesthesia at the mid-thoracic level (van Zundert et al. 2007). The implication is that other factors have to be involved

Table 4.1 Incidence of neurological complications after neuraxial blocks. (Data from Brull et al. 2007.)

Technique	Complication	Incidence (per 10,000 blocks)
Spinal anaesthesia	Radiculopathy/neuropathy	3.78
	Cauda equina syndrome	0.11
	Intracranial event	0.03
	Paraplegia	0.06
Epidural analgesia	Radiculopathy/neuropathy	2.19
	Cauda equina syndrome	0.23
	Intracranial event	0.07
	Paraplegia	0.09

for spinal cord damage to occur (Fettes & Wildsmith 2002), the most likely being over-vigorous insertion of the needle to too great a depth. One subsidiary factor may be the use of pencil-point needles; the opening in these is some 1–2 mm proximal to the tip so they have to be inserted that short distance further before CSF is obtained. Spinal stenosis may also mean that the space between the arachnoid mater and spinal cord is narrowed or even obliterated.

These subsidiary factors may also be relevant in cases in which an epidural needle or catheter damages the cord, accidental dural puncture probably being an associated event. Usually the ligamentum flavum provides an increased resistance to needle advancement, and thus indicates that the tip is about to reach the epidural space, but occasionally the ligaments on either side do not fuse, leaving a midline deficiency. This may occur at any level, but it is commoner in the upper thoracic and cervical regions (Hogan 1996). Lack of resistance to needle advancement may lead to excessive depth of insertion and cord damage, especially at the levels of the lumbar and cervical expansions.

Contact with the cord may result in pain, paraesthesiae, or other 'sensations', but it may also be silent, this depending on exactly which nerve tract is penetrated (Neal 2008). The spinal cord has no sensory receptors, and sensory input from the meninges is variable, this explaining cases in which spinal cord needle placement was not recognized even in awake patients (Jacob et al. 2004, Tsui & Armstrong 2005). Injection within the spinal cord seems to produce pain more consistently, and this may be related to stimulation of sensory neurones (Huntoon et al. 2004).

Nerve roots

Although the individual nerve roots in the cauda equina are somewhat more mobile than the cord, and present smaller 'targets', they can also be damaged if a needle is inserted too vigorously. There is good evidence that the incidence of paraesthesiae due to nerve root contact is greater when pencil-point needles are used (Hopkinson et al. 1997), particularly as part of a combined spinal/epidural technique (Turner & Reifenberg 1995). A nerve root may also be damaged in the region of the intervertebral foramen if the needle is inserted more laterally than intended, especially during the paramedian approach or in the presence of any kypho-scoliosis.

Chemical injury

Local anaesthetic neurotoxicity

Commercially available local anaesthetics from reputable manufacturers can be considered to be free of any risk of causing damage to nerves under normal use. However, the solutions used for neuraxial block should be *preservative-free* because these substances can injure nerves, certainly within the subarachnoid space where even the final protective layer of dura mater is missing (see discussion on chloroprocaine in Chapter 8). This means that multidose vials and commercial solutions containing adrenaline should not be used because they contain antibacterial agents or antioxidants. These substances cannot diffuse through the dura mater, but should not be used for epidural block because of the possibility of accidental subarachnoid injection. If a solution containing adrenaline is to be used, it should be mixed immediately prior to injection.

Another exception to the general view that local anaesthetic solutions are not neurotoxic is that the concentration should not exceed that supplied. Some years ago, when fine-gauge intrathecal

catheters first became available there were reports of the cauda equina syndrome following their use (Rigler et al. 1991). Investigation showed that the initial injection had produced a very limited block because the catheter was directing the solution caudally. The response was simply to inject more local anaesthetic with the result that very high concentrations accumulated around the cauda equina. Because lidocaine was involved in most of these cases it was assumed that this was a drug-specific problem, even though the original report included one patient who had received tetracaine (Rigler et al. 1991).

When spinal anaesthesia began to be used for day-care surgery lidocaine was often used because its short duration allows rapid mobilization. However, reports then began to appear of unusual postoperative symptoms: back pain and paraesthesiae radiating into the legs (Schneider et al. 1993). The question arose of whether this was further evidence of primary lidocaine neurotoxicity even though these *transient neurological symptoms* (TNS) regressed within 2–3 days (Hampl et al. 1995) and were described after other drugs as well. Some controversy remains, but the causative features seem to be surgery under spinal anaesthesia, extremes of posture (e.g. lithotomy), and early mobilization. The symptoms are commoner after lidocaine, probably because it produces very profound muscle relaxation which allows over-stretching of joints and ligaments. TNS are indicators of neuromuscular strain, *not* neurotoxicity.

Other substances

Chemicals other than local anaesthetics may be injected *therapeutically*. A wide range of drugs have been shown to have potentially useful analgesic actions at spinal cord level, and many have been used in neuraxial block. However, there are few stability or safety data relating to this practice (which is an 'off-licence' application of most of the drugs), particularly when there is more than one additive in the local anaesthetic solution.

Accidental contamination of equipment or injectate is most likely with the antiseptic used for skin preparation. Any substance which is designed to kill bacteria is bound to be toxic to nerves, and these agents have been alleged to cause adhesive arachnoiditis (Rice et al. 2004). Equally rare, but equally damaging, are the consequences of the injection of substances other than local anaesthetic by mistake.

Ischaemia

Basically, the blood supply to the spinal cord is autoregulated in the same way as that to the brain and should not, in essence, be compromised given an adequate perfusion pressure. However, a significant element of vulnerability is introduced by the dependence of the supply to the lower two-thirds of the anterior spinal artery on one lumbar feeding vessel (Chapter 12). If this fails, a painless paralysis of the lower half of the body will result: the anterior spinal artery syndrome. The feeding vessel is well protected from damage by anaesthetic (although not surgical) instrumentation, but cardiovascular collapse can lead to ischaemia, especially if there is local atheroma.

An increase in pressure within the vertebral canal, as with a haematoma or abscess, may impair blood flow, and such complications (see next two sections) can also cause arterial thrombosis. However, there are no data to suggest that the use of local anaesthetic solutions containing adrenaline has any adverse effect (Neal 2003).

Vertebral canal haematoma

The contents of the vertebral canal are vulnerable to injury when mass lesions compete for the limited space, either compressing the cord or increasing CSF pressure, eventually to impair blood flow and cause ischaemia or frank infarction. The effect of any haematoma will be further exaggerated by any other factor which decreases the volume of the canal, including degenerative disease such spinal stenosis and extremes of posture such as lithotomy or lordosis (Beloeil et al. 2003, Wills et al. 2004). However, there is no evidence that an epidural injection alone can increase pressure sufficiently to cause injury in the presence of stenosis (Neal 2008).

Spinal haematoma occurs most commonly in the epidural space because of the prominent venous plexus there, and may be spontaneous, about 25–33% of these cases being associated with either a disorder of coagulation or an episode of minor trauma (Groen & Ponssen 1990, Holtas et al. 1996). Vandermeulen and colleagues (1994) found that about two-thirds of the cases associated with neuraxial block had an abnormality of coagulation, the majority involving a drug with an antithrombotic or anticoagulant effect, and the rest a disease having similar effects. In the same review there was clear evidence of there being technical difficulty with the block in two-thirds of patients, and a quarter of the haematomas occurred shortly after the *removal* of an epidural catheter, most from a patient receiving therapeutic doses of heparin. What may fairly be described as an epidemic of cases associated with the use of enoxaparin in the USA during the late 1990s was almost certainly due to use of excessive doses of the drug, although other factors contributed (Checketts & Wildsmith 1999).

Infection

Epidural abscess

Epidural abscess is another condition which can occur spontaneously as well as in association with neuraxial block, and the predisposing factors are again common in both circumstances: compromised immunity, spinal column disruption, and a source of infection (Grewal et al. 2006). In more specific terms, the two commonest predisposing factors are diabetes mellitus and intravenous drug abuse, with remote infection providing a source in nearly half. The mass lesion can compress the cord and nerve roots, but the damage is out of proportion with the degree of compression (McLaurin 1966), suggesting that vascular injury is a major factor in pathogenesis.

Classically the condition presents with intense focal back pain, fever, and a neurological deficit, but modern evidence shows that this clear picture is relatively rare. Presentation is usually much vaguer, with fever and general malaise appearing first, and the neurological deficit being late. This vagueness contributes to diagnostic delay, and a high index of suspicion is required. Because the patients often present after discharge from hospital it has been argued that anaesthetists should work to raise awareness of the condition throughout the medical profession as a whole (Grewal et al. 2006).

Meningitis

Meningitis is a third complication which may occur postoperatively even when no neuraxial technique has been employed, and it has much the same predisposing complications as epidural abscess (see preceding section). Intriguingly, staphylococci (skin commensals) are the commonest organisms seen in meningitis after epidural block (suggesting spread along the catheter track), and streptococci (nasal commensals) after spinals (suggesting contamination from the operator's airway) (Report 2009). Although it is a condition which can lead to serious harm if untreated, meningitis is usually diagnosed and dealt with promptly

Incidence

The best assessment of the risks of serious harm from complications of neuraxial block was obtained in the Royal College of Anaesthetists Third UK-wide National Audit Project performed between 2006 and 2007 (Cook et al. 2009, Report 2009). After estimating the number of these techniques used in 12 months (>700,000) by extrapolating from a 2-week survey (Cook et al. 2008), information was collected on all such complications occurring over 12 months. The results were expressed as a range, with the low figure indicating an 'optimistic' assessment of final outcome in each case, and the high figure a 'pessimistic' one. The overall incidence of permanent injury was between 2 and 4.2 per 100,000 blocks, with the incidence of paraplegia or death being between 0.7 and 1.8 per 100,000. These overall figures (of permanent harm, not total incidence) are reassuring, as is the observation that two-thirds of the injuries reported to the audit resolved completely within 6 months.

However, the study did show that, rare though the events are, serious harm does still occasionally occur, with ischaemia having the worse potential for recovery, and meningitis the best (Table 4.2). The great majority of complications followed perioperative use in adults, primarily an elderly population, with the degree of instrumentation of the vertebral canal relating directly to the frequency of harm. Thus, in this group, the lowest incidence was with spinal anaesthesia (maximum of one case of permanent harm per 50,000 blocks) and the greatest with combined spinal-epidural block (one per 8,000). The findings of this audit are in line with an overview of earlier, less complete estimates of incidence (Cook et al. 2009).

Diagnosis and management

The rarity of these events is only one aspect which makes for difficulty in diagnosis, but all those involved in the postoperative care of patients who have received blocks should be aware that anything unexpected must trigger a rapid anaesthetic referral. The matters of most concern are back pain, paraesthesiae, increasing numbness, and lower limb paralysis, symptoms which have often been ascribed to an effect of the block, even when only a single

Table 4.2 Outcome of major complications of neuraxial block reported to the Royal College of Anaesthetists National Audit. (Data from Cook et al. 2009.)

Complication reviewed	Total reported	Good outcome	Percent recovery
Ischaemia	5	0	0
Abscess	12	7	58
Nerve injury	13	9	69
Haematoma	8	6	75
Meningitis	3	3	100

injection has been made (Report 2009). During a continuous epidural the symptoms are most often due to administration of excessive local anaesthetic, but they may also indicate migration of a catheter from the epidural to subarachnoid space and the onset of serious complications. No matter what the cause an anaesthetist must review the patient sooner rather than later, review the history and charts for features of the complications described earlier, and perform a full neurological examination. When a continuous epidural is being used the infusion should be stopped and signs of block regression sought closely. If recovery occurs, the infusion should be restarted at a lower dose rate and close monitoring continued.

In any situation there should be a low threshold for seeking a neurologist's opinion, and full consideration given to surgical factors which may be the cause of the neurological injury. A haematoma or abscess within the vertebral canal is an emergency which requires urgent diagnosis (usually magnetic resonance imaging scanning) and equally urgent surgery (well within 12 hours of onset) if the mass is to be drained before there is permanent neurological damage (Grewal et al. 2006). Mild deficits (e.g. due to nerve root damage) are treated conservatively and only investigated further if persisting 2–3 weeks beyond surgery. However, the further management of any patient will depend on the aetiology, scale, and nature of the injury, and the anaesthetist should play a full part in that process.

Prevention

Neurological injury after central neuraxial block is extremely rare, but the potentially devastating nature of the injuries means that every effort should be made to reduce the incidence to the lowest possible level. Prevention includes careful preoperative assessment and the identification of risk factors (Chapter 9), notably anatomical abnormality of the spine, drugs or diseases interfering with coagulation, conditions compromising immunity, and pre-existing neurological disease, the last of these requiring very careful assessment and recording of any existing neurological deficit. These conditions do not necessarily contraindicate regional anaesthesia, but its risk/benefit ratio will require detailed discussion and particular attention paid to that aspect of the patient's care to identify any problem as soon as possible.

Prevention also requires practising in a way which avoids the factors previously outlined, and close verbal contact with the patient allows warning features to be identified very readily. During block placement a strict antiseptic technique including skin preparation (preferably using a chlorhexidine containing solution (Hebl 2006)), gloves, hat, mask, and gown is mandatory. Careful attention to the technique of the block, with gentle manipulation of needle, catheter, and patient's posture is essential to minimize damage to the tissues, and every care should be taken to ensure that only what is intended is injected. This applies particularly to the antiseptic which must be allowed to dry before the skin is touched to avoid contamination of equipment or solutions.

The increasing availability of ultrasound looks set to minimize the risk of trauma by identifying the position of key structures. It can already be used to increase the accuracy of the estimation of vertebral level (Perlas 2010), and increases in capability mean that it may soon be used to identify other details as well. Paraesthesiae on insertion, while not to be equated with nerve damage, do indicate that there is direct contact so the needle (or catheter), whether it is in subarachnoid or epidural space, should be withdrawn until symptoms abate before anything is injected.

Level of insertion is not only important for spinal anaesthesia. When a catheter is inserted for a continuous epidural block it should be at the vertebral level equivalent to the nerve roots supplying the wound. This will ensure that the maximum concentration of drug is at those roots to optimize efficacy, but also leave the lower limbs unaffected after thoracic or abdominal surgery. This not only improves patient mobility, but also means that any complication impairing leg function should be identified early. If a continuous epidural is used after surgery to the legs, the concentration of the local anaesthetic infused must be low enough to preserve movement.

Peripheral nerve injury

Injury to peripheral nerves is not quite as catastrophic as to the neuraxis, but it can still result in considerable patient morbidity, and much of the previous discussion applies here. Peripheral nerves can be injured by all of the factors (direct trauma, chemicals, ischaemia, compression, and infection) described for the neuraxis and also by stretching. Many of these may affect the surgical patient without involving regional techniques, but the greatest concerns here are direct needle trauma and intraneural injection.

Direct trauma

Peripheral nerves are closely invested by three layers of tissue: the epineurium, perineurium, and endoneurium (see Chapter 6, Figure 6.1). Although needle placement or injection within any of these layers is undesirable, recent evidence suggests that it is injection within the perineurium which is most likely to cause significant injury (Hadzic et al. 2004). The epineurium is an external enveloping layer surrounding all fascicles and connective tissue within the nerve. The perineurium is a multilayered epithelial sheath that surrounds individual or groups of fascicles. Needle placement within the fascicle can cause injury directly or through pressure-related ischaemia after injection (Hadzic et al. 2004).

It has long been argued that short-bevel needles are less likely to injure nerves than those with long bevels (Selander et al. 1977), but there is little epidemiological evidence to support this assertion. What is more certain is that the injury is less severe if the needle is inserted with the bevel 'parallel' to the line of the axons, rather than at right angles when fascicles will be cut across rather than split longitudinally (Rice & McMahon 1992). Neurotmesis, complete disruption of axon and myelin sheath, is far more likely to cause permanent injury than neuropraxis due to compression or stretch because the myelin sheath is preserved.

Chemical injury

The peripheral nerves are reasonably well protected from chemical injury, but solutions containing preservatives and their accidental contamination should still be avoided. There is no evidence to suggest that local anaesthetics, in clinically used concentrations, have any more adverse effect on peripheral nerves than they do on the neuraxis. However, occasional laboratory studies, such as the observation (Johnson et al. 2002) that local anaesthetics have toxic effects on cell cultures, do raise questions. Such 'toxicity' is related to both concentration and duration of exposure, but the implications of these findings to man is unclear given the large numbers of patients who receive the drugs annually. However, it would seem prudent to use the lowest concentration of drug possible to achieve the desired effect, especially when an infusion technique is used (Lambert et al. 1994).

Other factors

Most local anaesthetic drugs have a slight vasoconstrictor effect at low concentrations, but there are no data to suggest that this contributes to injury, even when a solution containing an appropriate concentration of adrenaline is used. Many limb blocks will be performed in patients whose surgery will be performed under tourniquet and they can have a much more profound effect, especially if poorly applied so that there is mechanical distortion or excessive pressure. Compression due to haematoma or abscess is possible, these lesions having the same risk factors as after central blocks, but they tend to spread more readily through the peripheral tissues so high pressures are not generated.

It has been argued, in the context of nerve entrapment syndromes (Upton & McComas 1973), that patients with a pre-existing neurological problem are more likely to suffer injury if a second, more distant insult occurs: the 'double crush' phenomenon. However, the relevance of this to the risk of a patient with peripheral nerve disease (e.g. diabetic neuropathy) suffering injury from a peripheral block is unclear. Peripheral nerve injury requires disruption of the perineurium and, in practice, this is very difficult to accomplish, recent experience with ultrasound indicating that nerves are difficult to impale, tending to move away from approaching needles. Even if a nerve is pierced it is difficult to maintain the needle within the nerve, most of the solution leaking out of the epineurium after a small volume has been injected (Chan et al. 2007).

Incidence

Temporary sensory or motor impairment may occur in nearly 3% of patients after a peripheral nerve block, but most symptoms resolve within days or weeks of surgery (Brull et al. 2007). Permanent injury is much rarer, Auroy and colleagues (2002) reporting this in an average of only 2.4 instances per 10,000 blocks. There is quite marked variation in the incidence of both temporary (Table 4.3) and permanent syndromes, with popliteal block having the greatest incidence of the latter (31.5 per 10,000 patients). Risk factors can be patient, surgical, and anaesthetic. Patient factors include: pre-existing neurological disorder, diabetes mellitus, extremes of obesity, male gender, and extremes of age. Surgical factors include direct surgical trauma, compressive dressings, tourniquet pressure and/or time, compression by haematoma or abscess, and poor patient positioning (Neal et al. 2002).

Diagnosis and management

Symptoms suggesting postoperative neuropathy should prompt a full history to identify any predisposing risk factor or causative element in the anaesthetic or surgical technique, plus a detailed neurological examination to define the problem precisely. As noted earlier, most injuries have an excellent prognosis, but the symptoms of even a minor deficit can be distressing so considerable patient reassurance may be required. More severe deficits, or those which fail to resolve within 2–3 weeks, should be referred to a neurologist or neurosurgeon for further investigation and management. However, it is important that the anaesthetist is fully involved in

Table 4.3 Incidence of temporary neuropathy after peripheral nerve block. (Data from Brull et al. 2007.)

Block technique		Estimated rate of occurrence (%)
Brachial plexus	Interscalene	2.84
	Supraclavicular	0.03
	Axillary	1.48
	Midhumeral	0.02
Lumbar plexus	Posterior approach	0.19
	Anterior (femoral) approach	0.34
Sacral plexus	Sciatic nerve block	0.41
	Popliteal nerve block	0.24

this process because surgical colleagues (and patients) can, quite correctly, become irritated if the anaesthetist fails to follow up such problems. Conversely, the anaesthetist (or department) taking this seriously will build a relationship between colleagues that will, in turn, facilitate the future practice of regional anaesthesia.

Having made that point it is important that the evaluation of any postoperative neurological deficit includes a search for factors unrelated to anaesthesia technique. The incidence of nerve injury arising during surgery is several orders of magnitude greater than during regional anaesthesia so this must be considered before assigning responsibility to any one technique or practitioner. For example, the risk of nerve injury during total hip arthroplasty is as high as 1–2% (Dehart & Riley 1999), and similar estimates are quoted for other orthopaedic procedures. Surgery may predispose to nerve injury through direct trauma or stretching, tourniquet pressure, compressive dressings, haematoma or abscess formation, and improper patient positioning during surgery. However, some of these are considered to be the joint responsibility of surgeon and anaesthetist.

Prevention

As with central blocks thorough preoperative assessment and careful attention to the detail of block technique are essential in the prevention of neurological injury after peripheral blocks. It also seems advisable to use the lowest concentration of local anaesthetic possible, particularly when infusions are used for postoperative analgesia.

More specifically, a major factor predisposing to peripheral nerve injury is intraneural (or more accurately intrafascicular) needle placement or injection. Traditional teaching states that both of these produce severe pain and should therefore be easily detectable so that needle position can be corrected if it occurs. However, recent studies suggest that neither intraneural needle placement nor injection is always painful, with ultrasound suggesting that they have been performed unrecognized for many years. Robards and colleagues (2009) found that when typical final currents (0.2–0.4 mA) were achieved for popliteal nerve block the needle tip was intraneural in 100%. Similarly, Macaire and colleagues (2008), using nerve stimulation for median nerve block at the wrist, identified that the needle tip was intraneural on several occasions, with this placement explaining the faster block onset seen in their stimulation group.

Table 4.4 Factors which may indicate intraneural needle placement, and actions to reduce the risk of subsequent peripheral nerve injury.

Symptom/sign	Action
Pain on needle placement or injection	Withdraw needle, stop injection and redirect needle
High injection pressure (Hadzic et al. 2004)	Withdraw needle until pressure to inject decreases
Current threshold <0.4 mA (Chan et al. 2007)	Withdraw needle until threshold >0.4 mA
Sonographic visualization of nerve expansion (Chan et al. 2007)	Stop injecting. Redirect needle
High electrical impedance (Tsui et al. 2008)	Withdraw needle until impedance decreases

Such observations may have led to the suggestion that intentional intraneural injection might optimize success without invariably leading to injury (Bigeleisen 2006). However, there remains a paucity of evidence, even from animal models (Lupu et al. 2010), to support deliberate intraneural injection. Further, it is difficult to avoid the conclusion that the high incidence of neuropathy after popliteal block (Brull et al. 2007) is directly related to the ease with which intraneural needle placement occurs during this technique (Robards et al. 2009). Until there is much evidence to the contrary, intraneural needle placement and solution injection are practices to be avoided at all costs. Recent evidence suggests that several factors, apart from a gentle technique and inserting the needle with the bevel parallel to the nerve, may reduce the likelihood of severe injury, all of them aimed at preventing accidental intraneural injection (Table 4.4).

Many of the warning symptoms of direct nerve contact outlined here require a conscious, or only mildly sedated, patient to report them, and this would suggest that blocks should not be performed after administration of heavy sedation or anaesthesia. However, this is a matter of some controversy which is discussed further in Chapter 11.

Overview

Neurological complications occur rarely after regional anaesthesia, but can be devastating to all involved. Careful patient selection and gentle block performance reduce risks considerably, and recent advances such as ultrasound scanning may allow new strategies to further reduce risk. If symptoms of injury do develop, prompt and thorough clinical assessment, investigation, treatment, and follow-up are vital to minimize the final degree of disability.

Key references

Hogan QH (2008) Pathophysiology of peripheral nerve injury during spinal anesthesia. *Regional Anesthesia and Pain Medicine* 33: 435–41.
Neal JM (2008) Anatomy and pathophysiology of spinal cord injury associated with regional anesthesia and pain medicine. *Regional Anesthesia and Pain Medicine* 33: 423–34.
Neal JM, Bernards CM, Hadzic A, et al. (2008) ASRA practice advisory on neurologic complications in regional anesthesia and pain medicine. *Regional Anesthesia and Pain Medicine* 33: 404–15.

On-line resources

http://asra.com/publications-neurologic-complications-2008.php
http://www.rcoa.ac.uk/index.asp?PageID=717 Report 2009 Third National Audit Project of the Royal College of Anaesthetists

References

Auroy Y, Benhamou D, Bargues L, et al. (2002) Major complications of regional anesthesia in France: The SOS Regional Anesthesia Hotline Service. *Anesthesiology* 97: 1274–80.
Beloeil H, Albaladejo P, Hoen S, et al. (2003) Bilateral lower limb hypoesthesia after radical prostatectomy in the hyperlordotic position under general anesthesia. *Canadian Journal of Anesthesia* 50: 653–6.
Bigeleisen PE (2006) Nerve puncture and apparent intraneural injection during ultrasound-guided axillary block does not invariably result in neurologic injury. *Anesthesiology* 105: 779–83.
Brull R, McCartney CJ, Chan VW, El-Beheiry H (2007) Neurological complications after regional anesthesia: contemporary estimates of risk. *Anesthesia & Analgesia* 104: 965–74.
Chan VW, Brull R, McCartney CJ, et al. (2007) An ultrasonographic and histological study of intraneural injection and electrical stimulation in pigs. *Anesthesia & Analgesia* 104: 1281–4.
Checketts MR, Wildsmith JAW (1999) Editorial: Central nerve block and thromboprophylaxis—is there a problem? *British Journal of Anaesthesia* 82: 164–7.
Cope RW (1954) The Woolley and Rowe case. *Anaesthesia* 9: 249–70.
Cook TM, Mihai R, Wildsmith JAW (2008) A national census of central neuraxial block in the UK: results of the snapshot phase of the Third National Audit Project of the Royal College of Anaesthetists. *Anaesthesia* 63: 143–6.
Cook TM, Counsell D, Wildsmith JA (2009) Major complications of central neuraxial block: report on the Third National Audit Project of the Royal College of Anaesthetists. *British Journal of Anaesthesia* 102: 179–90.
Dehart MM, Riley LH Jr (1999) Nerve injuries in total hip arthroplasty. *Journal of the American Academy of Orthopaedic Surgeons* 7: 101–11.
Dripps RD, Vandam LD (1954) Longterm follow-up of patients who received 10,098 spinal anesthetics. I: failure to discover major neurological sequelae. *Journal of the American Medical Association* 156: 1486–91.
Fettes PDW, Wildsmith JAW (2002) Editorial: Somebody else's nervous system. *British Journal of Anaesthesia* 88: 760–3.
Furness G, Reilly MP, Kuchi S (2002) An evaluation of ultrasound imaging for identification of lumbar intervertebral level. *Anaesthesia* 57: 266–83.
Grewal S, Hocking G, Wildsmith JA (2006) Epidural abscess. *British Journal of Anaesthesia* 96: 292–302.
Groen RJ, Ponssen H (1990) The spontaneous spinal epidural haematoma. A study of the etiology (review). *Journal of Neurological Science* 98: 121–38.
Hadzic A, Dilberovic F, Shah S, et al. (2004) Combination of intraneural injection and high injection pressure leads to fascicular injury and neurologic deficit in dogs. *Regional Anesthesia and Pain Medicine* 29: 417–23.
Hampl KF, Schneider MC, Ummenhofer W, Drewe J (1995) Transient neurologic symptoms after spinal anesthesia. *Anesthesia & Analgesia* 81: 1148–53.
Hebl JR (2006) The importance and implications of aseptic techniques during regional anesthesia. *Regional Anesthesia and Pain Medicine* 31: 311–23.
Hogan QH (1996) Epidural anatomy examined by cryomicrotome section: Influence of age, vertebral level, and disease. *Regional Anesthesia and Pain Medicine* 21: 395–406.
Holtas S, Heiling M, Lonntoft M (1996) Spontaneous spinal epidural haematoma: findings at MR imaging and clinical correlation. *Radiology* 199: 409–13.

Hopkinson JM, Samaan AK, Russell IF, et al. (1997) A comparative multicentre trial of spinal needles for Caesarean section. *Anaesthesia* 52: 998–1014.

Horlocker TT, Abel MD, Messick JM Jr, Schroeder DR (2003) Small risk of serious neurologic complications related to lumbar epidural catheter placement in anesthetized patients. *Anesthesia & Analgesia* 96: 1547–52.

Huntoon MA, Hurdle M-FB, Marsh RW, Reeves RK (2004) Intrinsic spinal cord catheter placement: implications of new intractable pain in a patient with a spinal cord injury. *Anesthesia & Analgesia* 99: 1763–5.

Jacob AK, Borowiec JC, Long TR, et al. (2004) Transient profound neurologic deficits associated with thoracic epidural analgesia in an elderly patient. *Anesthesiology* 101: 1470–1.

Johnson ME, Saenz AJ, DaSilva AD, et al. (2002) Effect of local anesthetic on neuronal cytoplasmic calcium and plasma membrane lysis (necrosis) in a cell culture model. *Anesthesiology* 97: 1466–76.

Kennedy FG, Effron AS, Perry G (1950) The grave spinal cord paralyses caused by spinal anesthesia. *Sugery, Gynecology and Obstetrics* 91: 385–98.

Kim J, Bahk J, Sung J (2003) Influence of age and sex on the position of the conus medullaris and Tuffier's line in adults. *Anesthesiology* 99: 1359–63.

Lambert LA, Lambert DH, Strichartz GA (1994) Irreversible conduction block in isolated nerve by high concentrations of local anesthetics. *Anesthesiology* 80: 1082–93.

Lupu CM, Kiehl TR, Chan VW, et al. (2010) Nerve expansion seen on ultrasound predicts histologic but not functional nerve injury after intraneural injection in pigs. *Regional Anesthesia and Pain Medicine* 35: 132–9.

Macaire P, Singelyn F, Narchi P, Paqueron X (2008) Ultrasound- or nerve stimulation-guided wrist blocks for carpal tunnel release: a randomized prospective comparative study. *Regional Anesthesia and Pain Medicine* 33: 363–8.

McLaurin RL (1966) Spinal suppuration. *Clinical Neurosurgery* 14: 314–36.

Moen V, Dahlgren N, Irestedt L (2004) Severe neurological complications after central neuraxial blockades in Sweden 1990–1999. *Anesthesiology* 101: 950–9.

Neal JM (2003) Effects of epinephrine in local anesthetics on the central and peripheral nervous systems: neurotoxicity and neural blood flow. *Regional Anesthesia and Pain Medicine* 28: 124–34.

Neal JM (2008) Anatomy and pathophysiology of spinal cord injury associated with regional anesthesia and pain medicine. *Regional Anesthesia and Pain Medicine* 33: 423–34.

Neal JM, Hebl JR, Gerancher JC, Hogan QH (2002) Brachial plexus anesthesia: Essentials of our current understanding. *Regional Anesthesia and Pain Medicine* 27: 402–28.

Perlas A (2010) Evidence for the use of ultrasound in neuraxial blocks. *Regional Anesthesia and Pain Medicine* 35: S43–6.

Report (2009) Third National Audit Project of the Royal College of Anaesthetists. http://www.rcoa.ac.uk/index.asp?PageID=717

Reynolds F (2001) Damage to the conus medullaris following spinal anaesthesia. *Anaesthesia* 55: 238–49.

Rice AS, McMahon SB (1992) Peripheral nerve injury caused by injection needles used in regional anaesthesia: Influence of bevel configuration studied in a rat model. *British Journal of Anaesthesia* 69: 433–8.

Rice I, Wee MJ, Thomson K (2004) Obstetric epidurals and chronic adhesive arachnoiditis. *British Journal of Anaesthesia* 92: 109–20.

Rigler ML, Drasner K, Krejcie TC, et al. (1991) Cauda equine syndrome after continuous spinal anesthesia. *Anesthesia & Analgesia* 72: 275–81.

Robards C, Hadzic A, Somasundaram L, et al. (2009) Intraneural injection with low-current stimulation during popliteal sciatic nerve block. *Anesthesia & Analgesia* 109: 673–7.

Schneider M, Ettlin T, Kaufmann M, et al. (1993) Transient neurologic toxicity after hyperbaric subarachnoid anesthesia with 5% lidocaine. *Anesthesia & Analgesia* 76: 1154–7.

Selander D, Dhuner K-G, Lundborg G (1977) Peripheral nerve injury due to injection needles used for regional anaesthesia. *Acta Anaesthesiologica Scandinavica* 21: 182–8.

Selander D, Sjostrand J (1978) Longitudinal spread of intraneurally injected local anesthetics. An experimental study of the initial neural distribution following intraneural injections. *Acta Anaesthesiologica Scandinavica* 22: 622–34.

Tsui BC, Armstrong K (2005) Can direct spinal cord injury occur without paresthesia? A report of delayed spinal cord injury after epidural placement in an awake patient. *Anesthesia & Analgesia* 101: 1212–14.

Tsui BC, Li LX, Pillay JJ (2006) Compressed air injection technique to standardize block injection pressures. *Canadian Journal of Anesthesia* 53: 1098–102.

Tsui BC, Pillay JJ, Chu KT (2008) Electrical impedance to distinguish intraneural from extraneural needle placement in porcine nerves during direct exposure and ultrasound guidance. *Anesthesiology* 109: 479–83.

Turner MA, Reifenberg NA (1995) Combined spinal epidural anaesthesia. The single double-barrel technique. *International Journal of Obstetric Anaesthesia* 4: 158–60.

Upton AR, McComas AJ (1973) The double crush in nerve entrapment syndromes. *Lancet* 2: 359–62.

van Zundert AA, Stultiens G, Jakimowicz JJ, et al. (2007) Laparoscopic cholecystectomy under segmental thoracic spinal anaesthesia: a feasibility study. *British Journal of Anaesthesia* 98: 682–6.

Vandermeulen EP, Van Aken H, Vermylen J (1994) Anticoagulants and spinal-epidural anaesthesia. *Anesthesia & Analgesia* 79: 1165–77.

Wills JH, Wiesel S, Abram SE, Rupp FW (2004) Synovial cysts and the lithotomy position causing cauda equina syndrome. *Regional Anesthesia and Pain Medicine* 29: 234–6.

Wysowski DK, Talarico L, Balsanyi J, et al. (1998) Spinal and epidural hematoma and low molecular weight heparin. *New England Journal of Medicine* 338: 1774–5.

CHAPTER 5

Outcome issues

Susan Nimmo and Graeme McLeod

The debate on the benefit (or not) of using 'local' techniques for surgical anaesthesia is one which dates back to the middle of the 19th century, 'cold' having been proposed as 'safer' than ether or chloroform long before cocaine came into use (Arnott 1847). Refrigeration had limited application, as did cocaine, but improvements in drugs and their application made for better effectiveness and wider applicability so that topical, infiltration, and minor nerve block techniques are used widely today. General anaesthesia is not only unnecessary, but inappropriate for many minor dental and surgical procedures, local methods preserving both consciousness and the patient's protective reflexes to allow a single-handed practitioner to operate in safety. This approach also contributes to that most modern of healthcare outcomes, reduced expenditure, because drug and equipment costs are significantly less. That was always an issue in developing countries, but has become important everywhere. However, once surgery requires an anaesthetic team, the staff costs far outweigh all others and the economic difference between regional and general techniques is minimal (Kendell et al. 2000).

Refrigeration anaesthesia was advocated as a means of avoiding the major morbidity, and mortality, associated with early general anaesthesia, but regional techniques have their own risks. When central neuraxial block began to displace general anaesthesia in obstetrics 30–40 years ago, it was argued that unskilled use would be at least as dangerous, and not necessarily reduce the overall incidence of anaesthesia-related death. Obviously clinicians must be trained in all aspects of the methods which they are using, not forgetting the treatment of complications, but their ease of management is an issue also. Failure to intubate the trachea and aspiration of gastric content are, intuitively, much more difficult to manage than hypotension of sympathetic origin, no matter how skilled the anaesthetist (Rosen 1981). The reduction in the number of maternal deaths due to 'anaesthetic' factors recorded in both the UK and the USA with the progressive change to central nerve block for Caesarean section has proved this to be so (Hawkins et al. 1997, Reports 1952 to 2011).

Chapter 3 describes how regional methods offer other features (ablation of the surgical stress response, and a reduction in the incidence and severity of side effects) which may lead to patient benefit. However, when and where modern standards of care are available, any overall advantage in favour of regional techniques is not as obvious as in the two very different situations described previously. As a result many comparative studies, and subsequent meta-analyses, have been performed over the last 40 years to try and identify the 'best' approach. That the debate still continues is a clear indication that no definitive evidence has appeared, and the rest of this chapter aims to consider a range of 'outcomes' to provide a guide to clinical decision-making. First, three key points should be made, albeit with some qualification:

1. Not one study, whether of minor or major sequelae of anaesthesia and surgery, has even hinted that regional techniques are associated with more negative outcomes than general anaesthesia. The 'worst' that can be said is that there is no overall difference between them, although the pattern of sequelae may be different.

2. Conversely, every comparison has shown that regional methods are associated with a very obvious decrease in pain, certainly in the early postoperative period. Of course, the effect will regress and pain will develop eventually, but it is much less severe and more readily controlled than if a block is not used.

3. There is concern that this improved postoperative analgesia is offset by the risk of neurological complications of the block technique. These are considered in detail in Chapter 4 and, while they can be catastrophic for the individual patient, they are extremely rare.

Standard morbidity and mortality studies

The starting point for any consideration of this topic is the meta-analysis published at the turn of the century by Rodgers and colleagues (2000) who reviewed all the then available published prospective randomized studies and demonstrated a decrease in early morbidity and mortality in favour of regional anaesthesia. This prompted some to consider that the case was 'proven' (Harrop-Griffiths & Picard 2001), but that ignored a number of factors, including the cautious conclusions of the authors of the meta-analysis themselves. They said that 'our overview indicates that neuraxial blockade reduces major postoperative complications in a wide range of patients', but qualified this by noting that 'uncertainty about the net benefits of neuraxial blockade is likely to remain' and that 'it is unclear whether the differences that we observed reflect the benefits of regional anaesthesia alone'. Meta-analysis seeks to overcome the weaknesses of comparative studies, notably the relatively small numbers of patients involved in each, but it cannot overcome publication bias (only studies with positive outcomes are published), nor escape from the fact that advances in clinical practice may have rendered the findings obsolete.

Even accepting this more cautious interpretation, the 'Rodgers' paper did provide useful information supporting the case for wider use of neuraxial block techniques (it did not consider peripheral blocks, a point often ignored). Other meta-analyses have shown beneficial effects of epidural analgesia on pulmonary function (Ballantyne et al. 1998) and the duration of postoperative ileus (Jorgensen et al. 2000), but statistically the comparisons demonstrated only 'trends' rather than clear-cut benefits. Thus, any positive interpretation of the benefits of regional block was countered by the publication of what seemed initially to be a valid, large-scale assessment of postoperative analgesia in patients undergoing abdominal surgery (Rigg et al. 2002). Nearly 900 patients were recruited from 25 hospitals over a 5-year period and randomized to receive either thoracic epidural or patient-controlled intravenous analgesia, but there was no overall difference in morbidity or mortality.

This, together with the then growing concerns about the risk of major complications of postoperative epidural analgesia, led to a major change in attitudes to its benefit and use, but a number of important aspects require emphasis:

1. The authors conceded that the study was probably underpowered for a clinically meaningful evaluation of postoperative outcomes, and that the 'low numbers of participants could lead to a Type 1 error'. Subsequent recalculation using the primary endpoint, a baseline mortality of 4.3%, confirmed that in excess of 6,000 patients would have had to have been entered to provide a definitive conclusion (Rigg et al. 2002).

2. Regrettably, neither the general anaesthetic nor epidural regimens were standardized, and neither was the type of surgery performed, this ranging from appendectomy to major cancer resections. The complications of any operation are procedure specific, and the aim of anaesthesia is to maintain homeostasis during and after surgery, so the outcome will depend on the skill and experience of the clinicians involved. In any such comparative study, patients need to be stratified into single procedure sub-groups, and broad strategies for patient management must be agreed in advance.

3. Further, there was a very high epidural failure rate, something between 25% and 50% depending on the criteria used. The intention was to maintain the block for 96 hours, a challenging requirement, and others have found that block failure is not uncommon (15–35% of cases) (McLeod 2001, Ready 1999). Clearly, no benefit is going to accrue to the individual patient unless the block is effective, but it is noteworthy that, in spite of the failure rate, the epidural group as a whole still had better analgesia and (probably as a consequence) reduced pulmonary morbidity.

A more recent systematic review, while favouring regional methods, also concluded that the low incidence of major complications of surgery means that studies with what are probably impossibly large numbers of patients would be required (Liu & Wu 2007). Thus it has been argued that evidence is perhaps better sought from large-scale audits of outcome from routine practice (Wildsmith 2002), and one such (albeit retrospective) audit found no difference between general and regional (spinal or epidural) anaesthesia in over 9,000 patients undergoing hip fracture surgery (O'Hara et al. 2000). However, a more formal, and much larger (259,037 patients), population-based cohort study did produce results in favour of postoperative epidural analgesia (Wijeyisundra et al. 2008), and this may be the only methodology which can recruit the numbers needed for valid comparisons without formal randomization to one method or the other.

Pain control

For some, better postoperative pain control is reason alone for using regional methods; it is certainly a more relevant endpoint for making decisions about *anaesthetic* technique than the incidence of *surgical* complications, although those of anaesthesia must be factored into the equation as well (Wildsmith 2002). However, it is informative to compare the major sequelae of these two aspects of patient management. For example, the risk of death after elective cardiac surgery is about 1 in 50, and at least 1 in 20 after other major procedures such as lung and vascular surgery (Baudouin 2003, Leung et al. 2009). Arguing that considerable improvements in pain control are outweighed by the risk of major neurological complications is put into perspective when their incidence (see Chapter 4) is compared with these surgical figures; *and* there remains the likelihood that the block reduces those as well.

Consideration of individual, as opposed to population, outcomes provides further support for regional methods because effective pain control, with rapid postoperative recovery and early return to normal activity, can produce significant benefit for some patients (Wu et al. 2003). Maintaining such effective pain relief may be a challenge in up to 25% of cases, but for many others there is the potential for a virtually pain-free postoperative course (McLeod et al. 2001, 2006), so the aim should be to meet the challenge, not to deny the benefit to all. Blocks can 'fail' for reasons ranging from the simply technical (failure of the injection) to the near political (lack of adequate facilities for managing a continuous epidural), but all can be identified and addressed. Better training, especially with the wider use of increasingly sophisticated ultrasound scanning (Marhofer et al. 2010), should improve initial success rates, and the provision of Acute Pain Teams to manage patients postoperatively is recognized increasingly to be a major requirement (Report 2010). It is sometimes said that the facilities in a particular hospital are not appropriate for the management of continuous epidural block, especially at night, but does an epidural really add to the care requirement of a patient who has undergone major surgery?

Chronic postsurgical pain

Regional analgesia may have an impact on pain which extends beyond the immediate postoperative period: reduction in the incidence of chronic postsurgical pain. Defined as pain of at least two months' duration and related directly to the operative procedure, not to any pre-existing medical condition, its incidence varies according to the type of surgery. It follows 10–15% of all procedures, being severe in 2–10% of patients, and, perhaps because the aetiology is complex, it was ignored or unrecognized until relatively recently. Education of both healthcare staff and patients is needed to ensure that the problem is identified and addressed (Macrae 2008).

Developments in the understanding of pain physiology in the 1980s and since (see Chapter 2), especially recognition of neural plasticity, led to the concept of *pre-emptive analgesia*. The theory was that block of noxious input to the central nervous system would prevent the development of the abnormal neural connections which later generate sensations of pain in the absence of harmful stimuli. Positive animal studies and the attractiveness of the concept perhaps led to over-enthusiastic acceptance of early clinical results, particularly in relation to pain after amputation. A review of better controlled studies found no early benefit from performing a block before rather than after the surgical incision (Moiniche et al. 2002), although some limited data support the need for better, more procedure-specific investigation of the effect on the incidence and severity of chronic pain (Macrae 2008). There is some evidence that local anaesthetics need to be supplemented with agents (e.g. N-methyl-D-aspartate antagonists and α2 adrenergic agonists) which have a more specific effect on the development of hyperalgesia (Lavande'homme et al. 2005), but care needs to be exercised in the routine administration of drugs which are unlicensed for such use.

Enhanced recovery after surgery (ERAS)

The very positive influence which the analgesia produced by an effective block can have on a patient's condition in the early postoperative period poses the question (over and above the points raised already) of why it has been so difficult to demonstrate a reduction in morbidity and mortality. The answer is that pain control, while highly desirable in itself, will not have a wider impact unless those delivering postoperative care (surgeons, nurses, and physiotherapists) use the analgesia to introduce more proactive management regimens. Thus multidisciplinary, 'enhanced recovery' programmes have been developed to manipulate the features of regional techniques to meet the needs of specific procedures and patient groups.

Amelioration of the stress response, rapid mobilization, and early return of upper & lower gastrointestinal function are important components, as is the avoidance of large doses of systemic opioids, in speeding recovery, reducing morbidity, and shortening hospital stay. Anaesthetists have a role, not just in ensuring that the blocks continue to be effective, but also in teaching others how the care of that block is safely integrated with the other aspects of management. With this approach to postoperative care it has been possible to demonstrate positive benefit more definitely, almost certainly for two reasons: the clinical techniques used in the comparisons have been well defined and the studies have been procedure specific, both factors reducing variability.

Abdominal surgery

Some of the earliest work was in colorectal surgery, a Cochrane review and three meta-analyses now having shown that thoracic epidural analgesia improves outcome, particularly when part of an enhanced recovery programme (Eskicioglu et al. 2009, Gendall et al. 2007, Jorgensen et al. 2000, Marret et al. 2007,). That the epidural is important was shown by a comparison between opioid and non-opioid analgesia where all patients were managed proactively, the latter group doing significantly better (Omar et al. 2008).

Similarly positive results have been seen after hepato-biliary (van Dam et al. 2008), urological (Arumainayagam et al. 2008, Novotny et al. 2007), and major vascular (Muehling et al. 2009, Nishimori et al. 2006) surgery.

Intrathoracic surgery

Cardiac, pulmonary, and oesophageal procedures produce significant physiological derangement, much of which can be minimized by epidural block, but its application in this area is relatively recent because of anxiety about the consequences of extensive sympathetic nerve block. However, there is a growing body of evidence that even patients undergoing cardiac surgery can benefit through effects on both specific elements of the stress response (Gonca et al. 2007, Kilickan et al. 2005) and the inflammatory response to extracorporeal circulation (Kilickan et al. 2008). Crucially, epidural analgesia has been shown to reduce brain natriuretic peptide (Crescenzi et al. 2009, Suttner et al. 2005), high concentrations of which correlate with poor outcomes and increased mortality after coronary artery surgery (Bolliger et al. 2009). Large-scale reviews have shown not only that epidural analgesia is feasible for cardiac surgery (Chakravarthy et al. 2005) and reduces morbidity and mortality (Bignami et al. 2010), but that the systemic heparinization required does not increase the risk of vertebral canal haematoma (Braco & Hemmerling 2007).

Epidural analgesia has also been shown to reduce respiratory complications, mortality, and both intensive care and hospital stay after oesophagectomy (Cense et al. 2006, Munitiz et al. 2010, Saeki et al. 2009), with improved quality of life noted after 1 week (Ali et al. 2010). Studies on patients undergoing lung resection give a particular insight into the use of a whole package of care in enhanced recovery programmes. Patients who received epidural analgesia did better, but there was also emphasis on the use of minimally invasive surgical techniques, maintenance of normal physiology (normovolaemia, normothermia, good oxygenation & normoglycaemia), early ambulation and oral feeding, and avoidance of both systemic opioids and unnecessary antibiotics (Campos et al. 2009, Muehling et al. 2008, Zhao et al. 2010).

Major limb surgery

Some of the earliest claims that regional methods might reduce mortality after surgery resulted from retrospective reviews of patients who had undergone hip fracture surgery under spinal or general anaesthesia, but when more formal, randomized studies were performed the difference in outcome was nothing like as marked (McKenzie et al. 1984). However, as in other areas of practice, postoperative pain is much reduced, as are the complications associated with systemic opioid use (Block et al. 2003, Richman et al. 2006).

Many studies in the 1980s showed that neuraxial block reduced the incidence of thromboembolic complications (Kehlet 1998), but reviews of more modern research have questioned whether this is now the case after lower limb arthroplasty (Macfarlane et al. 2009a,b). The probable reason for the 'disappearance' of this benefit is that specific methods of thromboprophylaxis are now applied more widely and more consistently than in the past. Whether modern thromboprophylaxis and neuraxial block are additive, or even synergistic, in preventing thromboembolism would require a study which is unlikely to be performed for a variety of reasons, notably the ethical difficulty of having a group who do not receive standard preventive therapy.

The other feared major complication of arthroplasty is deep-seated infection, and a recent epidemiological study from Taiwan has suggested that its incidence is reduced by the use of both spinal and epidural anaesthesia, the magnitude of effect being equivalent to that of antibiotic prophylaxis (Chang et al. 2010). This study was not randomized, but involved survey of a population of 3,081 patients, and clearly needs confirmation, but several mechanisms could explain the effect:

1. The preservation of immunological function associated with regional block;

2. Reduced surgical bleeding resulting in less haematoma to act as a culture medium for infection; and

3. The vasodilation (or prevention of vasoconstriction) associated with regional block (Sessler 2010).

Restoration of function after arthroplasty requires early mobilization, which can be very painful, and many analgesic techniques have been tried to deal with this. The procedure specific postoperative pain management (PROSPECT) multidisciplinary review group recommended, within the framework of a multimodal approach, either general anaesthesia with peripheral nerve block or spinal anaesthesia with spinal opioid (Fischer & Simanski 2005; Fischer et al. 2008). These comprehensive reviews should be the starting point for any consideration of the subject, but that does not mean that the recommended techniques are fully effective or without side effects. Every possible analgesic technique has been tried, but has been found wanting in some regard, especially as the pressures for ever earlier mobilization and hospital discharge have increased.

Spinal opioids have a narrow risk/benefit profile and limited duration of effect, and routine use of continuous epidural analgesia, even after bilateral surgery, is probably not justified because it increases the level of care required and complicates mobilization. Continuous sciatic and femoral nerve blocks are effective, but too often result in muscle paralysis and loss of proprioception which actually delay mobilization, and occasionally result in patients falling (Kandasami et al. 2009). Two new techniques are at an early stage of evaluation in attempts to improve matters, especially after knee surgery: peripheral nerve block with low concentrations of local anaesthetic (e.g. ropivacaine 0.2%), and wound infiltration and infusion, usually initiated by the surgeon. Wound infusion has already become popular although the placing of a catheter near the joint may provide an avenue for the entry of infection, and there have been reports of chondrolysis after intra-articular injection of local anaesthetics (Chelly et al. 2010).

Further, the true efficacy of infiltration methods has been questioned (Kehlet & Andersen 2011, McCartney & McLeod 2011), and two comparisons with femoral block analgesia have produced interesting results. Mobilization was superior in the infiltration group when femoral block was instituted with ropivacaine 1% (Toftdahl et al. 2007), but better functional outcomes at 6 weeks were seen in a group in whom femoral block was instituted with ropivacaine 0.2% (Carli et al. 2010). Taking the two studies together suggests that femoral block with lower concentrations of drug than have been used previously has a place, but further specific studies are needed if only because recent work has shown that pain is not the only issue in functional recovery beyond the first postoperative night. It may be that early mobilization within an enhanced recovery programme is more important than the provision of total analgesia (Andersen et al. 2009, Holm et al. 2010), although that pain may have effects which extend beyond mobilization (Puolakka et al. 2010). Pain *after* hospital discharge (both subacute and chronic) is common, especially in relation to knee surgery, so there is a need to look at the balance between mobilization and pain relief, and the morbidity (*early and late*) which a technique prevents or causes.

Cancer recurrence

Another potential benefit of regional anaesthesia was identified when Exadaktylos and colleagues (2006) reported that the 3-year recurrence rate for breast cancer decreased from 24% to 6% after the introduction of paravertebral block for analgesia. The study was retrospective, but no difference between the groups, other than use of a block, was identified, and there are mechanisms which might explain the observation:

1. Reduction in the immunosuppressant components of the stress response;

2. Avoidance of systemic opioid drugs which, *in vitro* at least, have effects which may promote cancer cell survival (Farooqui et al. 2007, Gupta et al. 2002), and encourage neo-vascularization and tumour progression in angiogenesis-dependent tumours (Singleton et al. 2006);

3. Reduced requirement for general anaesthetic agents which also depress cell-mediated immunity; and

4. A direct cytotoxic effect of local anaesthetic drugs (Sakaguchi et al. 2006).

Great caution is needed in the interpretation of the data, even though similarly positive findings have been reported after the use of epidural analgesia for prostate cancer surgery (Biki et al. 2008), because several studies have found no benefit (Tsui & Green 2011). However, the effect might be specific to certain types of cancer so large, prospective randomized controlled clinical trials are needed to confirm or deny the other observations.

Conclusions

The early morbidity and mortality studies gave rise to the impression of a 'competition' between regional and general anaesthesia, with the decision being to use one or the other. In some circumstances it is a question of using one or the other, but for the great majority of surgical patients the real question is how a block can contribute to a 'better' outcome, this being very much the philosophy which gave rise to enhanced recovery programmes. Clearly, the case that regional anaesthesia produces better pain relief is proven, and good advice on incorporating appropriate techniques into routine practice is readily available, notably from the PROSPECT group. This is a unique collaboration between surgeons and anaesthetists which provides 'on-line' advice based on assessment of the quality, as well as the results, of published research. However, it is equally clear that there is 'insufficient evidence to conclude that analgesic technique (by itself) influences postoperative mortality or morbidity' (Liu & Wu 2007). Fortunately, there is growing evidence that outcome can be improved, but only by incorporating the improved analgesia into a novel approach to postoperative care.

This is not to deny that there are potential drawbacks to the wider use of local blocks. One very practical objection is that they may prolong significantly the operation list. This may be true for the occasional and inexperienced user because the block may take longer to perform than the induction of general anaesthesia, and this is particularly true if the theatre staff are not familiar with the routine of these procedures. Such delays may be quite justifiable in the interests of a particular patient, but soon become unacceptable if lists are prolonged repeatedly. However, proficiency, speed of induction, and success rate increase when blocks are practised regularly, and recovery time is usually decreased because the patient recovers consciousness rapidly and free of pain. If consecutive patients are to have local blocks it is possible, given the right circumstances (skilled assistance and careful planning), to save time by performing the second block while the first operation is being finished.

The major complications of regional anaesthesia are related to systemic toxicity (either from the local anaesthetic or adjuvants such as a vasoconstrictor), the systemic effects of the block itself, or local needle/catheter trauma. Drug toxicity is usually due to accidental intravascular injection or, more rarely, to the administration of an overdose. Both mishaps are avoidable, careful technique and the correct choice of drug, concentration, and volume virtually eliminating them as causes of complications. Arterial hypotension due to sympathetic paralysis is the commonest 'systemic' effect of central blocks. Choice of an appropriate technique should minimize unwanted spread of local anaesthetic solution to the upper thoracic dermatomes, but if this should occur, or if it is necessary for a particular patient, clear guidelines for management are available (Chapter 13). Local complications such as nerve damage or space-occupying lesions in the epidural space are minimized by good case selection and gentle insertion of needles and catheters (Chapter 11). Prolonged motor block can lead to patient injury and slow mobilization, but should be minimized by choice of technique and manipulation of the features of the solution used.

Choice of technique

As with all procedures in medicine the application of a particular technique requires a risk/benefit assessment for each patient for whom the technique is considered. The regional technique of choice will be the one most likely to achieve success with the least likelihood of complications for each individual patient and for the level of surgery being undertaken (Kehlet et al. 2007). Advances in surgical procedures such as the use of minimally invasive techniques will also significantly influence anaesthetic requirements and have an influence on the types of block which provide an optimal balance of risk and benefit.

Spinal, epidurals, paravertebral, intercostal, and transversus abdominis plane blocks may all be used to provide an effective if variable contribution to pain relief after abdominal and thoracic surgery. Even wound infiltration has been shown to improve analgesia and reduce opioid requirements after sternotomy and abdominal surgery (Liu and Wu, 2007), and its combination with joint infiltration may be useful after orthopaedic procedures. Patient management may be simpler with the more peripheral blocks, but

they are less effective and the more central techniques have the potential for contributing even more to patient care than the almost total elimination of pain. The challenge is to select the optimal block for each patient and then to manage that block to deliver the greatest benefit.

Key references

Rigg JR, Jamrozik K, Myles PS, et al. (2002) Epidural anaesthesia and analgesia and outcome of major surgery: a randomised trial. *Lancet* 359: 1276–82.

Rodgers A, Walker N, Schug S, et al. (2000) Reduction of postoperative mortality and morbidity with epidural or spinal anaesthesia: results from overview of randomised trials. *British Medical Journal* 321: 1493–6.

On-line resource

http://www.postoppain.org Procedure specific postoperative pain management (PROSPECT).

References

Ali M, Winter DC, Hanly AM, et al. (2010) Prospective, randomized, controlled trial of thoracic epidural or patient-controlled opiate analgesia on perioperative quality of life. *British Journal of Anaesthesia* 104: 292–7.

Andersen LO, Gaarn-Larsen L, Kristensen BB, et al. (2009) Subacute pain and function after fast-track hip and knee arthroplasty. *Anaesthesia* 64: 508–13.

Arnott J (1847) On cold as a means of producing local insensibility. *Lancet* ii: 98–9.

Arumainayagam N, McGrath J, Jefferson KP, Gillatt DA (2008) Introduction of an enhanced recovery protocol for radical cystectomy. *BJU International* 101: 698–701.

Ballantyne JC, Carr DB, deFerranti S, et al. (1998) The comparative effects of postoperative analgesic therapies on pulmonary outcome: cumulative meta-analyses of randomized, controlled trials. *Anesthesia & Analgesia* 86: 598–612.

Baudouin SV (2003) Lung injury after thoracotomy. *British Journal of Anaesthesia* 91: 132–42.

Bignami E, Landoni G, Biondi-Soccai GL, et al. (2010) Epidural analgesia improves outcome in cardiac surgery: A meta-analysis of randomized controlled trials. *Journal of Cardiovascular Anesthesia* 24: 586–97.

Biki B, Mascha E, Moriarty DC, et al. (2008) Anesthetic technique for radical prostatectomy surgery affects cancer recurrence: a retrospective analysis. *Anesthesiology* 109: 180–7.

Block BM, Liu SS, Rowlingson AY, et al. (2003) Efficacy of postoperative epidural analgesia: a meta-analysis. *Journal of the American Medical Association* 290: 2455–63.

Bolliger D, Manfred DS, Giovanna DL, et al. (2009) A preliminary report on the prognostic significance of preoperative brain natriuretic peptide and postoperative cardiac troponin in patients undergoing major vascular surgery. *Anesthesia & Analgesia* 108: 1069–75.

Bracco D, Hemmerling T (2007) Epidural analgesia in cardiac surgery: an updated risk assessment. *Heart Surgery Forum* 10: E334–7.

Campos JH (2009) Fast track in thoracic anesthesia and surgery. *Current Opinion in Anaesthesiology* 22: 1–3.

Carli F, Clemente A, Asenjo JF, et al. (2010) Analgesia and functional outcome after total knee arthroplasty: periarticular infiltration vs continuous femoral nerve block. *British Journal of Anaesthesia* 105: 185–95.

Cense HA, Lagarde SM, de Jong K, et al. (2006) Association of no epidural analgesia with postoperative morbidity and mortality after transthoracic esophageal cancer resection. *Journal of the American College of Surgeons* 202: 395–400.

Chakravarthy M, Thimmangowda P, Krishnamurhy J, et al. (2005) Thoracic epidural anesthesia in cardiac surgical patients: a prospective audit of 2,113 cases. *Journal of Cardiothoracic and Vascular Anesthesia* 119: 44–8.

Chang CC, Lin HC, Lin HW, Lin HC (2010) Anesthetic management and surgical site infections in total hip and knee replacement: a population-based study. *Anesthesiology* 113: 279–84.

Chelly JE, Ghisi D, Fanelli A (2010) Continuous peripheral nerve blocks in acute pain management. *British Journal of Anaesthesia* 105(Suppl 1): 86–96.

Crescenzi G, Landoni G, Monaco F, et al. (2009) Epidural anesthesia in elderly patients undergoing coronary artery bypass graft surgery. *Journal of Cardiothoracic & Vascular Anesthesia* 23: 807–12.

Eskicioglu C, Forbes SS, Aarts MA, et al. (2009) Enhanced recovery after surgery (ERAS) programs for patients having colorectal surgery: a meta-analysis of randomized trials. *Journal of Gastrointestinal Surgery* 13: 2321–9.

Exadaktylos AK, Buggy DJ, Moriarty DC, et al. (2006) Can anesthetic technique for primary breast cancer surgery affect recurrence or metastasis? *Anesthesiology* 105: 660–4.

Farooqui M, Li Y, Rogers T, et al. (2007) COX-2 inhibitor celecoxib prevents chronic morphine-induced promotion of angiogenesis, tumour growth, metastasis and mortality, without compromising analgesia. *British Journal of Cancer* 97: 1523–31.

Fischer HBJ, Simanski C (2005) A procedure-specific systematic review and consensus recommendations for analgesia after total hip replacement. *Anaesthesia* 60: 1189–202.

Fischer HBJ, Simanski CJ, Sharp C, et al. (2008) A procedure-specific systematic review and consensus recommendations for analgesia following total knee arthroplasty. *Anaesthesia* 63: 1105–23.

Gendall KA, Kennedy RR, Watson AJ, Frizelle FA (2007) The effect of epidural analgesia on postoperative outcome after colorectal surgery. *Colorectal Disease* 9: 584–98.

Gonca S, Kilickan L, Dalcik C, et al. (2007) The cardioprotective effects of thoracic epidural anesthesia are induced by the expression of vascular endothelial growth factor and inducible nitric oxygen synthase in cardiopulmonary bypass surgery. *Journal of Cardiovascular Surgery* 48: 93–102.

Gupta K, Kshirsagar S, Chang L, et al. (2002) Morphine stimulates angiogenesis by activating proangiogenic and survival-promoting signaling and promotes breast tumor growth. *Cancer Research* 62: 4491–8.

Harrop-Griffiths W, Picard J (2001) Editorial: continuous regional analgesia: can we afford not to use it? *Anaesthesia* 56: 299–301.

Hawkins JL, Koonin LM, Palmar SK, Gibbs CP (1997) Anesthesia-related deaths during obstetric delivery in the United States, 1979–1990. *Anesthesiology* 86: 277–84

Holm B, Kristensen MT, Myhrmann L, et al. (2010) The role of pain for early rehabilitation in fast track total knee arthroplasty. *Disability and Rehabilitation* 32: 300–6.

Jorgensen H, Wetterslev J, Moiniche S, Dahl JB (2000) Epidural local anaesthetics versus opioid-based analgesic regimens on postoperative gastrointestinal paralysis, PONV and pain after abdominal surgery. *Cochrane Database of Systematic Reviews* 4: CD001893.

Kandasami M, Kinninmonth AW, Sarungi M, et al. (2009) Femoral nerve block for total knee replacement—a word of caution. *Knee* 16: 98–100.

Kehlet H (1998) Modification of responses to surgery by neural blockade: clinical implications. In Cousins MJ, Bridenbaugh PO (Eds) *Neural blockade in clinical anesthesia and management of pain*, 3rd edn, pp. 129–78. Philadelphia, PA: Lippincott-Raven.

Kehlet H, Andersen LO (2011) Local infiltration analgesia in joint replacement: the evidence and recommendations for clinical practice. *Acta Anaesthesiologica Scandinavica* 55(7): 778–84.

Kehlet H, Wilkinson RC, Fischer HB, Camu F (2007) PROSPECT: evidence-based, procedure-specific postoperative pain management. *Best Practice Research in Clinical Anaesthesiology* 21: 149–59.

Kendell J, Wildsmith JAW, Gray IG (2000) Costing anaesthetic practice. An economic comparison of regional and general anaesthesia for varicose vein and inguinal hernia surgery. *Anaesthesia* 55: 1106–13.

Kilickan L, Solak M, Bayindir O (2005) Thoracic epidural anesthesia preserves myocardial function during intraoperative and postoperative period in coronary artery bypass grafting operation. *Journal of Cardiovascular Surgery* 46: 559–67.

Kilickan L, Yumuk Z, Bayindir O (2008) The effect of combined preinduction thoracic epidural anaesthesia and glucocorticoid administration on perioperative interleukin-10 levels and hyperglycemia. *Journal of Cardiovascular Surgery* 49: 87–93.

Lavand'homme P, De Kock M, Waterloos H (2005) Intraoperative epidural analgesia combined with ketamine provides effective preventive analgesia in patients undergoing major digestive surgery. *Anesthesiology* 103: 813–20.

Leung E, Ferjani AM, Stellard N, et al. (2009) Predicting post-operative mortality in patients undergoing colorectal surgery using P-POSSUM and CR-POSSUM scores: a prospective study. *Colorectal Disease* 24: 1459–64.

Liu SS, Wu CL (2007) The effect of analgesic technique on postoperative patient-reported outcomes including analgesia: a systematic review. *Anesthesia & Analgesia* 105: 789–808.

Macrae WA (2008) Chronic post-surgical pain: 10 years on. *British Journal of Anaesthesia* 101: 77–86.

Marhofer P, Harrop-Griffiths W, Kettner SC, Kirchmair L (2010) Fifteen years of ultrasound guidance in regional anaesthesia: part 1. *British Journal of Anaesthesia* 104: 538–46.

Marret E, Remy C, Bonnet F (Postoperative Pain Forum Group) (2007) Meta-analysis of epidural analgesia versus parenteral opioid analgesia after colorectal surgery. *British Journal of Surgery* 94: 665–73.

McCartney CJ, McLeod GA (2011) Local infiltration analgesia for total knee arthroplasty. *British Journal of Anaesthesia* 107: 487–9.

Macfarlane AJ, Prasad GA, Chan VW, Brull R (2009a) Does regional anaesthesia improve outcome after total hip arthroplasty? A systematic review. *British Journal of Anaesthesia* 103: 335–45.

Macfarlane AJ, Prasad GA, Chan VW, Brull R (2009b) Does regional anesthesia improve outcome after total knee arthroplasty? *Clinical Orthopaedics & Related Research* 467: 2379–402.

McKenzie PJ, Wishart HY, Dewar KMS, et al. (1984) Comparison of the effects of spinal anaesthesia and general anaesthesia on postoperative oxygenation and perioperative mortality. *British Journal of Anaesthesia* 52: 49–53.

McLeod GA, Davies H, Munnoch N, et al. (2001) Postoperative pain relief using thoracic epidural: outstanding success and disappointing failures. *Anaesthesia* 56: 75–81.

McLeod GA, Dell K, Smith C, Wildsmith JA (2006) Measuring the quality of continuous epidural block for abdominal surgery. *British Journal of Anaesthesia* 96: 633–9.

Moiniche S, Kehlet H, Dahl JB (2002) A qualitative and quantitative systematic review of preemptive analgesia for postoperative pain relief: the role of timing of analgesia. *Anesthesiology* 96: 725–41.

Muehling BM, Halter GL, Schelzig H, et al. (2008) Reduction of postoperative pulmonary complications after lung surgery using a fast track clinical pathway. *European Journal of Cardio-Thoracic Surgery* 34: 174–80.

Muehling BM, Schelzig H, Steffen P, et al. (2009) A prospective randomized trial comparing traditional and fast-track patient care in elective open infrarenal aneurysm repair. *World Journal of Surgery* 33: 577–85.

Munitiz V, Martinez-de-Haro LF, Ortiz A, et al. (2010) Effectiveness of a written clinical pathway for enhanced recovery after transthoracic (Ivor Lewis) oesophagectomy. *British Journal of Surgery* 97: 714–18.

Nishimori M, Ballantyne JC, Low JH (2006) Epidural pain relief versus systemic opioid-based pain relief for abdominal aortic surgery. *Cochrane Database of Systematic Review* 3:CD005059.

Novotny V, Hakenberg OW, Wiessner D, et al. (2007) Perioperative complications of radical cystectomy in a contemporary series. *European Urology* 51: 397–402.

O'Hara DA, Duff A, Berlin JA, et al. (2000) The effect of anesthetic technique on postoperative outcomes in hip fracture repair. *Anesthesiology* 92: 947–57.

Omar SH, Radwan KG, Youssif MA, et al. (2008) A non opioid fast track anesthetic regimen for colonic resection. *Journal of the Egyptian Society of Parasitology* 39: 849–64.

Puolakka PA, Rorarius MG, Roviola M (2010) Persistent pain following knee arthroplasty. *European Journal of Anaesthesiology* 27: 455–60.

Ready LB (1999) Acute pain: lessons learned from 25,000 patients. *Regional Anesthesia and Pain Medicine* 24: 499–505.

Report (2010) *An Age Old Problem. A review of the care received by elderly patients undergoing surgery*. A report by the National Confidential Enquiry into Patient Outcome and Death. http://www.ncepod.org.uk/2010eese.htm

Reports (1991–2011) *Confidential Enquiries into Maternal Deaths in the United Kingdom, 1985–87 (1991); 1988–90 (1994); 1991–93 (1996); 1994–96 (1998); 1997–1999 (2001); 2000–2002 (2004); 2003–2005 (2007); 2006–2008 (2011)*. London: HMSO & TSO.

Richman JM, Liu SS, Courpas G, et al. (2006) Does continuous peripheral nerve block provide superior pain control to opioids? A meta-analysis. *Anesthesia & Analgesia* 102: 248–57.

Rigg JR, Jamrozik K, Myles PS, et al. (2002) Epidural anaesthesia and analgesia and outcome of major surgery: a randomised trial. *Lancet* 359: 1276–82.

Rodgers A, Walker N, Schug S, et al. (2000) Reduction of postoperative mortality and morbidity with epidural or spinal anaesthesia: results from overview of randomised trials. *British Medical Journal* 321: 1493–6.

Rosen M (1981) Editorial comment. *Anaesthesia* 36: 36–7.

Saeki H, Ishimura H, Higashi H, et al. (2009) Postoperative management using intensive patient-controlled epidural analgesia and early rehabilitation after an esophagectomy. *Surgery Today* 39: 476–80.

Sakaguchi M, Kuroda Y, Hirose M (2006) The antiproliferative effect of lidocaine on human tongue cancer cells with inhibition of the activity of epidermal growth factor receptor. *Anesthesia & Analgesia* 102: 1103–7.

Sessler DI (2010) Neuraxial anesthesia and surgical site infection. *Anesthesiology* 113: 265–67.

Singleton PA, Lingen MW, Fekete MJ, et al. (2006) Methylnaltrexone inhibits opiate and VEGF-induced angiogenesis: Role of receptor transactivation. *Microvascular Research* 72: 3–11.

Suttner S, Lang K, Piper SN, et al. (2005) Continuous intra- and postoperative thoracic epidural analgesia attenuates brain natriuretic peptide release after major abdominal surgery. *Anesthesia & Analgesia* 101: 896–903.

Toftdahl K, Nikolajsen L, Haraldsted V, et al. (2007) Comparison of peri- and intraarticular analgesia with femoral nerve block after total knee arthroplasty: a randomized clinical trial. *Acta Orthopaedica* 78: 172–9.

Tsui BCH, Green JS (2011) Editorial: Types of anaesthesia for cancer surgery and cancer recurrence. *British Medical Journal* 342: 718–19.

van Dam RM, Hendry PO, Coolsen MM, et al. (2008) Enhanced Recovery After Surgery (ERAS) Group: Initial experience with a multimodal enhanced recovery programme in patients undergoing liver resection. *British Journal of Surgery* 95: 969–75.

Wijeysundera DN, Beattie WS, Austin PC, et al. (2008) Epidural anaesthesia and survival after intermediate-to-high risk non-cardiac surgery: a population-based cohort study. *Lancet* 372: 562–9.

Wildsmith JAW (2002) No sceptic me, but the long day's task is not yet done: The Gaston Labat Lecture. *Regional Anesthesia and Pain Management* 27: 503–8.

Wu CL, Naqibuddin M, Rowlingson AJ, et al. (2003) The effect of pain on health-related quality of life in the immediate postoperative period. *Anesthesia & Analgesia* 97: 1078–85.

Zhao G, Huang Y, Chen X, et al. (2010) Research on fast track surgery application in lung cancer surgery. *Chinese Journal of Lung Cancer* 13: 102–6.

CHAPTER 6

Peripheral nerve and local anaesthetic drugs

Cameron Weir and Gary Strichartz

Local anaesthetics are drugs which block reversibly the conduction of impulses in the peripheral nervous system. The fundamental mode of action is far from unique to peripheral nerves, explaining both the systemic toxicity of these drugs and their other clinical uses (e.g. cardiac arrhythmias and refractory epilepsy). However, this chapter will focus on their actions in blocking both afferent and efferent nerve impulses as a component of surgical anaesthesia.

'Local' anaesthesia may be achieved by simple surgical site infiltration, selective peripheral nerve block, or central neuraxial block. Whatever method is employed, optimal operating conditions and postoperative analgesia can only be provided if the clinician has a clear understanding of the anatomical, neurophysiological, and pharmacological aspects of neuronal function and local anaesthetic activity. For example, the anatomical arrangement of the nerves governs the distribution of a local anaesthetic block once an agent

has been applied at a particular site, with this impulse block having the same functional significance whatever factor (drug, temperature, surgery, etc.) is used to produce it. By contrast, micro-anatomical, in addition to neurophysiological and pharmacokinetic factors, affect the action of drugs, because they must be able to penetrate the often considerable coverings of a nerve before its function can be interrupted.

Structural components of nerve tissue

A considerable part of the substance of a peripheral nerve is connective tissue. Structurally and functionally, this may be divided into three separate layers (Figure 6.1). Bundles of nerve fibres—the fasciculi—are embedded in *endoneurium*. This consists mainly of longitudinally arranged collagen fibrils, with some condensation of

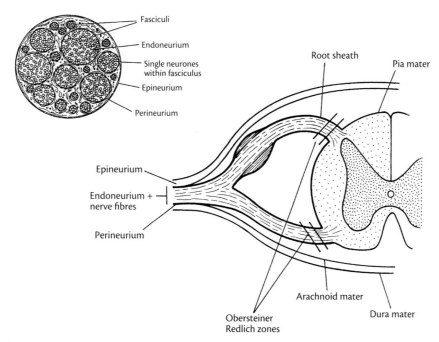

Figure 6.1 Cross-section (top) and structural components (below) of peripheral nerve. (Reproduced from J.A.W. Wildsmith, 'Peripheral nerve and local anaesthetic drugs', *British Journal of Anaesthesia*, 1986, 58, 7, pp. 692–700 by permission of Oxford University Press and the *British Journal of Anaesthesia*.)

the collagen around both the nerve fibres and the capillaries which supply them. Each fasciculus is surrounded by layers of flattened, overlapping or interdigitating fibroblasts, which are the major component of the *perineurium* (Shanthaveerappa & Bourne 1962). The larger the fasciculus, the thicker is this layer of cells. Finally, there is a condensation of areolar connective tissue around the perineurium that comprises the *epineurium*. Collagen and elastic fibrils are arranged longitudinally, and this layer also contains lymphatics and blood vessels. The epineurium attaches the nerve only loosely to surrounding structures, so that it is mobile except where branches and blood vessels tether it.

These structural components serve to bind the fibres together and to protect them. Peripheral nerves have considerable longitudinal strength, mainly a property of the epineurium, and the collagen in the perineurium is arranged in a lattice-work pattern to help prevent kinking when the nerve bends. Some nerves, particularly the human sciatic, contain a considerable amount of fat and this may help to cushion the nerve in the sitting position. The cellular component of the perineurium acts as a perifascicular diffusion barrier, preventing or slowing the diffusion of many substances, including local anaesthetics, into and out of the nerve (Feng & Liu 1949). In combination with the permeability properties of the endoneurial capillaries, this diffusion barrier maintains the composition of the extracellular fluid around the nerve fibres (Shanthaveerappa & Bourne 1962). Blood vessels enter the nerve at intervals and form anastomotic plexuses in both epineurium and perineurium. Within the endoneurium there are only capillaries, but (as in the other layers) these are arranged longitudinally.

Nerve root structure

The connective tissue components of the spinal nerve roots are essentially the same as those of the mixed peripheral nerves, although there is much less collagen. The endoneurium continues to the point of attachment of the root to the spinal cord, where there is a clearly defined transitional area, the Obersteiner–Redlich zone. In this zone the Schwann cell sheaths (see 'Functional components of peripheral nerve' section) are replaced by sheaths produced by oligodendrocytes, the supporting cells of the central nervous system. Perineural tissue is much thinner in the spinal roots and is present only as a thin root sheath. In fact, the mixed nerve perineurium divides to be continuous with both the arachnoid mater and the root sheath, while the epineurium merges into the dura mater (Figure 6.1). The nerve roots are thus less well protected by connective tissue than are the peripheral nerves, but they are of course bathed in cerebrospinal fluid and contained within the protection of the vertebral canal. The cell bodies of the sensory fibres are situated towards the periphery of the dorsal root ganglia and the fibres run uninterrupted through its centre.

Functional components of peripheral nerve

The functional unit of peripheral nerve is the *nerve fibre*. This term may be defined solely as the axon emanating from the cell body situated in the dorsal root ganglion or spinal cord, but it is more useful to widen the definition to include the Schwann cell sheath which surrounds every axon. This sheath has some structural and supportive roles, but its most significant effect is on the mode of impulse transmission in myelinated fibres although it has important 'metabolic' functions as well (Chapter 2).

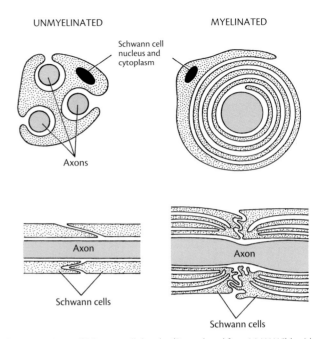

Figure 6.2 Types of Schwann cell sheaths. (Reproduced from J.A.W. Wildsmith, 'Peripheral nerve and local anaesthetic drugs', *British Journal of Anaesthesia*, 1986, 58, 7, pp. 692–700 by permission of Oxford University Press and the *British Journal of Anaesthesia*.)

Two distinct arrangements are recognized (Figure 6.2). In the simpler situation, projections from a single Schwann cell surround several axons, which are described as being *unmyelinated*. At junctions, the Schwann cells, which have a maximum length of 50 μm, simply overlap each other. The other arrangement is for the projection from each Schwann cell to wind itself many times around a single axon. Thus the axon is surrounded by a 'tube' formed of multiple double layers of phospholipid cell membrane, the *myelin sheath*. Each Schwann cell extends for 1 mm or more, but at junctions between them (the nodes of Ranvier) the myelin is absent (Figure 6.2). However, there is close interdigitation between processes of the adjacent cells, so that the axonal membrane still has considerable coverings. Fibres less than 1 μm total diameter are almost always unmyelinated (so called 'C-fibres'), while those greater than 1 μm are myelinated.

Nerve axoplasm contains the usual organelles, such as mitochondria and endoplasmic reticulum, which are required for normal cellular metabolism, but the most important structure for the transmission of nerve impulses is the axonal plasma membrane. Its basic structure (Figure 6.3) is a double layer of phospholipid arranged so that the polar, hydrophilic, phosphate-containing head groups are in contact with the interstitial or intracellular spaces. The hydrophobic lipid groups are opposed to one another in the centre of the membrane. Embedded in the membrane are large protein molecules, many of which function as enzymes, active transport 'pumps', receptors for hormones (and drugs), or as 'channels' for the passive movement of ions both into and out of the cell.

Sodium channel structure and function

In the present context the most important of these membrane proteins are the ion channels, especially those allowing the passage

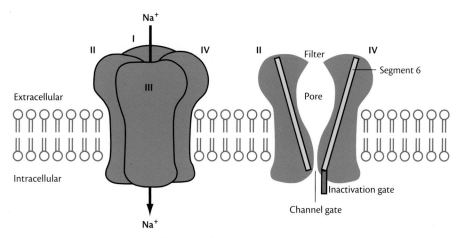

Figure 6.3 Overview of, and cross-section through, a neuronal sodium channel.

of sodium. These channels span the membrane and each has a central aqueous *pore* through which the ions can pass; most have some type of *filter* which makes the channel selective for one (or more) ions, this selectivity depending on the relative size and electrostatic properties of the ion and the channel pore. Many channels also have a *gate* which regulates the passage of ions through them. Associated with such a gate is a sensor mechanism which responds to changes in the membrane's electric field or potential (Stuhmer et al. 1989) and produces conformational changes within the protein, causing the gate to open or close. Channels which respond in this way are described as *voltage-gated*.

Voltage-gated sodium channels play a crucial role in the generation and conduction of impulses in excitable tissues, including nerve and muscle. Most are formed from a single glycoprotein of about 1,950 amino acids (the α subunit), which is shaped like an elongated 'doughnut' projecting into both extracellular and intracellular compartments (Figure 6.3). Each channel comprises four near identical sections, or *domains* (I–IV), each containing six transmembrane *segments* (1–6), and with intracellular and extracellular 'P' loops joining each domain and segment (Figure 6.4) (Catterall 2000). The segments are arranged so that numbers 5 and 6 from all four domains line the pore through the channel with the extracellular loops between these two segments acting together as a 'sieve' or filter to allow mainly sodium ions to pass during activation. Segment 4 in each domain contains many positively charged amino acid residues, these acting collectively as the voltage sensor to initiate channel activation (Catterall 2010). Changes in surrounding electrical potential cause each segment 4 to rotate, and

this distorts the protein so that the intracellular end of the associated segment 6, which projects into the pore at rest (Figure 6.3), moves 'outwards' to open the channel.

The nerve impulse

If a microelectrode is inserted into the axoplasm of a single nerve fibre it records a transmembrane potential in the region of –70 mV, the inside of the cell being negative relative to the outside. This is known as the *resting potential*. When the nerve is stimulated the electrode will record a transient *depolarization* to approximately + 40 mV, followed by *repolarization* back to the resting value. The entire process, which occupies 1–2 ms, is known as the *action potential* (Figure 6.5) and is associated with the longitudinal propagation of the nerve impulse.

Generation of the resting potential

The resting potential is the net result of many factors. The most important are the marked differences in ionic concentrations between intracellular and extracellular fluid, and the factors which tend to maintain those differences, particularly the semipermeable nature of the intervening membrane. For instance, sodium would normally diffuse down its concentration gradient into the cell, but cannot do so because the membrane is normally impermeable to it. Conversely, potassium can diffuse down its concentration gradient more easily, utilizing the *inward rectifier* channels in the membrane to do so. This outward diffusion of potassium leaves an excess of anions over cations within the cell and this imbalance

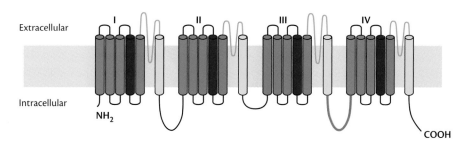

Figure 6.4 Expanded view of a neuronal sodium channel to show sub-components of each domain and the loops connecting them. The green coloured, extracellular segments, the 'P'-loops, fold into the pore to form an outer barrier which discriminates between ions, the 'selectivity filter'. The cytoplasmic loop between domains III and IV, coloured red, is the component which closes the channel during the inactivated state.

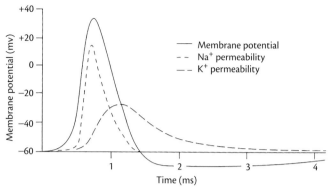

Figure 6.5 Relationship of the phases of a single action potential to the changes in membrane permeability to sodium and potassium associated with the opening and closing of their respective channels. The figures for, and changes in, membrane potential shown are less than those quoted in the text because of damage to the nerve during preparation of the specimen for the experiment. (Reproduced from A. L. Hodgkin and A. F. Huxley, 'A quantitative description of membrane current and its application to conduction and excitation in nerve', *Journal of Physiology*, 117, 4, pp. 500–44. Copyright 1952, Wiley, with permission. Personal communication: Sir Andrew Huxley.)

produces the negative intracellular potential. The electrical gradient so generated retards the further movement of positively charged potassium ions out of the axon and eventually near equilibrium is established between the concentration gradient (causing outward movement of potassium) and the electrochemical gradient (causing inward movement). If any factor causes the membrane potential to decrease, more potassium will diffuse out, but if the membrane tends to hyperpolarize, potassium will diffuse in. In each case the resting potential is restored, as long as the potassium gradient is maintained across the membrane. The generation and preservation of these ionic gradients is dependent on energy-coupled ionic pumps. In neuronal tissue, these pumps exchange proportionally more sodium than potassium (ionic ratio 3:2), each cycle utilizing one molecule of ATP. As well as maintaining the ionic gradients and the resting potential this process generates a pump-related current which tends to hyperpolarize the resting membrane potential.

Basis of the action potential

Depolarization (the steep, rising phase of the action potential) is caused by the movement into the axon of positive charge in the form of sodium ions, and repolarization (the falling phase) by the outward movement of an equivalent amount of positive charge in the form of potassium ions. The essential element of this 'regenerative' process is a sudden increase in the membrane's permeability to sodium during the initial depolarization (Hodgkin & Huxley 1952). Specific voltage-sensitive sodium channels in the membrane open (Figure 6.6), so allowing sodium ions to diffuse down both concentration and electrical gradients (Hille 1984, Moorman 1998).

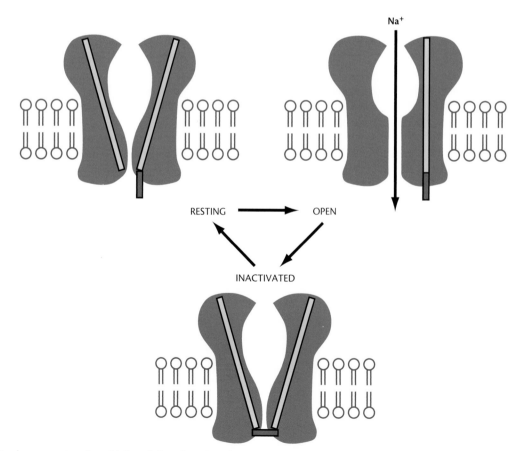

Figure 6.6 Functional components and possible 'states' of a sodium channel.

This influx, which swamps the tendency for potassium efflux to maintain the resting potential, stops when the membrane potential reaches about + 40 mV because of three factors:

1. The inward concentration gradient for sodium is almost balanced by the outward electrical gradient;

2. The open sodium channels slowly 'inactivate' (close) at depolarized potentials due to the loop between domains III and IV (Figure 6.4) closing off the inner end of the pore through the channel (Figure 6.6); and

3. A subset of voltage-gated potassium channels opens slowly (see following paragraph), leading eventually to a larger current of potassium outward than sodium inward. A small amount of potassium then diffuses out until the membrane potential is re-established.

Potassium can pass through the membrane by several routes. Voltage independent (sometimes called *leakage*) channels, of the *inward rectifier* type, are responsible for the background permeability to potassium that generates the resting potential. These channels are generally open at all times, but their state is subject to modification by biochemical processes, such as phosphorylation, triggered by activation of certain G-protein coupled receptors. In this way, the resting potential can be changed by transmitters and hormones (e.g. opioid peptides) acting on such G-protein regulated inward rectifier K$^+$ channels (GIRKs). In addition, several types of specific voltage-gated potassium channels open during depolarization. The sequence of depolarization followed by repolarization is produced because these gated K$^+$ channels open and close more slowly than those for sodium so that the changes in permeability are phased, one following the other (Figure 6.5). Relative to the total number of ions present, the number of ions involved in the exchange during one action potential is very small. The distribution of these ions across the membrane is restored during the resting phase by the sodium–potassium exchange pump. The use of adenosine triphosphate (ATP) to power this active transport process is the only point where energy is required to support impulse activity. By contrast, the ion fluxes that occur when channels open are examples of passive, facilitated diffusion.

Impulse propagation

When one segment of an axon is depolarized a potential difference exists between it and the adjacent sections. A local circuit current (Figure 6.7) will flow, making the membrane potential of the adjacent segment less negative and actuating the voltage sensors on the gates of the sodium channels there. Thus the local current causes some channels in the adjacent segment of the fibre to open and sodium permeability increases. The resulting inward sodium current further depolarizes the axon, spreading the action potential to the adjacent undepolarized region so that the impulse is propagated along the axon (Hodgkin & Huxley 1952).

Local currents also flow 'backwards' along the axon to the segment of nerve that has just repolarized, but it cannot fire an impulse again immediately for two reasons. First, the time course of the change in potassium permeability (Figure 6.5) due to the delay in closure of the voltage-dependent potassium channels ensures that any tendency for depolarization of the membrane potential is immediately counterbalanced by further outward movement of potassium. Second, the inherent properties of sodium channels act against further immediate depolarization. During an initial depolarization the channels change in *state* from 'closed' to 'open', but then (and at a slower rate) they close again—this time to an *inactivated* state (Figure 6.6) from which spontaneous opening cannot occur. Only when the membrane has repolarized does a further transition from the *closed-inactivated* to the *closed-resting* state take place, so eventually restoring the conditions present before the impulse. Thus nerve conduction is normally unidirectional.

An impulse in a non-myelinated fibre spreads almost like a continuous 'ripple' along the axon, but in a myelinated nerve this is not so because its sodium channels are situated almost exclusively in the region of the nodes of Ranvier. Thus the local currents have to flow from node to node, passively depolarizing the intervening section of axon. In fact, the local current from one node of Ranvier will affect more than the immediately adjacent one, and the length of axon depolarized by the action potential extends over several nodes. This *saltatory conduction* is much more rapid and accounts for the faster rate of impulse transmission in myelinated than in unmyelinated fibres.

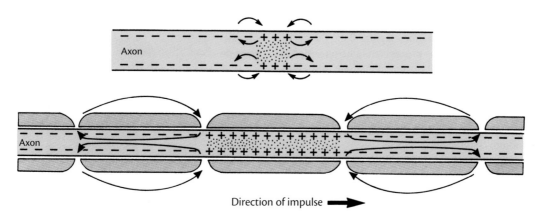

Direction of impulse ➡

Figure 6.7 Local current flows around depolarized segment (stippled area) in unmyelinated (top) and myelinated (bottom) axons. (Reproduced from J.A.W. Wildsmith, 'Peripheral nerve and local anaesthetic drugs', *British Journal of Anaesthesia*, 1986, 58, 7, pp. 692–700 by permission of Oxford University Press and the *British Journal of Anaesthesia*.)

Initiation of the action potential

Action potentials are initiated at peripheral nerve endings in much the same way that they are propagated, but with appropriate physiological stimuli producing the initial depolarization. Relatively little is known about the nature of the receptors which cause this, but it is obvious that each must be able to respond specifically to one of a range of stimuli as diverse as mechanical deformation, temperature, and neuroactive chemicals. Receptors for prostaglandins, and other inflammatory mediators, have an integral relationship with the endings of pain fibres and may have a role in maintaining certain classes of sodium channels in the activatable state, enhancing the fibres' excitability. Fibres so sensitized may also be more responsive to nucleotides or peptides, such as bradykinin, released by tissue damage. The initial opening of non-specific cation channels associated with these receptors allows some depolarization of the membrane. If the stimulus is inadequate, potassium leakage will stop the membrane from depolarizing sufficiently, but with an adequate stimulus the membrane potential will reach the threshold value which triggers the opening of other, voltage-sensitive channels, leading to the generation and propagation of a definitive action potential. In most healthy conditions the 'stimulus' afforded by the local circuit current (see 'Impulse propagation' section) from the adjacent, excited region is far more than adequate to bring the membrane to threshold, insuring robust impulse propagation.

Centrally, most nerves have connections to others that may cause excitation or inhibition by the release of a variety of neurotransmitters. Membrane receptors for these transmitters are associated with ion channels which are activated either directly by transmitter binding (they are *ligand-gated*), or indirectly by intracellular *second messengers* such as 'G' proteins. Excitatory transmitters are usually associated with non-selective cation channels which open under their influence and catalyse primarily sodium influx, thus leading to a degree of local depolarization. Inhibitory transmitters are usually associated with potassium or chloride selective channels, the opening of which will cause local hyperpolarization or at least maintain the membrane potential near its resting value. An action potential will only be generated when the effects of excitatory transmitters predominate to yield a net inward depolarizing current.

Conduction block

The transmission of nerve impulses is dependent upon a wave of depolarization, followed by repolarization, passing along the nerve membrane. Theoretically at least, the process could be interrupted in several ways, but it is obvious that the initial increase in sodium permeability produced by the opening of ion-selective channels is the key factor. Agents that interfere with the processes which underlie the other, subsequent phases of the action potential are known, but they do not have the same immediate effect on impulse transmission as sodium channel block.

A wide range of agents can be shown to block sodium channels when they are applied directly to neurophysiological preparations *in vitro*. They include many biotoxins (e.g. tetrodotoxin, saxitoxin), the phenothiazines, β-adrenergic blocking agents, and some opioids, in addition to the traditional local anaesthetic agents. Only the last are widely used clinically to block nerve conduction because they also have the ability to penetrate nerve coverings and are relatively free from local and systemic toxicity (Strichartz 1986). Fundamental to their mode of action is the chemistry of their behaviour in solution (Strichartz et al. 1990). All the clinically useful local anaesthetics have a common basic structure with an aromatic ring attached to an amine group by an intermediate chain (Table 6.1). In common with general anaesthetics they are more soluble in organic solvents than in aqueous ones, so to allow them to be administered by injection they are usually prepared in an acid solution of the hydrochloride salt in water. In this combination the amine group becomes protonated, albeit reversibly, the water solubility of the drug is increased considerably, and a preparation suitable for injection results.

The molecular mechanism of action of local anaesthetic drugs may be summarized as follows (Figure 6.8). After injection, tissue buffers increase the pH of the solution so that more of the lipid-soluble, base form of the drug is released. This is able to diffuse through the connective tissue barriers (Figure 6.1) and penetrate the nerve (Bernards & Hill 1992), eventually passing through the lipid cell membrane and into the axoplasm, where the molecules re-ionize and enter the sodium channel pore. Simplistically, local anaesthetics may be thought of as obstructing the pore of the channel, but evidence suggests that they bind to specific amino acids in segment 6 and alter channel kinetics, either inducing, or prolonging the duration of, the inactivated state (Figure 6.6) (Courtney 1980, Hille 1984).

The most convincing mechanistic evidence for this theory comes from *in vitro* experiments in which permanently ionized (and thus less lipid soluble) analogues of local anaesthetics were applied to either the inside or the outside of the axon of single nerve fibre preparations (Narahashi et al. 1970). Applied to the outside, these drugs have little effect because they cannot penetrate the cell membrane, but when perfused through the inside of the axon they have a potent action. By comparison, small non-ionizable (and thus water insoluble) local anaesthetics like benzocaine reach the same binding site primarily by diffusing into the sodium channel directly from the membrane. Such a mechanism may also be relevant to the action of the other, tertiary amine drugs, their un-ionized base forms also reaching the binding site from the membrane (Figure 6.8). These different routes of access are described as hydrophilic and hydrophobic pathways, respectively.

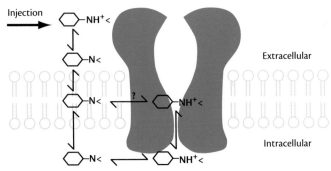

Figure 6.8 Access path of local anaesthetics to sodium channel. Intracellular fluid (ICF), extracellular fluid (ECF).

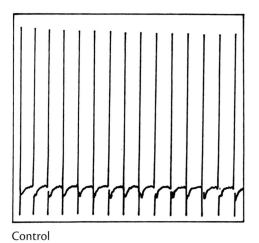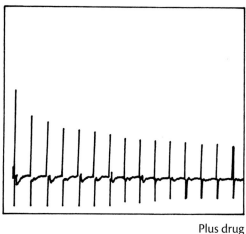

Control   Plus drug

Figure 6.9 Use-dependent block. 'A' fibre compound action potentials from rabbit vagus nerve stimulated at 30 Hz for 0.5 s before and after the application of tetracaine at 0.02 mmol l⁻¹. The decrease in 'spike' height between the control trace and the first spike of the second trace represents the degree of 'resting' block. The subsequent decrease in trace height is caused by 'phasic' block. Repetition of the stimulus train after a few seconds of rest would produce an identical trace. (Reproduced from J.A.W. Wildsmith, 'Peripheral nerve and local anaesthetic drugs', *British Journal of Anaesthesia*, 1986, 58, 7, pp. 692–700 by permission of Oxford University Press and the *British Journal of Anaesthesia*.)

Use-dependent block

The structural relationship between local anaesthetic drug and sodium channel receptor is the subject of much research, centred mostly on a combination of site-directed mutagenesis (Nau et al. 1999, Ragsdale et al. 1994) and the phenomenon known as *use-dependent block* (Courtney 1980). If an *in vitro* nerve preparation is stimulated at a very low frequency (<0.1 Hz) and exposed to a low concentration of a local anaesthetic, a minor decrease in impulse transmission develops. An increase in the stimulus frequency (to >5 Hz) will then appear to increase the degree of block (Figure 6.9), but a brief period of rest allows conduction to recover again (Schwarz et al. 1977).

The most likely explanation of the difference between *tonic* (or *resting*) block and *phasic* (*use-* or *frequency-dependent*) block is that the binding affinity of local anaesthetics differs among the various states of the sodium channels. Binding is weak to the resting state and stronger to open and inactivated states. Use-dependent block arises from this selective affinity, because depolarizations increase the population of open and inactivated channels. The phenomenon supports the theory that that at least part of local anaesthetic action is due to prolongation of sodium channel's inactivated state.

Whether or not this has any significant clinical relevance for nerve block is, at best, not proven, if only because the conditions of such experiments are so artificial. By contrast, the therapeutic actions of local anaesthetic-like Class 1 antiarrhythmic agents on cardiac impulses probably depend critically on this use-dependent mechanism. Concern over the cardiotoxicity of bupivacaine, coupled with the fact that drugs vary in the degree to which they produce phasic block, has led to suggestions that there may be a relationship between these, but the evidence is poor.

Structure–activity relationships

Local anaesthetics vary in their clinical profiles and these differences may be related to their chemical structures (Berde &

Strichartz 2010). Because certain physicochemical properties are related to activity, it is possible to quantify the differences between drugs. The factors usually quoted are pK_a, partition coefficient (an index of lipid solubility), and the degree of protein binding (Strichartz et al. 1990) (Table 6.1). It is important to appreciate that these features are not independent of one another, and even correlate with other pharmacological actions of the drugs, so that when two drugs with several structural differences are compared, the relationship of physicochemical property with clinical feature may not appear to be a direct one. The true relationship is only seen when a strictly homologous drug series is examined (Bokesch et al. 1986, Lee-Son et al. 1992, Wildsmith et al. 1989).

The local anaesthetic drugs in current use are classified into two groups according to the nature of the bond in the chain between the aromatic ring and the amine group. This may be either an ester linkage (procaine and its derivatives) or an amide linkage (lidocaine and its derivatives). These bonds have notable effects on the route of metabolism and the chemical stability of the compounds. Most esters are metabolized rapidly by plasma cholinesterase, so their systemic toxicity is less, but they also have relatively short shelf-lives when stored in solution without preservatives. The amides are very stable and cannot be hydrolysed by cholinesterase; therefore, they rely on hepatic detoxification mechanisms for breakdown.

The other important difference between the two groups is that the pK_a values of the esters are greater than those of the homologous amides. This means that the proportion of the lipid-soluble, un-ionized form of the drug present in solution at physiological pH is greater with amides. These differences in pK_a affect the overall rate of axonal membrane penetration and binding to sodium channels because the base form penetrates to the site more rapidly, yet the charged form stays there longer (Schwartz et al. 1977) (Figure 6.8). In addition, the coverings of nerves are essentially lipid membranes (Strichartz 1977) and the un-ionized, lipid-soluble form of the drug is required to penetrate them as well. Thus drugs

Table 6.1 Physicochemical properties of some local anaesthetics measured at 37°C.

Drug	Mol wt	pK_a	Distribution coefficient[a]	% protein bound
Procaine	236	8.9	3.1	5.8
Lidocaine	234	7.7	110	64
Prilocaine	220	7.7	25[b]	55
Mepivacine	260	7.7	42	77
Ropivacaine	288	8.1	115[b]	95
Bupivacaine	302	8.1	560 / 346[b]	95
Articaine	284	7.8	???	94

Notes: a = between water & octanol at pH 7.4; b = at 25°C.

with pK_a nearer to 7.4 may have a noticeably faster onset than those with pK_a greater than 8 when applied to nerves with considerable barriers to diffusion around them. Lidocaine has only a marginally lower pK_a than bupivacaine, but it is also a smaller molecule and this may aid its membrane penetrance (Bernards & Hill 1992). In addition, being less potent, lidocaine is applied at higher concentrations and therefore has a higher molecular gradient driving its diffusion into the nerve.

Addition of side chains to the basic local anaesthetic drug structure increases both lipid solubility and sodium channel affinity, and this is related directly to potency (compare lidocaine with bupivacaine, procaine with tetracaine) (Courtney 1980, Wildsmith et al. 1989). The third important physicochemical property, protein binding, also increases as side chains are added to the molecule. This measurement is related to the reaction with serum proteins, not with membrane targets, and any correlation between protein binding and duration of action is largely fortuitous.

Prilocaine presents an apparent contradiction to these rules. It is less lipid-soluble and less protein-bound than lidocaine, yet the two are equipotent in clinical use, and prilocaine has a longer duration of action. The apparent inconsistency relates to a difference in vasoactivity. Prilocaine does not have the vasodilator action of lidocaine, so it is removed from the site of injection more slowly. This more than compensates for its physicochemical disadvantage, because vascular flow removes more than 95% of the injected dose of local anaesthetic before it even enters the peripheral nerve. Similar factors may account for the finding that ropivacaine and bupivacaine produce almost equal degrees of sensory block.

Chirality and local anaesthetics

Chirality is derived from the Greek word, *chiros*, meaning 'handed'. A chiral compound is one that contains at least one atomic centre (usually a carbon atom) to which four different atoms or chemical groups are attached. If a molecule contains one such 'asymmetric' atom, two distinct, three-dimensional, mirror-image arrangements of the components, known as *stereo-isomers*, are possible. Although such isomers have identical atomic composition and chemical properties, the different spatial arrangement of the atoms means that, like our hands, they cannot be superimposed one upon the other. Matching stereo-isomers are called *enantiomers*, and a substance containing equal amounts of the two enantiomers is known as a 'racemate', or 'racemic' mixture. Enantiomers have identical physicochemical properties, and have the same pK_a and lipid solubility values (Tucker 1997), but there may be differences, qualitative and quantitative, in their pharmacokinetic and pharmacodynamic properties (Sidebotham & Schug 1997). This is because of stereoselective interactions (those due to differences in the three-dimensional structure) at drug receptor sites.

Stereo-isomers may be described and identified in a number of ways, with the current standard being the use of the 'Sequence Rule Notation' (Cahn et al. 1956). In this, the smallest of the four groups attached to the asymmetric atom is identified, and the molecule 'positioned' with this group directed away from the 'viewer', that is, on the 'far' side of the molecule. If the sequence of the sizes of the other three groups is 'clockwise' from smallest to largest, it is defined as an 'R' (from the Latin *rectus*—right) isomer, whereas if the sequence is 'anticlockwise' it is defined as an 'S' isomer (*sinister*—left) (Figure 6.10). These terms are described as the '*absolute*

descriptors', although the best known method of identifying isomers relates to their property of rotating plane-polarized light in equal degree, but in opposite directions, either clockwise (+) or anticlockwise (−). These are known as the '*relative* descriptors'. Unfortunately, there is no consistency between the absolute and relative descriptors and, within a homologous series of compounds, the S/R notation may change as the length of a particular side chain alters. This is seen in the 'bupivacaine' series of local anaesthetics where S-mepivacaine has the same spatial arrangement of atoms as R-bupivacaine. To deal with these complications it is common to quote both descriptors (e.g. S(−) bupivacaine) of a chiral compound.

With the exception of lidocaine, all the currently used amide local anaesthetics are chiral, and differences in the pharmacokinetic and pharmacodynamic properties of the isomers of each drug have been recognized for many years. Prilocaine was the first agent to be studied (Åckerman et al. 1967), but the differences between its isomers are of relatively little clinical impact. The local anaesthetic and toxic effects of the enantiomers of bupivacaine were first described by Aberg (1972), who showed that the S(−) enantiomer is less toxic than the R(+) form. However, the full significance of the difference was not apparent at that time, and it was not possible to produce a single isomer preparation in commercial quantities. It was only when clinical concerns about the cardiotoxicity of racemic bupivacaine became apparent that further development took place. The first single isomer local anaesthetic to reach clinical practice was ropivacaine, the 'S(−)' isomer of the propyl analogue of bupivacaine, chosen initially because it has a longer duration of action than the R(+) version (Åckerman et al. 1988). It was only later that it was shown that R(+)bupivacaine is the more cardiotoxic of the two isomers (Vanhoutte et al. 1991), a finding which led eventually to the development of S(−) bupivacaine, now known as levobupivacaine.

The stereoselectivity of the interactions of local anaesthetics at sodium channels is weak, but is probably of more significance when the channel is in the inactivated state (Nau et al. 1999), something that would explain the greater cardiotoxicity of the 'R' forms of bupivacaine and ropivacaine (see 'Use-dependent block' section). However, the issue is complicated by differences in vasoactivity, with both ropivacaine and levobupivacaine having a greater vasoconstrictor effect than their matching 'R' isomers. Thus, in a parallel to the differences between lidocaine and prilocaine (see 'Structure–activity relationships' section), ropivacaine appears, in clinical use at nerve blocking concentrations, to be equipotent to racemic bupivacaine even though its lipid solubility is less. For the same reason, levobupivacaine may be slightly more potent than the racemate, and there is some controversy about the relative potencies of the three agents (Whiteside & Wildsmith 2001), small though the differences may be. Unfortunately, clinical comparisons are further complicated by the 'weight per unit volume' method used to describe local anaesthetic drug concentrations in commercial preparations. Ropivacaine and bupivacaine are presented as mg ml^{-1} of the hydrochloride salt, but levobupivacaine as mg ml^{-1} of the local anaesthetic base, a result of changes in the regulations governing the labelling of new (but not older) drugs. Because the base has a lower molecular weight, levobupivacaine has about 11% more molecules of local anaesthetic than the racemic bupivacaine preparations of superficially the same concentration. This is a significant difference.

2-dimensional formula

COOH
CH$_3$-C-H
OH

3-dimensional formulae

R - Rectus   S - Sinister

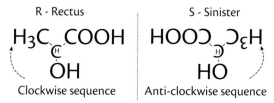

Clockwise sequence   Anti-clockwise sequence

Figure 6.10 Chemical formulae of lactic acid to illustrate absolute descriptor methodology. The smallest atom (−H) attached to the asymmetric carbon atom is positioned 'away' from the viewer. If the sequence of the other three atoms from largest to smallest is clockwise (here −OH, CH$_3$, −COOH), then it is an 'R' isomer. If the sequence is anticlockwise, it is an 'S' isomer. If, as is the case here, two of the atoms attached to the asymmetric carbon are the same, it is the next one in the sequence of each side chain that decides the rule.

Dynamics of nerve block

The effect of physiological factors on the performance of any particular drug is also seen in the way in which its clinical profile varies between injection sites. Each technique of local anaesthesia (spinal, epidural, plexus, major & minor nerve blocks) has its own particular rate of onset, duration, and risk of systemic toxicity (Winnie et al. 1977). These may be clearly related to the thickness of the coverings of the nerve at that point and the blood supply to the area of injection. The faster onset and lower dose requirement of spinal compared with epidural anaesthesia may be explained simply in terms of the considerable difference in the coverings of the nerves in the two spaces (Cohen 1968). After they have passed through the intervertebral foramina, the segmental nerves acquire further coverings, especially if they are involved in the formation of a plexus. These coverings become thinner as the nerve passes more peripherally so the rate of onset of block becomes faster.

The difference in diffusion barriers may also explain the greater susceptibility to chemical damage of nerves in the subarachnoid space. Reports of permanent neurological damage after the use of chloroprocaine for epidural block seem to have been related to the effects of the metabisulphite preservative which was once included in the solution. When injected correctly in the epidural space this preservative has minimal effect because it cannot penetrate the dural sheath, but accidental intrathecal injection of large quantities 'bypasses' that protection.

The pattern of onset of nerve block is further affected by the arrangement of fibres within the mixed nerve. Fibres to and from the most distal structures supplied by it are arranged at its core and those joining it more proximally are on the outside. As local anaesthetic diffuses into a nerve it affects the fibres at the core, that is those innervating the more distal regions, last (Winnie et al. 1977). This is one reason why anaesthesia of the hand may be slower to develop than that of the elbow during brachial plexus block, but this will, of course, depend also on the particular technique chosen and on gross anatomical factors such as which component (root, cord, trunk, branch) of the plexus is closest to the point of injection.

Differential nerve block

It is a common clinical observation that different modalities of nerve function are not blocked at the same rate (Catterall & Mackie 1996). The sequence depends on the site of injection and the drug used, but a typical order of development of block is sympathetic function first, followed by pin-prick sensation, touch, temperature, and finally motor. This phenomenon may be manipulated clinically. Adjustment of drug concentration and volume injected during continuous epidural techniques may produce sympathetic afferent block, with minimal sensory and motor block. The subarachnoid injection of increasing concentrations of procaine has been used to produce differential blocks in the diagnosis and treatment of chronic pain (but see Hogan & Abram 1997).

Peripheral nerve fibres are classified according to both the modality they subserve and their physiological properties. The most important of the latter is velocity of impulse transmission and this depends on both axon diameter and degree of myelination. These various factors may be correlated (see Table 2.1). Early laboratory work and clinical observations were often misinterpreted to conclude that the smallest nerve fibres were the most sensitive to local

anaesthetic block and the largest the least sensitive (Raymond & Gissen 1987). However, there is now a large amount of evidence against this oversimplified interpretation of the evidence. Laboratory studies *in vivo* on single functionally identified fibres show that B-fibres are most sensitive, followed by Aγ (motor) and Aδ (sensory) fibres, then Aβ (sensory) and Aα (motor) fibres, and finally C-fibres, which are the most resistant to block.

Clinically, loss of function is assessed rather than block of impulse transmission, and these two results may not be equivalent. For example, the average frequency of C-fibre discharge in response to pin-prick may fall from 10 Hz to 4 Hz due to use-dependent block by a local anaesthetic, but the perceived stimulus intensity would drop from noticeable to subliminal, because a minimal impulse frequency of about 5 Hz is required for this perception. In another example, partial block of small myelinated Aγ efferents will relax muscle spindles and thus attenuate firing of Ia-sensory fibres (muscle spindle afferents). This results in flaccid paralysis through the myotonic stretch reflex circuitry of the spinal cord. Clinicians often equate such paralysis or paresis with block of the large motor Aα fibres, although this is not required for 'motor block'. Thus, functional block observed clinically can arise for many reasons and it may not be directly apparent exactly which fibres are blocked.

Future developments

The currently available local anaesthetic drugs meet most requirements for local anaesthetic block during surgery, especially when their flexibility is extended by the use of catheter techniques for prolonged effect. What problems there are relate more to systemic toxicity than inadequacies in blocking characteristics, although a drug which could penetrate rapidly thick sheaths, as exist around the brachial plexus, and also have a long duration of action would be extremely useful. Arguably, a greater need is for an agent which specifically provides analgesia without affecting the other modalities of nerve function, so that the benefits of regional nerve block can be extended simply and safely into the postoperative period. The great wave of enthusiasm which followed the introduction to clinical practice of the spinal application of opioid drugs is clear evidence that many anaesthetists are aware of this need. In recent years the major research focus has been on the structure and function of the sodium channel, and this has increased dramatically our understanding of drug–channel interactions, with identification of the key amino acid residues in segment 6 which form the putative local anaesthetic binding site(s) (see 'Conduction block' section).

Some channel complexes, notably those at synapses, also include two auxiliary β-subunits (Alexander 2009), these having a range of functions, influencing channel positioning, manufacture, and gating dynamics (Caterall 2000). Voltage-gated sodium channels are ubiquitous so it is not surprising that subtypes exist to support the range of characteristics required for very diverse electrophysiological activity (e.g. primary afferent neurone versus cardiac myocyte). Nine isoforms of the α subunit, and four of the β, have been identified (England & de Groot 2009) and, while they are structurally similar, each isoform can be identified by its kinetics and sensitivity to tetrodotoxin (Table 6.2). For example, the neuronal isoforms $Na_V1.1$, $Na_V1.2$, $Na_V1.3$, and $Na_V1.7$ are highly sensitive to tetrodotoxin, whereas the cardiac isoform $Na_V1.5$ is relatively resistant. Differences in channel sensitivity may explain some of

Table 6.2 Voltage-gated sodium channel subtypes, their distribution and associated channelopathies. (Revised from England & de Groot 2009.)

Channel subtype	Tissue distribution	Tetrodotoxin sensitivity	Associated channelopathy
$Na_V1.1$	CNS/PNS	High (nM)	Epilepsy
$Na_V1.2$	CNS/PNS	High (nM)	Epilepsy
$Na_V1.3$	CNS/PNS	High (nM)	–
$Na_V1.4$	Skeletal muscle	High (nM)	Myotonia, periodic paralysis
$Na_V1.5$	Heart	Low (µM)	Long QT Brugada syndrome progressive familial heart block
$Na_V1.6$	CNS/PNS	High (nM)	Cerebellar atrophy
$Na_V1.7$	PNS/(SNS)	High (nM)	Altered pain sensitivity
$Na_V1.8$	PNS	Low (µM)	–
$Na_V1.9$	PNS	Low (µM)	–

Notes: CNS = central nervous system; PNS = peripheral nervous system; SNS = sympathetic nervous system.

the differential toxicity of clinically used local anaesthetic agents, bupivacaine showing greater binding to the cardiac $Na_V1.5$ channel (and indeed all others) than lidocaine. In addition, mutations in sodium channel genes have been identified in certain clinical conditions (the 'channelopathies') including epilepsy, long QT syndrome, and the condition of heightened pain known as 'erythromelalgia' (Sheets et al. 2007) (Table 6.2). These disorders provide valuable insights into channel function.

The development of drugs with actions limited to a specific channel isoform is a possible consequence of these discoveries. Obviously, any 'new' type of local anaesthetic must also be able to penetrate the nerve's coverings and have low systemic toxicity. The biotoxins, tetrodotoxin and saxitoxin, have long been known to produce potent block of neuronal sodium channels (by acting at the extracellular end of the pore), and they are 100–1000 times less potent at blocking cardiac Na^+ channels ($Na_V1.5$), but diffusion issues are one of the major reasons why these toxins have not been developed as new drugs. Potency and lower toxicity are often identified with greater specificity, but existing local anaesthetics, despite their safe profile, also inhibit mediators of neuronal function besides Na^+ channels (e.g. potassium and calcium channels, a range of G-protein-coupled receptors, and neurotransmitter release) (Scholz 2002). Voltage-gated sodium channels are the major target of local anaesthesia, yet the contribution made through these other mechanisms to either therapeutic or (probably more relevant) toxic effects is unknown. However, they are very relevant to the processing of impulses generated by noxious stimuli at both nerve endings and the synapse between primary and secondary neurones, points where aqueous pathways may be available for drug delivery.

Further reading

Catterall W (2010) Ion channel voltage sensors: Structure, function and pathophysiology. *Neuron* 67: 915–28.

Stricharz GR, Pastijn E, Sugimoto K (2009) Neural physiology and local anesthetic action. In Cousins MJ, Carr DB, Horlocker TT, Bridenbaugh PO (Eds) *Neural Blockade in Clinical Anesthesia and Pain Medicine*, pp. 26–47. Philadelphia, PA: Lippincott William & Wilkins.

On-line resource

http://onlinelibrary.wiley.com/doi/10.1111/j.1476-5381.2011.01649_1.x/pdf Alexander SPH, Mathie A, Peters JA (2011) *British Journal of Pharmacology*. Guide to Receptors and Channels (GRAC), 5th edn.

References

Aberg G (1972) Toxicological and local anaesthetic effects of optically active isomers of two local anaesthetic compounds. *Acta Pharmacologica et Toxicologica* 31: 444–50.

Åckerman B, Persson H, Tegner C (1967) Local anaesthetic properties of the optically active isomers of prilocaine (Citanest®). *Acta Pharmacologica et Toxicologica* 25: 233–41.

Åckerman B, Hellberg I-B, Trossvik C (1988) Primary evaluation of the local anaesthetic properties of the amino amide agent ropivacaine (LEA 103). *Acta Anaesthesiologica Scandinavica* 32: 571–8.

Alexander SPH, Mathie A, Peters JA (2009) Guide to Receptors and Channels (GRAC), 4th edn. *British Journal of Pharmacology* 158(Suppl. 1): S1–S254.

Berde CB, Strichartz GR (2010) *Local Anesthetics in Miller's Anesthesia*, 7th edn, pp. 913–40. Philadelphia, PA: Churchill-Livingstone/Elsevier.

Bernards CM, Hill HF (1992) Physical and chemical properties of drug molecules governing their diffusion through the spinal meninges. *Anesthesiology* 77: 750–6.

Bokesch PM, Post C, Strichartz, GR (1986) Structure-activity relationship of lidocaine homologues on tonic and frequency-dependent impulse blockade in nerve. *Journal of Pharmacology and Experimental Therapeutics* 237: 773–81.

Cahn RS, Ingold CK, Pelog V (1956) The specification of asymmetric configuration in organic chemistry. *Experientia* 12: 81–124.

Catterall WA (2000) From ionic currents to molecular mechanisms: The structure and function of voltage-gated sodium channels. *Neuron* 26: 13–25.

Catterall W, Mackie K (1996) Local anesthetics. In Hardman JG, Limbird LE, Molinoff PB, et al. (Eds) *Goodman and Gilman's The Pharmacological Basis of Therapeutics*, 9th edn, pp. 331–47. New York: McGraw Hill.

Cohen, EN (1968) Distribution of local anesthetic agents in the neuraxis of the dog. *Anesthesiology* 29: 1002–5.

Courtney KR (1980) Structure–activity relations for frequency-dependent sodium channel block in nerve by local anesthetics. *Journal of Pharmacology and Experimental Therapeutics* 213: 114–19.

England S, de Groot MJ (2009) Subtype-selective targeting of voltage-gated sodium channels. *British Journal of Pharmacology* 158: 1413–25.

Feng TP, Liu YM (1949) The connective tissue sheath of the nerve as effective diffusion barrier. *Journal of Cellular and Comparative Physiology* 34: 1–16.

Hille B (1984) *Ionic channels of excitable membranes.* Sunderland, MA: Sinauer Associates.

Hodgkin AL, Huxley AF (1952) A quantitative description of membrane current and its application to conduction and excitation in nerve. *Journal of Physiology* 117: 500–44.

Hogan QH, Abram SE (1997) Neural blockade for diagnosis and prognosis. A review. *Anesthesiology* 86: 216–41.

Lee-Son S, Wang GK, Concus A, Crill E, Strichartz GR (1992) Stereoselective inhibition of neuronal sodium channels by local anesthetics: evidence for two sites of action? *Anesthesiology* 77: 324–35.

Moorman JR (1998) Sodium channels. In Yaksh TL, Lynch C, Zapol WM, et al. (eds) *Anesthesia: biologic foundations*, pp. 145–62. Philadelphia, PA: Lippincott-Raven.

Narahashi T, Frazier D, Yamada M (1970) The site of action and active form of local anesthetics, 1. Theory and pH experiments with tertiary compounds. *Journal of Pharmacology and Experimental Therapeutics* 171: 32–44.

Nau C, Wang S-Y, Strichartz GR, Wang GK (1999) Point mutations at N434 in D1-S6 of mu-1 Na$^+$ channels modulate binding affinity and stereoselectivity of local anesthetic enantiomers. *Molecular Pharmacology* 56: 404–13.

Ragsdale DS, McPhee JC, Scheuer T, Catterall WA (1994) Molecular determinants of state-dependent block of Na$^+$ channels by local anesthetics. *Science* 265: 1724–30.

Raymond SA, Gissen, AJ (1987) Mechanisms of differential block. In Strichartz GR (Ed) *Handbook of experimental pharmacology*, Vol. 81, pp. 95–164. Berlin: Springer-Verlag.

Scholz A (2002) Mechanisms of (local) anaesthetics on voltage-gated sodium and other ion channels. *British Journal of Anaesthesia* 89: 52–61.

Schwarz W, Palade PT, Hille B (1977) Local anesthetics: effect of pH on use-dependent block of sodium channels in frog muscle. *Biophysics Journal* 20: 343–68.

Shanthaveerappa TR, Bourne GH (1962) The 'perineural epithelium', a metabolically active, continuous, protoplasmic cell barrier surrounding peripheral nerve fasiculi. *Journal of Anatomy, London* 96(4): 527–37.

Sheets PL, Jackson JO, Waxman SG, et al. (2007) A Na$_v$1.7 channel mutation associated with hereditary erythromelalgia contributes to neuronal hyperexcitability and displays reduced lidocaine sensitivity. *Journal of Physiology* 581: 1019–31.

Sidebotham DA, Schug SA (1997) Stereochemistry in anaesthesia. *Clinical and Experimental Pharmacology Physiology* 24: 126–30.

Strichartz GR (1977) The composition and structure of excitable nerve membrane. In Jamieson GA, Robinson DM (Eds) *Mammalian cell membranes*, vol 3, pp. 173–205. London: Butterworths.

Strichartz GR (Ed) (1986) *Handbook of Experimental Pharmacology, Vol 68: Local anesthetics.* Berlin: Springer-Verlag.

Strichartz GR, Sanchez V, Arthur GR, et al. (1990) Fundamental properties of local anesthetics, II. Measured octanol:buffer partition coefficients and pKa values of clinically-used drugs. *Anesthesia & Analgesia* 71: 158–70.

Stuhmer W, Conti F, Harukazu S, et al. (1989) Structural parts involved in activation and inactivation of the sodium channel. *Nature* 339: 597–603.

Tucker GT (1997) Ropivacaine: human pharmacokinetics. *American Journal of Anesthesiology* 24(Suppl 5): 8–13.

Vanhoutte F, Vereecke J, Verbeke N, Carmeliet E (1991) Stereoselective effects of the enantiomers of bupivacaine on electro-physiological properties of the guinea-pig papillary muscle. *British Journal of Pharmacology* 103: 1275–81.

Whiteside J, Wildsmith JAW (2001) Developments in local anaesthetic drugs. *British Journal of Anaesthesia* 87: 27–35.

Wildsmith JAW, Brown DT, Paul D, Johnson S (1989) Structure–activity relationships in differential nerve blockade at high and low frequency stimulation. *British Journal of Anaesthesia* 63: 444–52.

Winnie AP, Tay C-H, Patel KP, et al. (1977) Pharmacokinetics of local anesthetics during plexus blocks. *Anesthesia & Analgesia* 56: 852–61.

CHAPTER 7

Local anaesthetic kinetics

Jenny Porter and Geoff Tucker

Knowledge of the factors influencing the plasma drug concentration–time profiles (pharmacokinetics) of local anaesthetics (Figure 7.1) underpins their safe and effective use. The plasma drug concentration provides information not only on the margin of systemic safety, but also, indirectly, on the amount of dose yet to be absorbed and still available locally for anaesthetic effect. The relevant pharmacokinetic properties are determined by the physicochemical and structural features of the compounds. The former, in particular lipid solubility, have a major influence on systemic absorption rate and hence duration of activity. In concert with chemical structure, they determine how and at what rate the compound is removed from the body. In addition, stereochemical features (Chapter 6) can also modulate pharmacokinetic properties.

The key physicochemical properties of the main local anaesthetics are shown in Table 6.1. Of the amides, only lidocaine is achiral, the rest have an asymmetric carbon atom, giving rise to the possibility of two stereoisomers. Prilocaine and mepivacaine are available as racemates (50:50 mixtures of the two isomers), ropivacaine as the single S-isomer, and bupivacaine as either the racemate or the single S-isomer (levobupivacaine).

Consideration of the pharmacokinetics of local anaesthetic agents can be divided into three aspects: local disposition, systemic absorption, and systemic disposition.

Local disposition

Physiological and biochemical factors affecting the dispersion and distribution of local anaesthetics at and near the site of administration have been reviewed by Mather and Tucker (2009), and include bulk flow of the injected solution, regional blood flow and its distribution, and diffusion and binding of the agent. Local metabolic breakdown seems less important. There appears to be no stereoselectivity in the local membrane permeability of anaesthetics, as demonstrated by similar diffusion of the isomers of bupivacaine across excised monkey dura (Bernards et al. 2000). However, Mizogami and colleagues (2008) do report stereoselective interaction of bupivacaine enantiomers with lipid membranes. Clement and colleagues (1999), using microdialysis, found that access of lidocaine to cerebrospinal fluid after epidural injection in rabbits was about three times greater than that of bupivacaine. This probably reflects much greater sequestration of bupivacaine in epidural

fat (Mather & Tucker 2009). Sophisticated pharmacokinetic–pharmacodynamic models have been described to link local disposition and absorption of local anaesthetics after subarachnoid and epidural injection to changes in the extent and duration of analgesia (Schnider et al. 1996, Olofsen et al. 2008).

Of considerable interest is the possibility that new pharmaceutical formulations (e.g. microspheres and liposomal encapsulation) can be used to modify the clinical profile of local anaesthetics by providing a depot from which drug is released slowly. Compared to the use of equivalent doses in aqueous media, these systems have been shown to prolong duration of action and lower the risk of systemic toxicity when injected perineurally, epidurally, or intrathecally in experimental animals, and epidurally and subcutaneously in man (Grant & Bansinath 2001, Pedersen et al. 2004, Rose et al. 2005). Liposomal formulations increased intensity of effect as well as the durations of prilocaine, lidocaine, and mepivacaine in a rat model (Cereda et al. 2006), although plasma concentrations of bupivacaine were elevated for longer in the rabbit (Boogaerts & Lafont 1993). Complexing ropivacaine with a cyclodextrin has

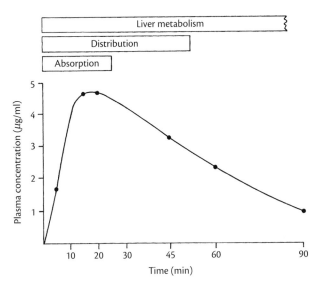

Figure 7.1 General factors affecting plasma concentrations of a local anaesthetic after injection.

been shown to decrease onset time and prolong duration and intensity of sensory block without influencing motor block in mice (Araujo et al. 2008). If lack of neurotoxicity from such vehicles can be guaranteed, they offer the promise of ultra-long duration (Dyhre et al. 2006), but bupivacaine *is* myotoxic and prolonged action may increase this risk (Padera et al. 2008).

Systemic absorption

Knowledge of the rates of systemic absorption of local anaesthetics helps to set confidence limits on the likelihood of systemic toxic reactions after different regional nerve block procedures. Indirectly, these rates give some indication of the relationship between neural block and the amount of drug remaining at or near the site of injection.

Plasma drug concentration and toxicity

To assess safety margins, blood or plasma drug concentrations measured after perineural injection are compared with estimates of the threshold values associated with the onset of significant central nervous system (CNS) toxicity. The latter are available from controlled studies involving intravenous infusion of the agents into healthy volunteers (Mather & Tucker 2009). Figures range from 5–10 mcg ml^{-1} of plasma for lidocaine, and from 2–4 mcg ml^{-1} for bupivacaine. Such intravenous tolerance studies have indicated that ropivacaine causes fewer CNS symptoms and cardiovascular changes than racemic bupivacaine, and is about 25% less toxic with regard to the maximum tolerated dose. At equal plasma concentrations ropivacaine is less toxic than bupivacaine (Knudsen et al. 1997, Scott et al. 1989).

Although 'threshold' levels associated with toxicity are useful guidelines for safe perineural dosage, they refer to the mythical 'average patient', and they should be interpreted in the light of a number of considerations. These include whether measurements are made of plasma or blood, total or unbound drug, ionized or unionized species, enantiomers, active drug metabolites, and, most importantly, the rate of drug administration. The values are most relevant when concentrations are not changing rapidly and there is time for equilibration between drug in plasma and tissue. The site of blood sampling (artery or vein) is critical for interpretation when drug concentrations are changing rapidly (Tucker 1986).

Determinants of systemic absorption

Because local anaesthetics are relatively lipid-soluble compounds, diffusion across the capillary endothelium is unlikely to limit rate of absorption which is related directly to local blood flow, and inversely to local tissue binding. Major determinants of these two include the properties of the agent, site of injection, dose, the presence of additives such as vasoconstrictors, other formulation factors intended to modify local drug residence and release, the influence of nerve block, and pathological features of the patient (Mather & Tucker 2009).

Agent

The extensive data on peak blood and plasma concentrations (C_{max}) of the amide local anaesthetics, and the times at which C_{max} occurs (t_{max}) after various routes of injection, have been tabulated elsewhere (Mather & Tucker 2009, Tucker & Mather 1979). For example, after single-dose epidural injection of plain solutions, the whole

blood drug concentration reaches a peak of about 0.9–1.0 mcg ml^{-1} for every 100 mg injected for lidocaine and mepivacaine, slightly less for prilocaine, and approximately half as much for bupivacaine. The figure for ropivacaine appears to be similar to that for bupivacaine (Katz et al. 1990).

Values of C_{max} and t_{max} for the isomers of mepivacaine and bupivacaine after epidural administration of the racemates are shown in Table 7.1. The enantiomeric differences reflect differences in systemic disposition rather than absorption, with sequestration in epidural fat of the more lipid-soluble bupivacaine having a rate-limiting effect on its systemic uptake and accounting for its much longer half-life. This has been confirmed by direct measurement of residual epidural fat drug concentrations in sheep (Mather & Tucker 2009), and by estimation of the time-course of systemic absorption from the epidural space in humans using the mathematical technique of deconvolution analysis (Burm et al. 1987, Tucker & Mather 1979). The latter calculations show that systemic drug uptake after epidural injection is a biphasic process, the contribution of the initial rapid phase being greater for short-acting agents than for long-acting ones. In the case of ropivacaine, a correlation has been noted between the duration of sensory block and the slower absorption half-life (Emanuelsson et al. 1997).

Differences in the absorption rates of the various agents after epidural injection have implications for their accumulation during repeated or continuous administration. Whereas systemic accumulation is most marked with the short-acting amides, extensive local accumulation is predicted for the longer-acting compounds despite longer dosage intervals (Inoue et al. 1985, Tucker & Mather 1975, Tucker et al. 1977). The slow absorption phase will determine the terminal plasma half-life and hence the rate of systemic accumulation.

The relatively low (in comparison to its toxic threshold) plasma concentrations of prilocaine after brachial plexus block (Figure 7.2) and intravenous regional anaesthesia (IVRA) support the claim that this compound should be the agent of choice for such single-dose procedures (Wildsmith et al. 1977). In this case, however, high systemic clearance, rather than slow absorption, is mainly responsible for the relatively low plasma drug concentrations.

Although the rate of systemic absorption of local anaesthetics is controlled largely by the extent of local binding, their *intrinsic vasoactive properties* may also modulate local perfusion and hence

Table 7.1 Mean pharmacokinetic parameters describing plasma concentration–time profiles of the R and S isomers of mepivacaine (460 mg) and bupivacaine (114 mg) after epidural injection of the racemates (Groen et al. 1998).

	Mepivacaine			Bupivacaine		
	R(−)	S(+)	R/S	R(+)	S(−)	R/S
C_{max} (ng ml^{-1})	1350	1740	0.77*	389	449	0.87*
Cu_{max} (ng ml^{-1})	485	460	1.00	20	15	1.36*
T_{max} (min)	18	18	1.00	8	8	1.00
$t_{1/2,z}$ (h)	2.0	2.2	0.96	7.3	6.9	1.05

C_{max} = maximum plasma drug concentration; Cu_{max} = maximum unbound plasma drug concentration; T_{max} = time to C_{max}; $t_{1/2,z}$ = terminal elimination half-life; R/S ratio of two isomers; * indicates statistically significant difference from unity.

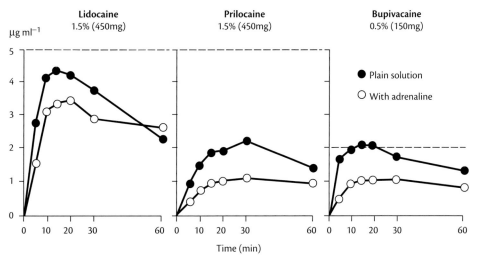

Figure 7.2 Mean plasma concentrations of amide-type local anaesthetics after interscalene brachial plexus block. Thirty millilitres of agent, with or without adrenaline, were injected. The broken lines indicate the putative thresholds for the onset of signs of toxicity. (Reproduced from J.A.W. Wildsmith et al., 'Plasma concentrations of local anaesthetics after interscalene brachial plexus block', *British Journal of Anaesthesia*, 1977, 49, 5, pp. 461–6 by permission of Oxford University Press and the *British Journal of Anaesthesia*.)

uptake. Thus, the greater vasoconstrictor potency of the S-isomers of amide agents may explain why they are longer acting than their 'R' equivalents after subcutaneous injection, despite lower intrinsic nerve blocking potency (Aps & Reynolds 1978).

Site of injection

Vascularity, and the presence of tissue and fat which can bind local anaesthetic, are primary influences on the rate of uptake from specific sites of injection. In general, and independent of the agent used, absorption rate decreases in the order: intercostal block > caudal block > epidural block > brachial plexus block > sciatic and femoral nerve block (Mather & Tucker 2009). Variations in anatomical approach or site of injection within particular block techniques are not associated with significant differences in local anaesthetic absorption rate (Maclean et al. 1988, Vester-Andersen et al. 1981, Yokoyama et al. 2001).

The greatest risk of producing excessive plasma drug concentrations is associated with intercostal nerve block, especially when supplementary bolus injections are superimposed on a continuous infusion (Safran et al. 1990), and with interpleural block, where large doses are applied to a relatively large surface area permitting rapid absorption (Kastrissios et al. 1991, van Kleef et al. 1990).

A pharmacokinetic analysis of plasma lidocaine concentrations after cuff-release during IVRA indicated that only about 20–30% of the dose is released immediately into the general circulation. About 50% still remains in the arm after 30 minutes, and longer application of the cuff further delays washout of drug from the arm (Tucker & Boas 1971).

Deconvolution analysis has shown significant differences in the pattern of systemic drug absorption after subarachnoid and epidural injection, and confirms that there is a slower net absorption of bupivacaine compared to lidocaine (Burm et al. 1987, 1988). Slower initial uptake from the subarachnoid space may reflect delay imposed by dural diffusion. The similarity of the slower phases of uptake after subarachnoid injection of bupivacaine (and the overall monoexponential uptake of subarachnoid lidocaine) to the corresponding slow phases of uptake after epidural bupivacaine suggests a common rate-limiting removal from epidural fat.

By far the largest doses of local anaesthetics are administered by subcutaneous infiltration as a component of the anaesthetic technique for liposuction. Klein (1990) considers that 35 mg kg^{-1} is a conservative estimate of the safe maximum dose of lidocaine, based on the observation that peak plasma drug concentrations are well below the toxic threshold 10–15 hours after injection. He emphasizes the importance of using a dilute solution with added adrenaline, and injecting slowly over 45 minutes. Injection of larger doses over less than 5 minutes results in dangerously rapid drug absorption. Nordstrom & Stange (2005) caution that at a dose of 35 mg kg^{-1} there is still a risk of subjective symptoms in association with peak concentrations of lidocaine that may develop after the patient is discharged. About 30% of the injected dose of lidocaine is removed with the subcutaneous fat (Klein 1990).

Adrenaline

The degree to which adrenaline decreases the systemic absorption rate of local anaesthetic is a complex function of the type, dose and concentration of local anaesthetic, and of the characteristics of the injection site (Mather & Tucker 2009). Although peak plasma concentrations of local anaesthetics are lowered by adrenaline after most types of block, it does not always prolong the time to peak (Mather & Tucker 2009). In general, its greatest effects are seen after intercostal block, and with short-acting rather than long-acting agents. This suggests that the greater local binding of the latter drugs has more influence on their duration of action than an added vasoconstrictor. In addition, the inherent vasoactivity of the local anaesthetic may modulate the effects of adrenaline. For example, its addition to ropivacaine not only has no effect on plasma concentrations after brachial plexus injection, but results in a tendency towards a shorter duration of nerve block (Hickey et al. 1990). Thus ropivacaine may actually be exerting an antagonistic, 'anti-adrenaline' effect.

Physical and pathophysiological factors

After nerve block, plasma concentrations of local anaesthetics are rather poorly correlated with body weight and height (Moore et al. 1976a,b, Pihlajamäki 1991, Scott et al. 1972, Tucker et al. 1977).

Increasing age (22–81 years) has been associated with an increase in the rate of the late phase of bupivacaine absorption after subarachnoid block, although no change was noted after epidural block (Veering et al. 1987, 1991, 1992). Simon and colleagues (2004) found both a smaller fraction absorbed and a shorter half-life for the early phase absorption of levobupivacaine after epidural injection in elderly compared to younger patients. Thus, these findings reinforce the view that an increased duration of analgesia in elderly patients has a pharmacodynamic rather than a pharmacokinetic basis. Limited data in children indicate a somewhat faster systemic absorption of local anaesthetics than in adults (Ecoffey et al. 1984, Eyres et al. 1978, 1983, Rothstein et al. 1986, Takasaki 1984). Pregnancy appears to have little influence on the plasma concentration–time profile of local anaesthetics after epidural injection (Pihlajamäki et al. 1990). Acute hypovolaemia slows lidocaine absorption after epidural injection in dogs (Morikawa et al. 1974). The hyperkinetic circulation associated with chronic renal failure does not appear to enhance the systemic uptake of local anaesthetic and does not, therefore, explain the decreased duration of brachial plexus block in these patients (Rice et al. 1991).

Systemic disposition

Systemic disposition refers to all processes occurring after absorption from the site of injection, and comprises distribution to other tissues (including placental transfer) and elimination, which is the combination of metabolic breakdown and excretion of unchanged drug.

Role of the lung

The lung is strategically placed to receive the entire dose of drug entering the systemic circulation. By acting as a 'capacitor', temporarily sequestering drug, it modulates the initial arterial drug concentration reaching the target organs of local anaesthetic toxicity, the brain and the heart (Jorfeldt et al. 1979, Lofström 1978, Tucker & Boas 1971). Lung uptake is dependent on binding within its tissues, and ion-trapping due to the pH gradient between plasma and the more acidic lung (Palazzo et al. 1991, Post & Eriksdotter-Behm 1982, Post et al. 1979). Thus, it may be altered by acid–base changes or by competition for uptake with other basic drugs (Rothstein et al. 1987). No stereoselectivity was observed in a study of the lung uptake of bupivacaine isomers in man (Sharrock et al. 1998), although uptake was greater for levobupivacaine than ropivacaine in rabbits (Ohmura et al. 2003).

Administration of local anaesthetics to patients with 'right-to-left' cardiac shunts (Bokesh et al. 1987), or inadvertent injection into the carotid or vertebral artery during attempted block of adjacent nerves, will by-pass this 'first-pass' lung uptake, and increase the probability of CNS toxicity.

Plasma binding

The extent of binding to plasma protein, principally to α_1-acid glycoprotein, is greater for the long-acting, more lipid-soluble agents (Table 7.2). Significant increases in plasma α_1-acid glycoprotein concentration, with increased drug binding, occur postoperatively and in association with many disease states, including cancer and arthritis (Jackson et al. 1982, Routledge et al. 1982). Conversely, low concentrations, with decreased drug binding, occur in neonates (Tucker et al. 1970).

Table 7.2 Mean plasma unbound fractions (fu) of amide-type local anaesthetics. (Data from Burm et al. 1994, 1997, Emanuelsson et al. 1995, Mather & Tucker 2009, van der Meer et al. 1999.)

Drug	Isomer	Fu
Prilocaine	R(−)	0.70
	S(+)	0.73
Mepivacaine	R(−)	0.36
	S(+)	0.25
Lidocaine	Achiral	0.30
Ropivacaine	S(−)	0.06
Bupivacaine	R(+)	0.07
	S(−)	0.05

The implications of changes in plasma binding, either because of disease or drug interactions, are widely misunderstood (Tucker 1986, 1994). It is essential to appreciate the difference between a change in the *fraction* bound or unbound, and a change in unbound drug *concentration*. A change in the former is rarely accompanied by change in the latter, and it is the unbound concentration which generally affects pharmacological activity. Thus, it is important to allow for plasma binding when interpreting measurements of total (bound plus free) drug concentrations. For example, there is marked accumulation of the total amount of local anaesthetic in plasma postoperatively, because the 'stress response' to surgery produces an increase in the concentrations of binding proteins, and therefore in the fraction of bound drug (Burm et al. 2000, Erichsen et al. 1996, Tucker & Mather 1975, Tucker 1986). However, unbound concentration, a better index of systemic effect, is relatively constant.

When systemic absorption is gradual, as after perineural injection, distribution of the drug is spread over time, and the large extravascular distribution space and extensive tissue binding ensure that only a small percentage remains in the blood at any time. In this situation, any change in plasma binding is buffered effectively by the high volume of distribution. Further, for drugs with relatively low hepatic extraction ratios, like bupivacaine and ropivacaine, any transient change in free drug concentration will be compensated rapidly by an increase in net plasma clearance.

In theory, plasma binding could limit the first-pass uptake of local anaesthetic into the brain and myocardium after rapid, inadvertent intravenous injection, and could thereby modulate toxicity. However, it is probable that a toxic dose would initially produce plasma drug concentrations high enough to overwhelm the limited binding capacity of α_1-acid glycoprotein during the first-pass through these organs (Mather & Tucker 2009, Tucker 1994). Although it is important to distinguish events during first-pass through an organ from those occurring after several recirculations, in neither case should it be assumed that plasma binding modulates tissue drug uptake and 'protects' against toxicity.

Tissue distribution

After passage through the lungs, local anaesthetics are distributed preferentially to those organs with a high blood supply, including the brain, heart, and liver (Figure 7.3). Concentrations in muscle and fat equilibrate with those in the blood more slowly. The time to

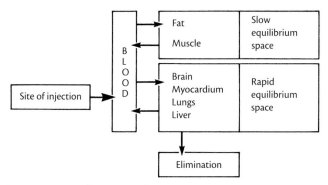

Figure 7.3 Pattern of distribution of local anaesthetics after absorption.

reach distribution equilibrium will be inversely proportional to tissue blood flow, and directly related to the capacity of the organ or tissue to take up the drug. In turn, the latter will depend on the volume of the organ and the affinity of drug for the tissue. Net tissue binding is reflected in the steady-state volume of distribution based on measurement of unbound drug in plasma (Vu_{ss}). The value of this parameter for amide-type local anaesthetics varies over a fivefold range, being greatest for the more lipid-soluble agents and exhibiting little or no stereoselectivity. Distribution volumes based on total plasma drug concentration (V_{ss}) vary less between agents, reflecting the balance between plasma and tissue binding (Table 7.3).

It is well established that the systemic toxicity of local anaesthetics is enhanced by acidosis and hypercapnia (Englesson 1974, Englesson & Grevsten 1974). In theory, increased brain and myocardial concentrations of free, un-ionized drug could be produced by haemodynamic changes and ion trapping. However, during metabolic acidosis of the type associated with convulsions there is no significant increase in the brain:blood partition coefficients of local anaesthetic, presumably because blood and tissue pH are lowered equally (Nancarrow et al. 1987, Simon et al. 1984). Nevertheless, data from rat studies suggest that treatment of convulsions by paralysis and artificial ventilation will actually tend to promote entry of local anaesthetic into the brain, because correction of the systemic acidosis promotes ion trapping of drug in the organ unless the cerebral acidosis is also corrected (Simon et al. 1984). Microdialysis studies in an awake, spontaneously breathing rat model indicate that adrenaline increases brain extracellular

lidocaine concentration in association with enhanced CNS toxicity (Ryota et al. 2006).

Excretion

Because local anaesthetics are relatively lipid-soluble compounds, extensive passive tubular re-absorption normally limits the renal excretion of unchanged drug to less than 1–6% of the dose (Tucker & Mather 1979). Although renal excretion of drug can be augmented by acidification of the urine to increase ionization, and thereby decrease re-absorption, the gain is insufficient to warrant using this procedure to treat systemic toxicity. Similarly, gastric lavage, to remove local anaesthetic 'ion-trapped' in the stomach contents, is not indicated because the percentage of dose recoverable is small.

Clearance

The amide linkage in the commonly used local anaesthetic agents is stable in blood, and most of their clearance is due to metabolism in the liver. Mean blood clearance values vary in the order: bupivacaine < ropivacaine < mepivacaine (reflecting the size of the N-methyl substituent in this homologous series) < lidocaine < prilocaine (Table 7.3) and show no relationship to anaesthetic potency or lipid solubility. Lidocaine clearance is partially dependent on liver blood flow, whereas that of bupivacaine and ropivacaine relates more to changes in intrinsic hepatic enzyme function (Tucker 1986). The relatively high clearance of prilocaine (in excess of liver blood flow) indicates that extrahepatic metabolism contributes significantly to the elimination of this agent. Significant differences in the clearance of R and S enantiomers have been observed (Table 7.3). For example, systemic exposure to unbound (active) concentrations of the intrinsically less toxic S(–)isomer of bupivacaine (levobupivacaine) is lower than that of the R-form.

Elimination half-life

The mean terminal elimination half-lives ($t_{1/2,z}$) of the amide local anaesthetics also show stereoselectivity, and vary between 1.5 and 3.6 hours, reflecting the balance between distribution and clearance characteristics (Table 7.3). Note that the figures obtained after bupivacaine is given intravenously are substantially less than after epidural injection (Table 7.1), reflecting rate-limiting absorption with the latter route of administration.

Table 7.3 Mean parameters describing the kinetics of amide-type local anaesthetic after intravenous injection in healthy individuals. (Data from Burm et al. 1994, 1997, Emanuelsson et al. 1995, Mather & Tucker 2009, van der Meer et al. 1999.)

	Prilocaine		Mepivacaine		Lidocaine	Ropivacaine	Bupivacaine	
	R(–)	S(+)	R(–)	S(+)	Achiral	S(–)	R(+)	S(–)
V_{ss} (l)	279	291	103	57*	73	54	84	54*
Vu_{ss} (l)	402	401	290	232*	253	900	1578	1498
CL (l min⁻¹)	2.6	1.9*	0.8	0.4*	1.2	0.5	0.4	0.3*
CLu (l min⁻¹)	3.5	2.7*	2.2	1.4*	3.7	7.9	6.6	8.7*
CL_B (l min⁻¹)	1.8	1.7*	0.9	0.4*	0.9	0.3	0.3	0.2*
$t_{1/2,z}$ (h)	1.5	2.1*	1.9	2.0*	1.6	1.9	3.6	2.6*

V_{ss} = steady-state volume of distribution; Vu_{ss} = steady-state unbound volume of distribution; CL = total drug plasma clearance; CLu = unbound drug clearance; CL_B = blood clearance; $t_{1/2,z}$ = terminal elimination half-life; all figures relate to measurements of drug in plasma except for CL_B = estimated clearance from whole blood based on plasma clearance and the blood/plasma drug concentration ratio; * indicates an R/S enantiomer ratio value significantly different from unity.

Accumulation

During continuous administration of a local anaesthetic its plasma concentration will increase over about four terminal half-lives until a steady-state concentration (C_{ss}), determined by the ratio of dosage rate and the systemic clearance, is reached. When assessing the safety of continuous dosage regimens, it is important to be sure that there is no time-dependent decrease in clearance that will result in systemic accumulation of drug greater than that predicted from single-dose data. Although there will be a progressive postoperative decrease in total clearance of local anaesthetic because of the increased protein level and binding, unbound clearance, as has been discussed, remains relatively stable. This certainly seems to be true for ropivacaine during postoperative epidural infusions lasting up to about 70 hours (Burm et al. 2000, Erichsen et al. 1996, Scott et al. 1997, Yokogama et al. 2007) (Figure 7.4). Beyond this time, both total and unbound ropivacaine concentrations appear to *decrease* in the face of a constant infusion, suggesting either recovery of drug metabolism after surgery and mobilization, or enzyme induction (Wiedemann et al. 2000).

Metabolites

Identification of the biotransformation products of the amide agents in urine indicates three main sites of metabolic attack: aromatic hydroxylation; *N*-de-alkylation; and amide hydrolysis (Figure 7.5; Table 7.4). With the exceptions of lidocaine and ropivacaine, net recoveries of the dose of drug actually administered are very low, leaving further metabolic products to be identified.

Various products have been measured in human plasma after the administration of different local anaesthetics: monoethylglycinexylidide (MEGX) and glycinexylidide (GX) from lidocaine; the 4-hydroxy products of lidocaine and bupivacaine; and pipecolylxylidide (PPX) from mepivacaine, ropivacaine, and bupivacaine. Significant accumulation of MEGX and PPX and, to a lesser extent of GX, occurs in the plasma during continuous epidural infusion of the relevant local anaesthetic. Such accumulation continues beyond the time when the parent drug concentration reaches a steady-state (Burm et al. 2000, Drayer et al. 1983, Fukuda et al. 2000, Kakiuchi et al. 1999, Kihara et al. 1999, Miyabe et al. 1998, Rosenberg et al. 1991). If systemic toxicity were to occur in patients on long-term dosage of local anaesthetics, it is likely that the presence of MEGX would contribute to CNS and cardiac effects (Blumer et al. 1973), whereas the unbound concentrations of PPX would probably be too low (Danielsson et al. 1997).

Studies using human liver microsomes and recombinant cytochromes P450 indicate that the *N*-de-ethylation of lidocaine to MEGX is mediated by the CYP1A2 isoform at low concentrations, and by CYP3A4 at higher concentrations. 3-hydroxylation,

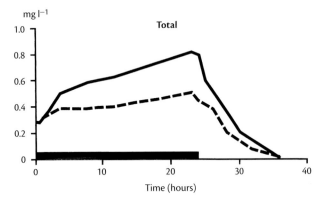

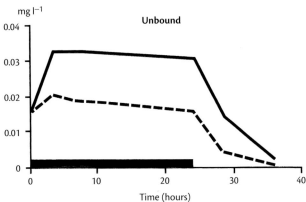

Figure 7.4 Mean total and unbound plasma concentrations of ropivacaine during 24-hour continuous epidural infusions for postoperative pain control in patients undergoing abdominal hysterectomy. Infusions were given at 10 mg h^{-1} (broken lines) and 20 mg h^{-1} (solid lines) in two groups of 10 patients after bolus epidural injections for surgical anaesthesia. (Reproduced with permission from Erichsen C-J, Sjövall J, Kehlet H et al., Pharmacokinetics and analgesic effect of ropivacaine during continuous epidural infusion for postoperative pain relief, *Anesthesiology*, 84, 4, pp. 834–42. Copyright Wolters Kluewer 1996.)

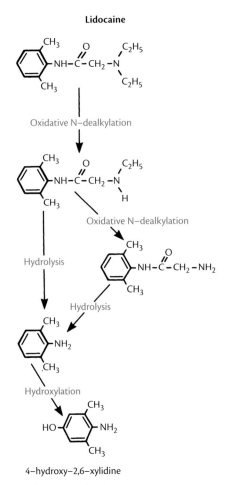

Figure 7.5 Metabolic pathways for lidocaine.

Table 7.4 Mean urinary recoveries (% dose) of amide-type local anaesthetics and their metabolites after intravenous or epidural administration to adults (ND = not determined). (Data from Burm et al. 2000, Halldin et al. 1996, Mather & Tucker 2009, Zhang et al. 1998.)

	Unchanged	Aromatic hydroxylation		N-dealkylation		Amide hydrolysis	
		3-OH	4-OH	Mono-	Di-	2,6-Xylidine	4-OH-Xylidine
Lidocaine	2	<1	<1	2	2	2	65
Mepivacaine	4	ND	ND	3	–	ND	ND
Ropivacaine	1	10–37	<1	2–10	–	ND	ND
Bupivacaine	0.3–3	2–4	2	5–20	–	~0	~0

which is a minor metabolic pathway for lidocaine and a major one for ropivacaine, is also mediated principally by CYP1A2. The *N*-de-alkylation of bupivacaine and ropivacaine to PPX is mediated mainly by CYP 3A4, as is formation of the 4-hydroxy and 2-hydroxymethyl products of ropivacaine (Bargetzi et al. 1989, Ekstrom & Gunnarsson 1996, Gantenbein et al. 2000, Imaoka et al. 1990, Wang et al. 1999, 2000).

Metabolism of prilocaine to *o*-toluidine, and subsequent *N*-hydroxylation of this product, is responsible for methaemoglobinaemia at doses above 600 mg (Hjelm & Holmdahl 1965). There is concern that this effect may become clinically significant in children less than 3 months of age receiving continuous applications of the cream containing prilocaine and lidocaine bases (Gajraj et al. 1994). Although methaemoglobinaemia has been reported after lidocaine (Deas 1956), its 2,6-xylidine metabolite is less potent in this respect than *o*-toluidine (McLean et al. 1969). The aromatic amine metabolites of lidocaine and prilocaine can generate DNA adducts in rats (Duan et al. 2008).

Effects of patient variables

Weight

The disposition kinetics of amide-type local anaesthetics do not appear to be related to body weight, surface area, or lean body mass in males with normal height:weight ratios (Tucker & Mather 1998). An increase in volume of distribution in obese patients of both sexes with minimal cardiac dysfunction may account for a 50% increase in the terminal elimination half-life of lidocaine (Abernethy & Greenblatt 1984a).

Age

In healthy people, increases in the elimination half-lives of lidocaine and bupivacaine with advancing age have been related to decreases in both clearance and distribution volume (Abernethy & Greenblatt 1984b, Cusack et al. 1980, Nation et al. 1977, Veering et al. 1987). Plasma concentration ratios of MEGX:lidocaine were found to be significantly lower in elderly patients during continuous epidural infusion of lidocaine (Fukuda et al. 2000).

Elimination half-lives of the amide-type local anaesthetics are prolonged two to three times in neonates, reflecting increased volume of distribution, decreased clearance, or both (Mather & Tucker 2009). In children over the age of 1 year, differences from adults are less marked, indicating similar or higher clearances and distribution volumes (Ecoffey et al. 1984, 1985, Finholt et al. 1986, Habre et al. 2000, Hansen et al. 2000, Lönnqvist et al. 2000, Mazoit et al. 1988). Urinary recoveries of the known metabolites of ropivacaine were found to be similar in children and adults (Halldin et al. 1996, Lönnqvist et al. 2000).

Sex

The terminal elimination half-life of lidocaine is reported to be up to 50% longer in women than men; this has been variously attributed to a difference in volume of distribution (Wing et al. 1984) or clearance (Abernethy & Greenblatt 1984b).

Race

White, oriental, and black subjects appear to exhibit similar disposition kinetics and plasma binding of lidocaine (Goldberg et al. 1982).

Posture

Although the clearance of lidocaine decreases on standing (Bennett et al. 1982), presumably because of reduced hepatic blood flow, prolonged recumbency appears to have no effect on kinetics (Kates et al. 1980).

Pregnancy

A trend to lower clearance of bupivacaine, accompanied by higher plasma concentrations of PPX, has been observed in healthy parturients (Pihlajamäki et al. 1990). The clearance of lidocaine is decreased, but its plasma binding is unchanged in pre-eclampsia (Bottorf et al. 1987, Ramanathan et al. 1986).

Disease

Studies of the kinetics of lidocaine after intravenous injection indicate that, on average, its clearance is halved in patients with heart failure and in those with severe cirrhosis of the liver. This is accompanied by a decrease in the volume of distribution in heart failure, and an increase in cirrhosis. As a result, the terminal elimination half-life of lidocaine is prolonged significantly in cirrhosis, but less so in heart failure (Thomson et al. 1973). Patients with chronic end-stage liver disease have, on average, 60% lower unbound plasma clearance of ropivacaine (Jokinen et al. 2007). Chronic hepatitis appears to be associated with a higher clearance of lidocaine than normal, and V_{ss} is also increased secondary to a decrease in plasma binding (Huet & LeLorier 1980, Huet et al. 1981).

The acute phase of viral hepatitis is accompanied by increases in lidocaine half-life and volume of distribution, with a trend to lower clearance, but no change in plasma binding (Williams et al. 1976). Patients undergoing hepatectomy have a marked decrease in lidocaine clearance during continuous epidural infusion (Yokoyama et al. 2001). The disposition kinetics of amide-type local anaesthetics are not influenced materially by mild to moderate renal disease (Thomson et al. 1973), although more polar metabolites tend to accumulate more than normally (Collinsworth et al. 1975). In patients with severe renal failure not receiving haemodialysis, the clearance of lidocaine was found to be half normal, reflecting downregulation of metabolizing enzymes and/or the accumulation of uraemic toxins (De Martin et al. 2006). Diabetes has been associated with a 60% lower total clearance of lidocaine, although some of this decrease may reflect higher plasma concentrations of α_1-acid glycoprotein, and hence increased plasma binding (Moises et al. 2008, Peeyush et al. 1992).

Drug interactions

Ideally, interpretation of pharmacokinetic data should be based on measurement of unbound drug concentration in plasma. Although displacement of local anaesthetics from plasma binding sites by other drugs alters the unbound fraction, theory indicates that this should have no pharmacological consequence. This is because it would be accompanied by only a transient increase in the concentration of unbound drug (Tucker 1994), at least for the relatively low extraction compounds (i.e. all except, to some extent, lidocaine).

Interactions of most concern will be those mediated through inhibition of metabolism of drugs with relatively low hepatic extraction (mepivacaine, ropivacaine, bupivacaine). No currently available agent has a high hepatic extraction susceptible to alteration in hepatic blood flow, but lidocaine is intermediate, and its clearance is dependent on both blood flow and enzyme activity. Mather & Tucker (2009) have summarized much of the data on kinetically-based drug interactions involving local anaesthetics. For example, halothane and propranolol both lower the clearance of lidocaine by about 40% through a combination of haemodynamic effects and enzyme inhibition.

Increasing knowledge of the specific isoforms of cytochrome P450 involved in local anaesthetic metabolism allows interactions with selective inhibitor drugs to be anticipated. For example, *in vitro* studies predicted that fluvoxamine, a potent inhibitor of CYP1A2, would decrease markedly the clearance of ropivacaine by blocking formation of its major 3-hydroxy metabolite, but that ketoconazole and erythromycin, selective inhibitors of CYP3A4, would have much less effect (Arlander et al. 1998, Jokinen et al. 2000, Olkkola et al. 2005). However, because these studies were carried out using small intravenous doses of ropivacaine, it is possible that at the higher and more prolonged systemic ropivacaine concentrations associated with regional anaesthesia, CYP1A2 might assume less importance with respect to net metabolism and drug interactions. Indeed, during continuous epidural infusion of ropivacaine the urinary excretion rate of its 3-hydroxy metabolite decreases while that of PPX increases, the latter being formed principally by CYP3A4 (Burm et al. 2000).

Placental transfer

The ratios of cord to maternal plasma concentrations of the amide drugs at delivery decrease in the order: prilocaine (1.0–1.1) > lidocaine ≈ mepivacaine (0.5–0.7) > ropivacaine, bupivacaine (0.2–0.4) (Datta et al. 1995, Tucker & Mather 1979), with no stereoselectivity detected for bupivacaine enantiomers (de Barros Duarte et al. 2007). These differences reflect, and can be predicted from, differential maternal and fetal plasma binding of drug secondary to relatively low fetal concentrations of α_1-acid glycoprotein, together with allowance for some ion trapping in the more acidic fetal plasma (Johnson et al. 1999, Kennedy et al. 1979, Tucker et al. 1970). As such, therefore, these ratios are not direct predictors of relative fetal toxicity, because the corresponding average ratios of unbound (active) drug across the placenta are, irrespective of the

drug, close to unity (other than at times when maternal concentrations are increasing or decreasing rapidly). This also indicates that passive distribution across the placenta is relatively rapid, irrespective of the lipid-solubility of the compounds (Johnson et al. 1999).

In theory, a high maternal to fetal plasma binding ratio should delay equilibration of drug in fetal tissues, despite rapid equilibrium across the placenta (Dawes 1973, Hamshaw-Thomas et al. 1984). However, the similar umbilical artery to umbilical vein concentration ratios observed with the various agents argue against large differences in their equilibration rates in the fetus, although this may be masked by shunting of blood in the placenta (Tucker et al. 1970). As a consequence of ion trapping, fetal acidosis increases both the cord:maternal ratio of unbound drug, and the rate of placental transfer of local anaesthetic (Biehl et al. 1978, Brown et al. 1976, Datta et al. 1981, Gaylard et al. 1990, Tucker et al. 1970).

Having entered the cord, drug is delivered directly to the fetal liver. Thus, significant first-pass metabolism in this organ may modulate fetal exposure to local anaesthetic. It may also have the effect of amplifying the transplacental gradient of drug. A significant net back-transfer of bupivacaine, but not of lidocaine, from fetus to mother was observed after short intravenous infusions of the agents into ewes (Kennedy et al. 1986, 1990). This might be explained by greater first-pass metabolism of lidocaine in fetal sheep liver, thereby maintaining the maternal to cord concentration gradient for longer. The extent of *in utero* metabolism of local anaesthetics in humans is unknown, but urinary metabolites have been measured in neonates after direct administration (Mather & Tucker 2009). Metabolites produced in the mother can pass across the placenta, and have been measured in fetal blood (Blankenbaker et al. 1975, Kuhnert et al. 1979, 1981). However, the toxicological significance of the presence of local anaesthetic metabolites in the fetus is unknown.

Toxicity and lipid resuscitation

Systemic toxicity from local anaesthetic overdose can occur from accidental intravascular injection, drug overdose, or rapid absorption from the administration site. Cardiovascular collapse caused by local anaesthetic overdose in humans is notoriously difficult to treat (Albright 1979, Long et al. 1989, Ruetsch et al. 2001). Guidelines endorsing lipid emulsion as therapy for local anaesthetic-induced cardiotoxicity are now prominently displayed anywhere regional anaesthesia is practised. There are conflicting reports in the literature regarding the efficacy of lipid emulsion in the treatment in the treatment of cardiac arrest caused by local anaesthetic toxicity. One hundred per cent survival was reported in rodent and canine models in which cardiac arrest was induced with a rapid bolus of intravenous bupivacaine and 100% mortality without lipid emulsion; no vasopressors were used in either group (Weinberg et al. 1998, 1999, 2003, 2008). These results contrast with findings in a swine model in which 100% of swine were resuscitated after treatment with chest compressions and vasopressors (Mayr et al. 2004, 2008). Several case reports suggest that lipid emulsion may be beneficial in the treatment of cardiac arrest associated with local anaesthetic toxicity (Litz et al. 2006, Ludot et al. 2008, Rosenblatt et al. 2006, Warren et al. 2008). Absolute scientific proof of the efficacy of lipid emulsion in reversing local anaesthetic-induced cardiac arrest in terms of prospective randomized controlled trials is as yet unavailable. The rapid transit of this therapy from bench to operating room has been in part driven by the absence of an alternative anti-dote to a feared complication of regional anaesthesia. Lipid emulsion appears to be effective in treating local anaesthetic cardiotoxicity secondary to bupivacaine, ropivacaine, and levobupivacaine (Foxall et al. 2007, Litz et al. 2008) and in reversing CNS toxicity (Litz et al. 2008, Spence et al. 2007).

The mechanism of action of lipid emulsions is not fully established. The 'lipid sink' has been forwarded as one potential explanation whereby the induction of an expanded plasma lipid phase sequesters hydrophobic drugs and accelerates their removal from the heart (Weinberg et al. 1998, 2003). The composition of the emulsion may be important as long-chain triglyceride emulsions (Intralipid) appear to be approximately 2.5 times more effective than a 50:50 medium chain/long chain emulsion (Medialipide) in binding bupivacaine, levobupivacaine, and ropivacaine (Mazoit et al. 2009). Pegylated liposomes have been shown to bind bupivacaine strongly in both buffer and in human serum and may represent another alternative for the treatment of bupivacaine toxicity (Howell et al. 2009). Alternative possibilities favour a metabolic mechanism with free fatty acids counteracting pharmacological inhibition to mitochondrial oxidative phosphorylation (Stehr et al. 2007) or by increasing intramyocyte calcium concentration (Huang et al. 1992). Infusion of free fatty acids is also known to modulate vascular reactivity. Infusion of lipid emulsion has been demonstrated to enhance α_1 adrenergic receptor-mediated pressor sensitivity (Haastrup et al. 1998, Stepmiakowski et al. 1995) and impair insulin-mediated vasodilation and nitric oxide production in humans.(Steinberg et al. 2000). Intralipid application has been shown to cause acute impairment of baroreceptor reflex sensitivity when administered to hypertensive patients (Gadegbeku et al. 2002). The role of lipid-induced vasoreactivity during cardiac arrest is unclear. All reported cases of successful resuscitation from local anaesthetic induced cardiac arrest have employed adrenaline, vasopressin, or a combination of both agents. Rapid infusion of lipid has been used to treat other forms of drug overdose in humans (bupropion, lamotrigine) and in animals (propranolol) (Sirianni et al. 2008, Weinberg et al. 2006). The role of additional agents used during cardiac arrest is unclear. Adrenaline (in a dose of over 10 mcg kg^{-1}) when co-administered with lipid emulsion in a rat model was associated with a poorer outcome (Hillier et al. 2009).

Key reference

Mather LE, Tucker GT (2009) Properties, absorption, and disposition of local anesthetic agents. In Cousins MJ, Carr DB, Horlocker TT, Bridenbaugh PO (Eds) *Neural blockade in clinical anesthesia and pain medicine*, 4th edn, pp. 48–95. Philadelphia, PA: Walters Kluwer/Lippincott Williams & Wilkins. [For a complete consideration of this topic the equivalent chapter in the 3rd edition of this text should be reviewed as well.]

References

Abernethy DR, Greenblatt DJ (1984a) Lidocaine disposition in obesity. *American Journal of Cardiology* 53: 1183–6.
Abernethy DR, Greenblatt DJ (1984b) Impairment of lidocaine clearance in elderly male subjects. *Journal of Cardiovascular Pharmacology* 5: 1093–6.
Aps C, Reynolds F (1978) An intradermal study of the local anaesthetic and vascular effects of the isomers of bupivacaine. *British Journal of Clinical Pharmacology* 6: 63–8.
Albright GA (1979) Cardiac arrest following regional anesthesia with etidocaine or bupivacaine. *Anesthesiology* 51: 285–7.

Araujo DR, Tsuneda SS, Ceredo CMS, et al. (2008) Development and pharmacological evaluation of ropivacaine-2 = hydroxypropyl-beta-cyclodextrin inclusion complex. *European Journal of Pharmaceutical Sciences* 33: 60–71.
Arlander E, Ekström G, Alm C, et al. (1998) Metabolism of ropivacaine in humans is mediated by CYP1A2 and to a minor extent by CYP3A4: an interaction study with fluvoxamine and ketoconazole as in vivo inhibitors. *Clinical Pharmacology and Therapeutics* 64: 484–91.
Bargetzi MJ, Aoyama T, Gonzalez FJ, et al. (1989) Lidocaine metabolism in human liver microsomes by cytochrome P. 450IIIA4. *Clinical Pharmacology and Therapeutics* 46: 521–7.
Bennett PN, Aarons LJ, Bending MR, et al. (1982) Pharmacokinetics of lidocaine and its deethylated metabolite: Dose and time dependency studies in man. *Journal of Pharmacokinetics and Biopharmacology* 10: 265–8.
Bernards CM, Ulma GA, Kopacz DJ (2000) The meningeal permeability of R- and S-bupivacaine are not different. *Anesthesiology* 93: 896–7.
Biehl D, Shnider SM, Levinson G, et al. (1978) Placental transfer of lidocaine: Effects of acidosis. *Anesthesiology* 48: 409–12.
Blankenbaker WL, Difazio CA, Berry FA (1975) Lidocaine and its metabolites in the newborn. *Anesthesiology* 42: 325–30.
Blumer J, Strong JM, Atkinson AJ (1973) The convulsant potency of lidocaine and its N-dealkylated metabolites. *Journal of Pharmacology and Experimental Therapeutics* 186: 31–6.
Bokesch PM, Castenada AR, Ziemer G, et al. (1987) The influence of right-to-left cardiac shunt on lidocaine pharmacokinetics. *Anesthesiology* 57: 739–74.
Boogaerts J, Lafont N, Luo H, Legros F (1993) Plasma concentrations of bupivacaine after brachial plexus administration of liposome-associated and plain solutions to rabbits. *Canadian Journal of Anesthesia* 12: 1201–4.
Bottorff MB, Pieper JA, Boucher BA, et al. (1987) Lidocaine protein binding in preeclampsia. *European Journal of Clinical Pharmacology* 31: 719–22.
Brown WU, Bell GC, Alper MH (1976) Acidosis, local anesthetics and the newborn. *Obstetrics and Gynecology* 48: 27–30.
Burm AGL, Vermeulen NPE, Van Kleef JW, et al. (1987) Pharmacokinetics of lidocaine and bupivacaine in surgical patients following epidural administration: Simultaneous investigation of absorption and disposition kinetics using stable isotopes. *Clinical Pharmacokinetics* 13: 191–203.
Burm AGL, Van Kleef JW, Vermeulen NPE, et al. (1988) Pharmacokinetics of lidocaine and bupivacaine following subarachnoid administration in surgical patients: Simultaneous investigation of absorption and disposition kinetics using stable isotopes. *Anesthesiology* 69: 584–92.
Burm AGL, Van der Meer AD, Van Kleef JW, et al. (1994) Pharmacokinetics of the enantiomers of bupivacaine following intravenous administration of the racemate. *British Journal of Clinical Pharmacology* 38: 125–9.
Burm AGL, Cohen IMC, Van Kleef JW, et al. (1997) Pharmacokinetics of the enantiomers of mepivacaine after intravenous administration of the racemate in volunteers. *Anesthesia & Analgesia* 84: 85–9.
Burm AGL, Stienstra R, Brouwer RP, et al. (2000) Epidural infusion of ropivacaine for postoperative analgesia after major orthopedic surgery. Pharmacokinetic evaluation. *Anesthesiology* 93: 395–430.
Cereda CMS, Brunetto GB, de Aranjo DR, de Paula E (2006) Liposomal formulations of prilocaine, lidocaine and mepivacaine prolong analgesic duration. *Canadian Journal of Anaesthesia* 53: 1092–7.
Clement R, Malinovsky J-M, Le Corre P, et al. (1999) Cerebrospinal fluid bioavailability and pharmacokinetics of bupivacaine and lidocaine after intrathecal and epidural administrations in rabbits using microdialysis. *Journal of Pharmacology and Experimental Therapeutics* 289: 1015–21.
Collinsworth KA, Strong JM, Atkinson AJ, et al. (1975) Pharmacokinetics and metabolism of lidocaine in patients with renal failure. *Clinical Pharmacology and Therapeutics* 18: 59–64.

Cusack B, Kelly JG, Lavan J, et al. (1980) Pharmacokinetics of lignocaine in the elderly. *British Journal of Clinical Pharmacology* 9: 293P.

Danielsson BRG, Danielsson MK, Lindström BE, et al. (1997) Toxicity of bupivacaine and ropivacaine in relation to free plasma concentrations in pregnant rats: A comparative study. *Pharmacology & Toxicology* 81: 90–6.

Datta S, Brown WU, Ostheimer GW, et al. (1981) Epidural anesthesia for Cesarean section in diabetic parturients: maternal and neonatal acid–base status and bupivacaine concentration. *Anesthesia & Analgesia* 60: 574–8.

Datta S, Camann W, Bader A, et al. (1995) Clinical effects and maternal and fetal plasma concentrations of epidural ropivacaine versus bupivacaine for Cesarean section. *Anesthesiology* 82: 1346–52.

Dawes GS. (1973) A theoretical analysis of fetal drug equilibrium. In Boreus L (Ed) *Fetal Pharmacology*, pp. 381–400. New York: Raven Press.

Deas TC (1956) Severe methemoglobinemia following dental extraction under lidocaine anesthesia. *Anesthesiology* 17: 204–8.

De Barros Duarte L, Moises ECD, Carvalho R, et al. (2007) Placental transfer of bupivacaine enantiomers in normal pregnant women receiving epidural anesthesia for cesarean section. *European Journal of Clinical Pharmacology* 63: 523–6.

De Martin S, Orlando R, Bertoli M, et al. (2006) Differential effect of chronic renal failure on the pharmacokinetics of lidocaine in patients receiving and not receiving hemodialysis. *Clinical Pharmacology and Therapeutics* 80: 597–606.

Drayer DE, Lorenzo B, Werns S, et al. (1983) Plasma levels, protein binding, and elimination data of lidocaine and active metabolites in cardiac patients of various ages. *Clinical Pharmacology and Therapeutics* 34: 14–22.

Duan J-D, Jeffrey AM, Williams GM (2008) Assessment of the medicines lidocaine, prilocaine and their metabolites, 2,6-dimethylaniline and 2-methylaniline for DNA adduct formation in rat tissues. *Drug Metabolism and Disposition* 36: 1470–5.

Dyhre H, Soderberg L, Bjorkman S, et al. (2006) Local anesthetics in lipid-depot formulations—Neurotoxicity in relation to duration of effect in a rat model. *Regional Anesthesia and Pain Medicine* 31: 401–8.

Ecoffey C, Desparmet J, Berdeaux A, et al. (1984) Pharmacokinetics of lignocaine in children following caudal anaesthesia. *British Journal of Anaesthesia* 56: 1399–402.

Ecoffey C, Desparmet J, Maury M, et al. (1985) Bupivacaine in children: pharmacokinetics following caudal anesthesia. *Anesthesiology* 63: 447–8.

Ekström G, Gunnarsson U-B (1996) Ropivacaine, a new amide-type local anesthetic agent, is metabolised by cytochromes P. 450 1A and 3A in human liver microsomes. *Drug Metabolism and Disposition* 24: 955–61.

Emanuelsson B-M, Dusanka Z, Nydahl P-A, et al. (1995) Pharmacokinetics of ropivacaine and bupivacaine during 21 hours of continuous epidural infusion in healthy male volunteers. *Anesthesia & Analgesia* 81: 1163–8.

Emanuelsson B-M, Persson J, Alm C, et al. (1997) Systemic absorption and block after epidural injection of ropivacaine in healthy volunteers. *Anesthesiology* 87: 1309–17.

Englesson S (1974) The influence of acid–base changes on central nervous system toxicity of local anaesthetic agents: I. An experimental study in cats. *Acta Anaesthesiologica Scandinavica* 18: 79–87.

Englesson S, Grevsten S (1974) The influence of acid–base changes on central nervous system toxicity of local anaesthetic agents: II. *Acta Anaesthesiologica Scandinavica* 18: 88–103.

Erichsen C-J, Sjövall J, Kehlet H, et al. (1996) Pharmacokinetics and analgesic effect of ropivacaine during continuous epidural infusion for postoperative pain relief. *Anesthesiology* 84: 834–42.

Eyres RL, Bishop W, Oppenheim RC, et al. (1983) Plasma bupivacaine concentrations in children during caudal epidural analgesia. *Anaesthesia and Intensive Care* 11: 20–2.

Eyres RL, Kidd J, Oppenheim RC, et al. (1978) Local anaesthetic plasma levels in children. *Anaesthesia and Intensive Care* 6: 243–7.

Finholt DA, Stirt JA, DiFazio CA, et al. (1986) Lidocaine pharmacokinetics in children. *Anesthesia & Analgesia* 65: 279–82.

Foxall G, McCahon R, Lamb J, et al. (2007) Levobupivacaine-induced seizures and cardiovascular collapse treated with Intralipid. *Anaesthesia* 62: 516–18.

Fukuda T, Kakiuchi Y, Miyabe M, et al. (2000) Plasma lidocaine, monoethylglycinexylidide, and glycinexylidide concentrations after epidural administration in geriatric patients. *Regional Anesthesia and Pain Medicine* 25: 268–73.

Gadegbeku C, Dhandayupani A, Sadler Z, Egan B (2002) Raising lipids acutely reduces baroreflex sensitivity. *American Journal of Hypertension* 15: 479–85.

Gajraj NM, Pennant JH, Watcha MF (1994) Eutectic mixture of local anesthetics (EMLA) cream. *Anesthesia & Analgesia* 78: 574–83.

Gantenbein M, Attolini L, Bruguerolle B, et al. (2000) Oxidative metabolism of bupivacaine into pipecolylxylidine in humans is mainly catalysed by CYP3A. *Drug Metabolism and Disposition* 28: 383–5.

Gaylard DG, Carson RJ, Reynolds F (1990) Effect of umbilical perfusate pH and controlled maternal hypotension on placental drug transfer in the rabbit. *Anesthesia & Analgesia* 71: 42–8.

Goldberg MJ, Spector R, Johnson GF (1982) Racial background and lidocaine pharmacokinetics. *Journal of Clinical Pharmacology* 22: 391–4.

Grant GJ, Bansinath M (2001) Liposomal delivery systems for local anesthetics. *Regional Anesthesia and Pain Medicine* 26: 61–3.

Groen K, Mantel M, Zeijlmans PW, et al. (1998) Pharmacokinetics of the enantiomers of bupivacaine and mepivacaine after administration of the racemates. *Anesthesia & Analgesia* 86: 361–6.

Haastrup A, Stepniakowski K, Goodfriend T, Egan B (1998) Intralipid enhances alpha1 adrenergic receptor mediated pressor sensitivity. *Hypertension* 32: 693–8.

Habre W, Bergesio R, Johnson C, et al. (2000) Pharmacokinetics of ropivacaine following caudal analgesia in children. *Paediatric Anaesthesia* 10: 143–7.

Halldin MM, Bredberg E, Angelin B, et al. (1996) Metabolism and excretion of ropivacaine in humans. *Drug Metabolism and Disposition* 24: 962–8.

Hamshaw-Thomas A, Rogerson N, Reynolds F (1984) Transfer of bupivacaine, lignocaine and pethidine across the rabbit placenta: Influence of maternal protein binding and fetal flow. *Placenta* 5: 61–70.

Hansen TG, Ilett KF, Lim SI, et al. (2000) Pharmacokinetics and clinical efficacy of long-term epidural ropivacaine infusion in children. *British Journal of Anaesthesia* 85: 347–53.

Hickey R, Blanchard J, Hoffman J, et al. (1990) Plasma concentrations of ropivacaine given with or without epinephrine for brachial plexus block. *Canadian Journal of Anaesthesia* 37: 878–82.

Hillier DB, Di Gregorio G, Ripper R, et al. (2009) Epinephrine impairs lipid resuscitation from bupivacaine overdose. A threshold effect. *Anesthesiology* 111: 498–505.

Hjelm M, Holmdahl MH (1965) Clinical chemistry of prilocaine and clinical evaluation of methaemoglobinaemia induced by this agent. *Acta Anaesthesiologica Scandinavica* 16: 161–70.

Howell BA, Chauhan A (2009) Bupivacaine binding to pegylated liposomes. *Anesthesia & Analgesia* 109: 678–82.

Huang JM, Xian H, Bacaner M (1992) Long-cahin fatty acids activate calcium channels in ventricular myocytes. *Proceedings of the National Academy of Sciences of the United States of America* 89: 6452–56.

Huet P-M, LeLorier J (1980) Effects of smoking and chronic hepatitis B on lidocaine and indocyanine green kinetics. *Clinical Pharmacology and Therapeutics* 28: 208–15.

Huet P-M, Arsene D, Richter D (1981) The volume of distribution of lidocaine in chronic hepatitis: relationship with serum alpha1-acid glycoprotein and serum protein binding. *Clinical Pharmacology and Therapeutics* 29: 252–8.

Imaoka S, Enomoto K, Oda Y, et al. (1990) Lidocaine metabolism by human cytochrome P-450s purified from hepatic microsomes: Comparison of those with rat hepatic cytochrome P-450s. *Journal of Pharmacology and Experimental Therapeutics* 255: 1385–91.

Inoue R, Suganuma T, Echizen H, et al. (1985) Plasma concentrations of lidocaine and its principal metabolites during intermittent epidural infusion. *Anesthesiology* 63: 304–10.

Jackson PR Tucker GT, Woods HF (1982) Altered plasma binding in cancer: Role of alpha1-acid glycoprotein and albumin. *Clinical Pharmacology and Therapeutics* 32: 295–302.

Johnson RF, Cahana A, Olenick M, et al. (1999) A comparison of the placental transfer of ropivacaine versus bupivacaine. *Anesthesia & Analgesia* 89: 703–8.

Jokinen MJ, Ahonen J, Neuvonen PJ, et al. (2000) The effect of erythromycin, fluvoxamine, and their combination on the pharmacokinetics of ropivacaine. *Anesthesia & Analgesia* 91: 1207–12.

Jokinen MJ, Neuvonen PJ, Lindgren L, et al. (2007) Pharmacokinetics of ropivacaine in patients with chronic end-stage liver disease. *Anesthesiology* 106: 43–55.

Jorfeldt L, Lewis DH, Lofström B, et al. (1979) Lung uptake of lidocaine in healthy volunteers. *Acta Anaesthesiologica Scandinavica* 23: 567–74

Kakiuchi Y, Kohda Y, Miyabe M, et al. (1999) Effect of plasma a1-acid glycoprotein concentration on the accumulation of lidocaine metabolites during continuous epidural anesthesia in infants and children. *International Journal of Clinical Pharmacology and Therapeutics* 37: 493–8.

Kastrissios H, Triggs EJ, Mogg GAG, et al. (1991) The disposition of bupivacaine following a 72 h interpleural infusion in cholecystectomy patients. *British Journal of Clinical Pharmacology* 32: 251–4.

Kates RE, Harapat SR, Keefe DLD, et al. (1980) Influence of prolonged recumbency on drug disposition. *Clinical Pharmacology and Therapeutics* 27: 624–8.

Katz JA, Bridenbaugh PO, Knarr DC, et al. (1990) Pharmacodynamics and pharmacokinetics of epidural ropivacaine in humans. *Anesthesia & Analgesia* 70: 16–21.

Kennedy RL, Erenberg A, Robilliard JE, et al. (1979) Effects of the changes in maternal-fetal pH on the transplacental equilibrium of bupivacaine. *Anesthesiology* 51: 50–4.

Kennedy RL, Miller RP, Bell JU, et al. (1986) Uptake and distribution of bupivacaine in fetal lambs. *Anesthesiology* 65: 247–53.

Kennedy RL, Bell JU, Miller RP, et al. (1990) Uptake and distribution of lidocaine in fetal lambs. *Anesthesiology* 72: 483–9.

Kihara S, Miyabe M, Kakiuchi Y, et al. (1999) Plasma concentrations of lidocaine and its principal metabolites during continuous epidural infusion of lidocaine with or without epinephrine. *Regional Anesthesia and Pain Medicine* 24: 529–33.

Klein JA (1990) Tumescent technique for regional anesthesia permits lidocaine doses of 35mg/kg for liposuction. *Journal of Dermatology and Surgical Oncology* 16: 248–63.

Knudsen K, Beckman-Suurküla SM, et al. (1997) Central nervous and cardiovascular effects of i.v. infusions of ropivacaine, bupivacaine and placebo in volunteers. *British Journal of Anaesthesia* 78: 507–14.

Kuhnert BR, Knapp DR, Kuhnert PM, et al. (1979) Maternal, fetal and neonatal metabolites of lidocaine. *Clinical Pharmacology and Therapeutics* 26: 213–20.

Kuhnert PM, Kuhnert BR, Stitts JM, et al. (1981) The use of selected ion monitoring technique to study the disposition of bupivacaine in mother, fetus, and neonate following epidural anesthesia for Cesarean section. *Anesthesiology* 55: 611–17.

Litz RJ, Popp M, Stehr SN, et al. (2006) Successful resuscitation of a patient with ropivacaine-induced asystole after axillary plexus block using lipid infusion. *Anesthesiology* 61: 800–1.

Litz RJ, Roessel T, Heller AR, et al. (2008) Reversal of central nervous system and cardiac toxicity after local anesthetic intoxication by lipid emulsion injection. *Anesthesia & Analgesia* 106: 1575–7.

Lofström B (1978) Tissue distribution of local anesthetics with special reference to the lung. *International Anesthesiology Clinics* 16: 53–8.

Long WB, Rosenblum S, Grady IP (1989) Successful resuscitation of bupivacaine-induced cardiac arrest using cardiopulmonary bypass. *Anesthesia & Analgesia* 69: 403–6.

Lönnqvist PA, Westrin P, Larsson BA, et al. (2000) Ropivacaine pharmacokinetics after caudal block in 1–8 year old children. *British Journal of Anaesthesia* 85: 506–11.

Ludot H, Tharin J-Y, Belouadah M, et al. (2008) Successful resuscitation after ropivacaine-induced ventricular arrhythmia following posterior lumbar plexus block in a child. *Anesthesia & Analgesia* 106: 1572–4.

Maclean D, Chambers WA, Tucker GT, Wildsmith JAW (1988) Plasma prilocaine concentrations after three techniques of brachial plexus blockade. *British Journal of Anaesthesia* 60: 136–9.

Mather LE, Tucker GT (2009) Properties, absorption, and disposition of local anesthetic agents. In Cousins MJ, Carr DB, Horlocker TT, Bridenbaugh PO (Eds) *Neural blockade in clinical anesthesia and pain medicine*, 4th edn, pp. 48–95. Philadelphia, PA: Walters Kluwer/ Lippincott Williams & Wilkins.

Mayr VD, Raedler C, Wenzel V, Lindner KH, Strohmenger HU (2004) A comparison of epinephrine and vasopressin in a porcine model of cardiac arrest after rapid intravenous injection of bupivacaine. *Anesthesia & Analgesia* 98: 1426–31.

Mayr VD, Mitterschiffthaler L, Neurauter A, et al. (2008) A comparison of the combination of epinephrine and vasopressin with lipid emulsion in a porcine model of asphyxia cardiac arrest after intravenous injection of bupivacaine. *Anesthesia & Analgesia* 106: 1566–71.

Mazoit J-X, Denson DD, Samii K (1988) Pharmacokinetics of bupivacaine following caudal anesthesia in infants. *Anesthesiology* 68: 387–9.

Mazoit J-X, Le Guen R, Beloeil H, et al. (2009) Binding of long-lasting local anesthetics to lipid emulsions. *Anesthesiology* 110: 380–6.

McLean S, Starmer GA, Thomas J (1969) Methaemoglobin formation by aromatic amines. *Journal of Pharmaceutics and Pharmacology* 21: 441–50.

Miyabe M, Kakiuchi Y, Kihara S, et al. (1998) The plasma concentration of lidocaine's principal metabolite increases during continuous epidural anesthesia in infants and children. *Anesthesia & Analgesia* 87: 1056–7.

Mizogami M, Tscuchiya H, Ueno T, et al. (2008) Stereospecific interaction of bupivacaine enantiomers with lipid membranes. *Regional Anesthesia and Pain Medicine* 33: 304–11.

Moises ECD, Duarte LB, Cavali RC, et al. (2008) Pharmacokinetics of lidocaine and its metabolite in peridural anesthesia administered to pregnant women with gestational diabetes mellitus. *European Journal of Clinical Pharmacology* 64: 1189–96.

Moore DC, Mather LE, Bridenbaugh PO, et al. (1976a) Arterial and venous plasma levels of bupivacaine following peripheral nerve blocks. *Anesthesia & Analgesia* 55: 763–8.

Moore DC, Mather LE, Bridenbaugh LD, et al. (1976b) Arterial and venous plasma levels of bupivacaine (Marcaine) following epidural and intercostals nerve blocks. *Anesthesiology* 4: 39–45.

Morikawa K-I, Bonica JJ, Tucker GT, et al. (1974) Effect of acute hypovolaemia on lignocaine absorption and cardiovascular response following epidural block in dogs. *British Journal of Anaesthesia* 46: 631–5.

Nancarrow C, Runciman WB, Mather LE, et al. (1987) The influence of acidosis on the distribution of lidocaine and bupivacaine into the myocardium and brain of the sheep. *Anesthesia & Analgesia* 66: 925–35.

Nation RL, Triggs EJ, Selig M (1977) Lignocaine kinetics in cardiac patients and aged subjects. *British Journal of Clinical Pharmacology* 4: 439–48.

Nordstrom H, Stange K (2005) Plasma lidocaine levels and risks after liposuction with tumescent anaesthesia. *Acta Anaesthesiologica Scandinavica* 49: 1487–90.

Ohmura S, Sugano S, Kawada M, Yamamoto K (2003) Pulmonary uptake of ropivacaine and levobupivacaine in rabbits. *Anesthesia & Analgesia* 97: 893–7.

Olkkola KT, Isohanni M, Hamunen K, et al. (2005) The effect of erythromycin and fluvoxamine on the pharmacokinetics of intravenous lidocaine. *Anesthesia & Analgesia* 100: 1352–6.

Olofsen E, Burm AGL, Simon MJG, et al. (2008) Population pharmacokinetic-pharmacodynamic modelling of epidural anesthesia. *Anesthesiology* 109: 664–74.

Padera, Belas E, Tse JY, et al. (2008) Local myotoxicity from sustained-release of bupivacaine from microparticles. *Anesthesiology* 108: 921–8.

Palazzo MGA, Kalso EA, Argiras E, et al. (1991) First-pass lung uptake of bupivacaine: effect of acidosis in an intact rabbit lung model. *British Journal of Anaesthesia* 67: 759–63.

Pedersen JL, Lilleso J, Hammer NA, et al. (2004) Bupivacaine in microcapsules prolongs analgesia after subcutaneous infiltration in humans: A dose-finding study. *Anesthesia & Analgesia* 99: 912–18.

Peeyush M, Ravishankar M, Adithan C, et al. (1992) Altered pharmacokinetics of lignocaine after epidural injection in Type II diabetics. *European Journal of Clinical Pharmacology* 43: 269–71.

Pihlajamaki KK (1991) Inverse correlation between the peak venous serum concentration of bupivacaine and the weight of the patient during interscalene brachial plexus block. *British Journal of Anaesthesia* 67: 621–2.

Pihlajamäki KK, Kanto J, Lindberg R, et al. (1990) Extradural administration of bupivacaine: pharmacokinetics and metabolism in pregnant and non-pregnant women. *British Journal of Anaesthesia* 64: 556–70.

Post C, Andersson RGG, Ryrfeldt A, et al. (1979) Physicochemical modification of lidocaine uptake in rat lung tissue. *Acta Pharmacologica et Toxicologica* 44: 103–9.

Post C, Eriksdotter-Behm K (1982) Dependence of lung uptake of lidocaine in vivo on blood pH. *Acta Pharmacologica et Toxicologica* 51: 136–40.

Ramanathan J, Bottorf M, Jeter JN, et al. (1986) The pharmacokinetics and maternal and neonatal effects of epidural lidocaine in preeclampsia. *Anesthesia & Analgesia* 65: 120–6.

Rice ASC, Pither CE, Tucker GT (1991) Plasma concentrations of bupivacaine after supraclavicular brachial plexus blockade in patients with chronic renal failure. *Anaesthesia* 46: 354–7.

Rose JS, Neal JM, Kopacz DJ (2005) Extended-duration analgesia: Update on microspheres and liposomes. *Regional Anesthesia and Pain Medicine* 30: 275–85.

Rosenberg PH, Pere P, Hekali R, Tuominen M (1991) Plasma concentrations of bupivacaine and two of its metabolites during continuous interscalene brachial plexus block. *British Journal of Anaesthesia* 66: 25–30.

Rosenblatt, MA, Abel M, Fischer GW, et al. (2006) Successful use of a 20% lipid emulsion to resuscitate a patient after a presumed bupivacaine related cardiac arrest. 105: 217–18.

Rothstein P, Arthur GR, Feldman H, et al. (1986) Bupivacaine for intercostal nerve blocks in children: blood concentrations and pharmacokinetics. *Anesthesia & Analgesia* 65: 625–32.

Rothstein P, Cole JS, Pitt BR (1987) Pulmonary extraction of (3H) bupivacaine: modification by dose, propranolol and interaction with (14C) 5-hydroxytryptamine. *Journal of Pharmacology and Experimental Therapeutics* 240: 410–14.

Routledge PA, Stargel WW, Barchowsky A, et al. (1982) Control of lidocaine therapy: new perspectives. *Therapeutic Drug Monitoring* 4: 265–70.

Safran D, Kuhlman G, Orhant EE, et al. (1990) Continuous intercostal blockade with lidocaine after thoracic surgery. Clinical and pharmacokinetic study. *Anesthesia & Analgesia* 70: 345–9.

Ruetsch YA, Boni T, Borgeat A (2001) From cocaine to ropivacaine: the history of local anesthetic drugs. *Current Topics in Medicinal Chemistry* 1: 175–82.

Ryota T, Yutaka O, Katsuaki T, et al. (2006) Epinephrine increases the extracellular lidocaine concentration in the brain: A possible mechanism for increased central nervous system toxicity. *Anesthesiology* 105: 984–9.

Schnider TW, Minto CF, Bruckert H, et al. (1996) Population pharmacodynamic modelling and covariance detection for central neural blockade. *Anesthesiology* 85: 502–12.

Scott DB, Jebson PJR, Braid DP, et al. (1972) Factors affecting plasma levels of lignocaine and prilocaine. *British Journal of Anaesthesia* 44: 1040–9

Scott DB, Lee A, Fagan D, et al. (1989) Acute toxicity of ropivacaine compared with that of bupivacaine. *Anesthesia & Analgesia* 69: 563–9.

Scott DA, Emanuelsson B-M, Mooney PH, et al. (1997) Pharmacokinetics and efficacy of long-term epidural ropivacaine infusion for postoperative analgesia. *Anesthesia & Analgesia* 85: 1322–30.

Sharrock NE, Mather LE, Go G, et al. (1998) Arterial and pulmonary arterial concentrations of the enantiomers of bupivacaine after epidural injection in elderly patients. *Anesthesia & Analgesia* 86: 812–17.

Simon MJG, Veering BT, Stienstra R, et al. (2004) Effect of age on the clinical profile and systemic absorption and disposition of levobupivacaine after epidural administration. *British Journal of Anaesthesia* 93: 512–20.

Simon RP, Benowitz NL, Culala S (1984) Motor paralysis increases brain uptake of lidocaine during status epilepticus. *Neurology* 34: 384–7.

Sirianni AJ, Osterhoudt KC, Calello DP, et al. (2008) Use of lipid emulsion in the resuscitation of a patient with prolonged cardiovascular collapse after overdose of bupropion and lamotrigine. *Annals of Emergency Medicine* 51: 412–15.

Spence AG (2007) Lipid reversal of central nervous system symptoms of bupivacaine toxicity. *Anesthesiology* 107: 516–17.

Stehr SN, Pexa A, Hannack S, et al. (2007) The effects of lipid infusion on myocardial function and bioenergetics in l-bupivacaine toxicity in the isolated rat heart. *Anesthesia & Analgesia* 104: 186–92.

Stepniakowski K, Goodfriend T, Egan B (1995) Fatty acids enhance vascular alpha-adrenergic sensitivity. *Hypertension* 25: 774–8.

Steinberg H, Paradisi G, Hook G, et al. (2000) Free fatty acid elevation impairs insulin- mediated vasodilation and nitric oxide production. *Diabetes* 49: 1231–8.

Takasaki M (1984) Blood concentrations of lidocaine, mepivacaine, and bupivacaine during caudal analgesia in children. *Acta Anaesthesiologica Scandinavica* 28: 211–14.

Thomson P, Melmon KL, Richardson JA, et al. (1973) Lidocaine pharmacokinetics in advanced heart failure, liver disease, and renal failure in humans. *Annals of Internal Medicine* 78: 499–508.

Tucker GT (1986) Pharmacokinetics of local anaesthetics. *British Journal of Anaesthesia* 58: 717–31.

Tucker GT (1994) Safety in 'numbers'. The role of pharmacokinetics in local anesthetic toxicity. *Regional Anesthesia* 19: 155–63.

Tucker GT, Boas RA (1971) Pharmacokinetic aspects of intravenous regional anesthesia. *Anesthesiology* 34: 538–49.

Tucker GT, Mather LE (1975) Pharmacokinetics of local anaesthetic agent. *British Journal of Anaesthesia* 47: 213–24.

Tucker GT, Mather LE (1979) Clinical pharmacokinetics of local anaesthetic agents. *Clinical Pharmacokinetics* 4: 241–78.

Tucker GT, Mather LE (1998) Properties, absorption, and disposition of local anesthetic agents. In Cousins MJ, Bridenbaugh PO (Eds) *Neural blockade in clinical anesthesia and management of pain*, 3rd edn, pp. 55–95. Philadelphia, PA: Lippincott-Raven.

Tucker GT, Boyes RN, Bridenbaugh PO, et al. (1970) Binding of anilide-type local anesthetics in human plasma. II: Implications in vivo with special reference to transplacental distribution. *Anesthesiology* 33: 304–14.

Tucker GT, Cooper S, Littlewood D, et al. (1977) Observed and predicted accumulation of local anaesthetic agents during continuous extradural analgesia. *British Journal of Anaesthesia* 49: 237–42.

Van der Meer AD, Burm AGL, Stienstra R, et al. (1999) Pharmacokinetics of prilocaine after intravenous administration in volunteers. *Anesthesiology* 90: 988–92.

Van Kleef JW, Burm AGL, Vletter AA (1990) Single dose interpleural versus intercostals blockade: nerve block characteristics and plasma concentration profiles after administration of 0.5% bupivacaine with epinephrine. *Anesthesia &Analgesia* 70: 484–8.

Veering BT, Burm AGL, Van Kleef JW, et al. (1987) Epidural anesthesia with bupivacaine: Effects of age on neural blockade and pharmacokinetics. *Anesthesia & Analgesia* 66: 589–93.

Veering BT, Burm AGL, Vletter AA, et al. (1991) The effect of age on systemic absorption and systemic disposition of bupivacaine after subarachnoid administration. *Anesthesiology* 74: 250–7.

Veering BT, Burm AGL, Vletter AA, et al. (1992) The effect of age on the systemic absorption, disposition and pharmacodynamics of bupivacaine after epidural administration. *Clinical Pharmacokinetics* 22: 75–84.

Vester-Andersen T, Christiansen C, Hansen A, et al. (1981) Interscalene brachial plexus block: Area of analgesia, complications and blood concentrations of local anesthetics. *Acta Anaesthesiologica Scandinavica* 25: 81–4.

Wang J-S, Backman JT, Wen X, et al. (1999) Fluvoxamine is a more potent inhibitor of lidocaine metabolism than ketoconazole and erythromycin in vitro. *Pharmacology & Toxicology* 85: 201–5.

Wang J-S, Backman JT, Taavitsainen P, et al. (2000) Involvement of CYP1A2 and CYP3A4 in lidocaine N-deethylation and 3-hydroxylation in humans. *Drug Metabolism and Disposition* 28: 959–65.

Warren JA, Thoma RB, Georgescu A, et al. (2008) Intravenous lipid infusion in the successful resuscitation of local anesthetic-induced cardiovascular collapse after supraclavicular brachial plexus block. *Anesthesia and Analgesis* 106: 1578–80.

Weinberg GL, Di Gregorio G, Ripper R, et al. (2008) Resuscitation with lipid versus epinephrine in a rat model of bupivacaine overdose. *Anesthesiology* 108: 907–13.

Weinberg GL, Hertz P (1999) Lipid emulsions in the treatment of systemic poisonimg. U.S. Patent 7261903 February 22, 1999.

Weidemann D, Mühlnickel B, Staroske E, Neumann W, Röse W (2000) Ropivacaine plasma concentrations during 120-hour epidural infusion. *British Journal of Anaesthesia* 85: 830–5.

Weinberg GL, VadeBoncouer T, Ramaraju GA, et al. (1998) Pretreatment of resuscitation with a lipid infusion shifts the dose-response to bupivacaine-induced asystole in rats. *Anesthesiology* 88: 1071–5.

Weinberg GL, Ripper R, Feinstein DL, et al. (2003) Lipid emulsion infusion rescues dogs from bupivacaine-induced cardiac toxicity. *Regional Anesthesia and Pain Medicine* 28: 198–202.

Weinberg GL, Ripper R, Murphy P, et al. (2006) Lipid infusion accelerates removal of bupivacaine and recovery from bupivacaine toxicity in the isolated heart. *Regional Anesthesia and Pain Medicine* 31: 296–303.

Wildsmith JAW, Tucker GT, Cooper S, et al. (1977) Plasma concentrations of local anaesthetics after interscalene brachial plexus block. *British Journal of Anaesthesia* 49: 461–6.

Williams R, Blaschke TF, Meffin PJ, et al. (1976) Influence of viral hepatitis on the disposition of two compounds with high hepatic clearance: Lidocaine and indocyanine green. *Clinical Pharmacology and Therapeutics* 20: 290–9.

Wing LMH, Miners JP, Birkett DJ, et al. (1984) Lidocaine disposition—sex differences and effects of cimetidine. *Clinical Pharmacology and Therapeutics* 35: 695–701.

Yokoyama M, Mizobuchi S, Nagano O, et al. (2001) The effect of epidural insertion site and surgical procedure on plasma lidocaine concentration. *Anesthesia & Analgesia* 92: 470–5.

Yokogama K, Shimomura S, Ishizaki J, et al. (2007) Involvement of alpha1-acid glycoprotein in inter-individual variation of disposition kinetics of ropivacaine following epidural infusion in off-pump coronary artery bypass grafting. *Journal of Pharmacy and Pharmacology* 59: 67–73.

Zhang AQ, Mitchell SC, Caldwell J (1998) The application of capillary gas chromatography selective ion mass spectroscopy for the separation, identification and quantification of phenolic metabolites of bupivacaine from human urine. *Journal of Pharmaceutical and Biomedical Analysis* 17: 1139–42.

CHAPTER 8

Drug toxicity and selection

Nigel Bedforth and Jonathan Hardman

The previous two chapters describe the pharmacodynamics and pharmacokinetics of local anaesthetic drugs, and this one uses that information as a basis for considering the clinical aspects of their pharmacology, particularly the prevention and treatment of systemic toxicity, and the principles of drug selection.

Systemic toxicity

Local anaesthetics stabilize all 'excitable' membranes so their effects are not confined to peripheral nerves, and increasing systemic concentrations affect the central nervous and cardiovascular systems. An appropriate dose delivered to the correct location is unlikely to produce concentrations sufficient to cause systemic effects, but rapid uptake, accidental overdosing, or predisposition to systemic effects may result in sudden and life-threatening side effects. However, most severe reactions result from accidental intravascular injection, although they may also follow prolonged or repeated administration during local anaesthetic administration for pain control.

Clinical features

As plasma concentrations of local anaesthetics increase, there is progressive depression of the central nervous and cardiovascular systems, neurological features predominating in most circumstances and virtually always preceding cardiovascular effects in the conscious subject. The early features are subjective, with patients noting tongue and circumoral numbness, light-headedness, or tinnitus before becoming anxious with slurred speech and skeletal muscle twitching. Drowsiness indicates the onset of severe systemic toxicity which may result in loss of consciousness, convulsions, and apnoea. Without immediate resuscitation, hypoxaemia and acidaemia will develop rapidly, with the risk of organ injury.

The cardiovascular system has long been thought to be less sensitive to the effects of local anaesthetic drugs than the central nervous system. As a result, circulatory collapse during a toxic reaction was considered to be more likely a consequence of hypoxaemia and acidosis (which increases the proportion of ionized, active drug present intracellularly) than a primary cardiac effect. In fact, local anaesthetic drugs have a primary depressant action on the myocardium that is proportional to their local anaesthetic potency, but the effect is of little significance at the systemic concentrations produced during uneventful regional anaesthesia or the therapy of arrhythmias (Covino & Vassallo 1976).

Low concentrations of most of the drugs tend to produce slight vasoconstriction, but vasodilation occurs at higher concentrations. These peripheral and myocardial effects are modified by central actions which result in an increase in sympathetic nerve activity (Bonica 1971), so that the intravenous injection of 1–2 mg kg^{-1} of lidocaine will produce measurable increases in blood pressure, heart rate, and cardiac output. However, the epidural injection of about 5 mg kg^{-1} of plain lidocaine will cause the expected decrease in these parameters (even though the systemic concentrations of drug are similar) because the effects of sympathetic nerve block predominate.

This relatively simple view of systemic toxicity had to change when Albright (1979) reported seven cases of primary ventricular fibrillation after administration of one of the longer acting agents. It may seem illogical that a class of drugs used for their antiarrhythmic action could actually cause such problems, but that was rapidly recognized to be the case. Under certain circumstances, racemic bupivacaine, in particular, was identified as a potent cause of severe ventricular arrhythmias which are very difficult to treat (Davis & de Jong 1982, Mallampati et al. 1984). Most such cases seem to have been associated with the rapid, accidental intravenous injection of a relatively large dose of bupivacaine, but as little as 50 mg has been known to produce ventricular fibrillation (Whiteside & Wildsmith 2001). Thus rapid, intravenous injection (of even a relatively modest dose) has the potential to produce convulsions and, possibly, cardiorespiratory collapse without any of the more minor manifestations of systemic toxicity appearing first.

Factors affecting toxicity

Systemic toxicity is related to the concentration of local anaesthetic agent reaching the brain and the heart. Many factors are relevant (Chapter 7), but a few are of crucial clinical importance.

Dose

The dose of drug administered for any procedure is the product of the volume injected and the concentration of the solution. However, neither volume nor concentration has any direct effect on the systemic concentrations which result. It is the *mass* of drug injected which is important: 20 ml of 2% lidocaine will produce virtually the same systemic concentration as 40 ml of 1%.

It has become common for 'safe' maximum dose recommendations to be proposed, but neither unqualified absolute, nor weight-related, maximum doses have any great scientific validity in adults. For example, the epidural administration of a fixed dose of lidocaine to adult patients with a considerable range in weight produced no correlation with maximum plasma concentrations (Scott & Cousins 1980). Scott (1989) convincingly argued the case against adherence to such maximum doses because it can result in the use of an inadequate amount of drug for the procedure. The anaesthetist should be aware of all the factors which affect systemic concentrations of local anaesthetics and relate these to the particular block, patient, and drug under consideration. For example, local anaesthetic drug requirements may be less in the pregnant patient. Although dosage information for children is limited, weight-related doses seem to be sensible in this age group.

Rate of absorption

Clearly, the most rapid rate of entry of drug into the circulation will be produced by direct intravascular administration. Absorption of a correctly placed dose from the site of injection depends on the blood flow; the larger the local blood flow the more rapid will be the increase, and the greater will be the peak in systemic drug concentration. There is also much circumstantial evidence that the rate of rise in plasma concentration is as important as the absolute figure for the production of toxic symptoms (Scott 1975), although this is difficult to quantify.

Basal blood flow is quite different among the various sites of local anaesthetic administration, so that the rate of absorption is greatest after intercostal and interpleural administration, followed by epidural, brachial plexus, and lower limb blocks. It is slowest after subcutaneous infiltration, but high concentrations may follow topical application to the upper respiratory and gastrointestinal tracts. Absorption may be reduced by the addition of a vasoconstrictor to the injected solution, and this will, in many cases, allow the safe dose to be increased by 50–100%, but use of a vasoconstrictor is not always appropriate.

Intravenous regional anaesthesia (Bier's block) is a special case. Premature tourniquet release will result in the rapid entry of a large dose of local anaesthetic into the circulation. However, when the tourniquet has been applied for a minimum of 20 minutes, much of the drug will have diffused into, and be sequestrated within, the tissues of the limb. Tourniquet release then results in slower increases in systemic concentrations than after brachial plexus block.

The overall state of the circulation will also affect the systemic concentration achieved. For example, 400 mg of drug injected intravenously over 1 minute into a patient with a cardiac output of $4 \, l \, min^{-1}$ will result (theoretically) in a peak concentration of $100 \, mcg \, ml^{-1}$. The resultant peak systemic concentration will increase directly with rate of injection, and inversely with cardiac output.

Distribution and metabolism

Although the clinician can control the factors which affect the rate of entry of drug into the circulation, there is not the same ability to influence the distribution and metabolism of drug once it has been injected. Nevertheless, an understanding of these processes is essential to the decision-making which underpins safe clinical practice.

Distribution throughout the body buffers the rise in systemic concentration as drug is absorbed. Before blood containing local anaesthetic reaches the systemic circulation it will pass through the right side of the heart, where it will have minimal effect, and then through the lungs, which are capable of temporarily sequestering, and possibly metabolizing, large amounts of drug. The percentage taken up by the lungs decreases as the dose increases, so their buffering capacity will be less able to prevent a toxic reaction should an intravenous injection be made rapidly.

After passage through the lungs, local anaesthetics are distributed to the organs of the body in proportion to their 'share' of cardiac output (see Figure 7.3). The organs with a high blood supply (brain, heart, liver) also have a high affinity for the drugs, and tissue concentrations will increase rapidly. Fat and muscle, having low blood supplies, equilibrate slowly, but the high affinity of fat for local anaesthetic drugs means that large amounts may be absorbed there temporarily during continuous infusion, prior to release back to the circulation before metabolism.

Generally, the *ester* drugs are metabolized by plasma cholinesterase so rapidly that it is very difficult to measure their concentrations in blood after a regional block. Because of this rapid metabolism systemic toxicity is very rare. Theoretically, an abnormal cholinesterase level could result in an increased risk of toxicity (as occurs with suxamethonium), but enzyme activity must be reduced dramatically to impair significantly the rate of hydrolysis of the ester drugs. One important situation in which this might occur is when an ester drug is administered *after* an amide because the latter drugs all inhibit plasma cholinesterase (see Chapter 7).

The *amide* local anaesthetics are metabolized in the liver, although it is likely that prilocaine undergoes some extrahepatic metabolism as well. Hepatocellular damage has to be severe before the rate of breakdown is affected, but because some amides (not bupivacaine) have relatively high hepatic extraction ratios, their rate of metabolism is more dependent on hepatic blood flow. This has practical relevance to the use of lidocaine as an anti-arrhythmic agent in cardiogenic shock, where liver blood flow will be reduced.

Protein binding

Like many other drugs, local anaesthetics bind to plasma proteins, primarily α1-acid glycoprotein and albumin, to varying degrees. The former binds the drugs avidly, but has a limited capacity for them, whereas albumin has a low affinity, but a large capacity. As a result, the greater proportion of a low concentration is bound, but once the binding sites on α1-acid glycoprotein are occupied the proportion that is bound decreases as the concentration increases (Table 8.1). The measurement of protein binding was originally undertaken to provide a physicochemical property which related to duration of action in the laboratory assessment of new compounds. It is often assumed that drugs with greater affinity for protein are less toxic because only a small part of the total amount present in

Table 8.1 Approximate percentages of amide local anaesthetics that are protein-bound at two different serum concentrations.

Drug	Serum concentration (mcg ml^{-1})	
	1	50
Bupivacaine	95	60
Ropivacaine	94	63
Mepivacaine	75	30
Lidocaine	70	35
Prilocaine	40	30

plasma is 'available' to diffuse into the tissues and produce toxic effects, but the analysis in Chapter 7 clearly refutes this argument. Finally, it is noteworthy that figures for protein binding do not correlate with acute systemic toxicity; in fact just the opposite is the case: prilocaine, the least protein-bound of all the amides, is the least toxic, whereas bupivacaine, the most protein-bound, is also the most toxic.

Prevention

The main causes of toxicity are overdose and accidental intravascular injection. The risk of overdose is virtually eliminated by careful attention to dose limits appropriate to the specific drug and the site of injection so the clinician must take note of the recommendations made in the later chapters. Inadvertent intravascular injection is more difficult to avoid, and several safeguards are required, starting with selection of appropriate equipment and performing very careful aspiration tests. These should be gentle (so that the vessel wall does not occlude the tip of the needle) and repeated after each 3–5 ml is injected or if the needle (or catheter) is moved. One of the advantages claimed for ultrasound guidance in regional anaesthesia is that it may help prevent accidental intravascular injection (Marhofer et al. 2005): the risk of vessel puncture may be reduced and lack of tissue distension during injection will alert to misplacement.

However, a negative test should not be regarded as absolute proof of extravascular placement, and all injections should be made slowly with verbal contact maintained with the subject wherever possible. After the first 5-ml increment there should be a very distinct pause in injection to allow time for features such as tinnitus or circumoral numbness to appear. In the elderly, this pause should last at least a minute in case a slow circulation time delays the onset of symptoms.

Particular vigilance is required with injections near the head and neck, and with intravenous regional anaesthesia. In the former, accidental intra-arterial injection of a very small dose of local anaesthetic can cause convulsions and in the latter, faulty equipment or erroneous slipshod technique may result in the rapid entry into the circulation of large amounts of drug.

Test doses

It is obvious that the needle or catheter has punctured a vessel or the dura when blood or cerebrospinal fluid appears spontaneously or after aspiration. Unfortunately, intravenous, intra-arterial, and subarachnoid injections can occur despite negative aspiration, and 'test doses' are commonly employed to help reduce this risk. The test solution will depend upon the hazards to be excluded, but three criteria must be satisfied:

1. The test solution should be capable of producing a prompt, predictable, easily observable and relatively innocuous effect if intravenous, intra-arterial, or subarachnoid injection has occurred;

2. There should be no detectable effect if the injection is correctly placed; and

3. Sufficient time must be allowed for any indication of misplacement to become apparent.

Many authorities advocate use of adrenaline (2–3 ml of 1:200,000 solution) in test doses, a step increase in heart rate during the next 1–2 minutes indicating an intravascular injection. However, the heart rate may vary considerably while a block is being established (particularly during labour), and adrenaline is not the safest of

drugs. In addition, no test dose can guarantee against subsequent migration of the catheter or needle into a vein.

Test doses are most commonly used after insertion of an epidural catheter, and are considered further in Chapter 14. However, they should be employed whenever a relatively large dose of local anaesthetic is used, and particularly in blocks in the head or neck. Intravascular injection into branches of the carotid and vertebral arteries will produce almost instantaneous cerebral effects, and quite small doses can produce dangerous reactions. In this area, much smaller test volumes (0.5–1 ml) should be injected slowly with close observation of the patient.

Alternatives to bupivacaine

Recognition of the potential for racemic bupivacaine to produce primary cardiac dysrhythmias led to the introduction of the single isomer drugs, ropivacaine and levobupivacaine. These have a wider safety margin than bupivacaine so that their use does reduce the risk of severe (especially primary cardiac toxicity) if an adverse event occurs. However, they are still capable of producing exactly the same effects if the primary safeguards described above are ignored (McLeod et al. 2009). They are only saf-*er*, not absolutely 'safe'.

Treatment

The early signs and symptoms of toxicity require no specific management other than cessation of local anaesthetic administration provided that consciousness, respiration and circulation are maintained. Thereafter, the primary requirement is to ensure oxygenation (clear airway, oxygen administration, encouragement to breathe or ventilatory support, and constant monitoring), but cardiac dysrhythmia and convulsions require urgent treatment to reduce the risk of organ injury. Cardiovascular depression should be treated by elevation of the legs, intravenous fluids, and administration of a vasopressor (e.g. ephedrine 6 mg as required). Major collapse will require cardiopulmonary resuscitation.

Control of convulsions

If convulsions occur, the aim is to stop them as soon as possible to prevent acidosis exaggerating the reaction, and to treat any accompanying depression of the cardiovascular or respiratory systems before hypoxia ensues. Convulsions may be treated as follows:

Intravenous induction agents (except ketamine) will rapidly abort local anaesthetic-induced convulsions and have the advantages of being short acting, readily available, and familiar to all anaesthetists. However, they may cause respiratory and cardiovascular depression and should be used in small, incremental doses (e.g. propofol 10–20 mg).

Benzodiazepines such as diazepam or midazolam have been shown to prevent/abort local anaesthetic-induced seizures. Again, incremental dosage should be small (e.g. midazolam 1–2 mg). Convulsions induced by the more potent, longer-acting agents (e.g. bupivacaine) appear to be more resistant to benzodiazepine treatment than those induced by short-acting, less potent drugs (e.g. lidocaine) (de Jong & De Rosa 1981).

Managing severe toxicity

Most cases of systemic toxicity are short in duration, even if convulsions occur, and can be managed successfully using the relatively simple interventions described in earlier sections. If this is not the case the first requirement is to ensure that hypoxia is not prolonging or complicating the reaction so the efficacy of the measures applied to support respiration and circulation must be confirmed. Repeated doses of anticonvulsant may be needed, and cardiotoxicity should be treated using advanced life support protocols. Over the years a number of drugs have been tried for bupivacaine-induced dysrhythmias (Eyres 1995), but none has been particularly effective for what is a very challenging clinical situation. Thus, the introduction of lipid emulsion therapy was a very welcome development.

Lipid therapy

The practice of using lipid in the management of severe local anaesthetic toxicity was developed from a series of animal studies which showed that it counters the primary cardiotoxic action of bupivacaine (Weinberg et al. 1998, 2003, 2006). Two mechanisms have been postulated for this effect (McLeod et al. 2009). The *lipid sink* theory proposes that lipophilic local anaesthetic molecules partition into lipid 'globules' formed in the plasma after lipid administration so that tissue concentrations decrease. The *metabolic* theory is derived from the observation that bupivacaine blocks the uptake of fatty acids into mitochondria, a process necessary for oxidative metabolism in the heart (Weinberg et al. 2000). Lipid infusion releases free fatty acids and their increased concentrations may, by a mass action effect, overcome the inhibitory effect of bupivacaine to restore oxidative metabolism.

A series of case reports of lipid treatment in humans developing severe local anaesthetic toxicity has suggested that it is an effective addition to the range of treatment options (Foxall et al. 2007, Litz et al. 2006, Rosenblatt et al. 2006) However, a number of caveats must be raised: it is an unlicensed indication for lipid emulsion and, although there are few complications related to acute infusion, allergic reactions are possible (Brull 2008). Thus it would seem wise to reserve its use for situations where all conventional treatment (as described earlier) has been commenced, but is not producing rapid resolution of the patient's condition. The Association of Anaesthetists of Great Britain & Ireland (2010) has published guidelines on the administration of 20% lipid emulsion in the management of severe local anaesthetic cardiotoxicity *after* institution of standard resuscitation measures (see 'On-line resources'). In spite of this development, local anaesthetic toxicity remains a frighteningly difficult complication to treat, and many of the case reports which support the use of lipid therapy *also* describe failure to follow the basic rules of safe local anaesthetic use. As ever, prevention is better than cure.

Aftercare

After successful treatment of a toxic reaction both patient and anaesthetist will need a little time for 'recovery', and an explanation should be given to all present. Trainees should involve a consultant colleague in subsequent decision-making, the starting point for this being an assessment of what extent of block has developed. If this is significant it is reasonable to assume that only a portion of the solution was misplaced, and that surgery may proceed, perhaps with more supplementation than was intended. However, if there is little or no block it is likely that most, if not all, of the injection was intravascular, and a difficult decision has to be made: repeat the block, choose another technique, or postpone the operation. The choice will depend on the urgency of surgery, the patient's ongoing condition, and the experience of the anaesthetist.

Other adverse drug reactions

Allergy

Allergy to the 'ester' local anaesthetics is relatively common, particularly with procaine, because p-aminobenzoic acid is produced when it is hydrolysed. Most reactions are dermal in personnel handling the drugs, but fatal anaphylaxis has been recorded in patients. True allergy to 'amide' drugs (rather than to a preservative in the solution) is very rare, although it has been reported (Brown et al. 1981). However, it is not uncommon to meet a patient who claims to be allergic to such drugs, or who has been so-diagnosed by a medical or dental attendant. Such patients merit close investigation because the diagnosis is usually wrong and can cause unnecessary difficulties in providing anaesthesia or analgesia. It also leaves the patient at risk of an even more major reaction on subsequent exposure if the original reaction was allergic in nature, but attributed to the wrong precipitant. Very often the history will identify the correct nature of the problem, but considerable investigation of past medical and dental treatments may be necessary. A proportion of patients will need to undergo challenge testing, usually where the history is equivocal or the events described are somewhat bizarre, the latter often an indicator of a patient's attempt at needle or dentist 'avoidance'. Challenge testing, although considered inappropriate with most drugs, is useful with local anaesthetics to demonstrate to the patient that they can be administered safely. However, the testing must be performed in a structured manner with all resuscitation facilities to hand (Wildsmith et al. 1998).

Anaphylaxis occurring during regional anaesthesia should be managed by reference to standard guidelines (Association of Anaesthetists of Great Britain and Ireland 2009).

Methaemoglobinaemia

One of the metabolites of prilocaine (see Chapter 7) can reduce haemoglobin, and 600 mg of prilocaine will produce a methaemoglobin concentration of 5.3% of circulating haemoglobin (Hjelm & Holmdahl 1965). This dose is greater than that usually used in clinical practice, but will lead to cyanosis which is just detectable clinically. In spite of this drawback, prilocaine remains the safest of the amide local anaesthetics and the cyanosis (which is not indicative of hypoxaemia) is of little significance in the healthy individual. Methaemoglobinaemia can be reversed within 30 minutes by the intravenous administration of methylene blue. A dose of $1–2$ mg kg^{-1} is often suggested, but significantly less is usually needed so it would be reasonable to titrate the dose. Clinically undetectable and insignificant concentrations of methaemoglobin can misleadingly reduce pulse oximetry readings.

Other systemic side effects

Drug interactions

Interactions with other drugs, particularly of a pharmacokinetic nature (see Chapter 7), are possible, but rarely give rise to clinical problems. All local anaesthetics have a weak neuromuscular blocking action and, in theory at least, might potentiate the definitive drugs with that action or cause problems in myasthenic patients, but there is no clear evidence that this happens. Therapy with anticholinesterases for myasthenia, or the concomitant administration of other drugs hydrolysed by plasma cholinesterase, could slow the metabolism of ester drugs. The amide local anaesthetics are potent inhibitors of plasma cholinesterase (Zsigmond et al. 1978) and the administration of an ester to a patient who has recently received an amide might have unexpectedly toxic effects.

The benzodiazepines can mask the early signs of systemic toxicity and may be used deliberately for that effect. Large doses given as premedication may even prevent convulsions, but cardiorespiratory collapse could then be the first sign of a toxic reaction. The dose of any anticonvulsant used to treat toxicity must be adjusted with care since it may exacerbate cardiorespiratory depression. Finally, the depressant action of drugs used in the treatment of cardiovascular disease might combine with the systemic effects of a local anaesthetic to precipitate cardiac failure.

Tissue toxicity

The local anaesthetic drugs in clinical use rarely produce nerve damage. Any neuropathy developing after surgery is more likely to be due to other factors such as faulty patient positioning or trauma from the needle, the catheter, or the operative procedure itself (Aitkenhead 1994). However, some years ago there were several reports in the American literature of neurological damage after the use of chloroprocaine. It would seem that this was caused by sodium bisulphite added to the solution as an antioxidant (Covino 1984). In the epidural space, the nerve sheath probably protected the nerve from the effects of this preservative, but when accidental intrathecal injection occurred (a feature common to most of the reported cases) the bisulphite had free access to the nerve tissue. This emphasizes the particular care which must be taken with intrathecal injection. Subsequently, renewed interest in continuous spinal anaesthesia was checked by the publication of several reports of cauda equina syndrome (Rigler et al. 1991). The common factor seems to have been the repeated injection of local anaesthetic (usually, but not always, lidocaine with glucose) in unsuccessful attempts to extend an initially restricted block. The solution would seem to have accumulated in the sacral section of the theca and exposed the unsheathed nerve roots to unusually high concentrations of drug. The proper response to the limited block would have been careful consideration of the position of the intrathecal catheter and the way in which this was influencing drug spread, not simply repeating a failed injection (Denny & Selander 1998).

More recently, concern about tissue toxicity of local anaesthetics has been associated again, but not uniformly, with the intrathecal injection of lidocaine. Reports of discomfort lasting 24–36 hours in the buttocks and thighs of patients who had received spinal anaesthesia, often as day cases in the lithotomy position, were labelled as 'transient radicular irritation' or 'transient neurological symptoms'. However, possibly neither term is appropriate as the actual cause may be overstretching of spinal ligaments by adoption of extremes of posture while the anaesthetic is effective (Selander 1999).

Antiplatelet activity

One side effect of local anaesthetic drugs may be looked upon as a benefit rather than a complication. Regional techniques can result in a reduction in the risk of the thromboembolic complications of surgery (see Chapter 3). One of the mechanisms explaining this is a direct pharmacological effect in decreasing both platelet aggregation and blood viscosity (Borg & Modig 1985, Henny et al. 1986). The relative importance of this, and the indirect effect of sympathetic block on lower limb blood flow, in reducing stasis has never been established.

Pharmacology of individual drugs

The available local anaesthetic drugs vary somewhat in their stability, potency, duration, and toxicity. Differences in these features relate to differences in physicochemical properties, and these in turn, to the underlying chemical structures (see Chapters 6 and 7).

Clinical factors affecting drug profile

Before making direct comparisons between the various local anaesthetic drugs, it is important to emphasize that several clinical factors affect rate of onset, potency, duration of action, and toxicity. Onset time will be decreased, and duration increased, by the use of a larger dose. Dose may be increased by increasing either volume or concentration, but given the same total dose, a large volume of a dilute solution will often produce a more extensive block than a small volume of a concentrated one. There are marked differences in onset time between the different types of block. Onset is almost immediate after infiltration and is progressively longer for spinal, peripheral nerve, epidural, and brachial plexus blocks. This order correlates with variations in diffusion barriers, both around and within the nerve trunks, at the different sites. In the cerebrospinal fluid the nerves are bare, but they acquire a sheath after piercing the dura mater. Further coverings are acquired as the nerves leave the intervertebral foramina, but these become progressively thinner as the nerves spread distally and become smaller. The dose of drug required for the different blocks and the likely duration of action also increases in much the same order as onset time.

Individual drug features

Because of the factors outlined earlier, comparisons between different agents should be made using only data collected for the same block. It is questionable whether there are any significant differences in onset time between agents if equipotent concentrations are used. However, there are real differences in potency, duration, and toxicity, and much of our understanding of the safe clinical use of local anaesthetics has come from studies of their pharmacokinetics as outlined in Chapter 7. The clinical features of the individual drugs are discussed in the following sections, but the definitive quantitative data on the more commonly used of these agents are to be found in Chapters 6 and 7.

The esters

Cocaine: because of its systemic toxicity, central nervous stimulant and addictive properties, and tendency to produce allergic reactions, cocaine has little if any place in modern anaesthesia. It is still used in ear, nose, and throat practice for its vasoconstrictor action, but is becoming very difficult to obtain legitimately at a reasonable price. In animals the main site of metabolism is thought to be the liver, but plasma esterases may be more important in man (Van Dyke et al. 1976).

Benzocaine: this ester does not contain the amine group common to all the other clinically useful agents. As a result it does not ionize and this has implications for our understanding of how local anaesthetic drugs act (see Chapter 6). Of more practical relevance, an inability to ionize means that benzocaine will not form water-soluble salts so it can only be applied topically, a use for which it is very effective. Benzocaine is hydrolysed very rapidly to p-aminobenzoic acid, and so it is of low toxicity, but may produce allergic reactions.

Procaine and chloroprocaine: the short shelf-life, brief duration of action, incidence of allergic reactions, and the introduction of better agents have all combined to limit the use of procaine. As its name suggests, chloroprocaine is structurally very similar. The simple addition of a chloride atom to the aromatic ring produces a drug which is hydrolysed even faster than procaine and is probably slightly more potent. Its metabolic product is 2-chloro-4-aminobenzoic acid which, from the lack of published reports, seems to be less likely to produce allergic reactions than p-aminobenzoic acid. The obvious advantages of this compound, which is used widely in the USA, were offset by reports of permanent neurological damage, probably due to the bisulphite included in the solution to prevent spontaneous hydrolysis (see 'Tissue toxicity' section). Chloroprocaine has become the subject of increased interest in the search for an agent with rapid offset for day-case spinal anaesthesia, but without lidocaine's disadvantage of producing transient neurologic symptoms (Casati et al. 2007).

Tetracaine: this is the most potent and longest acting of the ester drugs in clinical use. It is hydrolysed by plasma cholinesterase, but relatively slowly, so it is quite toxic. In small doses it can be used safely and is used either topically or for spinal anaesthesia.

The amides

Lidocaine: lidocaine is the standard agent against which all other local anaesthetics are compared. All the general features of the amides apply to it and it has no unusual properties. It has been used safely for all types of local anaesthesia and is also a standard antiarrhythmic agent. The use of lidocaine as a short acting agent for spinal anaesthesia has been limited by a higher incidence of transient neurologic symptoms (self-limiting slight to severe pain in the buttocks and legs lasting up to 2 days, discussed earlier) when compared to other agents (see Chapter 4).

Mepivacaine: although chemically somewhat different from lidocaine, mepivacaine is very similar clinically. It seems to have no particular advantage or disadvantage although it may be slightly less toxic.

Prilocaine: of all the amide drugs prilocaine has the lowest systemic toxicity. This is because it differs from lidocaine in several significant respects. It does not produce vasodilatation, is sequestered (or perhaps metabolized) by the lungs (Akerman et al. 1966a) in greater amounts, is distributed to the other tissues at a faster rate, and requires higher systemic concentrations to produce convulsions. As a result the safe dose of this agent is twice that of lidocaine. Because it is equipotent with lidocaine, and probably has a slightly longer duration of action, it is surprising that it is not more widely used.

Its lack of popularity is probably related to anxiety about producing methaemoglobinaemia, even though more than 600 mg are usually required to produce a noticeable effect (see 'Methaemoglobinaemia' section). This is in excess of the amount normally used for a single administration, and prilocaine is the agent of choice whenever the risk of systemic toxicity is high. However, *it should not be used during labour*, partly because 'top-up' injections may exceed the dose which will produce methaemoglobinaemia, but particularly because fetal haemoglobin is more sensitive to this transformation.

It would also seem wise to avoid using prilocaine in anaemic patients.

Bupivacaine: the introduction of bupivacaine was important because it is a long-acting agent and its acute toxicity is, relative to potency, much the same as lidocaine. Its duration makes it appropriate for single-shot blocks for more prolonged surgery, but more importantly, the risk of toxicity is less during catheter techniques because the intervals between injections are longer. The other advantage of bupivacaine for catheter techniques is that effective analgesia can be provided with less motor block than the agents previously available.

Unfortunately, bupivacaine was implicated in a series of very severe toxic reactions, some of which were fatal. In many of these instances the supervision of the patient was substandard, but evidence accumulated to suggest that the agent may occasionally produce cardiotoxicity before neurotoxicity, with primary ventricular fibrillation being described in both man and animals (see 'Clinical features' section, and Chapters 6 and 7). In some of the cases high concentrations were used for intravenous regional anaesthesia—a procedure for which this agent, in any concentration, is most unsuitable. Many of the other reactions were associated with the use of the higher concentration 0.75% solution and, should an accidental intravenous injection occur, this concentrated formulation allows the very rapid injection of a large dose into the circulation. Obviously, such serious reactions can be prevented if the drug is administered correctly, but concern about the problem led to a search for less cardiotoxic alternatives, and ropivacaine and levobupivacaine were the result.

Ropivacaine: chemically, this is intermediate in structure between mepivacaine and bupivacaine (Table 6.1), but unlike those drugs it is presented as a pure solution of a single 'S' isomer (see Chapter 6). In man, the pharmacokinetic properties of ropivacaine compare well with bupivacaine (Lee et al. 1989) and its cardiotoxicity is less (Scott et al. 1989). Early clinical studies suggested that it performs very similarly to bupivacaine (Reynolds 1991), but that it produces an even greater degree of 'separation' of motor and sensory block (Brockway et al. 1991). It is also more water soluble than bupivacaine so that higher concentrations can be made available for clinical use.

Subsequent clinical studies have confirmed the early promise (see McClure 1996 for a review). Continuous epidural infusions have been shown to produce less lower limb motor block than bupivacaine (Zaric et al. 1996), but to provide effective analgesia for up to 3 days after major surgery (Scott et al. 1999). A meta-analysis of obstetric epidural analgesia studies showed that the lower degree of motor block may translate into a reduced need for operative deliveries (Writer et al. 1998). Finally, the higher concentrations may provide more effective block of major nerve trunks, such as in the brachial plexus (Casati et al. 1999). However, the overall benefits of ropivacaine have been questioned on the grounds of both relative potency (Gautier et al. 1999, McDonald et al. 1999) and cost-effectiveness (D'Angelo 2000), although both claims have been refuted (Wildsmith 2000, 2001).

Levobupivacaine: this is the single 'S' isomer derivative of bupivacaine (see Chapter 6, and McLeod & Burke 2001 for review). Its clinical performance seems identical to that of bupivacaine, but it is less cardiotoxic in animals and man (Bardsley 1998, Morrison 2000). However, this benefit may not be achieved unless the consequences of changes in the regulations on labelling of new drugs are appreciated. As mentioned in Chapter 6, the older drugs (including ropivacaine) are presented in terms of the weight per unit volume of the hydrochloride salt, but for levobupivacaine it is base drug which is measured. This has a lower molecular weight so a solution of levobupivacaine '5 mg ml^{-1}' has 11% more drug in it than does bupivacaine '5 mg ml^{-1}'.

Articaine: this is a drug of limited use in the UK, being available only in a dental preparation. It is interesting chemically, the ring component of its structure being pentagonal, not hexagonal, and its side chain the same as prilocaine (see Table 6.1) with which it shares low systemic toxicity.

Additives

In addition to the active agent, local anaesthetic solutions often contain substances added to adjust factors such as pH, tonicity, and baricity. Solutions in multidose bottles, and those with adrenaline in single-use ampoules, will also contain a preservative, which can cause allergic reactions. Manufacturers usually recommend that solutions containing preservative should not be used for spinal and epidural injection because of the risk of nerve damage. Other additions may be made to the solution for pharmacological rather than pharmaceutical reasons.

Vasoconstrictors

Vasoconstrictors may reduce the toxicity, prolong the duration, and improve the quality of block resulting from the injection of a local anaesthetic, but they are not used universally. They are contraindicated for ring blocks and intravenous regional anaesthesia because they may produce tissue ischaemia, and the most commonly used agent, adrenaline, has its own systemic effects. It should be used cautiously, if at all, in patients with cardiac disease, concentrations greater than 1:200,000 should be avoided and the total dose should be limited, doses greater than 200 mcg having been shown to cause cardiovascular disturbances during brachial plexus block (Kennedy et al. 1966). Interactions with other sympathomimetic drugs, such as tricyclic antidepressants, may occur, especially when vasoconstrictors are used systemically to treat hypotension. Felypressin has less systemic effect, but it may cause coronary vasoconstriction and is usually only available for dental use.

There is also concern that vasoconstrictors increase the risk of neurological damage by producing nerve ischaemia. Their widespread use in the USA suggests that this is not a great concern, but many anaesthetists feel that they should be used only when there is no alternative method of reducing toxicity or prolonging duration. As with chloroprocaine, it might be that the preservative has been responsible for nerve damage, because most solutions of local anaesthetic marketed with adrenaline also contain the antioxidant sodium metabisulphite. The antioxidant can be avoided by adding pure adrenaline to the local anaesthetic just before use, but this needs to be done with great care to ensure that the correct concentration is produced.

Adrenaline overdose

If the described recommendations are not followed, a severe systemic reaction can follow, the treatment of which will depend upon the patient's cardiovascular state. Oxygen and sublingual glyceryl trinitrate should be administered if angina or severe hypertension develop, and β-adrenoceptor blocking agents may be needed to control tachycardia. However, these drugs should be avoided when hypertension is the presenting clinical sign, and a short-acting vasodilator (e.g. sodium nitroprusside) preferred, but given cautiously because the initial hypertension can be followed by a rapid decrease in blood pressure.

Other adjuvants

At various times solutions of local anaesthetics have been introduced containing substances which, it is claimed, may improve the block in some way. Some drugs have been prepared as the *carbonated* salt instead of the standard hydrochloride in an effort to speed the onset of block. Laboratory studies have consistently shown that this is effective due to a combination of direct axon depression by carbon dioxide, enhanced diffusion of the local anaesthetic and a decrease in intracellular pH favouring formation of the ionized form of the drug (Catchlove 1972). Clinical studies are less consistent in their results, but the evidence suggests that carbonated solutions produce some improvement in blocks of slower onset (McClure & Scott 1981).

The *alkalinization* of standard solutions of local anaesthetics by the addition of sodium bicarbonate has been employed to speed the onset of blocks. Theoretically an increase in the pH of the solution will increase the proportion of the drug in the non-ionized, membrane-permeant form and thus speed nerve penetration. The results of clinical studies have not been entirely consistent, and even where a positive effect has been demonstrated, doubt has been expressed about its clinical usefulness (Swann et al. 1991). There is always the risk that the pH change will cause the drug to precipitate before injection and the method has little to commend it.

A much older strategy for speeding onset is the addition of the tissue enzyme *hyaluronidase*. There is little objective evidence (Keeler et al. 1992) to support its use except in ophthalmology (Nicoll et al. 1986), where it continues to be popular.

Local anaesthetics have also been injected with *high-molecular-weight dextran* with the intention of prolonging their duration of action. Again the clinical results are inconclusive, but dextrans of very high molecular weight may be effective, especially in combination with adrenaline (Simpson et al. 1982).

A number of substances have been added to local anaesthetic preparations to try and improve their rate of penetration through intact skin. For many years these attempts were not very successful, but a significant development was the *eutectic mixture of local anaesthetics* (EMLA). This is an oil-in-water emulsion of equal amounts of the base forms of lidocaine and prilocaine. When crystals of these bases are mixed together at room temperature they assume a 'liquid' form, because this eutectic mixture has a lower melting point than either constituent. This allows the drugs to be prepared in a formulation suitable for topical application. The cream has to be applied to the skin for about an hour, but sufficient base does penetrate to allow relatively painless venepuncture and it is particularly useful in children. In some patients it may even allow the cutting of skin grafts. The topical preparation of tetracaine (Ametop) is similarly effective.

The addition of *opioids* to local anaesthetics for spinal and epidural use is now standard practice in both postoperative (Chapter 14) and obstetric (Chapter 21) pain control. Other substances with analgesic actions at spinal cord level, such α_2-adrenergic agonists (e.g. clonidine) and benzodiazepines (e.g. midazolam), have been used also. Great care must be taken when

Table 8.2 The clinical features of individual local anaesthetic drugs.

Drug	Potency[a]	Duration[a]	Toxicity	Main use in UK
The esters				
Cocaine	1	½	Very high	Nil
Benzocaine	NA	2	Low	Topical
Procaine	2	¾	Low	Not available
Chloroprocaine	1	¾	Low	Not available
Tetracaine	¼	2	High	Topical
The amides				
Lidocaine	1	1	Medium	Infiltration, nerve block, epidural
Mepivacaine	1	1	Medium	Not available
Prilocaine	1	1	Low	Infiltration, nerve block, IVRA[b]
Ropivacaine	¼	2–4	Medium	Infiltration, nerve block, epidural
Bupivacaine	¼	2–4	Medium	Extradural, spinal, nerve block
Levobupivacaine	¼	2–4	Medium	Extradural, spinal, nerve block
Articaine	I	1	Low	Dental preparation only

a = relative to lidocaine; b = intravenous regional anaesthesia.

making any such addition that the correct concentration is produced, and that the substance is safe for administration into the vertebral canal. None of these substances has a product licence for these applications, and there are few, if any, relevant safety data for many of them. Such additions should be made only when it is clear that there is benefit, and in line with agreed hospital policies.

Choice of local anaesthetic agent

One of the most important decisions to be made when performing a local anaesthetic technique is how much of which drug is to be injected. First, the solution has to be of adequate strength. For lidocaine (the relative potencies of the other agents are in Table 8.2) concentrations of 0.5% and less may not produce the density of block required for skin incision. Greater concentrations may be used to produce more profound blocks of faster onset and longer duration. The volume to be injected will depend on the particular technique and, once the required concentration and volume are known, an appropriate drug should be selected on the basis of the likely rate of absorption and expected duration of surgery at that site.

Some workers employ mixtures of drugs, usually in an attempt to overcome the somewhat slower onset of the longer-acting agents by adding a short-acting drug with a rapid onset. The evidence that this actually works is at best conflicting and it may be that pharmaceutical interactions between solutions are responsible for the failure of the technique to work (Covino 1986). In most situations it is simpler to insert a catheter and make sequential injections.

Further consideration of drug selection for particular blocks is given in the appropriate chapter of this book, but commercial factors may limit the availability of particular agents. However, it is often possible to arrange for a hospital pharmacy in Britain to import a supply of an otherwise unavailable drug from a country where it is on sale.

Key reference

McLeod GA, Butterworth J, Wildsmith JAW (2009) Clinical toxicity of local anaesthetic drugs. In Cousins MJ, Carr DB, Horlocker TT, Bridenbaugh PO (Eds) *Neural Blockade in Clinical Anesthesia and Pain Medicine*, 4th edn, pp. 114–32. Philadelphia, PA: Lippincott Williams & Wilkins.

On-line resources

http://www.aagbi.org/publications/guidelines/docs/la_toxicity_notes_2010.pdf AAGBI Safety Guideline: Management of Severe Local Anaesthetic Toxicity.
http://www.lipidrescue.org Lipid Rescue: Resuscitation for Cardiac Toxicity.

References

Aitkenhead AR (1994) The pattern of litigation against anaesthetists. *British Journal of Anaesthesia* 73: 10–21.
Akerman B, Astrom A, Ross S, Telc A (1966a) Studies on the absorption, distribution and metabolism of labelled prilocaine and lidocaine in some animal species. *Acta Pharmacologica et Toxicologica* 24: 389–403.
Akerman B, Peterson S A, Wistrand P (1966b) Methemoglobin forming metabolites of prilocaine. *Third International Pharmacological Congress* (Abstracts), p. 237. Sao Paolo, Brazil.
Albright GA (1979) Cardiac arrest following regional anesthesia with etidocaine or bupivacaine. *Anesthesiology* 51: 285–7.
Association of Anaesthetists of Great Britain and Ireland (2009) Suspected anaphylactic reactions associated with anaesthesia. *Anaesthesia* 64: 199–211.
Bardsley H, Gristwood R, Baker H, et al. (1998) A comparison of the cardiovascular effects of levobupivacaine and *rac*-bupivacaine following intravenous administration to healthy volunteers. *British Journal of Clinical Pharmacology* 46: 245–9.
Bonica JJ (1971) *Regional anesthesia: recent advances and current status*, pp. 69–70. Oxford: Blackwell.
Borg T, Modig J (1985) Potential antithrombotic effects of local anaesthetics due to their inhibition of platelet function. *Acta Anaesthesiologica Scandinavica* 29: 739–42.

Brockway MS, Bannister J, McClure JH, McKeown D, Wildsmith JAW (1991) Comparison of extradural ropivacaine and bupivacaine. *British Journal of Anaesthesia* 66: 31–7.

Brown DT, Beamish D, Wildsmith JAW (1981) Allergic reaction to an amide local anaesthetic. *British Journal of Anaesthesia* 53: 435–7.

Brull SJ (2008) Lipid emulsion for the treatment of local anesthetic toxicity: patient safety implications. *Anesthesia & Analgesia* 106: 1337–9.

Casati A, Fanelli G, Aldegheri G, et al. (1999) Interscalene brachial plexus anaesthesia with 0.5%, 0.75% or 1% ropivacaine: a double-blind comparison with 2% mepivacaine. *British Journal of Anaesthesia* 83: 872–5.

Casati A, Fanelli G, Danelli G, et al. (2007) Spinal anesthesia with lidocaine or preservative-free 2-chloroprocaine for outpatient knee arthroscopy: A prospective, randomized, double-blind comparison. *Anesthesia & Analgesia* 104: 959–64.

Catchlove RFH (1972) The influence of CO2 and pH on local anesthetic action. *Journal of Pharmacology and Experimental Therapeutics* 181: 298–309.

Covino BG (1984) Current controversies in local anaesthetics. In Scott DB, McClure JH, Wildsmith JAW (Eds) *Regional anaesthesia 1884–1984*, pp. 74–81. Sodertalje: ICM.

Covino BG (1986) Pharmacology of local anaesthetic agents. *British Journal of Anaesthesia* 58: 701–16.

Covino BG, Vassallo HG (1976) *Local anesthetics: mechanisms of action and clinical use*, pp. 131–40. New York: Grune and Stratton.

D'Angelo R (2000) Are the new local anaesthetics worth their cost? *Acta Anaesthesiologica Scandinavica* 44: 639–41.

Davis NL, de Jong RH (1982) Successful resuscitation following massive bupivacaine overdose. *Anesthesia & Analgesia* 61: 62–4.

de Jong RH, De Rosa RA (1981) Benzodiazepine treatment of seizures from supraconvulsant doses of local anesthetics. *Regional Anesthesia* 6: 51–4.

Denny NM, Selander DE (1998) Continuous spinal anaesthesia. *British Journal of Anaesthesia* 81: 590–7.

Eyres RL (1995) Local anaesthetoic agents in infancy. *Paediatric Anaesthesia* 5: 213–18.

Foxall G, McCahon R, Lamb J, et al. (2007) Levobupivacaine-induced seizures and cardiovascular collapse treated with Intralipid. *Anaesthesia* 62: 516–18.

Gautier PE, De Kock M, Van Steenberge A, et al. (1999) Intrathecal ropivacaine for ambulatory surgery: a comparison between intrathecal bupivacaine and intrathecal ropivacaine for knee arthroscopy. *Anesthesiology* 91: 1239–45.

Henny CP, Odoom JA, ten Cate H, et al. (1986) Effects of extradural bupivacaine on the haemostatic system. *British Journal of Anaesthesia* 58: 301–5.

Hjelm M, Holmdahl MH (1965) Biochemical effects of aromatic amines. II Cyanosis, methaemoglobinaemia and Heinz-body formation induced by a local anaesthetic agent (prilocaine). *Acta Anaesthesiologica Scandinavica* 9: 99–120.

Keeler JF, Simpson KH, Ellis FR, Kay SP (1992) Effect of addition of hyaluronidase to bupivacaine during axillary brachial plexus block. *British Journal of Anaesthesia* 68: 68–71.

Kennedy WF, Bonica JJ, Ward RJ, et al. (1966) Cardiovascular effects of epinephrine when used in regional anesthesia. *Acta Anaesthesiologica Scandinavica* 23: 320–33.

Lee A, Fagan D, Lamont M, et al. (1989) Disposition kinetics of ropivacaine in humans. *Anesthesia & Analgesia* 69: 736–8.

Litz RJ, Popp M, Stehr SN, Koch T (2006) Successful resuscitation of a patient with ropivacaine-induced asystole after axillary plexus block using lipid infusion. *Anaesthesia* 61: 800–1.

Mallampati SR, Liu PL, Knapp RM (1984) Convulsions and ventricular tachycardia from bupivacaine with epinephrine: successful resuscitation. *Anesthesia & Analgesia* 63: 856–9.

Marhofer P, Greher M, Kapral S (2005) Ultrasound guidance in regional anaesthesia. *British Journal of Anaesthesia* 94: 7–17.

McClure JH (1996) Ropivacaine: a review. *British Journal of Anaesthesia* 76: 300–7.

McClure JH, Scott DB (1981) Comparison of bupivacaine hydrochloride and carbonated bupivacaine in brachial plexus block by the interscalene technique. *British Journal of Anaesthesia* 53: 523–6.

McDonald SB, Liu SS, Kopacz DJ, Stephenson CA (1999) Hyperbaric spinal ropivacaine: a comparison to bupivacaine in volunteers. *Anesthesiology* 90: 971–7.

McLeod GA, Burke D (2001) Levobupivacaine. *Anaesthesia* 56: 331–41.

McLeod GA, Butterworth J, Wildsmith JAW (2009) Clinical toxicity of local anaesthetic drugs. In Cousins MJ, Carr DB, Horlocker TT, Bridenbaugh PO (Eds) *Neural Blockade in Clinical Anesthesia and Pain Medicine*, 4th edn, pp. 114–32. Philadelphia, PA: Lippincott Williams & Wilkins.

Morrison S, Dominguez J, Frascarolo P, Reiz S (2000) A comparison of the electrocardiographic cardiotoxic effects of racemic bupivacaine, levobupivacaine, and ropivacaine in anesthetized swine. *Anesthesia & Analgesia* 90: 1308–14.

Nicoll JMV, Trueren B, Acharya PA, et al. (1986) Retrobulbar anesthesia: the role of hyaluronidase. *Anesthesia & Analgesia* 65: 1324–8.

Reynolds F (1991) Editorial: ropivacaine. *Anaesthesia* 46: 339–40.

Rigler ML, Drasner K, Krejcie TC, et al. (1991) Cauda equina syndrome after continuous spinal anesthesia. *Anesthesia & Analgesia* 72: 275–81.

Rosenblatt MA, Abel M, Fischer GW, et al. (2006) Successful use of a 20% lipid emulsion to resuscitate a patient after a presumed bupivacaine-related cardiac arrest. *Anesthesiology* 105: 217–18.

Scott DA, Blake D, Buckland M, et al. (1999) A comparison of epidural ropivacaine infusion alone and in combination with 1, 2, and 4 microg/mL fentanyl for seventy-two hours of postoperative analgesia after major abdominal surgery. *Anesthesia & Analgesia* 88: 857–64.

Scott DB (1975) Evaluation of the clinical tolerance of local anaesthetic agents. *British Journal of Anaesthesia* 47: 328–31.

Scott DB (1989) Editorial: 'maximum recommended doses' of local anaesthetic drugs. *British Journal of Anaesthesia* 63: 373–4.

Scott DB, Cousins MJ (1980) Clinical pharmacology of local anesthetic drugs. In Cousins MJ, Bridenbaugh D (Eds) *Neural blockade in clinical anesthesia and management of pain*, pp. 86–127. Philadelphia, PA: Lippincott.

Scott DB, Lee A, Fagan D, et al. (1989) Acute toxicity of ropivacaine compared with that of bupivacaine. *Anesthesia and Analgesia* 69: 663–9.

Selander DE (1999) Transient lumbar pain (TLP) after lidocaine spinal anaesthesia is not neurotoxic. In Van Zundert A (Ed) *Highlights in regional anaesthesia and pain therapy VIII*, pp. 315–21. Limassol: Hadjigeorgiou.

Simpson PJ, Hughes DR, Long DH (1982) Prolonged local analgesia for inguinal herniorrhaphy with bupivacaine and dextran. *Annals of the Royal College of Surgeons of England* 64: 243–6.

Swann DG, Armstrong PJ, Douglas E, et al. (1991) The alkalinisation of bupivacaine for intercostal nerve blockade. *Anaesthesia* 46: 174–6.

Van Dyke C, Barash B, Jatlow P, Byck R (1976) Cocaine: plasma concentrations after intranasal application in man. *Science* 191: 859–61.

Weinberg GL (2008) Lipid infusion therapy: translation to clinical practice. *Anesthesia & Analgesia* 106: 1340–2.

Weinberg GL, VadeBoncouer T, Ramaraju GA, et al. (1998) Pretreatment or resuscitation with a lipid infusion shifts the dose-response to bupivacaine-induced asystole in rats. *Anesthesiology* 88: 1071–5.

Weinberg GL, Palmer JW, VadeBoncouer TR, et al. (2000) Bupivacaine inhibits acylcarnitine exchange in cardiac mitochondria. *Anesthesiology* 92: 523–8.

Weinberg G, Ripper R, Feinstein DL, Hoffman W (2003) Lipid emulsion infusion rescues dogs from bupivacaine-induced cardiac toxicity. *Regional Anesthesia and Pain Medicine* 28: 198–202.

Weinberg GL, Ripper R, Murphy P, et al. (2006) Lipid infusion accelerates removal of bupivacaine and recovery from bupivacaine toxicity in the isolated rat heart. *Regional Anesthesia and Pain Medicine* 31: 296–303.

Whiteside J, Wildsmith JAW (2001) Developments in local anaesthetic drugs. *British Journal of Anaesthesia* 87: 27–35.

Wildsmith JAW (2000) Correspondence: Relative potencies of ropivacaine and bupivacaine. *Anesthesiology* 92: 283.

Wildsmith JAW (2001) Letters: New local anaesthetics—how much is improved safety worth? *Acta Anaesthesiologica Scandinavica* 45: 652–3.

Wildsmith JAW, Mason A, McKinnon RP, Rae SM (1998) Alleged allergy to local anaesthetic drugs. *British Dental Journal* 184: 507–10.

Writer WDR, Stienstra R, Eddleston JM, et al. (1998) Neonatal outcome and mode of delivery after epidural analgesia for labour with ropivacaine and bupivacaine: a prospective meta-analysis. *British Journal of Anaesthesia* 81: 713–17.

Zaric D, Nydahl P, Philipson L, et al. (1996) The effect of continuous lumbar epidural infusion of ropivacaine (0.1%, 0.2% and 0.3%) and 0.25% bupivacaine on sensory and motor blockade in volunteers: a double-blind study. *Regional Anesthesia* 21: 14–25.

Zsigmond EK, Kothary SP, Flynn KB (1978 In vitro inhibitory effect of amide-type local analgesics on normal and atypical human plasma cholinesterases. *Regional Anesthesia* 3: 7–9.

CHAPTER 9

Preoperative considerations

Matthew Checketts

Regional anaesthesia, when skilfully administered, is a hugely satisfying experience for the patient, anaesthetist, and surgeon. It provides comfort for the patient, both during and after surgery, with little or no systemic upset, professional satisfaction for the anaesthetist, and, very often, better operating conditions for the surgeon. However, success depends crucially upon the skill and knowledge of the anaesthetist. Meticulous attention to detail is essential: the patient, the operation, and the surgeon must all be taken into consideration when planning each phase of care. Many factors have to be considered, including the patient's general health, the nature, site, and duration of the intended surgery, and the availability of appropriate equipment and facilities.

Preoperative assessment

Preoperative patient assessment should be identical to that carried out before general anaesthesia, if only because a decision on which technique is to be used cannot be made without the information gained from a medical history, physical examination, and the results of appropriate investigations. Review of the patient's case notes is also vital because it may provide important additional information on past medical history and previous anaesthetic difficulties (regional and general). The beginner, particularly, may find it useful to examine the site of any possible regional block injection to check for anatomical abnormality which may cause difficulty. Important aims of this process are the identification of potential technical anaesthetic difficulties and the need for further specialist investigation and treatment, both requiring good planning in advance of the procedure, although traditional hospital admission arrangements could make that difficult and lead to cancelled procedures.

The increasing use of out-patient assessment clinics overcomes such difficulties, and they provide good opportunities for patients to ask questions and express worries regarding the risks and benefits of different techniques to facilitate truly informed consent. Patients should also receive an outline account of what they will experience in regard to both surgical and anaesthetic procedures, and this verbal information can be supplemented with educational materials (leaflets, DVDs, website addresses, etc.) which have been shown to reduce preoperative anxiety (Bondy et al. 1999, Jlala et al. 2010). Copyright-free leaflets, explaining the use of neuraxial and the major peripheral nerve blocks are available on the Royal College of Anaesthetists website, as are others discussing the risks of both general and regional anaesthesia.

However, assessment clinics are not without problems so it is essential that anaesthetists are involved in setting them up to make sure that the right information is gathered, all co-morbidities are identified and treated optimally, and that suitable documentation, tailored to local circumstances, is used or problems will still only be identified at a late stage. A major source of potential difficulties is that the person conducting the clinic (often a nurse) is unlikely to be the anaesthetist responsible for the actual procedure so the clinic's routines and policies must be agreed at departmental level. Whether there has been a preliminary clinic visit or not, the patient's details should be confirmed at a preoperative visit (see 'The preoperative visit' section) near to the time of surgery. The anaesthetist should confirm the patient's medical status and also discuss and explain the planned technique to ensure that the patient knows what to expect.

Pre-existing disease

Most medical conditions have at least some implication for the practice of regional anaesthesia, and the significance of this must be appreciated if blocks are to be used safely and effectively.

Cardiovascular system

Regional anaesthesia for patients with ischaemic or valvular heart disease is challenging, and a careful risk–benefit analysis should be performed on each patient. There may be potential benefits in avoiding the generalized cardiovascular depressive effects of general anaesthesia, but there are potential pitfalls with regional anaesthesia which cannot be ignored. However, expertly managed regional anaesthesia may contribute much to the management of even the highest risk patients undergoing very complex surgical procedures.

Surgery on patients with *ischaemic heart disease* carries a higher risk than usual and this risk is increased markedly if there is any episode of prolonged hypotension (Mauney et al. 1970). In patients who had suffered a previous myocardial infarction, Steen and colleagues (1978) found a fivefold increase in re-infarction rate if the systolic pressure decreased by 30% or more for 10 minutes or longer, presumably because of a reduction in myocardial perfusion. Any situation which produces an imbalance between myocardial oxygen delivery and demand should be avoided, so hypoxaemia, tachycardia, hypertension, and hypotension are all likely to cause problems in the cardiac patient.

There is good evidence that regional anaesthesia can have a beneficial effect on the critical balance between myocardial oxygen supply and demand. Using the model of a dog with reduced coronary flow, Klassen and colleagues (1980) found that sympathetic block from an epidural caused a beneficial redistribution of coronary flow to the endocardium, probably due to alterations in the tone of transmural resistance vessels. Further, Davis and colleagues (1986), also working with dogs, found that thoracic epidural block reduced myocardial infarction size after coronary arterial occlusion. Human studies have shown that localized high thoracic epidural block (T_1–T_5) causes a decrease in systolic arterial pressure, heart rate, and pulmonary arterial and wedge pressures, without significant changes in coronary perfusion pressure, cardiac output, stroke volume, or systemic and pulmonary vascular resistances in patients with unstable angina (Blomberg et al. 1989). Thus, thoracic epidural block may reduce myocardial oxygen demand without jeopardizing coronary arterial supply.

Reiz (1989) reviewed understanding of the circulatory changes induced by epidural anaesthesia in cardiac patients. A high thoracic epidural block (T_1–T_5) improved left ventricular function during stress testing in patients with severe coronary artery disease (Kock et al. 1990), but myocardial ischaemic events are more likely to occur in such patients if there is more extensive block (T_1–T_{12}) (Reiz et al. 1980). However, thoracic epidural block has been found to be effective in patients with severe angina refractory to conventional medical therapy (Blomberg et al. 1989, Toft & Jorgensen 1989), and has been used successfully on a long-term (greater than 3 years) domiciliary basis in similar patients deemed unsuitable for coronary revascularization (Blomberg 1994). Despite these encouraging findings, only a handful of studies have demonstrated a clear beneficial effect of regional anaesthesia on cardiac outcome in surgical patients (Liu et al. 1995), although the evidence is stronger for high-risk patients (Tuman et al. 1991, Yeager et al. 1987). The early promise of perioperative β-adrenergic blockade as an alternative strategy to regional anaesthesia in these patients has not been fulfilled (Devereaux et al. 2008).

Central nerve block in patients with *valvular heart disease* is also controversial because such patients often have a reduced ability to increase cardiac output and, hence, to respond to physiological insults. As a result the vasodilatation produced by sympathetic paralysis during spinal or epidural block may result in an exaggerated degree of hypotension. In the presence of severe aortic stenosis (valve area <1.0 cm^2), the effect on coronary artery blood flow can be catastrophic because the pressure gradient across the narrowed aortic orifice means that left ventricular pressure remains elevated in the face of systemic hypotension.

Controlling the extent of sympathetic block will limit these problems, and a catheter technique will allow a central nerve block to be induced slowly and progressively. Any cardiovascular change will be similarly progressive and can be controlled with increments of appropriately chosen sympathomimetic agents, perhaps more readily than during the acute changes produced by induction of general anaesthesia. There are now several reports of uneventful spinal or epidural anaesthesia in patients with valvular disease (McDonald 2004), but the report of the death of a pre-eclamptic parturient with aortic incompetence serves as a reminder that the block has to be very carefully controlled in such patients (Alderson 1987). Careful

contemplation of the risks and benefits of the planned technique, as well as significant experience of managing both patients with cardiac disease and regional block are obviously essential.

Respiratory system

Patients with severe respiratory disease are among the most willing to accept regional anaesthesia for their operations. They are keenly aware of the limitations which their disease places upon their activity and of how local anaesthesia may be of benefit to them. For peripheral or lower abdominal surgery, neural block avoids the complications of both general anaesthesia and neuromuscular blocking agents, and enables patients to look after their own airway and ventilation. However, a supplementary general anaesthetic is usually necessary during upper abdominal and thoracic surgery, and block of at least some of the nerves supplying the respiratory muscles is inevitable (Freund et al. 1967). This may lead to a decrease in vital capacity, maximum breathing capacity, and the ability to cough and clear secretions.

The most important alteration in pulmonary function in patients undergoing surgery is an almost inevitable reduction in functional residual capacity which may result in atelectasis, ventilation perfusion mismatch, hypoxaemia, and pneumonia. Unfortunately, there is no evidence that any form of preoperative respiratory function testing can predict which patients may become compromised, but well-known risk factors are obesity, advanced age, pre-existing pulmonary disease, thoracic or abdominal incisions, and severe pain. The major advantage of regional anaesthetic techniques in upper abdominal and thoracic surgery is in the provision of postoperative analgesia. Published studies comparing the pulmonary sequelae of regional and systemic opioid analgesic techniques are conflicting, but it seems that the benefits of epidural analgesia on pulmonary complications are only apparent in high-risk patients and only when epidural block is maintained well into the postoperative period (Liu et al. 1995).

Most peripheral techniques are without respiratory impact, but the interscalene and supraclavicular approaches to the brachial plexus almost inevitably block the ipsilateral phrenic nerve and also carry a significant risk of pneumothorax. Either can lead to ventilatory failure in patients with severe lung disease, and require (embarrassingly for the anaesthetist) acute admission to the intensive care unit. It is essential to anticipate these hazards when such patients are scheduled for major upper limb surgery.

Nervous system

Pre-existing disease of the nervous system presents the anaesthetist with a most contentious problem. Bromage (1978) has reviewed possible causes of neurological damage during the performance of regional anaesthesia, especially near the spinal cord. These include direct trauma, haematoma, infection, vasoconstriction, and accidental injection of a neurotoxin. It is almost inevitable that, if a patient's neurological condition degenerates after a regional anaesthetic, the block will be blamed to the exclusion of all other possible causes. However, Bromage has elegantly shown that many peripheral nerve lesions occurring after extradural analgesia are not directly related to the technique itself. Marinacci and Courville (1958) carried out electromyography on 482 patients with neurological complications after subarachnoid anaesthesia and only in four cases were the complications considered to be due to the block.

Unfortunately, most of the literature relating to regional anaesthesia in patients with neurological disease is anecdotal. It is therefore difficult to define specific guidelines, but analysis of the few published series is helpful. There are several reports of permanent neurological deterioration after regional anaesthesia in patients with pre-existing problems (Ballin 1981, Chaudhari et al. 1978, Hirlekar 1980), but there are protagonists of regional anaesthesia who believe that it exerts no influence upon the clinical course of a wide range of neurological conditions (Crawford et al. 1981). Pre- and postoperative clinical evaluation and documentation are important regardless of the anaesthetic used, because changes in neurological status are common after surgery anyway. Accurate documentation is vital for medicolegal purposes also.

Patients with neurological conditions may be at risk from a number of complications which must be appreciated by the anaesthetist. A deterioration may not be due to the block itself, but a failure to recognize the implications of the existing condition. Respiratory compromise may occur secondary to musculoskeletal abnormalities or abnormal medullary control of ventilation. Autonomic hyper-reflexia is common and can result in unwelcome rapid and dramatic changes in haemodynamic status, or even in cardiac arrest. A state of relative hypovolaemia is well recognized after spinal-cord injury and in patients with multiple sclerosis. The combination of this pre-existing problem with the sympathectomy caused by a central nerve block may result in profound hypotension.

Multiple sclerosis (MS): stress, fatigue, infection, and hyperthermia are well documented as factors that can exacerbate MS. These factors are common in the perioperative period so it is usually impossible to specify the cause of a relapse after surgery. Most reports of MS patients receiving regional anaesthetic techniques are small, but Hebl and Horlocker (2006) published a series of 139 patients with pre-existing neurological disease who had undergone surgical procedures under central neuraxial block without suffering any exacerbation of their condition. Thirty-five of their patients had MS, 17 receiving a spinal anaesthetic and 18 an epidural. Typically, MS goes into remission during pregnancy, but may then relapse in the early postpartum period (Abramsky 1994). There are conflicting reports on whether central nerve block is associated with such a relapse; Samford and colleagues (1978) suggest that it is, but others refute this (Bader et al. 1988, Capdeville & Hoyt 1994, Crawford et al. 1981, Hebl & Horlocker 2006). It is important to consider carefully the risks and benefits of regional anaesthesia in MS, and to discuss the issues with the patient.

Spinal cord injury: the spinal cord redevelops reflex activity about 1 month after transection. Autonomic hyper-reflexia can be provoked by a skin incision or visceral stimulation such as a full bladder. These reflex responses may result in profound hypertension and bradycardia, and may be life threatening, especially if the transection level is above T_6. Procedures such as cystoscopy are particularly likely to provoke these reflexes and spinal anaesthesia can be employed with great benefit with the sole intention of blocking the reflex pathways (Lambert et al. 1982, Schonwald et al. 1981). However, there has been at least one report of such a mass reflex developing in the presence of an apparently adequate block (Lambert et al. 1982), but subarachnoid baclofen may further attenuate these reflexes (Muller et al. 1990) and central nerve block is probably the anaesthetic technique of choice in patients at risk of autonomic hyper-reflexia.

Peripheral neuropathy: the risks and benefits of regional techniques have to be considered carefully in patients with peripheral neuropathy, particularly if there is the possibility of autonomic involvement because it may be associated with greater cardiovascular morbidity (Burgos et al. 1989, Page & Watkins 1978). However, regional anaesthesia will offer clear advantages in many patients with this combination of problems, particularly diabetics (see 'Diabetes' section).

Other neuropathology: regional anaesthesia also has potential advantages in patients with other types of neurological disease. A clear example is the avoidance of neuromuscular blocking drugs in patients with myotonic dystrophy and myasthenia gravis so that the respiratory morbidity, to which they are particularly susceptible, is reduced.

An individual approach to the patient, the intercurrent disease, and the proposed surgery is necessary in order to decide on the most appropriate form of anaesthetic management.

Renal system

Bromage and Gertel (1972) alleged that patients with chronic renal failure are more susceptible than healthy patients to toxicity from local anaesthetic agents. These authors suggested that this might stem from a difference in drug binding due to the hypoproteinaemia associated with renal failure. They also noted that anaemia may cause a high output circulation and thus lead to rapid systemic absorption. On the other hand, the sympathetic block caused by regional anaesthesia may improve circulation and perfusion to the site of operation, whether this is the kidney itself, or a limb during the fashioning of an arteriovenous fistula. However, brachial plexus block, particularly by the axillary route, should be undertaken with great care in a patient with such a fistula because the associated venous distension will make accidental intravascular injection much more likely.

Obesity

There may be significant technical problems with the performance of regional anaesthesia in the morbidly obese patient. Fisher and colleagues (1975) suggested that difficulty in positioning, identifying landmarks, and needle location combine to make regional anaesthesia extremely difficult. Conversely, the benefits of combining light general anaesthesia with regional anaesthesia for upper abdominal surgery in these patients have been well documented by Buckley and colleagues (1983). Many of their patients also had cardiovascular and respiratory disease, and postoperative complications were less than in a similar (but unmatched) group given general anaesthesia alone.

Very obese patients appear to require less local anaesthetic than the non-obese to achieve the same block height during spinal (Taivainen 1990) or epidural anaesthesia (Hodgkinson and Husain 1980). The lower cerebrospinal fluid volume noted in very obese patients may partially explain these observations (Hogan et al. 1996).

Diabetes

Diabetic patients have an increased incidence of atherosclerosis and its attendant complications. They are particularly prone to episodes of painless myocardial ischaemia, and the cardiovascular system should be the focus of unremitting vigilance. In addition, diabetes is associated with microangiopathy, peripheral neuropathy, autonomic dysfunction, and predisposition to infection.

However, these problems are more than offset by the many occasions when regional anaesthesia allows surgery to be performed with minimal disruption to the diabetic patient's carbohydrate intake and insulin regimen, and with minimal activation of the 'stress' hormones, all of which act to increase blood sugar and destabilize its control.

Infection

Infection at or close to the site of injection is a major contraindication to the use of local anaesthetic techniques. Not only may it spread the infection, but the block is likely to be ineffective (Bieter 1936) because pH changes in the infected tissue will impair local anaesthetic action. It may be possible to block a nerve distant from the focus of infection, but this is not always effective, as many dental patients can confirm.

More distant foci of infection present more complicated challenges. Major infections such as meningitis, arachnoiditis, or epidural abscess are very rare after spinal or epidural anaesthesia and there is good epidemiological evidence that the incidence of meningitis after lumbar puncture is no higher than in the general population, even in bacteraemic patients (Eng & Seligman 1981). However, Carp and Bailey (1992) found that 12 out of 40 bacteraemic rats developed meningitis after cisternal puncture, although none of the comparative group, which had been given gentamicin, developed meningitis. This led Chestnut (1992) to recommend proceeding with central nerve block in bacteraemic patients provided that appropriate antibiotics have been given and that there is some evidence of clinical improvement (e.g. reduced pyrexia).

Placing an epidural catheter in a patient with systemic infection, even if this is being treated, is more controversial because, like any other foreign body, it may act as a focus for local infection so patients must be selected and monitored carefully (Carson & Wildsmith 1996). The belief that the caudal approach presents a greater risk than any other is unfounded as long as antiseptic precautions are adequate (Abouleish et al. 1980).

Muscle disease

Malignant hyperthermia is probably the best known example of a muscle disease with anaesthetic significance. Regional anaesthesia avoids the use of volatile agents and muscle relaxants, but may still be associated with increased temperature in susceptible individuals (Katz & Krich 1976, Wadhwa 1977). Amide agents such as lidocaine can release calcium from the sarcoplasmic reticulum and this would imply that they should be avoided, although prilocaine is used for muscle biopsy in the investigation of suspected patients (Hopkins 2000). Esters are probably safer (Gronert 1980), but there has been one report of a reaction in a susceptible individual (Katz & Krich 1976).

Sickle cell disease

Regional techniques are the methods of choice in sickle cell disease (Howells et al. 1972), although the usual precautions must still be taken to ensure good perfusion, maintain oxygenation, and avoid tourniquets. On theoretical grounds, prilocaine should not be used in these patients.

Allergy

Many patients claim to be 'allergic' to local anaesthetics, but the history usually reveals that a previous reaction was due to systemic toxicity, the effect of an added vasoconstrictor, or a psychological reaction. Most patients have only been exposed to local anaesthesia in the dental chair where fear and anxiety are relatively common, adrenaline is used in high concentration, and injections are made into vascular tissues. Allergy to local anaesthetics is rare, but each suspected case should be investigated (Wildsmith et al. 1998). Failure to do so may force the anaesthetist to avoid regional anaesthesia unnecessarily in the future and, if the reaction was truly allergic in nature, may result in subsequent administration of the real cause of the reaction again.

Intradermal injection is the usual method of testing for local anaesthetic sensitivity, but false positive responses are not infrequent (Fisher 1984). Full resuscitation facilities should be available and the initial injection should be 0.1 ml of solution. Complete investigation should include progressive injection of increasing doses of the local anaesthetic drug (Weiss et al. 1989). Cross-sensitivity is common between the ester drugs, but not between the amides, although the possibility that a reaction was due to a preservative should be kept in mind.

Psychological problems

Regional anaesthesia is not contraindicated by psychological illness, but its use must be assessed in the context of the patient's ability to understand and consent to the intended procedure. The patient must be able to cooperate fully with the block procedure, and it may be that the nature of the illness makes this impossible. Moore (1976) states that hysteria and malingering are both relative contraindications to the use of regional anaesthesia.

Coagulation considerations

Abnormalities of the coagulation process present particular problems for the regional anaesthetist. Even in the normal patient, there is the possibility of haematoma formation after regional anaesthesia where the nerve is so deeply placed that pressure cannot be used to control bleeding after needle insertion. The risk is obviously greater in cases where coagulation is deficient, and it has been argued that intercostal nerve block should be avoided in such patients (Nielsen 1989).

Disorders of coagulation may occasionally result from intercurrent disease, and the ideal solution is restoration of normal coagulation prior to the block, something which will usually require the help of a haematologist. If restoration of normal coagulation is not possible, clinical decisions should be based on the degree of disorder, and guidelines on a similar degree of drug-induced abnormality should be followed. Many surgical patients are at high risk of thromboembolism, and drug therapy is used commonly to reduce the risk. Regional anaesthesia in this situation is a complex issue which requires careful consideration. The 'simple' approach is to avoid regional block in any patient receiving pharmacological thromboprophylaxis, but this will deny many patients the benefits of a regional technique, often quite unnecessarily.

Vertebral canal haematoma

The extreme manifestation of this issue is vertebral canal haematoma formation after central nerve block. This is a potentially catastrophic complication because permanent paraplegia will ensue unless the haematoma is both diagnosed and evacuated rapidly, perhaps within as little as 8 hours. Anxiety about this happening can mean that the patient is denied *either* the benefits of the regional anaesthetic technique or appropriate prophylaxis against venous thromboembolic disease (VTE), even though vertebral canal haematoma is a very rare complication with an estimated incidence of 1 in 220,000 associated with spinals and 1 in 150,000 with epidurals (Tryba 1993). It is thus crucial that the concern does not lead to suboptimal management which may well have greater *total* risks for the patient. Appropriate advice on the use of spinal and epidural block in patients receiving pharmacological prophylaxis for thromboembolism was published some years ago (Wildsmith & McClure 1991), but the concerns were renewed by events in the USA in the late 1990s (Lumpkin 1998). The advice has now been updated (Horlocker & Wedel 2010) and the situation may be summarized as follows.

Most vertebral canal haematomas occur spontaneously, with an incidence estimated at one per million population per year (Holtas et al. 1996). Many are associated with *disordered coagulation* (Groen & Ponssen 1990), which has also been identified as one of the major factors in the cases reported after spinal and epidural block (Vandermeulen et al. 1994). *Technical difficulty* during instrumentation of the vertebral canal is another factor, with epidural block (especially with catheter insertion) carrying a greater risk than spinal. *Catheter removal* is an important time of further risk. To put the subject into perspective, it should be noted that the review highlighting these points was able to identify only 61 case reports published between 1906 and 1994 (Vandermeulen et al. 1994), but this was before the widespread use of low-molecular-weight heparin.

In 1998, a report appeared in the USA documenting over 40 cases of vertebral canal haematoma occurring in less than 5 years in patients receiving the low-molecular-weight heparin, enoxaparin (Lumpkin 1998). Most followed spinal or epidural block, although a few related to diagnostic lumbar puncture, and the report confirmed the other risk factors mentioned earlier in this section as well as noting an association with enoxaparin. This American series is in direct contrast to experience in Europe, where enoxaparin has been available for much longer, but where only two cases of vertebral canal haematoma have been reported. Its incidence after spinal or epidural block in patients receiving enoxaparin has been estimated at 1 in 2,250,000 in Europe, but at 1 in 14,000 in the USA (Tryba & Wedel 1997), a difference which has still to be explained.

Although there were other issues (Checketts & Wildsmith 1999), the major contributory factor seems to have been a difference in recommended dose of enoxaparin. In Europe the dose is 20–40 mg once daily, starting 12 hours before surgery, so that the peak effect of the drug (4–6 hours after administration) will be well past at the time of block administration and any risk will be minimal. In the USA, the recommended dose was 30 mg twice daily, starting 1 hour after surgery. Thus, there would be no effect at the time of institution of a block, but the long half-life of enoxaparin (10–12 hours) could lead to cumulation, particularly at the higher dose. The drug might well then produce an overt effect on coagulation and cause bleeding at the time of catheter removal. Even if dose were the major factor, other aspects provide lessons which will help to minimize the risk of this dreadful complication. The primary lesson is that surgeons and anaesthetists must communicate properly regarding policies for use of central nerve block and deep vein thrombosis prophylaxis. An overview of the more general points is that:

♦ Vertebral canal haematoma is a rare complication, but its serious nature requires that some precaution is taken to minimize the incidence.

♦ The risk seems to be related to the degree of coagulation disturbance, and interactions between drugs may be particularly important (Wysowski et al. 1998).

♦ Technical difficulty during block performance was reported in many cases, so technical skill and experience may be very relevant.

♦ Coagulation status at the time of catheter removal needs as much attention as at its insertion

Against this background, specific aspects of the various pharmacological agents used in thromboprophylaxis can be considered.

Specific factors

Warfarin: frank anticoagulation is the ultimate contraindication to spinal or epidural block, and most authorities recommend that the international normalized ratio (INR) should be 1.5 or lower for institution of a block or removal of a catheter (Horlocker et al. 1994, Odoom & Sih 1983, Wu & Perkins 1996). Patients who are taking warfarin should have it stopped 4–5 days before elective surgery, a manoeuvre which will usually result in an INR of <1.5, although this must be checked before regional anaesthesia and surgery. Very few patients need perioperative 'cover' with heparin because the risks of bleeding usually exceed the risks of thrombosis, but local hospital guidelines should be developed to guide this. Special provisions apply for ophthalmic surgery (see Chapter 20).

Unfractionated heparin: thromboprophylaxis with low-dose (5,000 units), subcutaneous heparin given two to three times daily does not usually prolong the activated partial thromboplastin time (APTT) and large numbers of such patients have received spinal or epidural block without sequelae (Schwander & Bachmann 1991). However, the numbers of patients involved in these studies are small relative to the risk of vertebral canal haematoma and a transient elevation of the APTT may occur (Cooke et al. 1976). Thus, some anaesthetists prefer not to institute spinal or epidural block within 4–6 hours of a dose of heparin, and they delay the next dose until after the block has been performed (Wildsmith & McClure 1991). Similar considerations would apply to catheter removal. Because of the risk of thrombocytopaenia with heparin, the platelet count should be checked before the block is performed, or the catheter removed, if the patient has been receiving the drug for more than 4 days.

Combining central neuraxial block with intravenous low-dose heparin (circa 5,000 units) for vascular surgical procedures is considered safe as long as the heparin is given at least 1 hour after the block. Indwelling regional anaesthetic catheters should be removed 2–4 hours after the heparin has been given.

Low-molecular-weight heparin (LMWH): LMWHs act by inhibiting factor Xa and have relatively little anti-IIa (thrombin) activity. They have a higher bioavailability and longer duration of action than unfractionated heparin. Peak anti-Xa activity occurs 2–4 hours after subcutaneous injection, but even at 12 hours the anti-Xa effect has only reduced by 50%. The effects of LMWHs are predictable and dose related, and their pharmacokinetics and dynamics have to be appreciated by the regional anaesthetist. The evidence suggests that the standard European thromboprophylactic dose regimen (e.g. enoxaparin 20–40 mg, once daily) is not associated with any increased risk as long as the block is instituted, or the catheter removed, 10–12 hours after drug administration. The next LMWH dose should not be given until 2 hours after block administration or catheter removal. Fortunately, postoperative administration (within 6 hours of surgery) has been shown to be as effective as preoperative for thromboprophylaxis after hip replacement (Hull & Pineo 2001), and will make life simpler for both surgeons and anaesthetists.

In patients on anticoagulant doses of LMWH, a minimum interval of 24 hours should elapse before performing central neuraxial or deep peripheral nerve blocks.

Antiplatelet agents: much concern has been expressed about the potential for the antiplatelet effect of aspirin and clopidogrel to increase the risk of vertebral canal haematoma in patients receiving spinal or epidural block. However, there is little or no evidence to support this concern, although interactions with other agents such as LMWH may occur (Horlocker et al. 1995, Wysowski et al. 1998). It is usual to stop clopidogrel a minimum of 7 days before elective surgery, if possible, to allow platelet function to return to normal, and local guidelines for the perioperative management of patients on this drug should be developed. The risk of vertebral canal haematoma in patients who have a spinal or epidural block and continue to take clopidogrel is unknown. The risks and benefits of performing the block should be assessed by the anaesthetist and discussed with the patient in such situations.

Platelet abnormalities: patients with disorders of platelet function or low platelet levels may present an increased risk of vertebral canal haematoma if they receive an epidural or spinal block. The risk is presumed to be high if there is clinical evidence of platelet dysfunction, that is, petechiae or spontaneous and easy bruising of the skin. Specialist advice may be useful if central neural block is considered appropriate because platelet therapy may be indicated before the patient undergoes surgery (Thomas 1997).

Direct oral thrombin blockers: rivaroxaban and dabigatran are now licensed for thromboprophylaxis in primary hip and knee arthroplasty. There are given once daily, starting within 6 hours of surgery and have elimination half-lives of 6–9 hours in healthy adults. Indwelling regional anaesthetic catheters should not be removed until two half-lives have elapsed since the last dose, and a further 2 hours allowed before the next dose is given.

Quantifying the risk

It is not unnatural to seek some numerical indicator of the actual risk in an individual patient. With warfarin and unfractionated heparin this is readily available in the clinical situation in the form of INR- and APTT-testing respectively. Unfortunately, testing for the activity of LMWH against factor Xa is not readily available *nor* predictive of the risk of bleeding, so it is necessary to rely on knowledge of the pharmacology of the agents. In platelet abnormalities a count may be of some use, but provides no information on the activity and effectiveness of those platelets. These difficulties have led to suggestions that the bleeding time can determine which patients are at risk, but this is a subjective screening test and not one on which to base clinical decisions. Thromboelastography (Sharma et al. 1999, Whitten & Greilich 2000) may be more objective, but as with bleeding time (Thomas 1997) there is no epidemiological evidence on what is, or is not, a 'safe' or 'dangerous' result. It may be that taking a careful bleeding history from the patient is the simplest and most cost-effective way of identifying the risk (Colon-Otero et al. 1991).

An overview

Definitive recommendations should be based on the results of randomized, double-blind studies, but none are available and, given the incidence of vertebral canal haematoma, it is unlikely that such evidence will appear. A common-sense approach, based on the evidence reviewed briefly here, is needed for practice within a framework of agreed local policies. It is particularly difficult to lay down guidelines for the patient in labour, or presenting for emergency surgery, who has already received a thromboprophylactic drug. The agent used, the dose, and the time interval since its last administration should be noted. Any decision should be based on the balance of risks and benefits, which will often require discussion with the patient as well as with the surgeon. These discussions should be documented fully. Trainees must understand the issues and seek advice from consultants if they are in any doubt.

Because many of the reported cases were associated with 'difficult' or 'traumatic' procedures, as well as with disordered coagulation *the need for a cautious, gentle technique is self-evident*. When there is difficulty or bleeding during the block procedure (or any other unusual risk factor) it is essential that this is recorded and greater vigilance maintained during the postoperative period. It may also be advisable to omit or delay the next dose of thromboprophylactic agent. In the face of difficulty occurring during a block it may even be appropriate to review the situation and switch to an alternative anaesthetic method. Finally, although this discussion of vertebral canal haematoma has dealt with the factors likely to predispose to the condition, it should be appreciated that a haematoma will only produce symptoms if it can exert pressure on the cord or cauda equina, and this will depend on the local anatomy of the epidural space at the point where the bleeding occurs. A small, loculated haematoma may therefore produce symptoms whereas one which can spread unimpeded may not.

Combinations of thromboprophylactic agents may cause greater disturbance of coagulation and require more caution.

The surgical procedure

Regional anaesthesia is not suitable for all types of surgery. In some cases, the appropriate block may be technically difficult with a high failure rate, or the operation may be so extensive that more than one block is required, and the problem of drug toxicity may arise. In many other cases though, regional anaesthesia can provide effective postoperative analgesia even if sedative or general anaesthetic supplementation is required for the operation itself. One of the chief advantages of regional anaesthesia in obstetrics is that the mother can be fully conscious and unsedated at the time of delivery.

Site and nature of the operation

Obviously, the chosen regional technique should provide anaesthesia over the area of the skin incision, but it must also be extensive enough to block stimuli arising from deeper structures manipulated during surgery. For example, a block limited to T_{11} and T_{12}, although adequate for an inguinal herniorrhaphy incision, will be inadequate when the surgeon handles the spermatic cord and hernial sac. Similarly, perineal anaesthesia alone will be inadequate for a vaginal hysterectomy. When a spinal or epidural block is used, particular care should be taken to ensure that the segmental block provided gives adequate anaesthesia for the surgical procedure.

Even if it is technically possible to supply complete anaesthesia for all stages of an operation, it is not always desirable that the patient should be fully aware throughout. Many patients prefer to be lightly sedated during surgery and the availability of short-acting intravenous drugs such as midazolam and propofol makes this possible with minimal postoperative after-effects. A controlled infusion of propofol allows the depth of sedation to be very carefully controlled with rapid wake up and virtually no 'hangover' effect.

Duration of surgery

This will have a major bearing on selection of the local anaesthetic drug and regional technique used. Insertion of a catheter allows increments of local anaesthetic to be given during surgery and should be used whenever there is the slightest risk that the operation may outlast the effect of a single dose. Single-injection techniques should be reserved for operations which are certain to be finished before a single dose has worn off, and do not require local analgesia for postoperative pain control.

The duration of the operation may also influence decisions regarding the choice of sedation or general anaesthesia. Operating tables are not designed for the comfort of the conscious patient, and lying on a firm surface for a long period can become an ordeal for even the most resilient and cooperative patient.

Anaesthetist and surgeon

The extent to which regional anaesthesia is deemed suitable in various cases depends on the attitude of both anaesthetist and surgeon. The main source of surgical prejudice against regional anaesthesia is the concern that the smooth running of the operating list will be impaired, but there is evidence that, in experienced hands, regional anaesthetic techniques take very little longer to perform than a general anaesthetic (Dexter 1998). The cooperation and enthusiasm of surgeons should be cultivated at all times and it is common courtesy to inform them in advance when regional anaesthesia is planned. When the clear benefits of regional anaesthesia are apparent in terms of a rapid and pain-free recovery, surgeons encourage rather than resist it.

Another area of surgical concern is the possibility that the operation might be compromised by inadequate anaesthesia or muscle relaxation. The surgeon expects the best possible operating conditions, and the anaesthetist requires skill, experience, and patience to provide these consistently. If a regional anaesthesia 'culture' is established in an institution in which surgeons, nurses, and patients are well informed about the many advantages, life becomes much easier for the anaesthetist. The atmosphere in the operating theatre should be relaxed and free of stress. There is wide variation among surgeons as to what constitutes an 'ideal' environment. Some enjoy the technical challenge and social contact provided by the conscious patient, whereas others value freedom of speech and prefer sedation or general anaesthesia. Many senior surgeons feel that surgical trainees should gain experience in operating on conscious patients. They point out that this refines surgical technique and tightens operating theatre discipline.

There is a similar variation in attitude towards regional anaesthesia among anaesthetists. Modern training requirements ensure that all trainee anaesthetists have some experience from an early stage, but not everyone is temperamentally suited to cope with the special challenges which regional anaesthesia presents. Such anaesthetists should aim to master one or two widely applicable blocks so that their repertoire is not restricted to general anaesthetic techniques, and their patients are not entirely denied the benefits of regional anaesthesia. At the other end of the scale, the enthusiast must make sure that his main concern is the patient's overall welfare, and not his own enthusiasm for regional block.

It is also crucial to accept readily failure of a regional technique should it occur and develop strategies to address such a failure, for example, additional peripheral regional block or general anaesthesia (Fettes & Wildsmith 2009). There are no guarantees in regional anaesthesia and anaesthetists should not promise 100% success to the patient or presume they can achieve it themselves.

Available facilities

Before proceeding further it is necessary to consider the equipment and drugs required for the safe and effective performance of the chosen technique.

Resuscitation

Intravenous access and fluids, a tipping trolley, an oxygen supply, and resuscitation drugs and equipment are all essential. The equipment must include an anaesthetic machine as a source of oxygen and means of lung ventilation, laryngoscopes, oropharyngeal airways, cuffed tracheal tubes, a stylet, and efficient suction. The full range of anaesthetic and resuscitation drugs (including a lipid preparation for the treatment of local anaesthetic toxicity) should be immediately available. A defibrillator must also be easily accessible and it is the anaesthetist's duty to be familiar with its function and to know the current guidelines on advanced cardiac life support.

Local anaesthetic drugs

The pharmacology of local anaesthetic drugs has been described in Chapters 6, 7, and 8. Obviously the appropriate drug for the planned procedure should be used. *Every care should be taken to avoid injection errors and ensure that the intended local anaesthetic solution is injected.*

The contents of single-use glass or plastic ampoules from a reputable drug company are guaranteed sterile and should be used for all central blocks. The ampoules themselves may be double wrapped and autoclaved for use within a sterile field. Multidose vials contain additional bacteriostatic agents and are certainly not suitable for spinal or epidural anaesthesia. It has been suggested that they should not be used for any regional technique (Henderson & Macrae 1983) because pathogens may have been introduced during previous use. These objections can be overcome by using a multidose vial once only and then discarding it. Generic local anaesthetics should be regarded with suspicion unless the exact contents are known.

All solutions should be drawn up through a micropore filter needle, to exclude problems due to particulate matter from ampoules (Somerville & Gibson 1973) and from disposable regional anaesthetic trays (Seltzer et al. 1977).

The preoperative visit

Explanation to the patient

It cannot be over-emphasized that the preoperative preparation of the patient is one of the keys to success with regional anaesthesia. It establishes rapport with the patient, ensures cooperation, and makes technical performance of the block easier. Patients with pre-existing medical conditions, such as chronic obstructive airway disease, are often keen to have regional anaesthesia, but may be encouraged if they are not. Healthier patients can be offered a choice of regional anaesthesia, general anaesthesia or a mixture of both. Many patients prefer to be asleep and their wishes should always be taken into account. It may be necessary occasionally to 'sell' the advantages of regional anaesthesia, but there should be no attempt at coercion.

An adequate explanation of what the patient can expect should be given in terms which are readily understood. Specific mention should be made of paraesthesiae if they are to be elicited or involuntary muscular twitching when a nerve stimulator is to be used. If the patient is to remain conscious during surgery, it is prudent to mention that some sensation may be preserved, and that feelings of pressure, movement, warmth or cold may be experienced; otherwise any stimulus may be interpreted as pain and this may result in unnecessary action being taken by the anaesthetist, although any truly painful sensation must be attended to immediately. Music can be a useful distraction during the procedure and patients can be encouraged to bring their favourite music to theatre if they wish. Recently, some anaesthetists have had DVD players installed in theatre in the patient's line of vision.

It is good practice to point out the advantages associated with the chosen technique—early recovery, lack of postoperative pain, reduced amount of nausea and vomiting, etc.—and to follow this with an explanation of what the patient will experience before, during, and after the block. An assurance that the patient will not see the operation is often required and the patient should be warned that motor block may outlast the sensory block postoperatively.

Preparation of the patient

Patients for major blocks should be treated in the same way as patients receiving general anaesthesia and standard protocols regarding fasting should be followed, remembering that there is evidence that these protocols do not need to be as stringent as they used to be (Strunin 1993). The urinary bladder should be empty preoperatively because a full bladder in a patient with a peripheral block can be both uncomfortable and disruptive, and over-distention increases significantly the need for catheterization after spinal or epidural block.

Premedication

Many patients require no more premedication than a preoperative visit and adequate explanation of the intended procedure by the anaesthetist. However, drug premedication may often be useful, and its aim should be the relief of pain and anxiety. Changes in the ways in which patients are managed (e.g. day and short stay surgery) may limit the opportunity for oral administration, but the judicious intravenous administration of sedatives and or analgesics prior to the block may increase patient comfort and facilitate the procedure.

Opioids

Pain relief may be necessary in patients with fractures or other painful conditions. This will allow the patient to be transported to the operating theatre and positioned for the block with the minimum of distress. In these circumstances, opioid analgesics are appropriate, although they possess many properties which are undesirable in patients having regional anaesthesia, including nausea, vomiting, respiratory depression, sedation, and delayed gastric emptying. However, opioid premedication prior to regional

anaesthesia does have the advantage of further reducing postoperative analgesic requirements (McQuay et al. 1988), although Grant and colleagues (1981) have suggested intramuscular ketamine (0.5 mg kg^{-1}) as an alternative.

Benzodiazepines

Anxiolytic drugs such as diazepam, lorazepam, and temazepam are useful premedicants for patients about to undergo surgery under regional anaesthesia. Oral temazepam (10–30 mg, 1–2 hours before surgery) is widely prescribed and is relatively short acting with minimal residual 'hangover' effect (Beechey et al. 1981). However, it does not produce amnesia and one of the other benzodiazepines, such as lorazepam (2–4 mg, 2 hours before surgery), should be used if this is required. Lorazepam has a slow onset and long duration of action, but these properties make it useful for night sedation or premedication of anxious patients who are towards the end of the operating list. Oral midazolam (0.5 mg kg^{-1}) has become popular for calming the very anxious or agitated child before anaesthesia, but its short duration means that it has to be administered approximately 30 minutes before the patient comes to theatre.

Other drugs

Before long operations, it can be useful to administer a long-acting non-steroidal anti-inflammatory drug (NSAID), not only as an analgesic adjunct, but also to minimize the discomfort caused by prolonged immobility. Even if a light general anaesthetic is to be administered, oral diclofenac given the night before surgery, or ibuprofen, 2–4 hours preoperatively, can be helpful. However, NSAIDs are contraindicated in patients with active peptic ulceration, renal impairment (including prerenal problems), or brittle asthma, and a small dose of an opioid may serve the same purpose.

The elderly patient

Heavy premedication should be avoided in older patients, and even the benzodiazepines may cause profound sedation, confusion, and restlessness. Many elderly patients present for fracture surgery, and premedication may be better provided with an analgesic.

Further reading

Horlocker TT, Wedel DJ, Rowlingson JC, et al. (2010) Regional anesthesia in the patient receiving antithrombotic or thrombolytic therapy. American Society of Regional Anesthesia and Pain Medicine Evidence-Based Guidelines (Third Edition). *Regional Anesthesia and Pain Medicine* 35: 64–101.

On-line resource

http://www.sign.ac.uk/guidelines/fulltext/122/index.html Scottish Intercollegiate Guidelines Network: Prevention and management of venous thromboembolism.

References

Abramsky C (1994) Pregnancy and multiple sclerosis. *Annals of Neurology* 36(suppl): S38–41.

Abouleish E, Orig T, Amortegui AJ (1980) Bacteriologic comparison between epidural and caudal techniques. *Anesthesiology* 53: 511–14.

Alderson JD (1987) Cardiovascular collapse following epidural anaesthesia for Caesarean section in a patient with aortic incompetence. *Anaesthesia* 42: 643–5.

Ballin NC (1981) Paraplegia following epidural analgesia. *Anaesthesia* 36: 952–3.

Bader AM, Hunt CO, Datta S (1988) Anesthesia for the obstetric patient with multiple sclerosis. *Journal of Clinical Anesthesiology* 1: 21.

Beechey APG, Eltringham RJ, Studd C (1981) Temazepam as premedication in day surgery. *Anaesthesia* 36: 10–16.

Bieter RN (1936) Applied pharmacology of local anaesthetics. *American Journal of Surgery* 34: 500–10.

Blomberg S, Emanuelsson H, Ricksten S-E (1989) Thoracic epidural anesthesia and central hemodynamics in patients with unstable angina pectoris. *Anesthesia & Analgesia* 69: 558–62.

Blomberg S (1994) Long term home self treatment with high thoracic epidural anesthesia in patients with severe coronary artery disease. *Anesthesia & Analgesia* 79: 413–21.

Bondy LR, Sims N, Schroeder DR, et al (1999) The effect of anesthetic patient education on preoperative patient anxiety. *Regional Anesthesia and Pain Medicine* 24: 158–64.

Bromage PR (1978) *Epidural analgesia*. Philadelphia, PA: WB Saunders.

Bromage PR, Gertel M (1972) Brachial plexus anesthesia in chronic renal failure. *Anesthesiology* 36: 488–93.

Buckley FP, Robinson NB, Simonowitz DA, Dellinger EP (1983) Anaesthesia in the morbidly obese. A comparison of anaesthetic and analgesic regimens for upper abdominal surgery. *Anaesthesia* 38: 840–51.

Burgos LG, Ebert TJ, Assiddao C, et al. (1989) Increased intraoperative cardiovascular morbidity in diabetics with autonomic neuropathy. *Anesthesiology* 70: 591–8.

Capdeville M, Hoyt MR (1994) Anesthesia and analgesia in the obstetric population with multiple sclerosis: A retrospective review. *Anesthesiology* 81: 1173–7.

Carp H, Bailey S (1992) The association between meningitis and dural puncture in bacteraemic rats. *Anesthesiology* 76: 739–42.

Carson D, Wildsmith JAW (1996) The risk of extradural abscess. *British Journal of Anaesthesia* 75: 520–1.

Chaudhari LS, Kop BR, Dhruva AJ (1978) Paraplegia and epidural analgesia. *Anaesthesia* 33: 722–5.

Checketts MR, Wildsmith JAW (1999) Central nerve block and thromboprophylaxis—is there a problem? *British Journal of Anaesthesia* 82: 164–7.

Chestnut DH (1992) Editorial view: Spinal anesthesia in the febrile patient. *Anesthesiology* 76: 667–9.

Colon-Otero G, Cockerill KJ, Bowie EJW (1991) How to diagnose bleeding disorders. *Postgraduate Medicine* 90: 145–50.

Cook TM, Counsel D, Wildsmith JAW (2009) Major complications of central neuraxial block: report on the third national audit project of the Royal College of Anaesthetists. *British Journal of Anaesthesia* 102: 179–90.

Cooke ED, Lloyd MJ, Bowcock SA, Pilcher MF (1976) Monitoring during low-dose heparin prophylaxis. *New England Journal of Medicine* 294: 1066–7.

Crawford JS, James FM, Nolte H, et al. (1981) Regional anaesthesia for patients with chronic neurological disease and similar conditions. *Anaesthesia* 36: 821.

Davis RF, DeBoer LWV, Maroko PR (1986) Thoracic epidural anaesthesia reduces myocardial infarct size after coronary artery occlusion in dogs. *Anesthesia & Analgesia* 65: 711–17.

Devereaux PJ, Yahng H, Yusuf S, et al. (2008) Effects of extended release metoprolol succinate in patients undergoing non-cardiac surgery (POISE trial): a randomised controlled trial. *Lancet* 372: 1962–76.

Dexter F (1998) Regional anesthesia does not significantly change surgical time versus general anesthesia—a meta-analysis of randomized studies. *Regional Anesthesia and Pain Medicine* 23: 439–43.

Eng RHK, Seligman SJ (1981) Lumbar puncture induced meningitis. *Journal of the American Medical Association* 245: 1456–9.

Fettes PDW, Jansson J-R, Wildsmith JAW (2009) Failed spinal anaesthesia: mechanisms, management and prevention. *British Journal of Anaesthesia* 102: 739–48.

Fisher A, Waterhouse TD, Adams AP (1975) Obesity: its relation to anaesthesia. *Anaesthesia* 24: 208–16.

Fisher MM (1984) Intradermal testing to anaesthetic drugs: practical aspects of performance and interpretation. *Anaesthesia and Intensive Care* 12: 115–20.

Freund FG, Bonica JJ, Ward RJ, et al. (1967) Ventilatory reserve and level of motor block during high spinal and epidural anesthesia. *Anesthesiology* 28: 834–7.

Grant IS, Nimmo WS, Clements JA (1981) Pharmacokinetics and analgesic effect of i.m. and oral ketamine. *British Journal of Anaesthesia* 53: 805–9.

Groen RJ, Ponssen H (1990) The spontaneous spinal epidural hematoma. A study of the etiology (review). *Journal of Neurological Science* 98: 121–38.

Gronert GA (1980) Malignant hyperthermia. *Anesthesiology* 53: 395–423.

Hebl JR, Horlocker TT, Schroeder DR (2006) Neuraxial anesthesia and analgesia in patients with pre-existing central nervous system disorder. *Anesthesia & Analgesia* 103: 223–8.

Henderson JJ, Macrae WA (1983) Complications. In Henderson JJ, Nimmo WS (eds) *Practical regional anaesthesia*, pp. 101–12. Oxford: Blackwell.

Hirlekar G (1980) Paraplegia after epidural analgesia associated with an extradural spinal tumour. *Anaesthesia* 35: 363–4.

Hodgkinson R, Husain FJ (1980) Obesity and the cephalad spread of analgesia following epidural administration of bupivacaine for Cesarean section. *Anesthesia & Analgesia* 59: 89–92.

Hogan QH, Prost R, Kulier A (1996) Magnetic resonance imaging of cerebrospinal fluid volume and the influence of body habitus and abdominal pressure. *Anesthesiology* 84: 1341–9.

Holtas S, Heiling M, Lonntoft M (1996) Spontaneous spinal epidural haematoma: findings at MR imaging and clinical correlation. *Radiology* 199: 409–13.

Hopkins PM (2000) Malignant hyperthermia: advances in clinical management and diagnosis. *British Journal of Anaesthesia* 85: 118–28.

Horlocker TT, Wedel DJ, Schlichting JL (1994) Postoperative epidural analgesia and oral anticoagulant therapy. *Anesthesia & Analgesia* 79: 89–93.

Horlocker TT, Wedel DJ, Schroeder DR, et al. (1995) Preoperative antiplatelet therapy does not increase the risk of spinal hematoma associated with regional anesthesia. *Anesthesia & Analgesia* 80: 303–9.

Howells TH, Huntsman RG, Boys JE, Mahmood A (1972) Anaesthesia and sickle-cell haemoglobin, with a case report. *British Journal of Anaesthesia* 44: 975–87.

Hull RD, Pineo GF (2001) Low molecular weight heparin prophylaxis: Preoperative versus postoperative intitiation in patients undergoing elective hip surgery. *Thrombosis Research* 101: V155–62.

Jlala HA, French JL, Foxall GL, et al (2010) Effect of preoperative multimedia information on perioperative anxiety in patients undergoing procedures under regional anaesthesia. *British Journal of Anaesthesia* 104: 369–74.

Katz JD, Krich LB (1976) Acute febrile reaction complicating spinal anaesthesia in a survivor of malignant hyperthermia. *Canadian Anaesthetists' Society Journal* 23: 285–9.

Klassen GA, Bramwell RS, Bromage PR, Zborowska-Sluis DT (1980) Effect of acute sympathectomy by epidural anesthesia on the canine coronary circulation. *Anesthesiology* 52: 8–15.

Kock M, Blomberg S, Emanuelsson H, et al. (1990) Thoracic epidural anesthesia improves global and regional ventricular function during stress-induced myocardial ischemia in patients with coronary artery disease. *Anesthesia & Analgesia* 71: 625–30.

Lambert DH, Deane RS, Mazuzan JE (1982) Anesthesia and the control of blood pressure in patients with spinal cord injury. *Anesthesia & Analgesia* 61: 344–8.

Liu S, Carpenter RL, Neal JM (1995) Epidural anesthesia and analgesia. Their role in postoperative outcome. *Anesthesiology* 82: 1474–506.

Lumpkin MM (1998) FDA Public Health Advisory: Reports of epidural or spinal hematomas with the concurrent use of low molecular weight heparin and with spinal/epidural anesthesia or spinal puncture. *Anesthesiology* 88: 27A–8A.

McDonald SB (2004) Is neuraxial blockade contraindicated in the patient with aortic stenosis? *Regional Anesthesia and Pain Medicine* 29: 496–502.

McQuay HJ, Carroll D, Moore RA (1988) Postoperative orthopaedic pain—the effect of opiate premedication and local anaesthetic blocks. *Pain* 33: 291–5.

Marinacci AA, Courville CB (1958) Electromyogram in evaluation of neurological complications of spinal anaesthesia. *Journal of the American Medical Association* 168: 1337–45.

Mauney FM, Ebert PA, Sabiston DC (1970) Postoperative myocardial infarction. A study of predisposing factors, diagnosis and mortality rate in a high risk group of surgical patients. *Annals of Surgery* 172: 497–502.

Moore DC (1976) *Regional block* (4th edn). Springfield, IL: CC Thomas.

Muller H, Sarges R, Jouaux J, Runte W, Lampante L (1990) Intraoperative suppression of spasticity by intrathecal baclofen. *Anaesthetist* 39: 22–9.

Nielsen CH (1989) Bleeding after intercostal nerve block in a patient anticoagulated with heparin. *Anesthesiology* 71: 162–4.

Odoom JA, Sih IL (1983) Epidural analgesia and anticoagulant therapy. Experience with one thousand cases of continuous epidurals. *Anaesthesia* 38: 254–9.

Page MM, Watkins PJ (1978) Cardiorespiratory arrest and diabetic autonomic neuropathy. *Lancet* i: 14–16.

Reiz S (1989) Circulatory effects of epidural anesthesia in patients with cardiac disease. *Acta Anaesthesiologica Belgica* 30: 21–7.

Reiz S, Nath S, Rais O (1980) Effects of thoracic epidural block and prenalterol on coronary vascular resistance and myocardial metabolism in patients with coronary artery disease. *Acta Anaesthesiologica Scandinavica* 24: 11–16.

Samford C, Sibley W, Laguna J (1978) Anesthesia in multiple sclerosis. *Canadian Journal of Neurological Science* 5: 41–8.

Schonwald G, Fish KJ, Perkash I (1981) Cardiovascular complications during anesthesia in chronic spinal cord injured patients. *Anesthesiology* 55: 550–8.

Schwander D, Bachmann F (1991) Heparin and spinal or epidural anesthesia. Decision analysis [review]. *Annales Françaises d'Anesthesie Reanimation* 10: 284–96.

Seltzer JL, Porretta JC, Jackson BG (1977) Plastic particulate contaminants in the medicine cups of disposable non-spinal regional anesthesia sets. *Anesthesiology* 47: 378–9.

Sharma SK, Philip J, Whitter CW, Udaya BP (1999) Assessment of changes in coagulation in parturients with preeclampsia using thromboelastography. *Anesthesiology* 90: 385–90.

Somerville TG, Gibson M (1973) Particulate contamination in ampoules: a comparative study. *Pharmaceutical Journal* 211: 128–31.

Steen PA, Tinker JH, Tarhan S (1978) Myocardial infarction after anesthesia and surgery. *Journal of the American Medical Association* 239: 2566–70.

Strunin L (1993) Editorial: How long should patients fast before surgery? Time for new guidelines. *British Journal of Anaesthesia* 70: 1–3.

Taivainen T, Tuominen M, Rosenberg PH (1990) Influence of obesity on the spread of spinal analgesia after injection of plain 0.5% bupivacaine at the L3–4 or L4–5 interspace. *British Journal of Anaesthesia* 64: 542–6.

Thomas DP (1997) Does low molecular weight heparin cause less bleeding? *Thrombosis and Haemostasis* 78: 1422–5.

Toft P, Jorgensen A (1989) Continuous thoracic epidural analgesia for the control of pain in myocardial infarction. *Intensive Care Medicine* 13: 388–9.

Tryba M (1993) Epidural anesthesia and low molecular weight heparin: Pro. *Anasthesiol Intensivmed Notfallmed Schmerzther* 28: 179–81.

Tryba M, Wedel DJ (1997) Central neuraxial block and low molecular weight heparin (enoxaparine): lessons learned from different dosage regimens in two continents. *Acta Anaesthesiologica Scandinavica* 41: 100–3.

Tuman KJ, McCarthy RJ, March RJ, et al. (1991) The effects of epidural anesthesia and analgesia on coagulation and outcome after major vascular surgery. *Anesthesia & Analgesia* 73: 696–704.

Vandermeulen EP, Van Aken H, Vermylen J (1994) Anticoagulants and spinal-epidural anaesthesia. *Anesthesia & Analgesia* 79: 1165–77.

Wadhwa RK (1977) Obstetric anesthesia for a patient with malignant hyperthermia susceptibility. *Anesthesiology* 46: 63–4.

Weiss MG, Adkinson NF, Hirshman CA (1989) Evaluation of allergic drug reactions in the peri-operative period. *Anesthesiology* 71: 483–6.

Whitten CW, Greilich PE (2000) Thromboelastography: Past, present and future. *Anesthesiology* 92: 1223–5.

Wildsmith JAW, McClure JH (1991) Editorial: anticoagulant drugs and central nerve blockade. *Anaesthesia* 46: 613–14.

Wildsmith JAW, Mason A, McKinnon RP, Rae SM (1998) Allergy to local anaesthetic drugs is rare but does occur. *British Dental Journal* 184: 507–10.

Wu CL, Perkins FM (1996) Oral anticoagulant prophylaxis and epidural catheter removal. *Regional Anesthesia* 21: 517–24.

Wysowski DK, Talarico L, Bacsanyi J, Botstein P (1998) Spinal and epidural hematoma and low-molecular-weight-heparin. *New England Journal of Medicine* 338: 1774–5.

Yeager MP, Glass DD, Neff RK, Brinck-Johnson T (1987) Epidural anaesthesia and analgesia in high risk surgical patients. *Anesthesiology* 66: 729–36.

CHAPTER 10

Peripheral nerve location techniques

George Corner and Calum Grant

Safe and effective peripheral block requires injection of an appropriate dose of local anaesthetic solution close to the target nerve, and the localization techniques described here allow the anaesthetist to position the needle tip correctly, either next to the nerve or in the correct fascial plane. Patient discomfort should be minimized and care taken to avoid trauma to surrounding structures (e.g. blood vessels and pleura) as well as to the nerves themselves.

A wide range of methods, from the solely anatomical to the technologically complex, is now available, but it must be stressed that a thorough understanding of the relevant anatomy is fundamental to *all* of the nerve localization techniques described in this chapter. No technological aid, ultrasound included, is a surrogate for knowledge of both the relevant anatomy and the specific block technique, nor is it an excuse for ignoring the principles of patient selection and management during (and after) block performance. The possible localization techniques are:

1. *Anatomical landmarks*: surface anatomy is used in conjunction with knowledge of the standard course of the nerve to identify where the local anaesthetic should be injected (e.g. saphenous block below the knee). The correct depth of injection may be further refined using tactile sensation: a 'pop' is noted as a short bevel needle penetrates the deep fascia covering the correct myofascial plane (e.g. ilio-inguinal nerve).

2. *Elicitation of paraesthesiae*: gentle contact of needle tip with nerve will generate paraesthesiae in its distribution.

3. *Electrical stimulation*: low current stimulation of the motor component of a mixed peripheral nerve will generate a 'twitch' in the muscles supplied by it.

4. *Ultrasound guidance*: the preceding two techniques rely on a knowledge of standard anatomy to identify the initial needle insertion point, but real-time ultrasound scanning allows the relevant nerves (and surrounding structures) to be identified first. Thus individual variation can be allowed for, and (often) both needle position and local anaesthetic spread visualized.

5. *Complex imaging*: modern radiological techniques have a key role in chronic pain practice (see Chapter 23), but their lack of 'portability' means that they are rarely used in anaesthesia. However, developments in operating theatre design and advances in technology may mean that this changes in the future.

The main focus of this chapter is on paraesthesiae, electrostimulation, and ultrasound guidance.

Paraesthesiae

Until the advent of nerve stimulators about 30 years ago, peripheral nerves could only be identified in conscious patients by eliciting paraesthesiae, an 'electrical' type of sensation radiating in the distribution of the nerve after direct contact by the needle. The position of the nerve is predicted from the anaesthetist's knowledge of anatomy and palpation of the relevant landmarks, and the needle advanced gently in its direction until the patient reports sensations, often described as 'pins and needles', in the distribution of the nerve.

The principal advantage of this technique is that the only equipment needed is a needle, but there are significant drawbacks. Contact between needle tip and nerve may cause discomfort, and several needle passes may be necessary due to operator inexperience or anatomical variation, so increasing the possibility of inadvertent damage to surrounding structures and subsequent neurological dysfunction (Selander et al. 1979). Further, it is not a suitable technique for children or adults unlikely or unwilling to tolerate a block procedure while conscious, and many patients have difficulty understanding what they should report as the needle is advanced. Finally, there has long been controversy regarding the risk of nerve damage as a consequence of deliberately making contact between needle and nerve.

Peripheral nerve stimulation

The pioneer of electrical stimulation in regional anaesthesia, as early as 1912, was the German surgeon, Georg Perthes (Goerg & Agarwal 2000), who identified nerves by eliciting a muscle response using a specially designed injection needle which incorporated a stimulating electrode. However, it was not until the development of more advanced and reliable portable devices from the 1960s onward that peripheral nerve stimulation gained any popularity. Thereafter, progressive increases in use led to it being considered the 'gold standard' for nerve localization by the end of the 20th century, although a thorough understanding of equipment requirements and function, as well as an appreciation of some of the technical limitations of the devices, are required.

Electrophysiological issues

In vivo application of an electrical current from the tip of an otherwise insulated regional block needle will elicit a response when the needle tip is in close proximity to the nerve. The clinical response may be either motor or sensory, depending on the function of the underlying nerve and the intensity of the electrical stimulus. The electrical charge applied to a nerve by a peripheral nerve stimulator (PNS) is a product of the current (milliamps) and the duration of the electrical impulse (milliseconds). The PNS should be designed to deliver a 'square wave' impulse to allow more precise delivery of the charge, an important issue because of the relationship between the total charge required and the distance between the tip of the stimulating needle and the target nerve. If less charge is required to produce a response it is reliable evidence that the needle tip has moved closer to the nerve. Thus a PNS allows the clinician to identify the location of a nerve or plexus and, most importantly, the point at which the needle tip is close enough to ensure a successful block.

There is a characteristic relationship between the strength and duration of the electrical stimulus required to depolarize a peripheral nerve (Pither et al. 1985). A plot of the two variables (Figure 10.1) can be used to obtain both the 'rheobase', the minimum current required to stimulate the nerve (note: this has a relatively long duration), and the 'chronaxie', the stimulus duration required to depolarize the nerve at twice the rheobase current. The chronaxie is used to compare the stimulation threshold of different nerves, and it has been shown that large myelinated fibres have a shorter chronaxie than small, unmyelinated pain fibres (Casey 1975, Koslow 1973, Shaefer 1940). In clinical practice this means that a mixed peripheral nerve can be located by using short duration pulses to stimulate the motor component preferentially. This produces involuntary muscle contraction without the pain which would result at higher currents, so making the procedure more acceptable to patients.

Discomfort is further minimized by using the correct polarity (configuration of cathode and anode) when establishing the electrical circuit because of the phenomenon of preferential cathodal stimulation (Pither et al. 1985). Because the exterior of the axon has a positive potential relative to the interior (Chapter 6), much less current is required to depolarize the nerve through a cathode than an anode, stimulation through the latter actually hyperpolarizing the membrane immediately adjacent to the needle. Thus the exploring needle should be attached to the cathode terminal of the stimulator and the anode (or ground electrode) to a standard electrocardiogram (ECG) skin electrode making good contact with the patient's skin a short distance away.

For routine clinical use a PNS (Figure 10.2) must be robust, portable, and designed to take the earlier mentioned points into account (stimulators for generating a muscle twitch for monitoring neuromuscular block are *not* suitable). As noted earlier, a square wave pulse is required, together with the means for both varying and displaying its strength. The pulse duration should be short ($\approx$ 1 msec), and its delivery frequency (usually 1–2 Hz) should allow ready identification of the resultant muscle twitch without disturbing the needle position or causing patient discomfort. Portability implies battery operation so there must be a facility for checking its status and an indicator (audible or visible) of pulse delivery. Finally, the terminals should be clearly marked as anode and cathode or (better still) the connecting leads should be configured so that only the cathode can be connected to the exploring needle.

Most of the relevant physical principles are important to the design and set-up of a PNS, but one, the inverse square law, is more relevant to its clinical use. This law means that the current required to depolarize a nerve is inversely proportional to the square of its distance from the needle or, more directly, that the current will increase fourfold if the distance doubles. Thus the clinician must still be able to place the needle reasonably close to the nerve using anatomical landmarks etc. if high currents and associated patient discomfort are to be avoided.

Needle selection

The aim of electrical stimulation is to identify that the needle tip is close to the nerve so that the local anaesthetic is deposited where its effect will be optimum. However, current can flow from any part of the needle shaft, not just the tip, and this can have consequences which may confuse the clinician. First, most block techniques involve needle insertion close to (or even through) skeletal muscle, electrical stimulation of which can cause depolarization and resultant twitch. Second, if the needle tip has been inserted too far initially the shaft may be in close proximity to the nerve and allow a depolarizing current to produce a muscle twitch in the expected

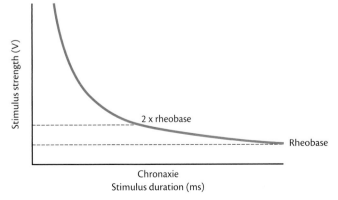

Figure 10.1 Strength duration curve for peripheral nerve stimulation.

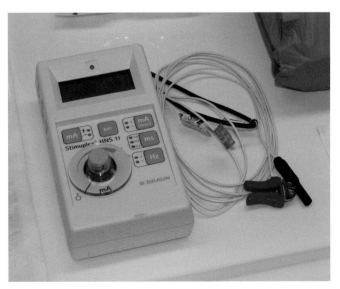

Figure 10.2 A typical nerve stimulator.

distribution. Unless these sources of error are recognized, the injection will be made in the wrong place.

To avoid these possibilities peripheral nerve block needles with all but the tip of the shaft coated with Teflon or a similar polymer are available, such 'insulation' meaning that any muscle twitch can only result from current flowing from the tip. Insulated needles are more expensive, and there is no definitive evidence of clinical benefit (e.g. improved block success rates or reduced complications) to support their use, but many practitioners feel more confident (an important consideration) when using them.

Using a peripheral nerve stimulator

If neurostimulation is to be used, a description of what will happen, especially involuntary muscle contraction, should be part of the explanation given to the patient, and this should be reinforced at intervals during the procedure. As with any other piece of equipment, the anaesthetist and assistant must be thoroughly familiar with the PNS in use; its proper function, including the fit of the connections, should be checked before the patient arrives—a stock of spare batteries is essential. Finally, all the routine preliminaries to a block (monitoring, intravenous access, patient position) should be established before stimulation starts.

The precise position of the ground electrode is not crucial, but it should not be too far from the block site and should ensure that the current path does not cross the myocardium or other peripheral nerves. It is essential that good (low-resistance) electrical contact is made by using a good quality adhesive ECG electrode for the anode, and placing it on an area of clean, dry skin where it will not be disturbed during the procedure. The aseptic preliminaries to the block are then completed, leaving the assistant to operate the controls thereafter. Where these functions are adjustable, pulse duration is usually set to 100 msec, frequency to 1 Hz, and the initial intensity to 1.5–2.0 mA.

The relevant anatomy is checked to confirm the needle insertion point, and the site is infiltrated with local anaesthetic (typically 1% lidocaine). The needle is inserted superficially and the indicator on the PNS used to confirm that the circuit is complete before the needle is advanced in the appropriate direction. If there is no muscle twitch, or it is not in the expected distribution, the needle tip is withdrawn to the subcutaneous tissues and its direction reassessed. Once the expected motor response has been elicited the current is reduced until it stops and the needle then advanced until it reappears. The process is repeated systematically until good muscle contractions are sustained at the 'optimum' current, usually considered to be 0.5 mA.

The needle should not be moved while each reduction in the stimulus current is being made, and it must be kept perfectly still once the desired end-point has been achieved at 0.5 mA, but the process does not end there. If a motor response occurs with a stimulus current below 0.5 mA the needle tip may be intraneural in position (Bigeleisen et al. 2009, Robards et al. 2009, Sala-Blanch et al. 2009) so it is worth confirming that the twitch *disappears* as the current is reduced below that figure. If it persists, the needle should be withdrawn very slightly and particular care taken during local anaesthetic injection that there is no evidence (e.g. excessive injection pressure or patient discomfort) of intraneural injection.

The final check of needle position is to inject 1–2 ml of local anaesthetic and observe that the motor twitches stops and then returns after a few seconds as the nerve is pushed away from the needle by the injected fluid, and then returns to is original position as the fluid dissipates. If the motor response persists after the initial injection, the possibilities of intraneural or intravascular injection should be considered and a check made that the output of the PNS is not inappropriately high.

Ultrasound guidance

The availability of conveniently sized portable ultrasound devices with an appropriate level of discrimination is the most significant innovation in regional anaesthesia during the past decade. Ultrasound is a very suitable method, with minimal safety issues, for imaging soft tissues for invasive procedures in the clinical setting, and its introduction has driven a major increase in the popularity of block techniques. Doppler ultrasound was first used to locate the subclavian artery during supraclavicular brachial plexus block well over 30 years ago (Lagrange et al. 1978), but a further 16 years elapsed before the first report of ultrasound guided nerve localization (also supraclavicular block) appeared (Kapral et al. 1994). Since then the applicability and availability of ultrasound equipment in anaesthesia have increased progressively, although the devices are expensive, and interpretation of the images requires training and experience. However, both cost and image quality are improving constantly, and many already consider it the 'gold standard' for peripheral nerve block techniques. It may not be too long before it is simply the 'standard'.

Perhaps the most outstanding potential benefit (Table 10.1) of using ultrasound guidance is that the clinician is no longer restricted by trying to make the individual patient's anatomy conform to the descriptions in the standard landmark based techniques. With ultrasound the relevant nerves can be visualized along their entire length, and the point of block chosen to ensure that surgical requirements are met, patient comfort maintained, and critical anatomical structures (often the source of complications) avoided. Once the injection point has been chosen, the spread of the solution can be monitored to ensure that it reaches all of the required nerves to produce a fully effective block. Initially, only the more superficial nerves could be visualized satisfactorily, but technical developments are overcoming this limitation, with even the central neuraxis starting to become accessible (Karmakar et al. 2009). Progressively smaller structures are also being visualized, although continued development is needed to improve identification of the needle within the field of view and observation of the spread of local anaesthetic.

Table 10.1 Potential benefits of ultrasound-guided nerve block.

◆ Accuracy of needle placement
◆ Visualization of local anaesthetic spread in real time
◆ Additional local anaesthetic deposition
◆ Compensation for anatomical variation
◆ Avoidance of intraneural/intravascular injection
◆ Reduced complications, e.g. pleural puncture
◆ Wide variety of approaches (not landmark dependent)
◆ Rapid block onset
◆ Reduced local anaesthetic dosage
◆ Avoidance of nerve stimulation-related fracture site pain

Basic principles

Ultrasound imaging in medicine was developed from the sonar range finding devices used at sea (Hill 2006). The technique relies on measuring the 'time of flight', the time taken for an ultrasonic pulse to return after being sent out in a known direction and reflected back from the target structures. From these time signals modern computing power can be used to construct an image for display (see Hoskins and colleagues (2010) for a comprehensive discussion).

Ultrasound is, by definition, sound of a frequency higher than the threshold of human hearing (<20 kHz). In general medical applications the frequencies used are 2–18 MHz, although 30 MHz and higher can be used in specialist work. Sound itself is a pressure wave in air, and longitudinal waves (where particles of the medium move in line with the direction of propagation of the wave) are used in ultrasound imaging as opposed to transverse or shear waves which vibrate at right angles to their direction.

Some basic physical attributes aid in the creation of an ultrasound image. The range of the speed of sound in different soft tissues is small enough for an average of 1540 m s^{-1} to be assumed in computations. This is important because distance is calculated, as noted earlier, from the time of flight. Some ultrasound energy is scattered at each change of acoustic impedance—effectively at each tissue boundary—with the energy reflected back to the receiver being detected and used to build up the image. Only part of the total energy is scattered at each tissue interface, the remainder passing on to allow visualization of underlying structures. The depth of such tissue penetration is greater with lower frequency signals, but higher frequencies produce better resolution between structures in the field. Thus, the precise frequency used (Table 10.2) depends on the depth of the target nerve.

Other physical properties work against the creation of a good image. Although the speed of sound is similar in different tissues, it is not the same—fat, in particular, can distort the image. A more diffuse distortion, the grainy appearance characteristic of ultrasound images and reducing their clarity, is known as 'speckle'. It is due to a simple physical phenomenon and does not represent the true surface appearance of the target structures. Ultrasound waves from the source are 'coherent', different points across the beam retain a constant phase (i.e. they remain 'in step'), but reflected signals are out of step and can interfere with each other. Sometimes this is additive, sometimes the reverse, but the overall effect is to degrade the sharpness of the image. Holograms produced by coherent laser light are due to the same effect.

Ultrasound signals are attenuated (reduced in amplitude) by all tissues (muscle more than fat and connective tissue) so that only very small signals are reflected back to be detected. Thus, very high gain amplification with a large dynamic range (to deal with the faintest signals from depth and stronger signals from near the surface) is needed, yet the background 'noise' level must be very low. Ultrasound is heavily attenuated in air and bone, and reflected strongly by both. Thus, although ultrasound is excellent for imaging soft tissues, it cannot image through bone and air-filled tissue (e.g. normal lung and intestine).

Because ultrasound waves of the frequency and intensity used in imaging do not penetrate bone it casts a 'shadow' in the image. It is by addressing these inherent problems that the vast improvements in image quality have been achieved over the last half century.

The transducer

In medical applications it is normal to use a single transmitter/receiver—the 'probe' or 'transducer'. The source of the ultrasound is made of 'piezo-electric' material, a substance which distorts when subjected to an electrical field and, conversely, generates an electric potential when distorted. The piezo-electric materials used over the years have been in single crystal, ceramic, and composite forms (Foster 2000), and the performance of an imaging system is fundamentally dependent on their properties and efficiencies. Early systems used a single element as both source and receiver, and it was scanned mechanically between each successive 'firing' to build up an image. The single element was either curved or an acoustic lens was fitted to focus the beam at an appropriate fixed distance.

Modern transducers (Figure 10.3) consist of an array (a single line) of piezo-electric elements, commonly 128 or 256 in number. A group of elements is activated, sends out a beam and the reflected signal is detected. Adjacent groups of elements are then activated in turn to produce a series of beams across the face of the transducer and complete the field of scan. During both transmit and receive modes, variable focusing of these beams can be applied '*in plane*' (that is in the line of the array) by applying a phase delay to the signals to or from individual elements nearer the centre of the probe. Focusing '*out of plane*' (at right angles to the array) is generally fixed and reliant on a lens. The piezo-electric material is set in a backing layer which does not resonate and keeps the ultrasound pulses short for optimal axial resolution. The matching layers are tuned for thickness and acoustic properties to maximize the two-way transfer of energy between the piezo-electric material and the tissues.

Table 10.2 Indicative frequencies for target depth with examples of use.

Frequency (MHz)	Target depth (mm)	Block example
10–14	10–40	Interscalene
7–10	40–50	Infraclavicular
4–8	60–150	Sciatic

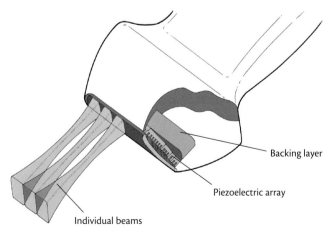

Figure 10.3 Components of a transducer head.

Image formation

Signals reflected back arrive at a time dependent on the depth from which they have come according to the equation

$$T = D/2v$$

where T = time, D = distance, and v = speed of sound. The factor of 2 is required because the signal has to travel to the reflection point and back again.

From the timing and known direction of the beam, the location of the source of the echo is calculated and stored. These data are then mapped to a display device or image file, each echo being located by its coordinates, and with its intensity recorded on a grey scale. This file is updated with each cycle of beam activations across the array, the frequency of this being known as the 'frame rate', and the dynamic store of information as the 'scan converter'. It takes a finite time to gather all the channels of data and 'refresh' the image, this refresh rate equalling the frame rate. It is commonly of the order of 100 Hz, but as long as it is above 4 Hz the eye will not detect any flickering in the image. The frame rate is affected by the depth of scan (it takes longer for signals to reach and return from deeper targets) and by the concurrent collection of other data (e.g. during Doppler scanning or when using compound imaging—see following section).

When the 'freeze' button on a scanner is operated, scanning stops (to reduce the energy emitted and avoid over-heating the transducer) and the data currently held in the scanner memory are displayed. It is usually possible to track back through a number of previous frames.

Doppler imaging

Doppler ultrasound detects motion by measuring the frequency change in the signal scattered from a moving target. In colour Doppler, different degrees of frequency shift are displayed as a range of colours superimposed over the grey-scale image in the region of interest. This facility is very useful for identifying blood vessels, distinguishing between pulsatile arteries and non-pulsatile veins, and also indicating direction of flow. However, modern scanners give such clear images that major blood vessels are identified easily without colour supplementation. Blood cells scatter ultrasound poorly so major vessels appear as distinct anechoic structures, although Doppler is useful for confirming whether a small structure is a vessel or not.

Refining the image

Basic ultrasound scans are fairly crude so a range of techniques is used to refine the image displayed.

Speckle reduction

Speckle is removed by image processing to enhance the signal to noise ratio, essentially by analysing the frequencies in the reflected signals rather than their spatial coordinates. Many algorithms (Abd-Elmonien et al. 2002, Achim et al. 2001, Gupta et al. 2004, Yongjian et al. 2002) are available, and each equipment manufacturer has its own approach. In some systems the amount of such processing can be adjusted so that the image varies from being highly speckled to rather diffuse when too much processing is applied.

Compound imaging

Compound images are constructed by combining signals obtained from various angles, commonly up to 10 or more, and not just those reflected straight back to the transmitting piezo-electric. The background noise signals (clutter) cancel each other out, but the signals from substantive features add up. Early systems used such scanning techniques, but when real-time imaging was introduced the scanners did not have the speed or computing power to process multiple images. However, increased computer power, and the introduction of electronic arrays, allowed the technique to be re-introduced in the 1990s. A particular variation of this is used when a specific angle is used for the additional scan to aid in identifying the inserted needle.

Harmonic imaging

Tissue behaves non-linearly—it does not compress in proportion to the stress applied—with the result that the sound wave is distorted as it passes through so that, instead of being a wave with a single frequency, harmonics (multiples of frequencies) are introduced. These harmonics are strongest in the centre of the beam where the useful energy is, they are less prevalent in the scattered energy from side sections or outside the beam. If harmonic signals are selectively deleted the result is a clearer image with improved resolution, but with tissue penetration maintained (Humphrey 2003). It is important to realize that the harmonic component is generated in the tissue, not by the transducer.

Time gain compensation and optimization

To balance the intensity of the image over the depth of the field of view the scanner automatically increases the gain during the receive window of each beam position. This is called 'time gain compensation' and can be fine tuned to the patient using slide controls. When scanning in the elderly or through muscle, which attenuates ultrasound more than other soft tissues, far gain (the amplification of signals from deeper structures) may have to be raised differentially compared to near gain. Conversely it may need to be lowered when scanning through less attenuating tissue such as fat. However, making such adjustments can be a distraction from the clinical procedure.

In fact, modern scanners readily produce acceptable images by having appropriate default settings for gain, depth, and other options selected by using customised pre-set figures, but many incorporate an 'optimization' facility which 'sharpens' the image. This can work in one of several different ways, but in general it analyses the image and optimizes electronically some property such as the gain or the grey scale used, and corrects for variations in the speed of sound.

Multidimensional imaging

Systems displaying data in three dimensions, basically produced by combining a longitudinal series of conventional ultrasound scans, have found use in obstetrics. Obviously, real-time scanning with a frame rate greater than 4 Hz is needed for regional block applications, but equipment with this capability is bulky, complex, and expensive. There are some reports assessing the applicability of these systems to both peripheral (Feinglass et al. 2007, Foxhall et al. 2007) and central neuraxial block (Belavy et al. 2011), but they do not yet seem to convey any overall advantage. The technical details of such advanced systems are beyond further consideration here.

Sono-anatomy

The essence of ultrasound-guided nerve localization is that each of the relevant tissues (nerve, blood vessels, muscle, pleura, and bone) each has a sufficiently characteristic appearance to enable them to be distinguished. Because of its high levels of reflection and acoustic impedance relative to the surrounding soft tissues, bone appears as a distinct hyperechoic line which casts a hypoechoic 'shadow' beyond the surface nearest to the transducer. Muscles are hypoechoic with hyperechoic flecks throughout, and are seen as circumscribed structures delineated in transverse section by the surrounding fascial planes. Blood scatters ultrasound weakly so vessel lumens are hypoechoic, but the walls are hyperechoic and are seen clearly; veins are compressible and non-pulsatile whereas arteries are relatively incompressible and pulsatile. Fascial planes (e.g. fascia iliaca) have a typically bright, hyperechoic appearance.

Tendons often have a similar ultrasound appearance to peripheral nerves, and it is clearly important to be able to differentiate between them. This can be achieved by scanning proximally; peripheral nerves generally increase in size, but tendons change in appearance, gradually merging with the muscle from which they arise and becoming less discreet. However, matters are complicated by the different appearance of nerves in the various anatomical areas of interest. Above the clavicle, in the interscalene groove and supraclavicular fossa, the nerves of the brachial plexus have a typical hypoechoic appearance, but in the infraclavicular fossa, the axilla, and more distally the nerves become hyperechoic with a characteristic 'honeycomb' appearance. This change in appearance is due to increasing amounts of connective tissue in the epineurium surrounding the fascicles as the plexus courses distally in the upper limb. The nerves of the lower limb are typically hyperechoic, but their deeper anatomical locations make the lumbar plexus and sciatic nerves challenging to visualize compared to the nerves of the brachial plexus. Lower frequency ultrasound is required for effective tissue penetration at these locations, but there is an associated loss of definition.

The echogenicity of peripheral nerve changes with the angle of incidence of the ultrasound beam, optimal clarity and definition usually being achieved when it is close to 90º. However, this will depend on the characteristics of the surface being imaged so the probe should be angled back and forth until the optimum picture is obtained. Imaging the sciatic nerve in the popliteal fossa provides a good example of this phenomenon because the nerve's course is from deep in the thigh to a more superficial position in the popliteal fossa. The image of the nerve can be improved significantly by making minor adjustments to the angle of the probe.

Challenges in ultrasound use

Needle location

While fine anatomical structures can be identified readily, needles are difficult to locate because a structure can only be 'seen' if it causes ultrasound to be reflected back to the receiving transducer. Tissue scatters the energy diffusely in all directions, but metal needles are polished to enable their easy passage through the tissues, and they act as 'specular' reflectors. In specular reflection the beam travels on at an angle equal to the angle of incidence with the surface (as in a mirror) and almost all of the energy is transmitted onwards into the body. Larger diameter needles (e.g. 18 g Tuohy)

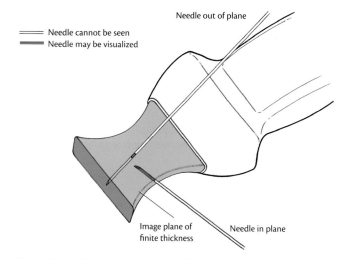

Figure 10.4 In-plane and out-of-plane needle positions.

are easier to visualize because they are more easily detected in the narrow ultrasound beam, but they produce greater tissue trauma than the smaller conventional peripheral block needles. The latter are more easily visualized if inserted at shallow angles in plane with the transducer, although the tip is better visualized using an out of plane approach at an angle of insertion greater than 60° (Figure 10.4) (Schafhalter-Zoppoth 2004).

Many different manufacturing techniques (coating, erosion (mechanical or chemical), and machining of the surface) have been tried to improve the ultrasonic 'visibility' of finer gauge needles, but the discontinuities in the surface must be smaller than the wavelength of the sound to produce significant scattering. Some new needles (Deam et al. 2007) have surfaces which are intended to improve ultrasound reflection at both superficial and steeper angles of insertion. Their reflecting surfaces have geometrically designed indentations circumferentially positioned around the needle shaft, just proximal to the needle tip and extending a variable length (typically 20 mm) from it (Figure 10.5). Evidence is emerging that

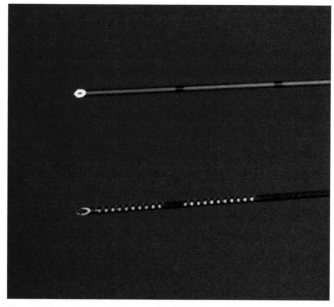

Figure 10.5 Standard and ultrasound 'visible' block needles.

visualization of such needles is superior at steeper angles of insertion (Munirama et al. 2012).

Transducer suitability

Most conventional transducers are designed for diagnostic imaging where they are the only equipment in the operator's hand and the image obtained is the main consideration. Consequently, they are not ergonomically well suited for use in regional anaesthesia where the needle and associated equipment must be manipulated concurrently. This is but one of the challenges in learning how to use ultrasound guidance for nerve block procedures.

As noted earlier, higher frequencies produce better images, but they are more heavily attenuated so there is a trade off between penetration and resolution. The probe frequency should be selected according to the depth of the target (Table 10.2), but lower frequencies may be needed in heavily muscled patients (e.g. athletes and manual workers) because muscle attenuates ultrasound more than fat and connective tissue.

Probe cables are connected using multipin plugs which are damaged easily, especially if changes are hurried, so a system which allows transducers to be switched without unplugging can be an advantage.

Equipment foot-print, cost, and ergonomics

Anaesthetic rooms are usually small and already crowded so finding room for an additional piece of equipment can be difficult. Ultrasound scanners come in a wide range of sizes and shapes, but the temptation to specify a small, very portable system should be resisted (the equipment used to guide central vein cannulation is inappropriate for regional anaesthesia). Equipment for this work should have as small a foot-print as possible to make it convenient to use, and be reasonably mobile to allow it to be moved from place to place, but there is no doubt that the bigger the screen (and thus the rest of the system), the better the image (and the greater the price!). Recently, some dedicated scanning systems, which can be wall or pole mounted, have been introduced in 'tablet' format with a touch screen, and have the great advantage of being easy to clean.

Neck strain injury is a constant risk for anaesthetists, and it is important that this is not exacerbated by using ultrasound. The screen should be placed where it is easily viewed with the minimum of head movement and certainly without twisting. It may be an advantage to have an assistant make any instrument adjustment required when seeking the optimum image.

Practical use of ultrasound scanning

The first step in the practical use of ultrasound is the recognition that this is an expensive and delicate piece of equipment which must be handled carefully, particularly the multiple pin connection between probe cable and instrument. Important preliminaries are making sure that the patient is comfortable and properly positioned, and aligning the probe to the monitor so that the orientation of the image is clear. Good contact between probe and patient must be ensured by the liberal application of lubricant jelly to exclude any air which might obscure the image.

Peripheral nerves can be imaged in both longitudinal and transverse section, but most ultrasound-guided block techniques use two-dimensional images of the target nerve in transverse section. This usually provides the most useful information on the surrounding anatomical structures (blood vessels, pleura, etc.) and allows assessment of the extent of local anaesthetic spread around the nerve.

However, scanning should be seen as a dynamic process. The user develops, perhaps over several minutes, a three-dimensional appreciation of the local anatomy by visualizing the block site longitudinally as well as transversely. Establishing the depth of the target nerve is a key aspect because over-insertion of the needle is a common error and an obvious cause of damage to deeper structures.

Once a clear picture has been obtained an aseptic field is created, the probe being covered by a sterile sheath. Thereafter, the details of technique will depend on the particular block being performed, a major issue being whether the needle is inserted in or out of plane with the transducer head. Good quality transducers produce a beam of no more than a few millimetres in thickness so the precision of in-plane alignment is critical, but it will allow the needle track to be seen if the angle of insertion is close to parallel with the transducer head. The view obtained should help avoid direct contact with nerves, arteries, and related structures such as the pleura. Out-of-plane approaches are technically simpler, and the needle tip may be visualized when it reaches the beam, but no information is obtained on structures in the needle's path. In practice, much additional information is obtained with both techniques by observing tissue deformation produced by the needle's advance or by the incremental injection of small aliquots (circa 1 ml) of local anaesthetic or 5% glucose ('hydro-localization').

Paraesthesiae, stimulation, or ultrasound?

Paraesthesiae

Despite the apparent shortcomings of using paraesthesiae for nerve identification, block success rates comparable to those achieved with nerve stimulation (>90%) were reported without any increased risk of subsequent neurological dysfunction (Liguori et al. 2006). Many expert practitioners of regional anaesthesia used paraesthesiae for nerve identification throughout their careers with high success rates and minimal sequelae, but that was at a time when there was no alternative and it was possible to acquire extensive experience in a relatively short period of time. Neither point applies today, with nerve stimulation and (even more so) ultrasonography providing more definitive indication of nerve location.

However, ultrasound imaging has, perhaps somewhat ironically, provided valuable insights into what can happen when using paraesthesiae. Using ultrasound as the determinant of outcome during axillary block, paraesthesiae were judged to be less than 40% (and neurostimulation only 75%) sensitive (Perlas et al. 2006). Further, the incidence of intraneural injection (observed with ultrasound) during axillary block after nerve identification with paraesthesiae was reported to be as high as 81% (Bigeliesen 2006). Interestingly, despite this apparently high incidence of intraneural injection no neurological sequelae were reported, although the investigators were able to reposition the needle if subepineural injection was suspected.

Nerve stimulation

Nerve stimulation superseded elicitation of paraesthesia for nerve localization and, theoretically at least, allowed the user to confirm needle tip position *on*, rather than *in*, the nerve. It provides a more objective indication of nerve position, specific motor responses, for example, allowing the user to identify the musculocutaneous and radial nerves far more reliably in axillary block (Coventry et al. 2001). Perhaps the main advantage is that it provides an indication of the nerve's position, and the required needle angulation, *before* the nerve has actually been reached. The safeguards outlined earlier should make intraneural injection less likely, and it is a technique which can be used in anaesthetized patients, children in particular.

However, stimulation has limitations as a technique for nerve localization. The output from different instruments can be variable (Jochum et al. 2006) and poor anode connection can result in excessive voltage being applied (Hadzic & Vloka 2000). Variation in the electrical impedance of human tissue can influence the current required (Sauter et al. 2009), and the stimulation current can be significantly greater in patients with peripheral neuropathy (Sites et al. 2003). Some patients find the involuntary motor responses uncomfortable, and the twitches can cause severe pain in patients with limb injuries. Finally, the technique provides no information about other structures (e.g. blood vessels, pleura) which the needle may contact with the risk of complications.

Peripheral nerve simulation is still widely used (Brull et al. 2008), but it is being superseded by ultrasound, to an extent because the latter is, as with paraesthesiae, questioning long-held beliefs about the older technique. Studies have shown that a needle placed close to the nerve produces an appropriate motor response at 0.5 mA in only 75% of axillary (Perlas et al. 2006) and no more than 46% of popliteal blocks (Perlas et al. 2008). Further, the median stimulation thresholds for intra- and extraneural needle placements during ultrasound-guided supraclavicular block were 0.3 and 0.6 mA respectively (Bigeleisen et al. 2009), although it is difficult to exclude bias due to subjective ultrasound interpretation in such studies.

Ultrasound guidance

Ultrasound guidance avoids many of the problems of using paraesthesiae or nerve stimulation, has no inherent side effects, and has aspects which are not available with the other methods. However, suitable equipment is very expensive, and the cost must be justified, yet some published comparisons have not shown any clear improvements in block success rates (Liguori et al. 2006, Liu et al. 2009, Walker et al. 2009) or the incidence of neurological complications (Abrahams et al. 2009, Liguori et al. 2006, Liu et al. 2009, Walker et al. 2009). However, those results are perhaps as much a testament to the skills and experience of those trained in the older techniques as to the methods themselves. Like any other new technique ultrasound guidance has been greeted with enthusiasm, but this must be tempered by thoughtful consideration of its clinical utility and appropriate clinical implementation, together with proper training. Excellent guidelines on these issues have been produced by the societies of regional anaesthesia (Ivani & Ferrante 2009, Sites et al. 2009a).

Being able to visualize both target nerves and related structures which must be avoided is an invaluable facility, but there is a widely held view that the most significant benefit is the ability to visualize the spread of local anaesthetic around the nerve (Denny & Harrop-Griffiths 2005, Griffin & Nichols 2010). The potential consequences of these two aspects, acting together or separately, are considerable:

1. Improved efficacy because of accuracy of placement, with local anaesthetic being seen to have surrounded the target nerve(s);

2. Less physical trauma because fewer needle 'passes' are needed and nerves, blood vessels, and other structures can be identified and avoided;

3. Shorter procedural times because of accurate placement and subsequent faster onset;

4. Less patient discomfort because of shorter procedures and fewer needle insertions; and

5. Reduced risk of local anaesthetic toxicity because accurate placement will allow reduced doses, and accidental intravenous injection should be avoided.

The results of an increasing number of clinical trials support these claims, especially in comparison with stimulator based techniques (Chan et al. 2007, Fredrickson et al. 2009, Kapal et al. 2008, Marhofer et al. 1997, Perlas et al. 2008, Weintraud et al. 2008). Relatively small numbers of patients were involved in these studies, but larger-scale reviews have reported improved success rates with ultrasound (Abrahams et al. 2009) and shorter block performance and onset times (Abrahams et al. 2009, Liu et al. 2009). Given the background low incidence of neurological (Chapter 4) and other complications, data on very large number of patients will need to be collected before any firm statistical comments can be made on the risk with ultrasound.

Arguably some of the most interesting aspects of the introduction of ultrasound guidance are the early demonstrations of ability of much reduced volumes of local anaesthetic to produce effective neural block and/or reduce side effects. For instance, the incidence of phrenic nerve block after interscalene injection was only 45% with 5 ml of ropivacaine 0.5% compared to 100% with 20 ml (Riazi et al. 2008). Again, as little as 1 ml of lidocaine 2% was used successfully to block each component of the brachial plexus during ultrasound-guided axillary block (O'Donnell et al. 2010). There is a very strong implication that the much larger doses used traditionally for many peripheral blocks were needed, in essence, to overcome relative inaccuracy of placement.

Finally, there are the training benefits. The trainer can see exactly where the trainee has placed the needle and made the injection so assessment can be far more objective. It also means that misplacement can be noted immediately without waiting for it to become apparent because no block develops. The benefits for both the individual patient and patient throughput are obvious.

Combining ultrasound with stimulation

An area of ongoing debate and research is whether combining stimulation with ultrasound for nerve localization improves block performance and outcome. Supporters argue that it improves the accuracy of both nerve identification and needle positioning (Jochum et al. 2009). In addition, nerve stimulation can (as described earlier) identify intraneural placement *before* any injection is made. However, other workers have found that the combination does not improve efficacy (Beach et al. 2006, Dingemans et al. 2007), increases the number of needle passes (which may result in inadvertent neurological injury), prolongs procedural time (Sites et al. 2009b), increases patient discomfort (Abrahams et al. 2009) and increases cost because a nerve stimulator and nerve stimulator compatible needles are needed. They argue that the two techniques, when used simultaneously, detract from rather than enhance one another.

Many anaesthetists have found the continued use of a peripheral nerve stimulator reassuring when making the transition to ultrasound guidance, and it useful when starting to see where the needle tip lies when apparently 'optimized' with stimulation. However, most find, relatively quickly, that stimulation adds little to most superficial block techniques, although for more deeply sited nerves, such as the proximal sciatic and the posterior lumbar plexus, stimulation retains a role because they are much harder to define with ultrasound.

Other modalities

Computed tomography (CT) and magnetic resonance imaging (MRI) allow visualization of interventional techniques, but have severe limitations in nerve block practice because both suffer from high capital cost, limited availability, lack of portability, and inability to produce 'real-time' images. Only 20 years ago not even ultrasound was a feasible technique for nerve localization, and who knows what technical developments may occur in the future. However, CT will always involve ionizing radiation and MRI requires the exclusion of ferrous and conducting materials from the vicinity. Non-ferrous needles would be required, and are already available for biopsy use, but is hard to see the size of equipment required fitting into the average anaesthetic room!

Key reference

Hoskins PR, Martin K, Thrush A (2010) *Diagnostic Ultrasound: Physics and Equipment*. Cambridge: Cambridge Medicine.

On-line resources

http://www.usra.ca/
http://www.nysora.com

References

Abd-Elmoniem KZ, Youssef A, Kadah YM (2002) Real-time speckle reduction and coherence enhancement in ultrsound imaging via non-anisotropic diffusion *IEEE Transactions of Bio-medical Engineering* 49: 997–1014.

Abrahams MS, Aziz MF, Fu RF, Horn JL (2009) Ultrasound guidance compared with electrical neurostimulation for peripheral nerve block: a systematic review and meta-analysis of randomized controlled trials. *British Journal of Anaesthesia* 102: 408–17.

Achim A, Bezerianos A, Tsakalides P (2001) Novel Bayesian multiscale method for speckle removal in medical ultrasound images. *IEEE Transaction of Medical Imaging* 20: 772–83.

Abrahams M, Aziz M, JL Horn (2009) Author Reply. *British Journal of Anaesthesia* 103: 773–4.

Beach ML, Sites BD, Gallagher JD (2006) Use of a nerve stimulator does not improve the efficacy of ultrasound –guided supraclavicular nerve blocks. *Journal of Clinical Anesthesia* 18: 580–4.

Belavy D, Ruitenberg MJ, Brijball RB (2011) Feasibility study of real-time three/four dimensional ultrasound for epidural catheter insertion. *British Journal of Anaesthesia* 107: 438–45.

Bigeleisen PE (2006) Nerve puncture and apparent intraneural injection during ultrasound guided axillary block does not invariably result in neurologic injury. *Anesthesiology* 105: 779–83.

Bigeleisen PE, Moayeri N, Groen GJ (2009) Extraneural versus intraneural stimulation thresholds during ultrasound-guided supraclavicular block. *Anesthesiology* 110: 1235–43.

Brull R, Wijayatilake DS, Perlas A, et al. (2008) Practice patterns related to block selection, nerve localization and risk disclosure: A survey of the American Society of Regional Anesthesia and Pain Medicine. *Regional Anesthesia and Pain Medicine* 33: 395–403.

Casey KL (1975) Which elements are excited in electrical stimulation of mammalian central nervous system: a review. *Brain Research* 98: 417–40.

Chan VW, Perlas A, McCartney CJ, et al. (2007) Ultrasound guidance improves success rate of axillary brachial plexus block. *Canadian Journal of Anaesthesia* 54: 176–82.

Coventry DM, Barker KF, Thomson M (2001) Comparison of two neurostimulation techniques for axillary brachial plexus blockade. *British Journal of Anaesthesia* 86: 80–3.

Deam RK, Kluger R, Barrington MJ, McCutcheon CA (2007) Investigation of a new echogenic needle for use with ultrasound peripheral nerve blocks. Anaesthesia & Intensive Care 35: 582–6.

Denny NM, Harrop-Griffiths W (2005) Location, location, location! Ultrasound imaging in regional anaesthesia. *British Journal of Anaesthesia* 94: 1–2.

Dingemans E, Williams SR, Arcand G, et al. (2007) Neurostimulation in ultrasound-guided infraclavicular block: a prospective randomized trial. *Anesthesia & Analgesia* 104: 1275–80.

Feinglass NG, Clendenen SR, Torp KD (2007) Real-time three-dimensional ultrasound for continuous popliteal blockade: a case report and image description. *Anesthesia & Analgesia* 105: 272–4.

Foster FS (2000) Transducer materials and probe construction. *Ultrasound in Medicine & Biology 26 (Suppl 1):* 2–5.

Foxall GL, Hardmann JG, Bedforth NM (2007) Three–dimensional, multiplanar, ultrasound guided, radial nerve block. *Regional Anesthesia and Pain Medicine* 32: 512–21.

Fredrickson MJ, Ball CM, Dalgleish AJ, et al. (2009) A prospective randomized comparison of ultrasound and neurostimulation as needle end points for interscalene catheter placement. *Anesthesia & Analgesia* 108: 1695–700.

Goerig M, Agarwal K (2000) Georg Perthes—The man behind the technique of Nerve-Tracer technology. *Regional Anesthesia and Pain Medicine* 25: 296–301.

Griffin J, Nicholls B (2010) Ultrasound in regional anaesthesia. *Anaesthesia 65 (Suppl 1):* 1–12.

Gupta S, Chesan RC, Sexana SC (2004) Wavelet-based statistical approach for speckle reduction in medical ultrasound images. *Medical & Biological Engineering & Computing* 42: 186–92.

Hadzic A, Vloka JD (2000) Peripheral nerve stimulators for regional anesthesia can generate excessive voltage output with poor ground connection. *Anesthesia & Analgesia* 91: 1306.

Hebard S, Hocking G (2011) Echogenic technology can improve needle visibility during ultrasound-guided regional anaesthesia. *Regional Anesthesia and Pain Medicine* 36: 185–9.

Hill CR (2006) Ultrasound for cancer investigation: An anecdotal history. *Ultrasound* 14: 78–86.

Hoskins PR, Martin K, Thrush A (2010) *Diagnostic Ultrasound: Physics and Equipment*. Cambridge: Cambridge Medicine.

Humphrey VF (2003) *Non-Linear Propagation for Medical Imaging*. Paris: WCU.

Ivani G, Ferrante FM (2009) The American Society of Regional Anesthesia and Pain Medicine and the European Society of Regional Anaesthesia and Pain Therapy Joint Committee recommendations for education and training in ultrasound guided regional anesthesia. *Regional Anesthesia and Pain Medicine* 34: 8–9.

Jochum D, Iohom G, Diarra DP, et al. (2006) An objective assessment of nerve stimulators used for peripheral nerve blockade. *Anaesthesia* 61: 557–64.

Jochum D, Bondar A, Delaunay L, et al. (2009) One size does not fit all: proposed algorithm for ultrasonography in combination with nerve stimulation for peripheral nerve blockade. *British Journal of Anaesthesia* 103: 771–3.

Kapral S, Krafft P, Eibenberger K, et al. (1994) Ultrasound-guided supraclavicular approach for regional anaesthesia of the brachial plexus. *Anesthesia & Analgesia* 78: 507–13.

Karmakar MK, Li X, Ho AM, et al. (2009) Real-time ultrasound-guided paramedian epidural access: evaluation of a novel in-plane technique. *British Journal of Anaesthesia* 102: 845–54.

Kapral S, Greher M, Huber G, et al. (2008) Ultrasonographic guidance improves the success rate of interscalene brachial plexus blockade. *Regional Anesthesia and Pain Medicine* 33: 253–8.

Koslow M, Bak A, Li CL (1973) C fiber excitability in the cat. *Experimental Neurology* 41: 745–53.

LaGrange P, Foster PA, Pretorius LK (1978) Application of Doppler ultrasound bloodflow detector in supraclavicular brachial plexus block. *British Journal of Anaesthesia* 50: 965–7.

Liguori GA, Zayas VM, YaDeau JT, et al. (2006) Nerve localization techniques for interscalene brachial plexus blockade: A prospective, randomized comparison of mechanical paraesthesia versus electrical stimulation. *Anesthesia & Analgesia* 103: 761–7.

Liu SS, Ngeow JE, YaDeau JT (2009) Ultrasound-guided regional anaesthesia and analgesia: A qualitative systematic review. *Regional Anesthesia and Pain Medicine* 34: 47–59.

Marhofer P, Schrogendorfer K, Koinig H, et al. (1997) Ultrasonographic guidance improves sensory block and onset time of three-in-one blocks. *Anesthesia & Analgesia* 85: 854–7.

Munirama S, Joy J, Habeshaw R, et al. (2012) Visibility of echogenic Tuohy needles in the Thiel cadaver. *British Journal of Anaesthesia* In press.

O'Donnell B, Riordan J, Ahmad I, Iohom G (2010) Brief reports: a clinical evaluation of block characteristics using one millilitre 2% lidocaine in ultrasound-guided axillary brachial plexus block. *Anesthesia & Analgesia* 111: 808–10.

Perlas A, Niazi A, McCartney CJ, et al. (2006) The sensitivity of motor response to nerve stimulation and paraesthesia for nerve localization as evaluated by ultrasound. *Regional Anesthesia and Pain Medicine* 31:445–50.

Perlas A, Brull R, Chan VW, et al. (2008) Ultrasound guidance improves the success of sciatic nerve block at the popliteal fossa. *Regional Anesthesia and Pain Medicine* 33: 259–65.

Pither CE, Raj PP, Ford DJ (1985) The use of peripheral nerve stimulators for regional anaesthesia: A review of experimental characteristics, technique and clinical applications. *Regional Anesthesia and Pain Medicine* 10: 49–58.

Riazi S, Carmichael N, Awad I, et al. (2008) Effect of local anaesthetic volume (20 vs 5ml) on the efficacy and respiratory consequences of ultrasound-guided interscalene brachial plexus block. *British Journal of Anaesthesia* 101: 549–56.

Robards C, Hadzic A, Somasundaram L, et al. (2009) Intraneural injection with low-current stimulation during popliteal sciatic nerve block. *Anesthesia & Analgesia* 109: 673–7.

Sala-Blanch X, Lopez AM, Carazo J, et al. (2009) Intraneural injection during nerve stimulator-guided sciatic nerve block at the popliteal fossa. *British Journal of Anaesthesia* 102: 855–61.

Sandhu NS, Sidhu DS, Levon LM (2004) The cost comparison of infraclavicular brachial plexus block by nerve stimulator and ultrasound guidance. *Anesthesia & Analgesia* 98: 267–8.

Sauter AR, Dodgson MS, Kalvoy H, et al. (2009) Current threshold for nerve stimulation depends on electrical impedance of the tissue: a study of ultrasound-guided electrical nerve stimulation of the median nerve. *Anesthesia & Analgesia* 108: 1338–43.

Schafhalter-Zoppoth I, McCulloch CE, Gray AT (2004) Ultrasound visibility of needles used for regional nerve block: an in-vitro study. *Regional Anesthesia and Pain Medicine* 29: 480–8.

Selander D, Edshage S, Wolff T (1979 Paresthesiae or no paresthesiae? *Acta Anaesthesiologica Scandinavica* 23: 27–33.

Sites BD, Gallagher J, Sparks M (2003) Ultrasound-guided popliteal block demonstrates an atypical motor response to nerve stimulation in 2 patients with diabetes mellitus. *Regional Anesthesia and Pain Medicine* 28: 479–82.

Sites BD, Chan VW, Neal JM, et al. (2009a) The American Society of Regional Anesthesia and Pain Medicine and the European Society of Regional Anaesthesia and Pain Therapy Joint Committee recommendations for education and training in ultrasound guided regional anesthesia. *Regional Anesthesia and Pain Medicine* 34: 40–6.

Sites BD, Beach ML, Chinn CD, et al. (2009b) A comparison of sensory and motor loss after a femoral nerve block conducted with ultrasound versus ultrasound and nerve stimulation. *Regional Anesthesia and Pain Medicine* 34: 508–13.

Shaefer J (1940 *Elektrophysiologie 1*. Germany: Wein Franz Deufficke.

Walker KJ, McGrattan K, Aas-Eng K, Smith AF (2009) Ultrasound guidance for peripheral nerve blockade (Review). *Cochrane Database of Systematic Reviews* 4: CD006459.

Weintraud M, Marhofer P, Bosenberg A, et al. (2008) Ilioinguinal/iliohypogastric blocks in children: Where do we administer the local anaesthetic without direct visualization? *Anesthesia & Analgesia* 106: 89–93.

Yongjian Yu, Acton DT (2002) Speckle reducing anisotropic diffusion. *IEEE Transactions in Image Processing* 11: 1260–70.

CHAPTER 11

Principles of patient management

Barrie Fischer

Regional anaesthesia offers considerable potential benefit to high-risk patients undergoing major surgery but, perversely, these patients are also more likely to suffer serious adverse events from its use. In a major prospective study, central neuraxial complications (especially epidural) were reported more commonly in the subgroup of elderly patients undergoing major abdominal surgery for cancer than other subgroups (Cook et al. 2009a). A large retrospective study of the adverse events associated with central neuraxial block found an increased risk of epidural haematoma in elderly females undergoing major orthopaedic procedures, compared to other subsets of patients and procedures (Moen et al. 2004).

There are four important aspects of providing safe and successful regional anaesthesia.

1. Patient assessment and preoperative preparation;

2. Selection of the most appropriate block for the intended surgical procedure;

3. Performance of that block; and

4. Management of the patient thereafter.

While the patient and the anaesthetist are the main individuals involved, best practice in regional anaesthesia can only be achieved if all the staff involved with the patient's care (surgical team, anaesthesia and recovery staff, ward nurses, acute pain team, and rehabilitation staff) are fully engaged with the process. Staff training and education are important components of safe patient care, and these require significant time and resources to establish and maintain.

Patient assessment and preparation

The preliminary aspects of the management of patients presenting for surgery which may involve the use of regional anaesthesia have been considered in Chapter 9. The great majority of patients do not pose particular concerns and can be managed using agreed treatment plans for the common co-morbid states, but is important that those with rare or extreme problems are identified for more specific assessment at as early a stage as possible. The discussions in Chapters 3 and 5 have emphasized the considerable benefits which regional techniques may provide, but the risk of major complications seems, almost perversely, to be greatest in those with most to benefit (Chapter 4). Elderly patients with significant co-morbidity can gain much from continuous epidural analgesia after major surgery, but minimizing the risks requires careful initial assessment of any predisposing factors as well as careful planning and delivery of their care.

Consent

There is, as yet, no need for written consent for any aspect of anaesthesia in the UK, but all aspects of the technique(s) to be used, potential complications as well as benefits, must be discussed according to the level of information desired by the individual patient. Identifying which side is to be operated on in 'handed' procedures is a key component of the preoperative visit and a responsibility shared by all involved. Unfortunately, a number of cases has come to light where the block was performed on the wrong side, with a range of causative factors (primarily distraction and inattention to detail) being identified (Safe Anaesthesia Liaison Group 2010). Marking of the operative site is a surgical responsibility, but this does not absolve the anaesthetist from taking every precaution to ensure that the block is performed on the correct side.

Block selection

Selecting the most appropriate block, or combination of blocks, can be a complex process because all regional techniques are capable of causing side effects and complications ranging from the trivial to the life threatening. Thus the selection process should balance the difficulty of the intended block and its potential complications against the anticipated benefits. The underlying principle is to select the method most likely to benefit the individual patient undergoing a particular surgical procedure so patient- and procedure-specific factors will have to be considered as well.

The severity of the surgery and its associated stress responses, the duration and intensity of the anticipated postoperative pain, and the postoperative recovery and rehabilitation requirements are major determinants of which block(s) to use. Patient co-morbidities and specific surgical and anaesthetic needs will also influence the ultimate choice so that the balance between benefits and risk can be optimized (Fischer & Simanski 2005, Fischer et al. 2008, Joshi et al. 2008). Surgical and anaesthetic practices continue to evolve, and regional blocks which were appropriate for a procedure a few years ago may not offer the same benefits today. Minimal access or laparoscopically-assisted techniques, together with other developments aimed at early mobility, accelerated rehabilitation, and shorter hospital stay (PROSPECT web site, Kehlet et al. 2007), mean that operations which once required in-patient care are now performed on an ambulatory (day-case) basis. The regional techniques used must ensure rapid recovery, minimal side effects, and early mobilization to allow discharge home.

Performance of the block

General principles

Regional anaesthesia places specific demands on the patient (especially one in pain) so the staff involved must appreciate that particular support and care are needed during block performance. It is a matter of individual choice whether this is done with the patient on their bed, a trolley, or the operating table, but the chosen vehicle should provide the patient with reasonable comfort and support, allow for accurate positioning, and be capable of being adjusted for height *and* tilt. All the necessary equipment, including a foot stool and pillows if required for the sitting position, must be ready in advance to reduce both patient anxiety and delay.

Suitable surroundings are required: the room should be well lit, maintained at a comfortable temperature for the lightly clad patient, and have a quiet, calm atmosphere to minimize patient anxiety, and maintain cooperation and dignity. Unnecessary distraction must be discouraged. There should be enough space for the patient, the trolley to provide a sterile field for block performance, other equipment (e.g. an ultrasound machine), and for staff to circulate to support the patient and assist the anaesthetist. Careful thought should be given to how the various items of equipment are arranged around the patient and anaesthetist. The anaesthetist may sit or stand according to preference, but the posture used should avoid any straining during block performance and keep the various items of equipment comfortably within the field of vision (Figure 11.1).

In the UK, anaesthetic induction rooms are commonplace and normally fulfil this requirement; elsewhere, such rooms may not be available and a specific area (the 'block' room) should be provided instead. Suitably trained and experienced staff are essential: one person assists the anaesthetist, passing the equipment, solutions, and drugs required; another is wholly responsible for looking after the patient. The number of personnel not directly involved should be kept to a minimum, but those who are present to learn should introduce themselves to the patient and then be as unobtrusive as possible.

After the initial patient checks, venous access is secured, appropriate monitoring (non-invasive blood pressure, oxygen saturation, electrocardiogram) instituted, and intravenous fluids and oxygen therapy started as necessary. Dialogue, to remind patients what is to happen and what they might experience, helps to keep them engaged with the procedure and reduce anxiety. Preoperative explanation should have warned the patient what to expect, but a reminder at each stage is good practice and avoids surprises. Proper patient positioning is vital and should be undertaken by the anaesthetist, *not* an assistant, this also being the stage for confirming that the correct side is to be blocked. The relevant landmarks are identified and the key features marked, not only for teaching purposes, but because the anatomy may be less clear after skin preparation and draping.

All manoeuvres, including the preliminaries just discussed, should be carried out as calmly and gently as possible to build the patient's confidence. This is easy when things are going well, but not so if the unexpected occurs; remaining calm will keep the mind clear to help overcome difficulties as well as continuing to reassure the patient. Be constantly aware that there is 'Someone else's nervous system' at the 'sharp end' of the needle (Fettes and Wildsmith 2002).

Awake or asleep?

Regional anaesthesia may be used alone (with or without sedation) or combined with general anaesthesia. In the latter situation a decision has to be made on whether the block is instituted before or after induction, there being arguments in favour of each approach.

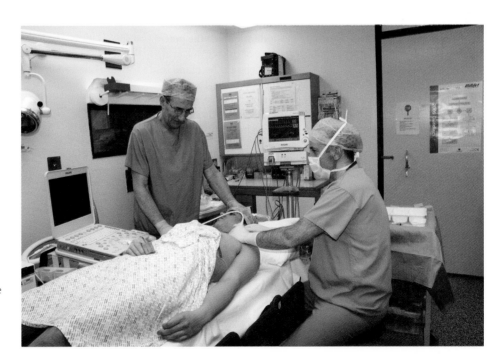

Figure 11.1 Arrangement of equipment around patient and anaesthetist. Note that the sterile tray is convenient for his dominant (right) hand and that patient, monitors, and ultrasound screen are within his comfortable field of vision.

In the unconscious patient the risk of complications may be increased (Bromage & Benumof 1998), the patient being unable to report needle/catheter contact with nerves or the early signs of systemic toxicity. However, there is little definitive, as opposed to anecdotal, evidence to support or refute this claim apart from one study of epidural block (Horlocker et al. 2003).

Although properly conducted regional techniques should cause little discomfort, it is claimed that they are easier to perform in the unconscious patient, and there have been impassioned pleas for the prior administration of general anaesthesia, especially in children (Krane et al. 1998). Debate on this topic has raged for over a decade (Fischer 1998, Wildsmith & Fischer 1999), with practice determined by the wishes of the patient and the anaesthetist's preference, training, and experience. In the continuing absence of accurate data on the relative incidence of harm, the performance of major regional blocks on anaesthetized patients cannot be considered unacceptable practice, although consensus recommendations from the American Society of Regional Anesthesia (Neal et al. 2008a) may change this.

Aseptic technique

Although infective complications of regional techniques may be more common than once assumed (Grewel et al. 2006), they are still rare, but can have catastrophic effects. Thus, prevention is essential, with central and major peripheral blocks requiring the same standards of asepsis as equivalent surgical procedures. For central blocks, full asepsis (hat, mask, surgical scrub, gown, gloves, and a 'no-touch' technique) is considered essential, the skin being cleaned with a bactericidal antiseptic and the area draped with sterile towels. Some argue against the need for surgical facemasks, but they reduce bacterial contamination of the site (Phillips et al. 1992). The sterile area provided for preparation must be large enough to allow manipulation of equipment (especially a catheter) without it accidentally touching something which is not sterile.

The optimum antiseptic is 0.5% chlorhexidine in 70% alcohol, iodine-based preparations being less effective (Darouiche 2010). Chlorhexidine (like any bactericide) is neurotoxic, and its use before regional anaesthesia is an 'off-label' indication, but the practice has been defended as an acceptable balance of risks (Cook et al. 2009b). However, it is clear that every effort should be made to avoid contamination of equipment and drug solutions. The disinfectant should be placed nearest the patient on the block tray so that it cannot drip onto other items, and it should be removed once cleaning is complete. The risk may be further reduced by having an assistant apply the solution, ideally with a spray, but it is still essential to allow it to dry before touching the area: first to allow it to work; second to avoid glove contamination.

For major peripheral blocks, many anaesthetists do not wear a gown, but the evidence to support this is lacking. Maintaining sterility remains vital, especially when a catheter technique is employed, if not for single injection procedures (Hebl 2006).

Equipment

Modern sterile, disposable equipment is of a very high standard, but faults may be found occasionally: a non-patent catheter, a leaking syringe, or a bad fit between devices. Thus it is wise to check and assemble as much as is possible, including priming the catheter with normal saline, before starting.

Currently, compatibility of equipment is assured by the use of 'Luer' connections, the international standard, for syringes, needles, and associated devices. However, soon this may no longer be the case in the UK because of severe patient harm resulting from injection errors, preparations destined for the vertebral canal having been given intravenously, and vice versa. Each case has had, at its heart, failure to check labels properly, but instructions were issued that, from April 2011, all devices for intrathecal procedures must be fitted with connectors which are 'Luer' incompatible (National Patient Safety Agency 2009). The same was to apply to epidural and other regional block procedures by April 2013, but the difficulties in designing and producing acceptable alternative equipment has meant that the change has been delayed (Walker et al. 2010). It seemed, for a while, inevitable that there would be a change eventually, but concerns about the possible adverse consequences have grown so it is not clear currently what is to happen. However, if new connections are introduced it will mean that the careful checking of the compatibility of items provided for a procedure will assume even greater importance. A 'mechanical' safeguard may reduce some risks, but the availability of two distinct sets of equipment in the same clinical area may introduce other problems.

In the interim, and because 'wrong route' injections continue to cause avoidable adverse events (Cranshaw et al. 2009), every precaution (labelling, checking, double checking) must be used to prevent them.

Block packs

Regional anaesthesia requires an area large enough for the preparatory work to be carried out safely for reasons already indicated, and the pack should be opened on a suitably sized trolley. A variety of sterile block packs are commercially available, each containing the relevant needles, syringes, and other items; the most comprehensive (and expensive) can be used for a range of blocks, but contain much that may be surplus to specific requirements. The alternative is to use a basic preparation pack and add whatever is needed for each procedure. In the interests of consistency, and reducing errors due to unfamiliarity, there is merit in having the same equipment in all areas of the hospital. A regional block trolley is useful in this regard (Figure 11.2); stocked with an agreed list of equipment etc., it is kept separate from all other anaesthetic equipment and fluid storage trolleys.

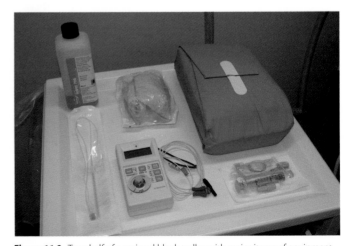

Figure 11.2 Top shelf of a regional block trolley with major items of equipment ready for use.

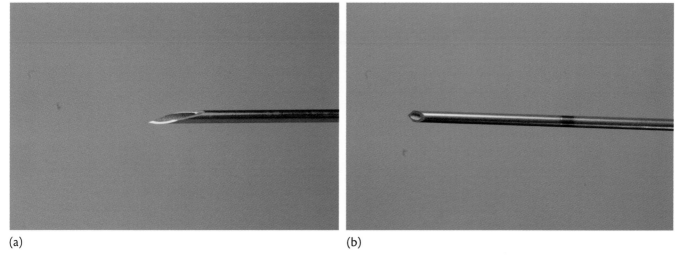

(a)   (b)

Figure 11.3 Long (a) and short (b) bevelled needle tips.

Needles

Specialized, sterile, disposable needles are available for both central and peripheral techniques, there being three broad types available in a range of lengths and gauges:

1. *Uninsulated*: for central blocks and infiltration;

2. *Insulated*: used with peripheral nerve stimulators; and

3. *Hyperechoic*: for use with ultrasound.

Needles for central blocks are discussed in the appropriate chapters, but are also used for other blocks where insulation is not necessary (e.g. paravertebral, transversus abdominis, rectus sheath, fascia iliaca, infiltration).

Most specialist block needles have a short bevel (Figure 11.3), although the exact bevel angle varies between designs. A short bevel needle gives more positive 'feedback' as the tip passes through tissue planes, and may be less traumatic when paraesthesiae are sought (Selander et al. 1977), but can cause more damage if inadvertent nerve penetration occurs (Rice et al. 1992, Sala-Blanch et al. 2009). Winnie (1983) was the first to advocate the use of a length of small bore tubing between syringe and needle, and most devices now incorporate this feature (Figure 11.4). This allows the anaesthetist to maintain the needle in the correct position during an aspiration test or when the syringe is being changed by an assistant. This should be standard practice when large volumes of drug are injected.

If a needle bends during insertion, it should be changed; the same applies if, after firm bony contact, there is a 'burr' on the tip because it will tear tissue subsequently.

Catheters

Catheter techniques allow extension of the duration of blocks by intermittent bolus injection or continuous infusion. The material should be biochemically inert, easy to sterilize, have a low coefficient of friction with a high tensile strength, and be flexible yet kink-resistant. External markings should allow accurate placement. Spinal and epidural catheters are considered further in Chapters 13 and 14. Peripheral nerve catheters are available in a range of lengths and gauges and should, ideally, be radio-opaque

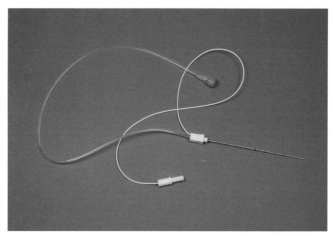

Figure 11.4 An 'immobile' needle set. Note that this needle has an insulated covering and that there is an integral attachment for a nerve stimulator.

and 'visible' with ultrasound. Catheters with a fine stimulating electrode running through them are said to allow precise placement because the precise position can be monitored by the changing pattern of muscle twitch, but they do not actually offer any significant advantage and are considerably more expensive (Dauri et al. 2007, Salinas et al. 2004).

Peripheral nerve catheter techniques are more demanding than single bolus injections and there is an increased risk of failure, both primary (no block initially) and secondary (late failure due to catheter displacement, migration, or disconnection). There is no evidence of increased risk of nerve injury or infection when catheters are used for limited periods (<72 hours), but they require close attention to detail and frequent monitoring to ensure that the intended benefits are achieved and the risks are minimized. Inadvertent removal, obstruction, and accidental disconnection may all occur, and fixation can be difficult, especially where the tissues are mobile (neck, axilla, inguinal area) or subject to pressure (gluteal area). Tunnelling or fixation using tissue glue can improve fixation, simplify nursing care, and thus prolong utilization.

Syringes

Standard, disposable plastic syringes are perfectly adequate for most indications, but specific types may be preferred (e.g. 'loss of resistance' devices for epidural and other blocks). Although it may seem that the choice of syringe size will depend only on the volume to be injected, it may be easier to control aspiration and injection with a small one. Using a standard size syringe for all injections will also aid recognition of greater than usual resistance to injection (see 'Needle insertion' section).

Needle insertion

All equipment and drugs should be checked and prepared before the procedure starts, and kept out of the patient's line of sight, if at all possible. As already noted, dialogue is important at all stages, especially when working behind the patient, but is vital during needle insertion to aid success and identify problems. Other personnel looking after the patient can reassure and support the patient, but should refrain from commenting about the block itself because they may not entirely understand any difficulties the anaesthetist is experiencing.

Most needles used for regional anaesthesia are quite large or have relatively flat bevels, and preliminary skin infiltration is essential. This should start with an intradermal injection (to ensure that skin puncture is painless) and continue with infiltration along the projected needle path. Sufficient local anaesthetic should be used to ensure patient comfort, but not to obscure landmarks. Using a small aliquot of the block solution for this demonstrates its efficacy. If a blunt needle (e.g. Tuohy) is being used, a small 'nick' in the skin with a sharp needle will ease insertion and reduce the risk of sudden penetration causing the needle to pass to a greater depth than intended.

Every attempt should be made to avoid touching the shaft of the needle. This can be difficult when long, flexible needles are used, but the shaft should be gripped as near to the hub as possible. The needle can be steadied by placing the back of the non-dominant hand against the patient, and using its thumb and index finger to grasp the hub. This will give excellent control while the needle is advanced with the dominant hand.

Good technique should ensure that the first pass of the needle will be successful in a high proportion of cases, but realignment will be necessary on occasion. However, the needle should always be withdrawn somewhat before changing its direction. If the tip remains in the denser tissues, there will either be no change in direction or the needle will bend. At best, any curvature will cause the needle to deviate further from the intended route as it is advanced and, at worst, it risks breakage.

The overall goal is to place the needle tip close to the target nerves without damaging them or associated structures. The risk of such damage can be minimized by combining a high degree of attention to detail with subtlety of touch and finesse ('fingerspitzengefühl') during needle placement and subsequent drug injection. Paraesthesiae and/or pain at any stage are warning signs, although not invariable ones, of impending nerve injury; they may not occur even though evidence of nerve damage appears subsequently.

Paraesthesiae and pain

Effective local anaesthetic infiltration and a gentle technique should ensure that regional block procedures cause only minimal discomfort (local pressure or mild, localized irritation). Even when paraesthesiae are being sought deliberately in traditional nerve location techniques, the sensation should be no more than mild 'pins and needles'. Any other complaint demands immediate attention, and cessation of all further action, until the distribution, nature (pain, paraesthesiae, or motor response) and intensity of the patient's reaction have each been assessed. This analysis should identify which structure the needle (or catheter, the same principles apply) has come into contact with to inform the most appropriate course of further action.

A mild reaction in the distribution of the target nerve(s) should be taken as an indication that the needle tip is in the correct location; it should be withdrawn very slightly (about 1 mm), but no injection made until symptoms have subsided. Severe reactions require immediate partial withdrawal of the needle. If the features are in the distribution of the target nerve, the implication is that the needle has been advanced too vigorously, and this experience should inform future practice. Any other distribution of symptoms obviously requires reassessment of the direction and depth of insertion. Clearly, close and continuing dialogue with the patient is essential, both for explanation and assessment.

The greatest difficulty comes when symptoms persist or recur. There are reports of pain without subsequent damage (and damage without any warning features), but the mantra that 'discomfort (let alone pain) equals damage until proved otherwise' must be kept in mind. Abandoning the procedure may undermine the patient's confidence, but must always be an option, although an alternative approach to the same nerves might be tried. The ultimate decision will depend on the particular clinical situation, with the experience of the anaesthetist being perhaps the most important issue.

Symptoms during local anaesthetic injection are less common. Occasionally a patient may complain of a dull, aching sensation thought to be due to the combination of the cold temperature of the solution and local compression of the nerve. It is usually associated with over-'vigorous' injection rates and can be minimized by a more cautious approach. Anything else implies that there is a serious problem, either contamination of the solution or intraneural injection. Only meticulous preparation will prevent the former, but withdrawal of needle or catheter may deal with the latter. However, persistence of symptoms may, as mentioned earlier, mean that discretion is the safer option.

The significance of low resistance to injection

Most major nerves are contained within compliant compartments which allow free dispersion of the injectate. Therefore, one of the principal characteristics of any technique is that there should be little resistance to the flow of local anaesthetic during injection. Increased resistance is a cardinal sign that the needle or catheter tip is in the wrong tissue plane and, if accompanied by significant pain or reflex movement, is almost certainly due to intraneural injection (see Chapter 4). The resistance of any injection system depends on the diameters and lengths of its components; being familiar with the force needed to produce flow before insertion will mean that any difficulty can be more readily appreciated thereafter.

Aspiration and test doses

Systemic local anaesthetic drug toxicity is a life-threatening complication, with most cases being due to accidental intravenous injection. The details are dealt with elsewhere (Chapter 8), but a few general practical points may be made here.

Once the needle (or catheter) is in place, a gentle aspiration test must be performed to eliminate intravascular placement (or subarachnoid in epidural block). The aspiration must be gentle or tissue may be 'sucked' onto the needle tip and prevent any fluid backflow. A further test with a catheter is to hold the proximal end below the level of the patient to see if anything 'siphons' along it.

If blood or cerebrospinal fluid (CSF) appear it is obvious that a vessel or the dura has been punctured, but intravenous, intra-arterial, and subarachnoid injection can occur despite a (false) negative test, so 'test doses' are commonly employed to further exclude these possibilities. The precise nature of the test solution will depend on the clinical situation, but three criteria must be satisfied:

1. The test solution must be capable of producing unequivocal and easily verifiable evidence of intravascular or subarachnoid injection within a few seconds of injection;

2. The solution used for the test dose should be unlikely to produce any detectable effect if injected into the correct place; and

3. Sufficient time must be allowed for the test dose to produce an effect before the full dose is administered.

Test doses are most commonly used during epidural block, and are considered in more detail in Chapter 14. However, they should be used in all situations where relatively large doses of local anaesthetic are needed, and particularly in blocks of the head and neck. Intravascular injection into branches of the carotid and vertebral arteries will produce almost instantaneous cerebral signs, and quite small doses can produce major reactions. Small volumes (0.5–1 ml) should be injected slowly with close observation of the patient to avoid serious complications.

Unfortunately, not even the combination of aspiration with test dose can guarantee that intravascular injection will not occur. Thus all large volumes of local anaesthetic should be injected in 5-ml increments, with a pause of 60 seconds after the first increment and repeat aspiration tests performed between each one.

Defining the block

Once the local anaesthetic has been injected, the focus changes sequentially to monitoring the onset of action, managing the primary and secondary effects, and caring for the patient during and after the operation, with the process documented throughout. Monitoring should be intense for the first 15–20 minutes after injection.

Testing

Monitoring the onset of a block aims to show that it is adequate for the proposed surgery, and will also warn of complications (such as hypotension) if spread is excessive. Superficially, it may seem a straightforward process, but a number of factors mean that it is not. First, the innervations of superficial and deep structures are often from different dermatomes or through different nerves, meaning that skin numbness does not guarantee anaesthesia of underlying viscera, muscles, or bones. Second, no single test of neurological function provides an accurate indication of either extent or quality of block. Third, assessing the extent of block, especially in the anxious patient, is not always easy, and judging its quality can be even more difficult. Fourth, even spinal anaesthesia takes a finite time to develop, and other blocks are much slower in onset.

The broad modalities of nerve function are obtunded at different rates with, in most techniques, sympathetic block appearing first, motor weakness second, and numbness last. Thus, observation should start with noting sympathetic block (vasodilatation in the limb or a decrease in blood pressure), progress to assessment of muscle power, and finish with testing of sensation. Pain is blocked fairly quickly so the onset of analgesia is the perfect indicator in acute situations (e.g. the patient in labour or with a fracture). It takes experience and confidence to take an expectant approach to block onset, but too much testing too soon can raise serious doubt in the patient's mind about effectiveness and cause significant anxiety.

For medicolegal, as well as humanitarian reasons, very formal testing of the block is mandatory before surgery is allowed to commence in the conscious patient. Indicators of the extent and degree of both motor and sensory block are needed, with motor block being a little easier to assess. In the lower limb the ability to straight leg raise, extend the knee, and flex the ankle can be graded using a modified Bromage scale where 'zero' equals full power and 'four' equals complete paralysis (Fischer 2009). In the upper limb similar tests can be applied at shoulder, elbow, and wrist. However, the different modalities of sensation make its testing more complex, with the added complication that numbness may not equate to surgical anaesthesia.

Clinically, pin-prick testing allows discrimination between touch and 'sharp' sensation, with abolition of touch usually equating to surgical anaesthesia. However, repeated testing can lead to skin damage, although this may be minimized by using a blunt neurological pin (an unfolded paper clip is a makeshift alternative), and many use temperature testing as a less traumatic method. A spirit-soaked swab or an ice-cube wrapped in gauze will demonstrate loss of cold sensation, but repeated spraying of ethyl chloride is not recommended. It is a flammable, highly volatile general anaesthetic which also acts as a local anaesthetic so it is a dangerous atmospheric pollutant which can confuse the assessment. Loss of temperature sensitivity does not equate as well with surgical anaesthesia as does loss of touch sensation.

During a spinal anaesthetic it is usual to record the upper level of dermatomal block bilaterally, but an extensive block is not necessarily an effective one, this being better assessed by the degree of leg weakness. The same applies to epidural block, although the lower level may need to be assessed also because of the different pattern of onset (see Chapter 14). For plexus blocks testing needs to establish that both the dermatomes and terminal nerves supplying the operative area, including the tourniquet site, are anaesthetized.

Overall, testing helps define that the required effect has been produced, but it does not guarantee it. The ultimate test is the surgeon's knife, and it is good practice for the surgeon to test the operative site by pinching the skin surreptitiously with a pair of forceps before any incision is made. Even with a perfect block the conscious patient should be warned about movement and other 'sensations' from the operative field, especially during intra-abdominal surgery because the viscera are supplied by the vagus nerve. The skills of the surgical team (gentle tissue handling, careful packing of abdominal organs, working within the area of block) are vital in minimizing such sensations, and dialogue with the patient should allow any issue to be dealt with before it causes distress.

Dealing with failure

Failure can be minimized by having a thorough knowledge of the procedure, careful case selection, meticulous attention to detail, and seeking assistance from a more experienced colleague whenever a new problem is encountered. However, despite everybody's best efforts success is not always achieved so that an effective alternative is needed, but the only true failure is a failure to learn something from the experience. A block may be slow in onset, inadequate in extent or intensity or it may fail completely, but the (somewhat humbling) explanation is virtually always a failure of technique. Even when the endpoint (appearance of CSF) is as clear as it is in spinal anaesthesia, there are many reasons for failure, and each must be avoided (Fettes et al. 2009).

Slow onset

Time for the block to develop must be factored into its performance, and the anaesthetist should never be rushed into abandoning a block: 'tincture of time' is often as effective a supplement as anything. A spinal usually reaches maximum effect within 15 minutes, but can take 30; epidural and major peripheral blocks may take 45 minutes, especially with long-acting drugs. Careful observation of the extent of the developing block will inform the actions which may be taken to improve matters such as changes in posture during a spinal, adjustment of an epidural catheter before administration of a top-up, and more peripheral supplementation of a plexus block.

Inadequate block

Patient discomfort during a block which appears to be extensive enough may be dealt with in a similar fashion, but this situation often results (because the operation has already started) in the rapid induction of general anaesthesia. This can upset the patient, who may well prefer to remain awake despite the discomfort, and a better approach is to seek and address the cause (e.g. over-vigorous surgery, discomfort of lying on an operating table, patient anxiety).

Sedation can help, but may disinhibit the patient so a small dose of opioid can be more appropriate, and inhalation of nitrous oxide (50% in oxygen from a facemask) provides both sedation and analgesia although it raises concerns about contamination of the working environment. Remaining wide awake during surgery is a test of both the quality of the block and the patient's courage, and careful sedation can do much for both! However, large doses of sedative and opioid drugs, especially the longer acting drugs, may delay recovery meaning that a general anaesthetic would have been a better option.

Complete failure

Total absence of block leaves two stark alternatives: repeat the block or induce general anaesthesia. The latter progresses the operating list, but undermines (with both patient and surgeon) the original reason for the block. Further, it is a common experience to find that, after recovery of consciousness, a satisfactory block has developed: 'tincture of time' may have been the answer!

Repeat injections

Total failure of a spinal anaesthetic can probably be dealt with safely by repeating the procedure, but the situation is different when an inadequate block has developed (Fettes et al. 2009). The same factor which limited intrathecal spread may still be operating and result in the local accumulation of a high, and potentially neurotoxic, concentration of drug. Careful analysis is needed before a decision is made.

With other techniques both supplementary and repeat injections may lead to cumulative toxicity of the local anaesthetic. Many factors (see Chapter 7) affect its plasma concentration and each must be taken into account before further injections are made. If a block requiring a large dose of drug is considered worthy of repeating, it may be necessary to delay the procedure to allow time for the risk of toxicity to subside. In this, and indeed, in all of these difficult situations, full explanations must be offered to the patient and one's colleagues.

Care during surgery

Positioning

The patient should be made comfortable on the operating table with all anaesthetized areas padded and supported for protection without impeding surgical access. The patient is shown how much movement is allowed and a final assessment made of tolerance to remaining conscious throughout the procedure; it is easier to induce a general anaesthetic before surgery starts rather than once the patient is draped and surgery under way. All the theatre staff must be aware that the patient is conscious, that this can be stressful, and that all movement and comments must be guarded. At times when the anaesthetist is busy, the assistant must be deputed to continue the dialogue with the patient.

Monitoring

Monitoring should be continued, as during general anaesthesia, at a level appropriate to the effects of both anaesthetic and surgery, right through to recovery, remembering that verbal contact may give early warning of complications. When top-up injections of local anaesthetic are made, or infusions started, observations should be as intense as after the initial injection. Shivering is common after central blocks because vasodilatation increases heat loss so temperature should be monitored and active warming devices employed (Frank et al. 1999).

Awake, sedated, or 'asleep'?

During surgery, regional blocks may be used alone, with conscious sedation or with a supplement (deep sedation or general anaesthesia) which guarantees unconsciousness. The decision should be made during the preoperative discussion, as part of the informed consent process, and many factors influence it: patient preference, the presence of systemic disease or an airway problem, the block to be used, the type & duration of surgery, and the experience of the anaesthetist.

Most of the difficulties of having the patient fully conscious during surgery have been mentioned or implied already, but basically they relate to the need for a complete block of all input before surgical preparation can begin, and continuation of that state thereafter. This can be extremely difficult, arguably impossible, to achieve in some settings, yet there are very few procedures during which full consciousness is in any way necessary. The judicious use of systemic supplements can make the procedure much more relaxing for all involved.

Sedation

Any sedative, anxiolytic, and analgesic might be used to supplement regional anaesthesia, but intravenous increments of midazolam (1–2 mg), propofol (10–20 mg—or a slow infusion), and fentanyl (25 mcg), or the inhalation of nitrous oxide (25–50%), are the most widely used. They induce light sedation with minimal hangover, and can be used in combination according to the patient's needs. The patient should be able to respond to question and command, although many will fall asleep once surgery is in progress. If sedation is used to produce loss of consciousness, very close watch will need to be kept for airway obstruction and respiratory depression.

General anaesthesia

An important factor in deciding whether or not to use general anaesthesia is the flexibility of purpose which regional techniques provide. A peripheral block, or a segmental epidural, would not be sufficient for surgery, but can provide the analgesic component of a balanced anaesthetic technique. This is particularly useful during abdominal surgery where stimulation of unblocked viscera may cause distress, as may lying on an operating table for long periods of time. The benefits of both methods are obtained, but the disadvantages are minimal. However, adding a general anaesthetic to a more extensive central block, which would be sufficient in itself, combines two sources of physiological depression and risks major side effects (see 'Hypotension and regional anaesthesia' section). There may be situations (e.g. induced hypotension) where this has benefit, but very careful patient management is required.

Hypotension and regional anaesthesia

Sympathetic block

Hypotension may complicate central and, less commonly, thoracic paravertebral (due to epidural spread) block, the risk being proportional to the extent of sympathetic block. A block to T_{10} results in little effect, but further cephalad spread results in progressive depression of the thoraco-lumbar sympathetic outflow and increased likelihood of significant hypotension—generally accepted as a 25–30% decrease in systolic pressure from the normal, resting (*not* the immediate preanaesthetic) figure (Carpenter et al. 1992). Epidural anaesthesia usually develops more slowly than spinal anaesthesia, and there is time for compensation to occur, so the initial decrease in blood pressure may be less dramatic. The effects of an epidural may also be modified by the systemic actions of vasoconstrictors and the larger doses of drugs required, but the basic cardiovascular effects are the same.

Peripheral arterial dilatation decreases systemic vascular resistance and left ventricular afterload; venous dilatation decreases venous return and hence cardiac output, but *only* if the denervated vessels are below the right atrium. Mean arterial pressure decreases in proportion to the change in cardiac output, but less so to the reduction in peripheral vascular resistance. Very extensive sympathetic block is not necessarily accompanied by hypotension, but there is a reduction in coronary blood flow if the mean arterial pressure decreases. However, hypotension is accompanied by a decrease in myocardial oxygen requirement because of coronary artery dilatation, reduced heart rate, and decreases in both left ventricular afterload and preload (Meissner et al. 1997).

Sympathetic block to T_4 dilates splanchnic, pelvic, and lower limb vessels, but compensatory vasoconstriction above that level is mediated by unblocked fibres (T_1–T_4) and systemic release of catecholamines from the adrenal medulla. Block above T_4 reduces or abolishes compensatory vasoconstriction in the head, neck, and upper limb, as well as the ability of the cardiac sympathetic fibres to stimulate the heart. However, the cardiovascular consequences of a limited, upper thoracic block are relatively modest (15–20% reduction in cardiac output and an increase in central venous pressure) because the lower sympathetic chain is spared.

Secondary factors

The cardiovascular consequences of an extensive central block can be minimal in the supine subject, especially one in a slight headdown tilt to maintain venous return. However, a wide range of patient and anaesthetic factors can exaggerate the effect, notably hypovolaemia, vena caval compression (by gravid uterus, packs, or retractors), drug-induced central depression, sudden movement, and autonomic dysfunction (as in old age, diabetes mellitus, alcoholism, rheumatoid arthritis, and rare conditions such as the Riley–Day and Shy–Drager syndromes). Each impairs the ability of the circulation to compensate for sympathetic block and increases the severity of any change in blood pressure.

The combination of general anaesthesia and epidural block will cause more cardiovascular depression than the epidural alone (Borghi et al. 2002). Artificial lung ventilation may exaggerate the effect because it reduces venous return and the sympathetic block prevents the usual compensation. Sympathetic block is particularly dangerous in the hypovolaemic patient and central block should not be instituted in a hypovolaemic patient. Correction of pre-existing fluid losses, with carefully monitoring to avoid overtransfusion, is even more vital than before general anaesthesia and fluid lost during surgery must be replaced immediately.

Significance of hypotension

Some consider any decrease in blood pressure undesirable, or even dangerous, but that accompanying uncomplicated regional anaesthesia can have beneficial effects such as decreased blood loss, improved operating conditions, and decreased myocardial workload. Even patients with cardiac disease may benefit, especially if the block is accompanied by the usual gentle decrease in heart rate.

However, the circulation must be monitored carefully, particularly the state of the peripheral circulation, and a proactive approach should be taken to the various factors noted previously which may increase the risk of severe hypotension. Before the block is instituted a decision should be made on what constitutes an acceptable blood pressure to guide management. In the healthy patient treatment is rarely required before mean arterial pressure decreases by more than 30%, but earlier intervention may be required in the presence of risk factors. In the conscious patient nausea demands immediate attention because it may be an indication that blood pressure is inadequate.

Nausea and bradycardia

The progressive slowing in heart rate which usually accompanies central block is a normal response which, as noted, has its own benefits. However, sudden bradycardia (heart rate <45), often preceded or accompanied by nausea (and even vomiting) is a much more serious condition. It may be due to the Bainbridge reflex (right atrial pressure receptors responding to decreased venous return), this implying that venous return has failed for some reason, but it may also be an indirect result of block of the cardioaccelerator nerves.

As an extreme example, the normal response to hypoxaemia is tachycardia, but if the sympathetic outflow is blocked the direct effects of oxygen lack on the heart (bradycardia) will predominate. Another possibility is that, in the presence of cardioaccelerator nerve block, any vagal activity is unopposed. Extreme bradycardia, with gross circulatory inadequacy, can occur and has been associated with cardiac arrest, and even death, in healthy patients (Caplan et al. 1988). Further, studies have confirmed that this sudden bradycardia is associated with reduced preload, increased vagal tone, and extensive sympathetic block (Auroy 1997, 2002, Kopp 2005).

However, sudden, although not quite so severe, bradycardia can occur in the absence of extensive sympathetic block (Burke & Wildsmith 2000). Basically, the patient simply faints, a seemingly unlikely event in a supine subject, but one which suggests that patients are not always as free from anxiety as they seem.

Prevention and treatment of hypotension

Hypotension is not a universal accompaniment of even extensive central nerve blocks, but fluid loading and, to a much lesser extent, prophylactic vasopressor therapy are used widely to try and prevent it. There are occasions when such proactive management is appropriate, but its routine application risks complications in those patients who would not have become hypotensive. It is better to take an expectant approach, monitor the circulation closely, and treat the patient on the basis of the changes observed once the pressure reaches the threshold figure for intervention (see 'Significance of hypotension' section).

Oxygen

Oxygen therapy is not essential during uncomplicated regional anaesthesia, but should be given to all patients receiving sedation, and those at risk of developing, or being treated for, hypotension.

Posture

Hypotension during central block is almost invariably due to decreased venous return reducing cardiac output. The simplest way to correct this is to raise the legs above the level of the heart. A steep head-down tilt does the same, but can cause the conscious patient some discomfort although it has minimal effect on cephalad spread of local anaesthetic. However, placing any patient with a central block in a slight head-down tilt is a useful prophylactic manoeuvre with no adverse features.

Intravenous fluids

The rapid infusion of 500–1000 ml of crystalloid or colloid is used widely to prevent or treat hypotension due to central block despite a wealth of published data providing little evidence in its favour. Not only is this *preloading* minimally ineffective, it can cause problems. Most central blocks regress from above downwards so sympathetic tone returns before bladder sensation, and catheterization is often necessary. In the elderly patient there is also the risk that the fluid may overload the pulmonary circulation and produce haemodilution (Holte et al. 2004).

However, it is good practice, no matter what type of anaesthetic is being given, to anticipate blood loss and pre-empt its effects. Thus, *co-loading* (colloid infused as the spinal develops), with increments of ephedrine, can minimize hypotension and reduce the need for subsequent intervention, at least during spinal anaesthesia for Caesarean section (Cyna et al. 2006).

Vasopressors

Prophylactic vasopressor therapy can lead to hypertension and tachycardia, and is unnecessary except in specific circumstances such as during deliberately extensive epidural block for major orthopaedic surgery. The aim is to produce induced hypotension, and titrated infusions of adrenaline are used to maintain the circulation, not to increase blood pressure (Sharrock et al. 1990).

Otherwise vasopressors should be used sparingly in small, incremental doses until the vasomotor tone is restored. The most commonly used drugs are ephedrine, metaraminol, and phenylephrine. Methoxamine is no longer available.

Ephedrine is both a direct and an indirectly acting α- and β-adrenoceptor agonist. It increases heart rate, stroke volume, cardiac output, and, less reliably, peripheral vascular resistance. It is more effective at restoring systolic blood pressure than crystalloid infusion (Wright & Fee 1992), and is probably the drug of choice in obstetric practice because it has less effect on uterine blood flow than other vasopressors (Ralston et al. 1974). Intravenously, increments of 3–6 mg are satisfactory (larger doses may cause tachycardia and hypertension), but relatively short acting. If repeated doses are needed, an intramuscular injection (15–30 mg) may have a more sustained action.

Metaraminol is an α-adrenoceptor agonist with minimal beta activity so its primary action is to increase peripheral vascular resistance. Increases in systolic and diastolic pressures are often accompanied by slowing in pulse rate; cardiac output may remain unchanged or be reduced and this agent is better reserved for treatment (0.5-mg incremental boluses intravenously) of hypotension with tachycardia.

Phenylephrine is a pure α-adrenoceptor agonist with a very short duration of action. It may be given intravenously by infusion of a 2-mcg ml^{-1} concentration or in 20–40-mcg boluses. It is very potent and must be used with care to avoid rebound hypertension.

Vagolytics

A heart rate of less than 60 bpm may be associated with an inadequate cardiac output, but vagolytic treatment (intravenous atropine 0.3 mg or glycopyrrolate 200–300 mcg) is advised only if there is hypotension as well or a tachycardia results. However, increasing the heart rate before administering a vasopressor often reduces the dose needed, or may avoid the need altogether.

Treatment of sudden, extreme bradycardia as described earlier (see 'Nausea and bradycardia' section) is difficult, and may require oxygen, head-down tilt, and combinations of chronotropic drugs. Given that vagal overactivity (which is often driven by anxiety) seems to be a crucial factor, there is some logic in the view that sedation may have an important prophylactic role (Burke & Wildsmith 2000).

Respiratory effects

The majority of peripheral blocks, and central blocks below T_{10}, do not affect respiratory function, but more extensive epidural and spinal spread may impair respiratory (primarily expiratory) effort, making it difficult for the patient to exhale and cough effectively. In patients with pre-existing respiratory disease (those in whom regional anaesthesia may be most suitable) this may lead to an unpleasant sense of dyspnoea. Interscalene brachial plexus block reduces respiratory effort by producing phrenic nerve palsy (Urmey 1991, 1993), and other brachial plexus approaches can also impair respiration in patients with borderline respiratory reserve (Rettig et al. 2005). Pneumothorax (a recognized risk with intercostal, paravertebral, interpleural, supraclavicular, infraclavicular, and stellate ganglion blocks) must always be considered when sudden respiratory distress occurs.

Postoperative care

Regional anaesthesia usually results in a much better quality of recovery than general anaesthesia, with better analgesia and avoidance of opioid side effects. This means that specific recovery targets are reached sooner and allows earlier discharge from the recovery ward. However, the quality of personnel and facilities must remain high because there are still side effects which require specific attention in the early postoperative period.

Cardiorespiratory effects

Hypotension may recur in the recovery period because sympathetic block will persist for some time, requiring close circulatory monitoring. Sudden postural change or continued fluid loss may destabilize the circulation, especially as the effect of earlier vasopressor treatment regresses. After spinal and epidural block the patient should be kept supine, preferably with a slight head-down tilt, until the blood pressure starts to increase and allows for progressive mobilization. Hypotension should be treated as outlined in the 'Prevention and treatment of hypotension' section, but it is vital that all staff looking after the patient realize that the block is not the only explanation for hypotension, especially when epidural infusions are continued on the surgical ward. Surgical bleeding is the most likely cause, and must be sought whenever hypotension occurs.

Respiratory depression is rare after regional techniques, but is a risk after the use of neuraxial opioids (see Chapter 14).

Written guidelines, setting out threshold levels for concern and the actions to be taken are useful for both recovery area and surgical ward staff. These guidelines should include instructions on oxygen and fluid therapy, the management of epidural top-ups & infusions, and the indications for naloxone to combat respiratory depression and pruritis in patients who have had neuraxial opioids.

Care of anaesthetized areas

Until the block regresses completely, the patient is at risk of complications resulting from the continued lack of sensation, muscle power, and proprioception. Hyperextension or flexion injuries at joints, stretching or compression of nerves, and skin damage can all occur unless the nursing staff take appropriate care. This becomes even more important when a block is continued into the postoperative period. Again these points should be in the written guidelines for staff, and in instructions given to patients and their carers if they are discharged home before full block regression.

Urinary retention

The bladder is innervated by the sacral autonomic fibres and these are among the last to regain function after central block. Any patient who has received large volumes of fluid during surgery, and who does not have a catheter in place, is at risk of urinary retention. There is no need to leave the catheter in place if prompt block regression is expected, but if epidural analgesia is continued into the postoperative period, an indwelling urinary catheter will be needed.

After spinal anaesthesia the incidence of retention requiring catheterization is directly related to the duration of the agent used; lidocaine produces a lower incidence than bupivacaine (Baldini et al. 2009).

Regression of the block

Ward staff should be given an approximate indication of how long the block will last, and the anticipated duration of a catheter infusion, so that any obvious variation will trigger a review. The patient should also be encouraged to report any strange subjective feelings, especially the *return* of numbness or motor weakness. The concern is that the features of a major complication, such as an epidural haematoma, will simply be ascribed to the block so that diagnosis and treatment are delayed.

The concentration of local anaesthetic solution used for infusions should be that which produces analgesia without immobility (e.g. bupivacaine 0.125–0.15% and ropivacaine 0.2%). Dense motor block is unnecessary, increases the risk of complications, and is avoidable. If an intense block has been produced for surgery it is good practice to allow (and document) return of voluntary muscle movement before starting the postoperative infusion. Thereafter, any increase in motor block should trigger immediate anaesthetic review to exclude a serious adverse event.

Good rapport between the patient and staff aids both detection of genuine complications and tolerance of minor discomforts unrelated to the block so that potentially serious side effects do not go unnoticed.

Sequential postoperative analgesia

The provision of excellent analgesia during the early postoperative period is a major benefit of regional anaesthesia. However, small doses of conventional analgesics must be available for discomforts outside the field of the block, and to encourage the sleep which all patients need after major surgery. At some stage, however, even when an infusion prolongs its duration, the block will regress; it is essential that additional analgesics are not only prescribed, but administered in advance of the return of pain.

The combination of drugs with different modes of action (*multimodal analgesia*) takes advantage of the synergism between them to reduce doses and allow earlier recovery with more rapid mobilization. This is a key component of *Enhanced Recovery Programmes* being developed for a number of surgical procedures (see Chapter 5).

Documentation

All regional block techniques should be properly documented in the patient's notes, either on the standard anaesthetic chart or on a specific record (Gerancher et al. 2005). The detail recorded should meet the requirements of good clinical practice, fulfil clinical risk management needs (including the need to audit personal and departmental practice), and be sufficient to defend potential medico-legal claims. A suggested minimum dataset includes:

◆ Named technique and approach;

◆ Needle insertion site and number of attempts;

◆ Type of needle (including length) and any catheter used;

◆ Nerve location technique used (stimulation, ultrasound, loss of resistance, etc.);

◆ Stimulator settings and minimum current;

◆ Local anaesthetic, concentration, volume, and adjuvants;

◆ Objective evidence of motor and sensory onset; and

◆ Adverse events during needle and catheter insertion and withdrawal.

With the development of acute pain teams and clinical guidelines for the care of patients using different analgesic regimens, all areas caring for postoperative patients should have standardized documentation for recording vital signs, sedation, and pain scores. During infusions, additional observations are required:

◆ Sensory level;

◆ Degree of motor block;

◆ Infusion rates (hourly and cumulative); and

◆ For peripheral blocks performed close to the neuraxis (interscalene, psoas sheath, paravertebral), check for bilateral spread periodically.

Observation intervals vary to reflect individual patient factors, the time since surgery, and the duration of the infusion, but with more frequent recordings after bolus injections and changes in infusion rate.

Teaching and training

Anatomy is the foundation upon which the entire concept of regional anesthesia is built.

(Gaston Labat 1922)

Training in regional anaesthesia was, like its practice, patchy, and this has only begun to change recently. Those fortunate enough to work in a department with relevant expertise, would learn from the experts, but in an unstructured, often lengthy process, sometimes at the expense of the patient. Others had little exposure, not even to central blocks, until these became widely used in obstetrics. Even in countries where a core curriculum existed, the emphasis was on performing a certain number of blocks (50 spinals, 50 epidurals, and 50 peripheral blocks is typical) rather than achieving competency, something which may need larger numbers. In one study trainees required 70 spinals to achieve 90% success, 90 epidurals for 80% success, and 60 brachial plexus blocks for 80% success (Konrad et al. 1998). Others have found similarly steep learning curves for spinals and epidurals (Kopacz et al. 1996), and particular problems with training in peripheral blocks (Kopacz and Neal 2002).

Training in regional anaesthesia requires a structured approach to learning with close supervision of the trainee (whether training or career grade) within a system which monitors the acquisition of

knowledge and skills while ensuring patient safety and little risk of failure. The theoretical aspects are relatively easy to provide: classroom-based teaching and self-directed learning from textbooks, multimedia programmes, and internet resources can be incorporated into training programmes with periodic assessment of progress. There are some excellent on-line (see reading list) and published (Enneking et al. 2005, Neal et al. 2008b) educational resources.

Basic skills can be taught in small-group sessions using simple simulators of block technique and the use of nerve location devices. Video feedback (Friedman et al. 2006), virtual reality animation (Lim et al. 2005), and simulation (Friedman et al. 2009, Grottke et al. 2009) techniques are being developed to provide for both knowledge and skill acquisition as well as assessment, although they are not yet widely available. Cadaver workshops are an excellent resource for understanding nerve location using both landmarks and ultrasound (Tsui et al. 2008), and offer practical experience of probe and needle handling. Modern ultrasound scanning devices provide further understanding of anatomy and its importance in regional anaesthesia. A block attempted without detailed knowledge of the relevant anatomy is more likely to fail than succeed.

However, the final stage of learning requires supervised practice on patients in the busy clinical setting, the aspect of training which is most difficult to deliver. Increased use of regional methods, driven in part by the introduction of new technologies, has coincided with changes in medical training and hospital practices that make the traditional training model unsustainable. Major factors are:

◆ Shorter working hours: typically 40–48 hours per week, including on-call;

◆ More flexible and part-time training, with shorter rotations between hospitals;

◆ Reduction in annual case load per trainee;

◆ Pressures on theatre throughput and utilization (less time to teach per case);

◆ Ethical and medico-legal concerns about the patient as a 'training tool';

◆ Conflict between the obligation to train and the delivery of safe and timely care to patients;

◆ Lack of individuals able to deliver the training requirements.

New training strategies must allow assessment of basic skills (including the preoperative aspects) while maintaining safety, efficacy, and outcome in a limited number of blocks because no trainee will acquire wide experience of the full range. Formal assessment on a selection of blocks at basic, intermediate, and advanced levels will be a more practical means of identifying competence, but with the onus remaining on the individual trainee to seek out the opportunities for learning. Such an approach will also allow for the wide variation between centres in the techniques used, a crucial issue because the trainers must be skilled and experienced users.

Quality assurance and personal development require that all anaesthetists keep a record of the blocks performed and their outcomes (good and adverse). Objective scoring systems are available, but currently little used. Cumulative sum analysis (CUSUM) (Kestin 1995) and Anaesthetic Competence Evaluation (ACE), a modified form of CUSUM (Harrison 2001), are easily incorporated into routine practice for both individual and departmental purposes. They plot progress during learning and can be used to demonstrate that standards are maintained.

If the current claims for the potential of ultrasound-guided nerve identification are fulfilled it may simplify training for, and the performance of, regional anaesthesia, but has its own competency requirements. A joint committee of the American and European Societies of Regional Anaesthesia has produced recommendations for the relevant education and training based on four skill sets (Sites et al. 2009):

- Understanding the ultrasound machine;
- Image optimization (probe handling skills);
- Image interpretation and visualization of the needle; and
- Spread of local anaesthetic.

Each can be taught and assessed individually before a specific block procedure is considered, thus minimizing both the time spent on training requiring patient contact and clinical risk. However, the use of ultrasound guidance still requires the other competencies outlined earlier in this chapter: patient assessment and preparation; gentle handling of patient, needle, and probe; an effective aseptic technique; and quality care during and after the procedure.

Key references

Bernards CM, Hadzic A, Suresh S, Neal JM (2008) Regional anesthesia in anesthetized or heavily sedated patients. *Regional Anesthesia and Pain Medicine* 33: 449–60.

Fettes PD, Jansson JR, Wildsmith JA (2009) Failed spinal anaesthesia: mechanisms, management, and prevention. *British Journal of Anaesthesia* 102: 739–48.

Hebl JR (2006) The importance and implications of aseptic techniques during regional anaesthesia. *Regional Anesthesia and Pain Management* 31: 311–23.

Sites BD, Chan VW, Neal JM, et al. (2009) The American Society of Regional Anesthesia and Pain Medicine and the European Society of Regional Anaesthesia and Pain Therapy Joint Committee recommendations for education and training in ultrasound-guided regional anesthesia. *Regional Anesthesia and Pain Medicine* 34: 40–6.

On-line resources

http://www.postoppain.org Procedure specific postoperative pain management (PROSPECT) information.

http://www.asra.com and http://www.esraeurope.org Educational material.

References

Auroy Y, Narchi P, Messiah A, et al. (1997) Serious complications related to regional anesthesia. *Anesthesiology* 87: 479–86.

Auroy Y, Benhamou D, Bargues L, et al. (2002) Major complications of regional anesthesia in France. *Anesthesiology* 97: 1274–80.

Baldini G, Bagry H, Aprikian A, Carli F (2009) Postoperative urinary retention: anesthetic and perioperative considerations. *Anesthesiology* 110: 1139–57.

Borghi B, Casati A, Iuorio S, et al. (2002) Frequency of hypotension and bradycardia during general anesthesia, epidural anesthesia or integrated epidural-general anesthesia for total hip replacement. *Journal of Clinical Anesthesia* 14: 102–6.

Bromage PR, Benumof JL (1998) Paraplegia following intracord injection during attempted epidural anesthesia under general anesthesia. *Regional Anesthesia and Pain Medicine* 23: 104–7.

Burke D, Wildsmith JAW (2000) Severe vasovagal attack during regional anaesthesia for Caesarean section. *British Journal of Anaesthesia* 84: 824–3.

Caplan RA, Ward RJ, Posner K, Cheney FW (1988) Unexpected cardiac arrest during spinal anesthesia: a closed claims analysis of predisposing factors. *Anesthesiology* 68: 5–11.

Carpenter RL, Caplan RA, Brown DL (1992) Incidence and risk factors for side effects of spinal anesthesia. *Anesthesiology* 76: 906–16.

Cook TM, Counsell D, Wildsmith JA (2009a) Royal College of Anaesthetists Third National Audit Project. Major complications of central neuraxial block: report on the Third National Audit Project of the Royal College of Anaesthetists. *British Journal of Anaesthesia* 102: 179–90.

Cook TM, Fischer B, Bogod D, et al. (2009b) Antiseptic solutions for central neuraxial blockade: which concentration of chlorhexidine should we use? *British Journal of Anaesthesia* 103: 456–7.

Cranshaw J, Gupta KJ, Cook TM (2009) Litigation related to drug errors in anaesthesia: an analysis of claims against the NHS in England 1995–2007. *Anaesthesia* 64: 1317–23.

Cyna AM, Andrew M, Emmett RS, et al. (2006) Techniques for preventing hypotension during spinal anaesthesia for caesarean section. *Cochrane Database Systematic Reviews* 18: CD002251.

Darouiche RO, Wall MJ Jr, Itani KM, et al. (2010) Chlorhexidine-Alcohol versus Povidone-Iodine for Surgical-Site Antisepsis. *New England Journal of Medicine* 362:18–26.

Dauri M, Sidiropoulou T, Fabbi E, et al. (2007) Efficacy of continuous femoral nerve block with stimulating catheters versus nonstimulating catheters for anterior cruciate ligament reconstruction. *Regional Anesthesia and Pain Medicine* 32: 282–7.

Enneking FK, Chan V, Greger J, et al. (2005) Lower-extremity peripheral nerve blockade: essentials of our current understanding. *Regional Anesthesia and Pain Medicine* 30: 4–35.

Fettes PD, Wildsmith JA (2002) Somebody else's nervous system. *British Journal of Anaesthesia* 88: 760–3.

Fischer HBJ (1998) Editorial: Regional anaesthesia—before or after general anaesthesia? *Anaesthesia* 53: 727–9.

Fischer HBJ (2009) Regional anaesthesia and analgesia. In Smith T, Pinnock C, Lin T (Eds) *Fundamentals of Anaesthesia*, 3rd edn, p. 119. Cambridge: Cambridge University Press.

Fischer HBJ, Simanski C (2005) A procedure-specific systematic review and consensus recommendations for analgesia after total hip replacement. *Anaesthesia* 60: 1189–202.

Fischer HBJ, Simanski CJ, Sharp C, et al. (2008) A procedure-specific systematic review and consensus recommendations for postoperative analgesia following total knee arthroplasty. *Anaesthesia* 63: 1105–23.

Frank SM, Nguyen JM, Garcia CM, Barnes RA (1999) Temperature monitoring practices during regional anesthesia. *Anesthesia & Analgesia* 88: 373–7.

Friedman Z, Katznelson R, Devito I, et al. (2006) Objective assessment of manual skills and proficiency in performing epidural anesthesia—video-assisted validation. *Regional Anesthesia and Pain Medicine* 31: 304–10.

Friedman Z, Saddiqui N, Katznelson R, et al. (2009) Clinical impact of epidural anesthesia simulation on short and long-term learning curve: High versus low-fidelity model training. *Regional Anesthesia and Pain Medicine* 34: 229–32.

Gerancher JC, Viscusi ER, Liguori GA, et al. (2005) Development of a standardized peripheral nerve block procedure note form. *Regional Anesthesia and Pain Medicine* 30: 67–71.

Grewal S, Hocking G, Wildsmith JA (2006) Epidural abscesses. *British Journal of Anaesthesia* 96: 292–302.

Grottke O, Ntouba A, Ullrich S, et al. (2009) Virtual reality-based simulator for training in regional anaesthesia. *British Journal of Anaesthesia* 103: 594–600.

Hadzic A, Dilberovic F, Shah S, et al. (2004) Combination of intraneural injection and high injection pressure leads to fascicular injury and neurologic deficits in dogs. *Regional Anesthesia and Pain Medicine* 29: 417–23.

Harrison MJ (2001) Tracking the early acquisition of skills by trainees. *Anaesthesia* 56: 995–8.

Holte K, Foss NB, Svensen C (2004) Epidural anesthesia, hypotension and changes in intravascular volume. *Anesthesiology* 100: 281–6.

Horlocker TT, Abel MD, Messick JM Jr, Schroeder DR (2003) Small risk of serious neurologic complications related to lumbar epidural catheter placement in anesthetized patients. *Anesthesia & Analgesia* 96: 1547–52.

Joshi GP, Bonnet F, Shah R, et al. (2008) A systematic review of randomized trials evaluating regional techniques for post-thoracotomy analgesia. *Anesthesia & Analgesia* 107: 1026–40.

Kehlet H, Wilkinson R, Fischer HBJ, Camu F (2007) Evidence-based, procedure-specific postoperative pain management. *Best Practice and Research: Clinical Anaesthesiology* 21: 149–59.

Kestin IG (1995) A statistical approach to measuring the competence of anaesthetic trainees at practical procedures. *British Journal of Anaesthesia* 75: 805–9.

Konrad C (1998) Learning manual skills in anaesthesiology: is there a recommended number of cases for anaesthetic procedures? *Anesthesia & Analgesia* 86: 635–9.

Kopacz DJ, Neal JM, Pollock JE (1996) The anesthesia learning curve. What is the minimum number of epidural and spinal blocks to reach consistency? *Regional Anesthesia and Pain Medicine* 21: 182–90.

Kopacz DJ, Neal JM (2002) Regional anesthesia and pain medicine: residency training—The year 2000. *Regional Anesthesia and Pain Medicine* 27: 9–14.

Kopp SL, Horlocker TT, Warner ME, et al. (2005) Cardiac arrest during neuraxial anaesthesia: frequency and predisposing factors associated with survival. *Anesthesia & Analgesia* 100: 855–65.

Krane EJ, Dalens BJ, Murat I, Murrell D (1998) The safety of epidurals placed during general anesthesia. *Regional Anesthesia and Pain Medicine* 23: 433–8.

Lim MW, Burt G, Rutter SV (2005) Use of three dimensional animation for regional anaesthesia teaching: application to interscalene brachial plexus blockade. *British Journal of Anaesthesia* 94: 372–7.

Meissner A, Rolf N, Van Aken H (1997) Thoracic epidural anesthesia and the patient with heart disease: benefits, risks and controversies *Anesthesia & Analgesia* 85: 517–28.

Moen V, Dahlgren N, Irestedt L (2004) Severe neurological complications after central neuraxial blockades in Sweden 1990–1999. *Anesthesiology* 101: 950–9.

National Patient Safety Agency (2009) *Safer spinal (intrathecal), epidural and regional devices—Part A and Part B.* http://www.nrls.npsa.nhs.uk/alerts/?entryid45 = 65259. (Accessed 31 January 2010.)

Neal JM, Bernards CM, Hadzic A, et al. (2008a) ASRA Practice Advisory on Neurologic Complications in Regional Anesthesia and Pain Medicine. *Regional Anesthesia and Pain Medicine* 33: 404–15.

Neal JM, Gerancher JC, Hebl JR, et al. (2008b) Upper extremity regional anesthesia: essentials of our current understanding. *Regional Anesthesia and Pain Medicine* 34: 134–70.

Philips BJ, Ferguson S, Armstrong P, et al (1992) Surgical facemasks are effective in reducing bacterial contamination caused in dispersal from the upper airway. *British Journal of Anaesthesia* 69: 407–8.

Ralston DH, Shnider SM, De Lorimier AA (1974) Effects of equipotent ephedrine, metaraminol, mephentermine and methoxamine on uterine blood flow in the pregnant ewe. *Anesthesiology* 40: 354–70.

Rettig HC, Gielen MJ, Boersma E, et al. (2005) Vertical infraclavicular block of the brachial plexus: effects on hemidiaphragmatic movement and ventilatory function. *Regional Anesthesia and Pain Medicine* 30: 529–35.

Rice AS, McMahon SB (1992) Peripheral nerve injury caused by injection needles used in regional anaesthesia: influence of bevel configuration, studied in a rat model. *British Journal of Anaesthesia* 69: 433–8.

Safe Anaesthesia Liaison Group (2010) *Wrong site blocks during surgery.* (Safety notice.) http://www.rcoa.ac.uk/docs/SALG-Statement-WSB.pdf

Sala-Blanch X, Ribalta T, Rivas E, et al. (2009) Structural injury to the human sciatic nerve after intraneural needle insertion. *Regional Anesthesia and Pain Medicine* 34: 201–5.

Salinas FV, Neal JM, Sueda LA, et al. (2004) Prospective comparison of continuous femoral nerve block with nonstimulating catheter placement versus stimulating catheter-guided perineural placement in volunteers. *Regional Anesthesia and Pain Medicine* 29: 212–20.

Selander D, Dhuner K-G, Lunbdborg G (1977) Peripheral nerve injury due to injection needles used for regional anaesthesia. *Acta Anaesthesiologica Scandinavica* 21: 182–8.

Sharrock NE, Mineo R, Urquhart B (1990) Hemodynamic response to low-dose epinephrine infusion during hypotensive epidural anesthesia for total hip replacement. *Regional Anesthesia* 15: 295–9.

Tsui BC, Dillane D, Pillay J, Walji A (2008) Ultrasound imaging in cadavers: training in imaging for regional blockade at the trunk. *Canadian Journal of Anaesthesia* 55: 105–11.

Urmey WF, Gloeggler PJ (1993) Pulmonary function changes during interscalene brachial plexus block: effects of decreasing local anesthetic injection volume. *Regional Anesthesia* 18: 244–9.

Urmey WF, Talts KH, Sharrock NE (1991) One hundred percent incidence of hemidiaphragmatic paresis associated with interscalene brachial plexus anesthesia as diagnosed by ultrasonography. *Anesthesia & Analgesia* 72: 498–503.

Walker IA, Griffiths R, Wilson IH (2010) Replacing Luer connectors: still work in progress. *Anaesthesia* 65: 1059–62.

Wildsmith JAW, Fischer HBJ (1999) Correspondence: Regional anaesthesia—before or after general anaesthesia? *Anaesthesia* 54: 86.

Winnie AP (1983) *Plexus anesthesia*, vol 1, p. 211. Edinburgh: Churchill Livingstone.

Wright PM, Fee JP (1992) Cardiovascular support during combined extradural and general anaesthesia. *British Journal of Anaesthesia* 68: 585–9.

PART 2

Anatomy and techniques

CHAPTER 12

Anatomy and physiology of the vertebral canal

Ian Parkin and Alastair Chambers

The vertebral column

The vertebral column is a strong curved pillar, which extends from the base of the skull to the pelvis in the midline (Figure 12.1). It is formed by a series of vertebrae which contribute about three-quarters of its length, the remainder deriving from the intervening fibrocartilaginous discs. Only a small degree of movement occurs between any two adjacent vertebrae, but the cumulative effect results in a column of considerable flexibility that is strong and stable. The vertebral column has three major functions.

1. It transmits the upper body weight to the pelvis and then to the lower limbs and the ground;

2. It provides the sites of attachment of the muscles of posture and locomotion; and

3. It forms a protective canal for the spinal cord and its covering meninges.

Typically, there are 24 'true' vertebrae, making up the cervical (7), thoracic (12), and lumbar (5) regions of the column. There are normally 9 'false' vertebrae which fuse to constitute the sacrum (5) and coccyx (4).

In the embryo, the spine is curved into a 'C' shape, concave forwards. This primary curvature persists throughout life in the thoracic and sacral regions, and may return to some extent in the lumbar and cervical region with ageing. Extension of the head when it is held up, and of the lower limbs when standing erect, produces secondary curvatures in the cervical and lumbar regions which are concave backwards (Figure 12.1). All of these curves are produced predominantly by moulding of the intervertebral discs, with the 'high' points in the supine position being C_4–C_5 and L_2–L_4, and the 'low' points T_5–T_7 and S_2. The lumbar curve is more marked in women, particularly during pregnancy, while the cervical curve usually includes the first two thoracic vertebrae. Most curvature occurs in the anterior/posterior plane, but minor lateral curves may also occur. In the thoracic region the column may deviate somewhat laterally, usually towards the right, and be compensated for by curves above or below.

The vertebrae

A typical vertebra

The general features of vertebrae change gradually between regions, but are similar enough to be considered together (Figure 12.2).

Viewed from above, the 'typical' vertebra has an anterior body through which the weight of the person is transmitted. This body increases in size down the column to accommodate the increase in transmitted weight. The flat superior and inferior surfaces are the sites of attachment of the intervertebral discs which separate adjacent vertebrae and act as shock absorbers to dissipate the forces placed on the column. The posterior surface of the body is flat (but may display a small midline ridge), while the anterior and lateral faces are curved. Posteriorly, there is a vertebral or neural arch

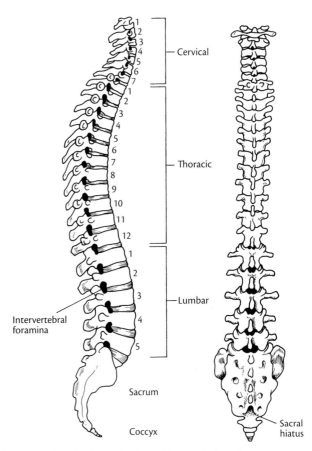

Figure 12.1 Lateral and posterior views of the vertebral canal.

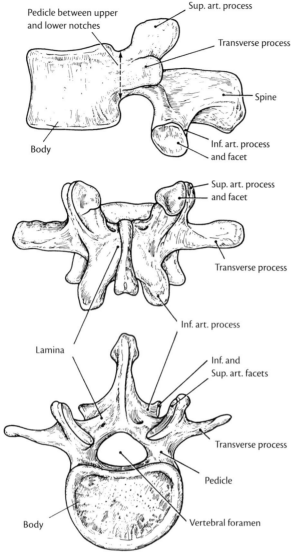

Pedicle between upper and lower notches

Sup. art. process

Transverse process

Spine

Body

Inf. art. process and facet

Sup. art. process and facet

Transverse process

Inf. art. process

Lamina

Inf. and Sup. art. facets

Transverse process

Pedicle

Vertebral foramen

Body

Figure 12.2 Lateral, posterior, and superior views of a 'typical' vertebra.

which completes the boundaries of the vertebral foramen. Anterolaterally, this arch is formed by two stout pedicles and is completed posteriorly by two laminae which unite in the midline to form the base of the spinous process. The pedicles attach to the upper, posterolateral surfaces of the vertebral body—a feature which allows confirmation of vertebral orientation. When viewed laterally, each pedicle carries two notches of uneven depth, the inferior notch usually being deeper than the superior. Articulation of two neighbouring vertebrae forms the intervertebral foramina, through which the roots of spinal nerves and the vascular structures supplying the spinal cord pass.

An articular pillar of paired superior and inferior articular processes lies behind the pedicles. The superior articular processes of one vertebra articulate with the inferior articular processes of the vertebra above to form the synovial zygapophysial joints. The spinous process projects posteriorly, while left and right transverse processes project posterolaterally, from the neural arch. The laminae and spinous process together form a large surface area for muscle and ligament attachment.

Cervical vertebrae

The typical cervical vertebrae have relatively small bodies and are found in the middle of this region: the C_1 (atlas), C_2 (axis), and C_7 (vertebra prominens) are atypical. The transverse processes contain the foramen transversarium for the passage of the vertebral artery, and have grooves superiorly that house the emerging spinal nerves. The spinous processes are short, bifid, and horizontal. The laminae are flat, long, and increase in depth from C_3 downwards. The vertebral foramina are triangular and relatively large to accommodate the cervical enlargement of the spinal cord.

The atlas (C_1) is essentially a ring of bone, formed from the two lateral masses which are united by an anterior (shorter) and posterior (longer) arch. Superior facets articulate with the occipital condyles to allow flexion and extension of the head.

The axis (C_2) has the dens or odontoid peg extending from its body and articulating with the posterior aspect of the anterior arch of the atlas. Consequently the axis is the pivot for rotatory movements of the head.

The seventh cervical vertebra (C_7) is essentially transitional, having some of the characteristics of the cervical vertebrae above, and others of the thoracic vertebrae below. Its spine is not bifid, but longer and forms a palpable landmark—the *vertebra prominens*.

Thoracic vertebrae

The vertebral bodies of the thoracic region are more or less circular, although in the upper and lower regions they are transitional from cervical and lumbar vertebral bodies respectively. From T_1–T_8 the bodies bear superior and inferior articular surfaces (demifacets), the upper articulating with the head of the corresponding rib and the lower with the head of the rib below. A similar surface on the large transverse process articulates with the rib tubercle. T_1 and the last two to four thoracic vertebrae have complete articular surfaces for the corresponding rib only. The vertebral foramina are circular in shape. The pedicles pass directly backwards carrying deep inferior notches and virtually no superior notch (T_1 excepted). The laminae are broad, thick, and overlap. The spinous processes are long and generally angled caudally to overlap the spine below. The intervertebral discs are thin in comparison with other regions and this, together with the overlap of the spinous processes and the presence of the ribs, greatly restricts movement in the thoracic region.

Lumbar vertebrae

In the lumbar region the vertebral bodies are large and kidney shaped, the pedicles are short and stout with shallow superior notches, and the transverse processes are generally quite long and slender except for L_5 where they are short, thick, strong, and arise from the vertebral body as well as the neural arch. The laminae are deep, short, and tend not to overlap as they do in the thoracic region. The spinous processes are horizontal, thick, and square. The vertebral foramina are triangular and are larger than in the thoracic region, but smaller than in the cervical region. The body of L_5 is wedge shaped, being thicker anteriorly and forming the characteristic lumbosacral angle.

The sacrum

In the adult, the five (sometimes six) vertebrae below the lumbar segment fuse to form the sacrum (Figure 12.3), the central part of the pelvic girdle. It is a wedge-shaped bone, wider above than

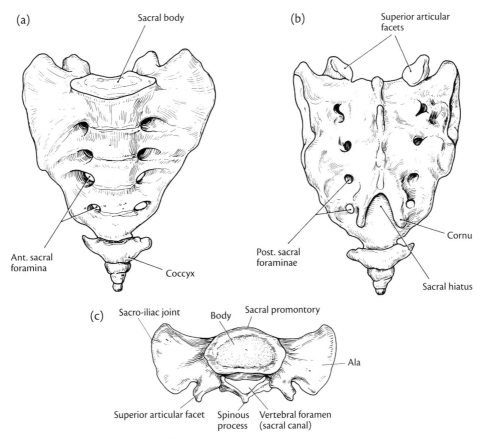

Figure 12.3 Anterior (a), posterior (b), and superior (c) views of the sacrum.

below, and concave anteriorly, both from above downwards and from side to side. The central part of the sacrum is formed by the fusion of the vertebral bodies, and there are four transverse ridges on the anterior surface representing the obliterated intervertebral discs. At the lateral ends of these ridges are the four anterior sacral foramina, the remnants of the anterior ends of the intervertebral foramina, through which pass the ventral rami of the sacral spinal nerves. The posterior surface of the sacrum is formed by the fusion of the neural arches. A midline crest derives from the laminae and has three or four tubercles on it, these representing the fused spinous processes. Lateral to this is the intermediate crest (the fused articular process) and, directly opposite the anterior foramina, the four posterior foramina for the posterior rami of the sacral nerves. The lateral crest is the result of fusion of the transverse processes.

The sacral canal is triangular in cross section. The dural sac usually ends opposite S_2. Inferiorly, the laminae of the last sacral arch, and occasionally those of the adjacent arch, fail to meet and leave a roughly triangular sacral hiatus, bounded by the cornua which are the remnants of the lowest articular process. The sacral hiatus shows considerable variation in both length and width, but can usually be found approximately 5 cm above the tip of the coccyx, directly above the uppermost limit of the natal cleft. The hiatus is traversed by the fifth sacral nerves.

Vertebral anomalies

Variations in the bony anatomy of the spine are of more than passing interest because they may make the performance of spinal

or epidural block difficult or impossible. Common anomalies include fusion of two or more vertebrae (particularly the fifth lumbar vertebra to the sacrum), separation of the first sacral segment, and absent or additional vertebrae. Grossly abnormal development can result in hemi-vertebra, or even in spina bifida occulta, caused by failure of fusion of two developmental centres in the neural arch. This is not usually associated with any neurological defect, although there may be an overlying dimple, lipoma, or tuft of hair, but only rarely is there a gross defect of one or more arches with protrusion of the cord or its coverings. Variations in the structure of the sacrum are dealt with in Chapter 15.

Intervertebral joints and ligaments

The individual vertebrae articulate with each other through the column of bodies and intervertebral discs. Additionally, the neural arches articulate through the superior and inferior processes on each side at the zygapophysial joints. The vertebrae are linked to each other by groups of ligaments, with only the pedicles not being connected directly to a ligament.

Ligaments of the vertebral bodies

A number of ligaments (Figure 12.4) connect the vertebrae.

The *anterior longitudinal ligament* attaches to the occipital bone and the anterior arch of the atlas. It then runs along the front of the vertebral bodies from C_2 to the upper sacrum, becoming wider as it descends. It is attached primarily to the superior and inferior margins of the vertebral bodies and secondarily (loosely) to their

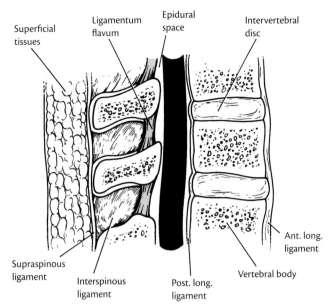

Figure 12.4 Sagittal section of lumbar vertebrae to the show the principal ligaments.

curved anterior surfaces. Over the intervertebral discs it is firmly attached to the annuli fibrosi. The ligament has a number of layers, its deepest fibres are unisegmental whereas the most superficial ones may cover four or five segments.

The *posterior longitudinal ligament* runs over the posterior surfaces of the vertebral bodies and discs, being attached mainly to the annuli fibrosi, but also to the margins of the adjacent vertebral bodies. It extends from C_2 to the sacrum, but is continuous superiorly with the membrana tectoria. It is wider cranially, but narrower inferiorly, where it appears denticulate—the 'teeth' extending laterally as the attachments to the intervertebral discs. The ligament displays an anterior (deep) layer and a posterior (superficial) layer over the vertebral bodies, but these are fused and indistinguishable at the attachments to the discs and vertebral margins. The shortest fibres of the anterior layer of the ligament extend across two spinal segments, that is, from the disc or superior margin of one vertebral body to the inferior margin or disc of the body two above. The longer fibres, of the posterior layer may extend over four or five segments. These longitudinal ligaments, plus the fan-like fibres attaching to the discs, combine to resist forward flexion, lateral flexion, and rotation.

Both layers attach to a midline, bony septum on the posterior aspect of the vertebral bodies, although the septum may not be present in the mid-one-third of the vertebra. This midline attachment may direct infection or tumour spread to the right or left. It appears that the peridural membrane (see 'Epidural space' section) extends laterally from the posterior longitudinal ligament (Loughenbury et al. 2006).

The *annuli fibrosi of the intervertebral discs* are structurally and functionally the principal ligaments of the vertebral bodies. They lie in the peripheral part of the intervertebral disc, the collagen fibres running from the disc of one vertebral body to the next in a series of concentric lamellae which are often deficient posterolaterally. These fibres act to resist movement between the vertebrae.

Ligaments of the neural arches, spines, and transverse processes

The *ligamenta flava* are a series of paired ligaments arising from the lower border and adjacent inner surface of one lamina plus the inferior aspect of the pedicle (Figure 12.4) and then dividing into medial and lateral components. The medial component attaches to the upper border and outer surface of the lamina below, while the lateral part attaches and contributes to the facet joint capsule. The thickness of the ligament varies considerably (2–10 mm), and increases from above downwards. It is 80% elastin in young adults, but its elasticity decreases with increasing age and it may calcify. The ligamenta flava probably add a gradual control to vertebral flexion, and assist in returning to the erect position. Their elasticity may serve to prevent buckling and encroachment on to other structures, as well as providing protection to the intervertebral discs. Each pair of ligaments may meet in the midline at an attenuated junction, but fail to do so in approximately 50% of segments. Any deficiency is usually filled by small veins and the anterior surface of the interspinous ligament, although this may be deficient also (Harrison 1999, Hogan 1996, Westbrook et al. 1993). It is theoretically possible therefore that a needle inserted in the midline could enter the epidural space without traversing the ligamentum flavum or interspinous ligament, and therefore without any loss of resistance.

The *interspinous ligaments* run between the shafts of adjacent spines. They are thin except in the lumbar region where they are thick, quadrangular, and usually in left and right halves, with a potential cleft between. Dorsally the ligaments are augmented by the tendinous insertions of the erector spinae musculature.

The *supraspinous ligament* is a powerful fibrous structure attaching to the posterior edges of the vertebral spines from C_7 downwards. It reaches L_3 in 20%, L_4 in 75%, and L_5 or the sacrum in 5% of individuals. Although called a ligament, this structure consists mainly of the tendinous attachments of the long back muscles, with only the most superficial (posterior) layers lacking any continuity with muscle. The supraspinous ligament offers little resistance to the separation of spinous processes and may become ossified in old age, so making penetration with a fine needle difficult or impossible. Above C_7 the supraspinous ligament is continuous with the ligamentum nuchae, which is essentially an intermuscular septum spanning the spinous processes from C_7 to the external occipital protruberance.

The *intertransverse ligaments* pass between the transverse processes of the vertebrae and are variable in size and thickness, but often blend with adjacent muscles.

The intervertebral discs

Whatever an individual's height, the vertebral column is about 70 cm in length in the male and 60 cm in the female, with the intervertebral discs accounting for 20–25% of this. With ageing, atrophy of the discs and osteoporosis of the vertebrae lead to kyphotic deformity and a decrease in height. The discs allow some rotation, and a 'rocking' between adjacent vertebrae during flexion, extension, and lateral flexion (a ball and socket joint in this position would compromise weight bearing ability).

An intervertebral disc requires to be:

◆ Strong, in order to sustain body weight without collapsing;

◆ Deformable enough to allow the movements outlined earlier;

◆ Resilient enough to avoid damage during those movements.

To achieve these properties the disc is formed in two parts. The ligamentous annulus fibrosus (see 'Ligaments of the vertebral bodies' section) surrounds the nucleus pulposus, a semifluid, mucoid mass which will deform, but not compress, under pressure. These properties result in applied pressure being transmitted in all directions, as when a water-filled balloon is compressed. With ageing, the nucleus gradually changes until it cannot be distinguished from the annulus fibrosus, the disc becoming thinner and less resilient.

Movement of the spine

Movement between individual vertebrae is limited, but summates through the vertebral column to provide relatively free flexion, extension, and lateral flexion in the cervical and lumbar regions. The thoracic movements are limited by the ribs and respiration, but a small amount of rotation is available. It should be noted that natural forward bending is largely flexion at the hip joints rather than flexion of the vertebral column. The ligamentum flavum stretches freely on flexion and its elastic recoil avoids the formation of folds which might be caught between bones on extension.

If the vertebral column is viewed from behind, the laminae and spines can be seen to overlap each other so that the spinal canal is completely hidden except in the lower lumbar region. The gap between the lumbar spinous processes can be widened by flexion of the spine (Figure 12.5), but this manoeuvre has a more limited effect in the thoracic region. Rotation may distort the bony structures so that a direct approach to the vertebral canal is not possible from the midline. This is more likely to be a problem in the thoracic region where, as noted earlier, a greater degree of rotation is possible.

The vertebral canal

The vertebral canal extends from the foramen magnum to the sacral hiatus. It is formed by the neural arches, the posterior surfaces of the vertebral bodies, and the ligaments and other structures that link them. The curves of the vertebral column are mirrored in the canal, which has a roughly triangular cross-sectional shape with the apex posteriorly, although it is more circular in cross section in the thoracic region. The volume of the canal is largest in the cervical region to house the cervical enlargement of the spinal cord. It is smaller in the thoracic region, but increases again in the lower thoracic and upper lumbar region (to house the lumbar enlargement) before narrowing progressively through the remaining lumbar and sacral regions.

The most notable openings of the canal are the pairs of *intervertebral foramina*, which are formed by the inferior and superior notches of the adjacent pedicles together with contributions from the vertebral bodies and discs anteriorly, and the laminae and zygapophyseal joints posteriorly. Each foramen is lined by the periosteal, perichondrial, and capsular fibrous coverings of its boundaries, as well as being crossed by small, fibrous bands or transforaminal ligaments.

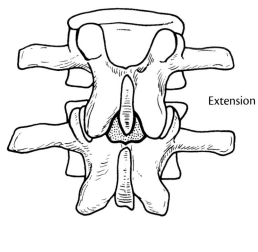

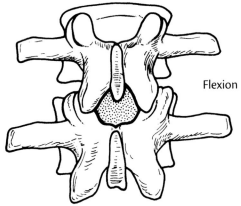

Figure 12.5 Effect of flexion and extension on the interspinous space in the lumbar region.

Twenty-four of the intervertebral foramina face laterally (although the cervical ones are slightly anterolateral) whereas four (sacral) face anteroposteriorly. They tend to increase in diameter from above downwards, although the L_5/S_1 foramen is relatively small. The larger spinal nerves which supply the upper and lower limbs pass between $C_5–T_1$ and $L_2–S_1$. The vertebral canal communicates with the thoracic and abdominal cavities through these foramina, and with the cranial cavity through the foramen magnum.

As well as the mixed spinal nerves with their coverings, the intervertebral foramina also contain spinal arteries, a plexiform arrangement of veins which connect the internal and external vertebral venous plexuses, and tiny meningeal (sinuvertebral) nerves.

The sacrococcygeal ligament usually seals the sacral hiatus completely.

The meninges and dural sac

The spinal cord has three covering membranes or meninges—the *dura*, *arachnoid*, and *pia maters*—which divide the vertebral canal into three compartments: the *epidural*, *subdural*, and *subarachnoid* 'spaces'. The potential epidural space (see 'Epidural space' section) lies between the dura mater and the margins of the spinal canal. The subdural compartment is definitely only a potential space between the dura and the arachnoid mater, which is approximated to the inner surface of the dural sac and separated from it by only a thin film of serous fluid. The subarachnoid space contains cerebrospinal fluid (CSF), and the spinal cord with its emerging nerve roots which are intimately covered by pia mater.

The dura mater is a continuation of the inner layer of cerebral dura and is composed of dense longitudinally orientated fibrous tissue. The outer, periosteal layer of cerebral dura is continued as the periosteal lining of the vertebral canal.

Extensions of the dura mater and the applied arachnoid continue along each spinal nerve root as far as the ganglion on the dorsal root and sometimes further, progressively thinning to become continuous with the coverings of the peripheral nerves (see Figure 6.1). These extensions of the subarachnoid space, known as dural 'cuffs', contain a pocket of CSF and are pierced by numerous veins, arteries, and lymphatics as they pass between the subarachnoid and epidural spaces. Additionally, arachnoid granulations protrude through the dura to communicate with the epidural veins and lymphatics, thus facilitating drainage of CSF and the removal of foreign material. The pia mater, the innermost membrane, is a vascular sheath which closely invests the spinal cord and continues caudally, closely invested with dura, as the *filum terminale* to attach to periosteum on the posterior surface of the coccyx. The blood vessels supplying the spinal cord lie within the tissue of the pia mater (see 'Spinal cord blood supply' section).

Dural sac

The dural sac extends from the foramen magnum to the second, or occasionally third, sacral segment where it continues distally as a covering of the filum terminale. However, there is some variation. The termination of the sac is lower in children, and in some adults it may be as high as the fifth lumbar segment. The sac lies within the vertebral canal, being attached to the edge of the foramen magnum above, the posterior longitudinal ligament anteriorly, the ligamentum flavum and laminae posteriorly, the pedicles laterally, and the coccyx by the filum terminale inferiorly. These attachments, together with the continuation of dura laterally along each spinal nerve root, stabilize both the dural sac and the spinal cord. Along with the CSF pressure, they also ensure that the sac adapts to the shape of the overlying vertebral canal.

Subarachnoid space and spinal cord

The subarachnoid space lies deep to the arachnoid mater. It contains the spinal cord, dorsal and ventral nerve roots, and CSF. The space tends to be symmetrical on the left and right sides, averaging 2.5 mm. However, it is variable both anteriorly and posteriorly, ranging from 1–5 mm. The spinal cord extends from the medulla oblongata, with which it is continuous, to end as the *conus medullaris* near the lower border of the first lumbar vertebra. The exact level is variable (Figure 12.6). The pia mater continues caudally as a thread-like filum terminale, ultimately attaching to the coccyx. The adult cord has an average length of 45 cm and weight of 30 g in the adult male, is elliptical in cross-section (with a greater transverse diameter at all levels), and tapers caudally except for two distinct expansions. The first, and larger of these, is the cervicothoracic enlargement which reaches maximum width at the level of C_5 and reflects the extensive upper limb innervation. The second, lumbosacral, enlargement innervates the lower limbs, and is situated between the ninth and twelfth thoracic vertebrae. There are 31 pairs of spinal nerves (8 cervical, 12 thoracic, 5 lumbar, 5 sacral, and 1 coccygeal), each formed from a dorsal and a ventral

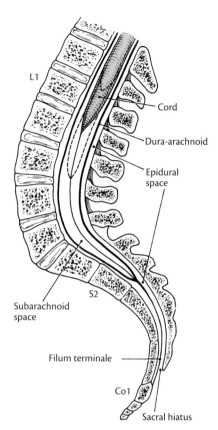

Figure 12.6 Sagittal section of lumbar and sacral regions of the spine. The dotted lines indicate the range for the termination of the spinal cord.

root. These roots are formed from several smaller rootlets or fibrils, and every dorsal root has a ganglion where the cell bodies of the sensory nerves are situated.

Up to the third month of intrauterine life the cord extends the full length of the canal, but thereafter the vertebrae grow much more rapidly, and this results in the neonatal conus medullaris being at the third lumbar level. The differential growth means that, in the adult, there is increasing obliquity of the nerve roots from above downwards, so that the lumbar and sacral roots lie freely within CSF below the level of the conus medullaris to form the *cauda equina*.

Numerous delicate trabeculations run between the arachnoid and pia maters, the pattern varying between individuals, with more to be found along the dorsal aspect of the cord than ventrally (Nauta et al. 1983) (Figures 12.7 and 12.8). A midline dorsal septum, the *septum posticum* (Di Chiro & Timins 1974, Nauta et al. 1983) typically extends from the midcervical to lumbar regions. Generally, it is attached to the pia mater along the course of the dorsal vein of the spinal cord (Nauta et al. 1983) and has irregular perforations, particularly towards its upper and lower ends. Lateral to the septum posticum, two other septae extend from the region of the dorsal rootlets and attach to the dorsolateral arachnoid mater. These dorsolateral septae tend to be more irregular, more densely fenestrated, to atrophy with age, and to extend further rostrally and caudally than the septum posticum; they probably serve to tether the dorsal rootlets, keeping them clear of the lateral parts of the spinal cord (Nauta et al. 1983). Ventrally, there are similar fenestrated septae, but they are less marked than the dorsolateral septae

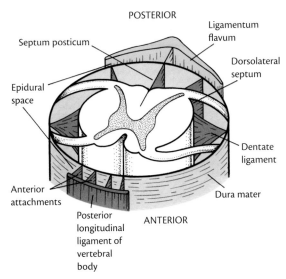

Figure 12.7 Transverse section of spinal cord to show its attachments.

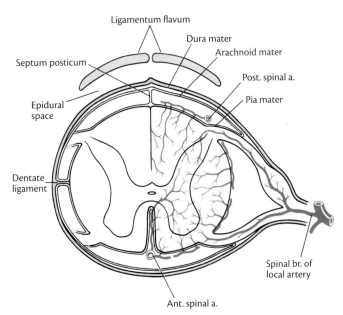

Figure 12.8 Transverse section to show the spinal meninges and arterial blood supply. The nerve roots have been omitted on the left for clarity.

and there is no ventral midline septum. Substantial lateral projections from the pia mater, known as *denticulate* or *dentate ligaments*, attach to the dura mater and act to support the spinal cord. There are no attachments anterior to the dentate ligaments.

Spinal cord blood supply

The spinal cord is supplied by an *anterior* and two *posterior spinal arteries* (Figure 12.8), all of which run within the pia mater. The anterior spinal artery is a single midline vessel, formed at the foramen magnum from a branch of each vertebral artery. It is the largest of the spinal vessels and supplies a substantial portion of the anterior cord. There is one posterior spinal artery (occasionally two) on each side, each derived from the posterior inferior cerebellar artery. Spinal branches of the vertebral, ascending cervical, posterior intercostal, lumbar, and lateral sacral arteries pass through the intervertebral foramina to augment blood supply. Most of these are insignificant, but some contribute substantially, especially those at T_4 and T_{11}. The arterial supply to the cord is vulnerable to the consequences of occlusion, such as may follow trauma, hypotension, or the use of vasoconstrictors. Blockage of a posterior vessel may have little effect, but occlusion of the anterior spinal artery usually leads to ischaemia of a large section of the spinal cord. Venous drainage is through a plexus of anterior and posterior veins which drain along the nerve roots into epidural and segmental veins.

Epidural space

The epidural space has been studied frequently in live, cadaveric, human, and animal subjects by methods including dissection, imaging, epiduroscopy, and microscopy. The results are conflicting and there is scope for further work, particularly as this so-called space is an important and frequently used route for anaesthetic administration. Of course, the normal range of human variation, and changes with age, may explain some of the variable results, particularly in relation to meningovertebral ligaments, the shape of the epidural space and dural sac dorsally, and the amounts of epidural fat. Such variations may well cause inexplicable, individual variation in anaesthetic efficacy. However, there is evidence that the topography of the space is not appreciably altered by

putting a patient in either the supine or the lateral position (Harrison 1999).

It must be stated at the outset that this compartment between the lining of the vertebral canal and the dural sac is a potential space. Ordinarily, the CSF pressure presses the arachnoid and overlying dura against the canal walls, turning the epidural space into a 'sandwich' of the intervening fibrous strands (meningovertebral ligaments), any fat that is present, and veins, arteries, and lymphatics. The balance between the pressure created in the epidural space by injecting solution, and the pressure of the CSF in the subarachnoid space is likely to be a major cause of the unpredictable distribution of epidural block (Harrison 1999).

In the thorax and abdomen the potential spaces between the visceral and parietal layers of the pleura or peritoneum that line the cavities allow movement of the viscera in relation to each other and to the overlying thoracic and abdominal walls. In the same way, the (potential) epidural space may be seen as a (potential) epidural cavity (similar to the pleural cavity) which allows for movement between the elements of the vertebral column and the underlying dura and spinal cord, and also allows epidural venous engorgement (Newell 1999). However, excessive movement of the cord and meninges must be prevented (fibrous strands) and buffered (fat).

Newell's review, 'The spinal epidural space', indicates that the spinal dura has an external, smooth and translucent layer of cells, which are probably mesothelial (but possibly endothelial) in origin. Similarly, the ligamentous and osseous elements of the vertebral canal are internally clothed by a thin membrane that also has a mesothelial lining. The latter is likely to be the *peridural membrane* (Loughenbury et al. 2006) which extends laterally from the midline septum on the posterior aspect of the vertebral bodies, into the intervertebral foramina with the emerging nerves, and probably fuses with the fibrous tissue overlying the ligamentous, cartilaginous (perichondrial) and bony (periosteal) elements of the vertebral canal, in the same way that the dura within the skull is said to have an inner, meningeal layer and an outer layer which becomes the periosteum of the overlying bone. The peridural membrane may be considered a homologue of the vertebral periosteum (Wiltse 2000). At the foramen magnum the spinal dura is continuous with the meningeal dura, but fuses with the cranial, periosteal dura, sealing the upper limit of the epidural space. Inferiorly, the sacral hiatus is closed by the posterior sacrococcygeal ligament.

The epidural 'space' has been described as having a small anterior compartment (roughly 10% of the total) and a much larger posterolateral compartment (90%). The distance from the posterior border of the vertebral canal to the dura varies according to spinal segment, being as little as 0.5 mm in the cervical region and up to 9 mm in the lumbar (Hirabayashi et al. 1997). The space itself is largest in the lower sacral region after the dural sac has ended, whereas in the cervical region the relative thickness of the spinal cord may obliterate the epidural space altogether, because the dura lies opposed to the lining of the vertebral canal (peridural membrane) with little intervening tissue. Similarly, the thoracic vertebral canal is smaller and at the site of the lumbar cord enlargement (lower two or three thoracic vertebrae) the epidural space is minimal and the cord itself may be at risk during thoracic epidural injection. In the lumbar region the epidural space has a mean distance from the skin of about 5 cm, but this is subject to considerable individual variation and ranges from 3–8 cm.

The shape of the vertebral canal dictates the shape of the epidural space at any given level. Magnetic resonance imaging (MRI) shows that the dorsal epidural compartment is triangular in cross section in the lumbar region, but more crescent shaped in the thoracic region (Hirabayashi et al. 1997), with an oval transition zone in the upper lumbar region (Harrison 1999). The ventral epidural space varies in depth, being larger behind the vertebral body and smaller behind the protruding intervertebral disc (Luyendijk 1963). MRI and cryomicrotomy have revealed that the widest section is that nearest the cephalad lamina (Hogan 1996, Igarashi et al. 1998). Computerized axial tomography (CAT) has shown that the dorsal part of the epidural space, in sagittal section, has a 'sawtooth' outline because of the attachment, position, and bulk of the ligamenta flava. When these ligaments are separate in the midline, the space is variably filled by the interspinous ligament, and epidural fat may extend into the residual recess, contributing to the sawtooth appearance.

The thecal sac is stabilized within the epidural space by extremely variable *fibrous strands or meningovertebral ligaments*. The posterior longitudinal ligament has numerous connections to the anterior dural sac and some authors have found that the two are often fused at the level of the discs in the lumbar region. This close opposition and even attachment of the dural sac to the anterior canal wall may serve to separate the ventral epidural compartment (Harrison et al. 1985, Savolaine et al. 1988). Other, more recent authors believe that such connections are inconsistent and unlikely to prevent the spread of injectate from side to side, or laterally out to the intervertebral foramina, where the dorsal root ganglia and nerve roots may be readily bathed by anaesthetic solution (Hogan 2002, Hogan & Toth 1999). This belief tends to be supported in a study (Greers et al. 2003) that found irregular and incomplete, thin fibro-elastic meningovertebral ligaments in ventral, lateral, and posterior positions within the epidural space.

Previously, periduroscopy has also demonstrated the existence of dorsal midline strands connecting the dura mater to the ligamentum flavum, a finding confirmed later by epiduroscopy (Blomberg 1986, Savolaine et al. 1988). These strands have been described as producing a fold in the dura mater termed the plica mediana dorsalis (Luyendijk 1976), which narrows the epidural space in the midline to its point of attachment to the ligamentum flavum (Figure 12.8). These authors found that the strands are particularly well developed in the region of the vertebral arches and, in some cases, may alter epidural catheter direction, especially as the amount of catheter in the space increases. On occasion the strands may form a complete membrane capable of preventing a catheter crossing from one side to the other (Blomberg 1986). CAT and MRI studies confirmed this midline division of the posterior epidural space (Hirabayashi et al. 1997, Savolaine et al. 1988). Other connective tissue bands have been described, originating from the plica mediana dorsalis and extending laterally, subdividing further the posterolateral compartment of the epidural space into lateral and posterior sections (Savolaine et al. 1988).

On the contrary, it has been found by other researchers, and some more recently, that the dural folding, or plica mediana dorsalis is an artefact caused by epidural fat in the dorsal midline, or by dural compression caused by the injectate (Harrison 1999, Hogan 1996, 1999) and it has been argued that any fibrous strands represent simple distortions of the septa responsible for loculating fat in the lateral compartment (Hogan 1991). The posterolateral space is split into posterior and lateral compartments at the level of each neural arch by the opposition of the dura with the laminae. The posterior and lateral compartments themselves are generally discontinuous longitudinally, being separated by intervening laminae and pedicles, though this is less marked in the thoracic region (Westbrook et al. 1993).

The *nerve roots* on either side cross the posterolateral part of the epidural space to the two intervertebral foramina present at each segmental level. Inferiorly, their course is increasingly oblique, and they may lie in channels, known as radicular canals, leading to the foramina. The nerves of the cauda equina are arranged in bundles which diverge slightly in the epidural space before expanding and fusing with the dorsal root ganglion. Each bundle is surrounded by a tiny extension of the subarachnoid space. This multifascicular topography increases the surface area, allowing easier 'access' for both local anaesthetics and neurotoxins. Similarly, the very thin extension of the subarachnoid space means less anaesthetic dilution by CSF, augmenting its effect (Hogan & Toth 1999). At the foramina the nerves, together with fat and blood vessels, are tethered to the canal walls by connective tissue structures known as *Charpy's ligaments*. With increasing age the foramina tend to occlude (Atkinson et al. 1987, Reynolds 1985), although this is not the case with the anterior sacral foramina (Luyendijk 1963, Luyendijk & Van Voorthuisen 1966).

The *epidural fat*, which inconsistently and variably lies within the rest of the space, is very vascular and has a semifluid consistency. It is found predominantly in the dorsal midline and only sparsely ventrally. This dorsal fat may form tenuous, focal connections between the midline dura and the overlying vertebral canal, allowing movement between the structures, but causing apparent tenting of dura when air or solutions are injected into the epidural space and the (probably erroneous) impression of a plica mediana dorsalis (Hogan & Toth 1999). This dorsal midline fat may offer some impediment to anaesthetic spread, but elsewhere in the epidural space the fat is unlikely to do so. Conversely, others believe that with age the nature of the fat changes so that it offers progressively more resistance to injection (Cousins & Bromage 1988), although the amount present may decrease (Igarashi et al. 1997). More fat is found in the lumbar than the thoracic region, and this may be one of the reasons for enhanced spread of local anaesthetic at the thoracic level (Hogan 1996, Igarashi et al. 1998). MRI has shown that there is virtually no fat in the cervical region (Hirabayashi et al. 1997). Interestingly, the fat is discontinuous in the lumbar region, being present only at the levels of the intervertebral discs, whereas it is continuous in the thoracic region, even though there is less of it (Hirabayashi et al. 1997, Hogan 1996).

The *epidural veins*, known as the plexus of Batson, are large, valveless vessels which lie in the anterolateral part of the space and run vertically in four principal trunks. These communicate freely, through a venous ring at each vertebral level, with the basivertebral veins, with the sacral (and hence iliac and uterine) venous plexus, and with the abdominal and thoracic veins. Thus pressure changes within the body's cavities are reflected in the epidural veins, most notably in pregnancy when the veins are distended and the effective volume of the epidural space is decreased. It has also been suggested that such engorgement transfers to veins in the intervertebral foramina, effectively narrowing the foramina and preventing the escape of anaesthetic (Takiguchi et al. 2006). *Lymphatics and arteries*, which are relatively small, lie mainly in the lateral part of the space, pass through the intervertebral foramina to supply adjacent vertebrae and ligaments, and contribute to the supply of the spinal cord. Cryomicrotomy has revealed that a vein often enters the posterior epidural space, in the midline between the pair of ligamenta flava. Less commonly, this vein is found more laterally, actually piercing the ligament (Hogan 1996). In general, there appear to be more vessels posterolaterally than in the dorsal midline, emphasizing that the needle should enter the epidural space in the midline with both median and paramedian approaches to the canal.

Physiology of the vertebral canal

Cerebrospinal fluid

The CSF is normally clear and colourless with a specific gravity of approximately 1.005 at 37°C, though this may be increased slightly in old age, uraemia, hyperglycaemia, and hypothermia, but decreased during pregnancy (Richardson & Wissler 1996). It fills all the cavities in, and spaces around, the central nervous system and its function is to support and protect it. CSF is isotonic with plasma (280–290 mOsmol l^{-1}) and has similar constituents except that it contains only traces of protein (Table 12.1). Small numbers of blood cells are present in healthy CSF. It is produced in the choroid plexuses (small tufts of capillaries in direct contact with the ventricular lining) of the lateral ventricles, and also by plexuses in the third and fourth ventricles and on the surface of the brain. The differences between CSF and plasma imply that it is actively secreted rather than an ultrafiltrate. This is confirmed by the effects of drugs which influence sodium transport (such as acetazolamide) on CSF composition and rate of formation. The total volume is approximately 130 ml in the adult, with a daily production of approximately 150 ml, although this may decrease when the pressure is high, and increase up to threefold should the volume be low. Spinal CSF accounts for about 35 ml of the total, the majority being in the area of the cauda equina. CSF formation varies linearly with serum osmolality, decreasing when this is increased.

Table 12.1 Constituents of cerebrospinal fluid (CSF) and plasma.

Constituent	CSF	Plasma
H$^+$ mmol l^{-1}	32–36	36–44
Na$^+$ mmol l^{-1}	140	142
Cl$^-$ mmol l^{-1}	115	98
K$^+$ mmol l^{-1}	2.9	4.5
Urea mmol l^{-1}	5.0	5.0
Glucose mmol l^{-1}	4.5	5.0
HCO$^-_3$ mmol l^{-1}	22	25
Ca^{2+} mmol l^{-1}	1.2	2.3
Mg^{2+} mmol l^{-1}	1.0	0.8
Protein mg ml^{-1}	20–40	6,000–8,000

After secretion the fluid passes from the lateral ventricles into the third and then fourth ventricles through the interventricular foramen of Munro and the aqueduct of Sylvius respectively. It reaches the cisterna magna and cerebral subarachnoid space through the foramina of Luschka and Magendie (Figure 12.9). Most flows upwards over the brain to be reabsorbed through the arachnoid villi (herniations of arachnoid mater through the dura that come to lie in contact with the vascular endothelium) into the superior sagittal and transverse sinuses and other sinuses to a lesser extent. There is very little active CSF flow within the vertebral canal, the character of the fluid being maintained by a combination of diffusion and the bulk flow produced by alterations in posture. Most of the spinal CSF returns to the cranial cavity, but some is absorbed by the arachnoid granulations in the dural cuffs (see 'The meninges and dural sac' section). Normal pressure in the lumbar region is 60–100 mmH$_2$O in the lateral position and 200–250 mmH$_2$O when sitting, and it oscillates in time with both arterial pulsation and respiration. Respiration can cause pressure changes of up to 30 mmH$_2$O (a decrease with inspiration, an increase with expiration), while the arterial waves may have an

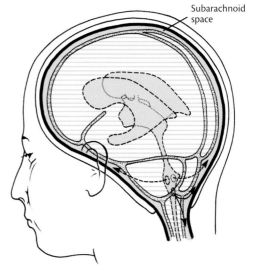

Figure 12.9 Circulation of CSF. The arrows show the movement of CSF through the foramina of Lushka and Magendie.

amplitude of 2–15 mmH$_2$O (Usubiaga et al. 1967a). These pressure variations are consistent throughout the CSF, unlike the situation in the epidural space (see 'Epidural pressure' section).

Epidural pressure

The presence of a subatmospheric pressure in the epidural space was first reported in 1926 (Janzen 1926), and the 'hanging drop' sign as a method of utilizing this pressure to identify the space, in 1932 (Gutierrez 1933). Pressure as low as –10 cmH$_2$O on deep inspiration (Bryce-Smith 1950, Usubiaga et al. 1967b) has been recorded in the upper and middle thoracic regions where it is due largely to transmission of the negative intrathoracic pressure through the intervertebral foramina. Pressure increases with distance from the thorax so that it is least negative (if negative at all) in the lumbar and sacral regions (Usubiaga et al. 1967a,b). The negative pressure in the thoracic and cervical regions is enhanced when sitting and when the spine is flexed (Usubiaga et al. 1967a) whereas in chronic obstructive airways disease it may cease to be negative. Coughing and the Valsalva manoeuvre have been shown to increase the epidural pressure in all regions (Usubiaga et al. 1967a,b).

Cyclical variations in epidural pressure have been demonstrated. Small pressure waves, synchronous with arterial pulsation, are found in the thoracic and cervical regions, but less consistently in lumbar pressure traces and never in sacral recordings. Larger amplitude pressure variations, synchronous with respiration, also occur. In the cervical and thoracic regions, pressure decreases with inspiration and increases with expiration, whereas in the lumbar region the reverse is found. This is unlike the pattern of pressure changes in CSF discussed earlier. These respiratory patterns are also found in the superior and inferior venae cavae respectively (Usubiaga et al. 1967a). When the pressure in each venous system is elevated independently, for example, by the Queckenstedt manoeuvre or abdominal compression, epidural pressure changes are largely confined to the adjoining space. A Valsalva manoeuvre or cough results in increased epidural pressure except in the sacral region. These observations led to the conclusion that the epidural space has three functional compartments: (a) cervicothoracic, which is the largest, and is influenced by pressure changes in the superior vena cava; (b) the lumbar, which is influenced by intra-abdominal pressure; and (c) the sacral canal, which has no negative pressure, no pressure oscillations, and does not respond to abdominal compression. It is thought (Usubiaga et al. 1967a) that the lipid tissues of the epidural space serve to isolate the regions (Hirabayashi et al. 1997, Hogan 1996), allowing them to reflect the pressure changes in the cavities with which they communicate most directly.

During pregnancy there is an increase in intra-abdominal pressure, and consequent venous engorgement of the epidural space results in an increase in baseline epidural pressure, especially during uterine contractions, such that a negative pressure in the epidural space can no longer be demonstrated (Usubiaga et al. 1967b). This pressure increase is more marked when the patient is supine during the second stage of labour (Galbert & Marx 1974).

Key references

Hogan QH, Toth J (1999) Anatomy of soft tissues of the spinal canal. *Regional Anaesthesia and Pain Medicine* 24(4): 303–10.

Newell RLM (1999) The spinal epidural space. *Clinical Anatomy* 12: 375–9.

On-line resource

http://www.instantanatomy.net Illustrations of human anatomy.

References

Atkinson RS, Rushman GB, Lee JA (1987) *Spinal analgesia: intradural; epidural. A synopsis of anaesthesia*, 10th edn, pp. 662–721. Bristol: John Wright.

Blomberg R (1986) The dorsomedian connective tissue band in the lumbar epidural space of humans: an anatomical study using epiduroscopy in autopsy cases. *Anesthesia & Analgesia* 65: 747–52.

Bryce-Smith R (1950) Pressures in the extra-dural space. *Anaesthesia* 5: 213–16.

Cousins MJ, Bromage PR (1988) Epidural neural blockade. In Cousins MJ, Bridenbaugh PO. *Neural blockade in clinical anesthesia and management of pain*, 2nd edn, pp. 253–360. Philadelphia, PA: Lippincott.

Di Chiro G, Timins EL (1974) Spinal myelography and the septum posticum. *Radiology* 111: 319–27

Galbert MW, Marx GF (1974) Extradural pressures in the parturient patient. *Anesthesiology* 40: 499–502.

Greers C, Lecouvet FE, Behets C, et al. (2003) Polygonal deformation of the dural sac in lumbar epidural lipomatosis: Anatomic explanation by the presence of meningovertebral ligaments. *American Journal of Neuroradiology* 24: 1276–82.

Gutierrez A (1933) Valor de la aspiracion liquida en el espacio peridural en Ia anestesia peridural. *Revue Circulation, Buenos Aires* 12: 225.

Harrison GR (1999) Topographical anatomy of the lumbar epidural region: an *in vivo* study using computised axial tomography. *British Journal of Anaesthesia* 83 (2): 229–34.

Harrison GR, Parkin IG, Shah JL (1985) Resin injection of the lumbar extradural space. *British Journal of Anaesthesia* 57: 333–6.

Hirabayashi Y, Saitoh K, Fukuda H, et al. (1997) Magnetic resonance imaging of the extradural space of the thoracic spine. *British Journal of Anaesthesia* 79: 563–6.

Hogan QH (1991) Lumbar epidural anatomy. A new look by cryomicrotome section. *Anesthesiology* 75: 767–75.

Hogan QH (1996) Epidural anatomy examined by cryomicrotome section. *Regional Anesthesia* 21: 395–406.

Hogan QH (2002) Distribution of solution in the epidural space: Examination by cryomicrotome section. *Regional Anaesthesia and Pain Medicine* 27 (2): 150–6.

Janzen E (1926) Der negative vorschlag bei lumbalpunktion. *Deutsche Z Nerven Heilk* 94: 280–92.

Igarashi T, Hirabayashi Y, Shimizu R, et al. (1997) The lumbar extradural structure changes with increasing age. *British Journal of Anaesthesia* 78: 149–52.

Igarashi T, Hirabayashi Y, Shimizu R, et al. (1998) Thoracic and lumbar extradural structure examined by extraduroscope. *British Journal of Anaesthesia* 81: 121–5.

Loughenbury PR, Wadhwani S, Soames RW (2006) The posterior longitudinal ligament and peridural (epidural) membrane. *Clinical Anatomy* 19: 487–92.

Luyendijk W (1963) Canalography. *Journal Belge de Radiologie* 46: 236–54.

Luyendijk W (1976) The plica mediana dorsalis of the dura mater and its relation to lumbar peridurography. *Neuroradiology* 11: 147–9.

Luyendijk W, Van Voorthuisen AE (1966) Contrast examination of the spinal epidural space. *Acta Scandinavica Radiologica* 5: 105–66.

Nauta HJE, Dolan E, Yasargil MG (1983) Microsurgical anatomy of the spinal subarachnoid space. *Surgical Neurology* 19: 431–7.

Reynolds AF Jr, Roberts PA, Pollay M, Stratemeier PH (1985) Quantitative anatomy of the thoracolumbar epidural space. *Neurosurgery* 17: 905–7.

Richardson MG, Wissler RN (1996) Density of lumbar cerebrospinal fluid in pregnant and nonpregnant humans. *Anesthesiology* 85: 326–30.

Savolaine ER, Pandaya JB, Greenblatt SH, Conover SR (1988) Anatomy of the human lumbar epidural space: new insights using CT-epidurography. *Anesthesiology* 68: 217–20.

Standring S (Ed) (2008) *Gray's Anatomy: The Anatomical Basis of Clinical Practice*, 40th edn. London: Churchill Livingstone, Elsevier Health.

Takiguchi T, Yamaguchi S, Tezuka M, et al. (2006) Compression of the subarachnoid space by the engorged epidural venous plexus in pregnant women. *Anaesthesiology* 105(4): 848–51.

Usubiaga JE, Moya F, Usubiaga LE (1967a) Effect of thoracic and abdominal pressure changes on the epidural space pressure. *British Journal of Anaesthesia* 39: 612–18.

Usubiaga JE, Wikinski JA, Usubiaga LE (1967b) Epidural pressure and its relation to spread of anesthetic solutions in the epidural space. *Anesthesia & Analgesia* 46: 440–6.

Westbrook JL, Renowden SA, Carrie LES (1993) A study of the anatomy of the extradural region using magnetic resonance imaging. *British Journal of Anaesthesia* 71: 495–8.

Wiltse LL (2000) Anatomy of the extradural compartments of the lumbar spinal canal. Peridural membrane and circumneural sheath. *Radiologic Clinics of North America* 38 (6): 1177–206.

CHAPTER 13

Spinal anaesthesia

Jonathan Whiteside and Tony Wildsmith

Spinal anaesthesia is induced by the injection of local anaesthetic into the subarachnoid space, and is generally regarded as one of the most reliable of regional block methods. It has the particular advantage that very small doses of local anaesthetic produce profound effects so that systemic toxicity is not a problem. However, other drugs, such as opioids, co-administered by the same route to produce more prolonged pain control may have systemic effects. The second major advantage is that needle insertion is relatively straightforward with cerebrospinal fluid (CSF) providing both a clear indication of successful needle placement and a medium through which local anaesthetic solution usually spreads readily.

The popularity of the technique has waxed and waned since its introduction by August Bier in 1898. Widespread use in the 1930s and 1940s was followed by a sharp decline in the 1950s, coinciding with improvements in general anaesthetic techniques (notably the introduction of the neuromuscular blocking drugs) and the adverse publicity regarding neurological sequelae in the Woolley and Roe case (Cope 1954, Hutter 1990). However, the technique has regained a significant place in anaesthetic practice over the last four decades, having been used in all age groups from premature neonates to the most elderly, and in a wide range of clinical situations.

Lumbar puncture is usually performed below the termination of the spinal cord, which is at or about L_1 in the adult, the subarachnoid space ending at the level of the second sacral vertebra (Chapter 12). The tough dura mater and flimsy arachnoid are closely applied to each other, but there remains a potential (subdural) space between them. If the whole bevel of the spinal needle is not within the subarachnoid space, some of the solution may be deposited within the subdural space and this can account for some failures (Fettes et al. 2009). The posterior subarachnoid space contains several membranous structures (see Figure 12.7) and, in the lumbar region particularly, the septicum posticum may be well developed. These structures can lead to maldistribution of solutions, and account not only for failure to achieve adequate block, but also for neurotoxicity and the development of the cauda equina syndrome (CES).

The site of action is primarily the nerve roots, but the dorsal root ganglia and the superficial parts of the cord may be affected also (Greene & Brull 1993). Differential effects may result in wide differences in the rostral levels of different types of block: up to seven segments between sympathetic and sensory block (Chamberlain &

Chamberlain 1986), and 2.5 segments between sensory and motor block (Freund et al. 1967).

Indications and contraindications

Spinal anaesthesia is restricted largely to operations performed below the level of the umbilicus. The likely duration of surgery is important, because spinal anaesthesia will not reliably produce surgical anaesthesia for longer than 2–3 hours unless a catheter technique is used. It is particularly indicated for older and some poor-risk patients, such as those suffering from chronic respiratory, diffuse hepatic and renal disease, diabetes mellitus, and some forms of cardiovascular disease. The higher the sensory block, the more extensive will be the sympathetic block and the greater the degree of vasodilatation produced. Sympathetic block, with reduced afterload and cardiac work, may be beneficial in patients with congestive cardiac failure or ischaemic heart disease, but reduced perfusion pressure could be disastrous in a patient with a fixed cardiac output.

The advantages and disadvantages to the individual patient must be balanced, and only when the risks outweigh the benefits is the technique contraindicated, although many of the contraindications to spinal anaesthesia apply equally to other forms of regional block. These include anticoagulant therapy and other coagulation disorders, refusal by the patient, disease or severe deformity of the spinal column, active neurological disease, localized or systemic infection, severe hypovolaemia and other forms of shock. Lumbar puncture is contraindicated in the presence of raised intracranial pressure because it may lead to escape of CSF and coning of the brainstem. A history of headache does not contraindicate spinal anaesthesia, but may give rise to diagnostic difficulty in the postoperative period.

For many years, day-care surgery was thought to be a contraindication to spinal anaesthesia because of the risks of postdural puncture headache (PDPH), the effect on bladder function, and the delay in recovery of motor function. However, a wider range of day-care surgery is now performed on patients who are increasingly elderly, and the balance of risk has changed. The use of fine gauge, pencil-point needles has reduced the incidence of PDPH considerably (Turnbull & Shepherd 2003), and it is claimed that techniques using low doses of the longer acting agents maintain rapid onset and reliable efficacy, but reduce duration so allowing early discharge

(Whiteside & Wildsmith 2005). Lower rates of nausea and vomiting than with general anaesthesia are a particular advantage.

However, using a low dose reduces the margin for error if any local anaesthetic is misplaced and so increases the risk of the block being inadequate in some way, especially if a glucose-free solution is used (Fettes et al. 2009). Therefore some clinicians favour the continuous spinal or combined spinal–epidural (CSE) technique to increase flexibility (Burnell & Byrne 2001, Rawal 2001). A shorter acting drug might avoid such complicated methods, but concerns about transient neurological symptoms (TNS) inhibit wider use of lidocaine (see 'Transient neurological symptoms' section), and prilocaine is difficult to source in preservative-free solution, although preservative-free chloroprocaine is increasingly popular where available (Wiles & Nathanson 2010). The general aspects of regional anaesthesia in day-care surgery, including discharge criteria, are considered in Chapter 24.

Technique of lumbar puncture

The patient should be on a firm surface on a tilting table or trolley. Intravenous access must be established, and oxygen saturation, blood pressure, and electrocardiogram monitored. Resuscitation equipment must be available and checked. An understanding of the anatomy of the spine (Chapter 12) and a scrupulous aseptic technique (Chapter 11) are essential.

Position

In choosing the position for lumbar puncture, various factors should be considered, notably the patient's general condition, level of sedation, girth, spinal anatomy, and the baricity of the solution to be used.

Lateral horizontal position

This is the usual position because it is easily adopted and maintained, and is easier in less cooperative or sedated patients. The patient is placed in the lateral position, with the back vertical and level with the edge of the trolley (Figure 13.1). It is very important to avoid rotation of the spine by ensuring that both hips and shoulders remain vertical. Maximum flexion of the lumbar spine, produced by flexing the legs acutely at the hips and knees, is essential to open the spaces between the spines and laminae in order to facilitate the passage of the needle through the ligaments and into the vertebral canal. The needle entering in the midline will continue in the midline if it is kept at right angles to the back and parallel to the top of the trolley.

Sitting position

This position is helpful in the obese patient and in others in whom the spines are difficult to palpate, because it may be easier to identify the midline and assess the angles. However, it may be more dangerous in the sedated or anxious patient because vasovagal effects or pooling of blood in the lower limbs may precipitate a sudden bradycardia with marked hypotension.

The patient is placed with the buttocks near to the edge of the trolley, and the legs over the opposite side with feet supported on a stool. The patient rests the elbows on the thighs, or folds the arms forwards over pillows, to flex the spine (Figure 13.2). An assistant should support the patient from the front and ensure that the patient remains vertical when viewed in the sagittal plane.

The midline approach

The midline approach is recommended because the angles are easier to identify, and the ligaments are less sensitive than the paraspinal muscles. A line drawn between the highest points of the iliac crests (Tuffier's line) will usually cross the spine at the level of the fourth lumbar spine, although this line may be as high as the third lumbar spine or as low as the L_5/S_1 interspace (Broadbent et al. 2000, Reynolds 2000). Other vertebral levels may be identified from this line. Because the spinal cord ends at approximately the first lumbar interspace in the adult, the needle is usually inserted below this level. The widest appropriate interspace is usually selected, although the intended area of block may influence the choice because a higher level of injection will usually result in greater spread (Tuominen et al. 1989). However, using a higher

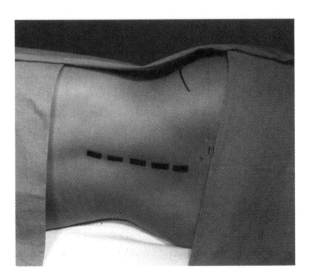

Figure 13.1 Position for lumbar puncture in the lateral horizontal position. The hips and shoulders are vertical to eliminate rotation. A sandbag has been placed beneath the patient's loin to prevent lateral curvature of the spine.

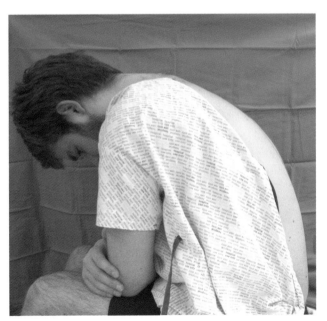

Figure 13.2 Position for lumbar puncture in the sitting position.

level does increase the risk of needle insertion being above the termination of the spinal cord.

The area is prepared carefully with antiseptic, which should be allowed to dry so that it is effective and to eliminate any risk of it being carried into the epidural or subarachnoid spaces. Sterile drapes are applied over a wide area to allow palpation of the relevant spines and iliac crests without compromising the aseptic technique. Local anaesthetic for infiltration of the skin and subcutaneous tissues is drawn up into one syringe, and the exact volume of solution for the spinal injection drawn into a *different* size syringe to avoid confusion. It is essential that the preliminary infiltration includes the dermis as well as the subcutaneous tissues and the deeper ligaments. The index and middle fingers of the non-dominant hand are placed on either side of the midline so that only the spines, supraspinous ligament, and interspace remain between the fingers to ensure that the infiltration is made in the midline (Figure 13.3). Sufficient local anaesthetic should be injected to allow painless insertion of the introducer and spinal needle, but not to obscure the bony landmarks of the interspace. Care should be taken to ensure that the spinal needle passes through the anaesthetized area by keeping the 'straddling' fingers in place throughout.

Lateral and paramedian approaches

Both these approaches involve insertion of the needle about a centimetre from the midline. In the *lateral approach*, the needle is inserted lateral to the midpoint of the interspace, and is angled medially only. In the *paramedian approach*, the needle is inserted about 2 cm caudal and 1 cm lateral to the selected interspace, and the needle has cephalad as well as medial angulation. These approaches may be used if there is little space in the midline, the ligaments are calcified, or the anaesthetist prefers one of them. It is important to recognize that these approaches are only lateral or paramedian at the skin because the angulation of the needle ensures that it still enters the vertebral canal in the midline. Determining the precise angles required makes these approaches more difficult to understand and practise. The paramedian approach is considered further in Chapter 14.

Spinal needles

Spinal needles (Figure 13.4) are usually 9 cm long, and should have a close-fitting stylet, a smooth lining, and a transparent hub, so that the flow of CSF is fast and can be identified quickly. The needle should produce minimal trauma with the smallest hole in the dura mater, and developments in needle design have been driven largely by the need to reduce the incidence of PDPH (Hoskin 1998). Reduction in needle size reduced significantly the incidence of PDPH, but technical difficulties leading to failure of spinal anaesthesia are common when needles of 29 g or smaller are used. Fortunately, development of atraumatic 'pencil-point' needles also led to a reduction in the incidence of PDPH (Turnbull & Shepherd 2003), and their use has become widespread, although they are not without problems.

The terminal opening of a pencil-point needle is a finite distance from the actual tip (Figure 13.4) so the needle has to be inserted a little further through the dura before CSF flow is appreciated, and the blunt nature of the tip also means that entry into the theca can be a little precipitate. These two factors may facilitate accidental needle tip contact with either the spinal cord or the cauda equina and increase the risk of nerve injury (Turner & Shaw 1993).

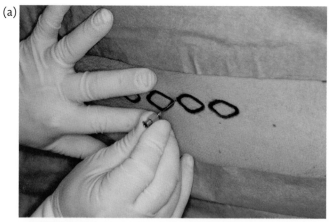

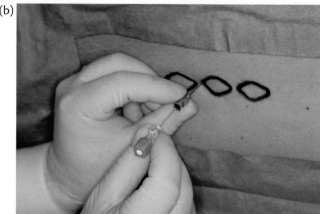

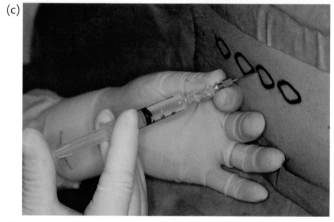

Figure 13.3 Midline insertion of a 25-g spinal needle. The fingers of the left hand straddle the spine as an introducer needle is inserted into the supraspinous ligament with a very slight cephalad angulation (a). The guide needle is then held steady and the spinal needle passed through it (b). Once the dura has been punctured, the spinal needle assembly is immobilized between thumb and fingers, and a syringe attached (c).

It is also possible for the terminal opening to 'straddle' the dura, allowing CSF to flow back through the needle on insertion, but then for the flow of the injectate to displace the dura so that solution enters the epidural or subdural spaces (Figure 13.5), and the block fails (Crone & Vogel 1991, Fettes et al. 2009). The 'Atraucan' needle, having a more distal opening (Figure 13.4), was introduced to try and overcome these problems, but some studies have found that it produces a greater incidence of PDPH (Vallejo et al. 2000).

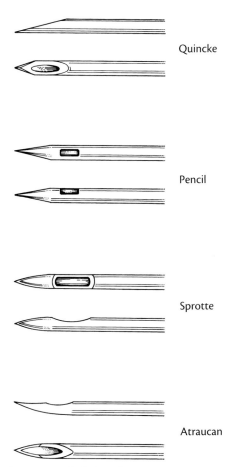

Figure 13.4 Four patterns of spinal needles.

As with any device, the clinician must be aware of the features of the particular type of spinal needle in use and practise appropriately.

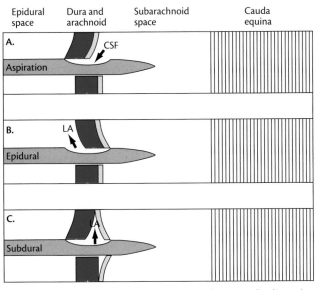

Figure 13.5 Misplaced injection possibilities with pencil-point needles. (Reproduced from P.D.W. Fettes et al., 'Failed spinal anaesthesia: mechanisms, management, and prevention', *British Journal of Anaesthesia*, 2009, 102, 6, pp. 739–48, by permission of Oxford University Press and the *British Journal of Anaesthesia*.)

The issue of syringe/needle connections for central nerve block techniques is considered in Chapter 11.

Needle insertion

A fine needle (≤24 g) should be inserted through an 'introducer needle' to avoid bacterial contamination from the skin, implantation of skin into the deeper structures, and to act as a guide to keep the needle on the desired path. Most modern disposable sets include a suitable introducer, which should be short to avoid traversing the ligaments completely. The needle with stylet in place, and the bevel facing laterally if it has a Quincke tip, is inserted through the introducer needle. It is advanced at right angles to the back or in a slightly cephalad direction, because the interlaminar space may be at a slight cephalad angle to the interspinous space, especially in the older patient. If the needle leaves the midline, it enters the paraspinal muscles and will tend to drop rather than be gripped and held by the midline ligaments. Once this 'grip' is identified, the midline position and the degree of cephalad angulation should be confirmed, and the needle advanced further.

The tissues between the skin and the subarachnoid space offer different degrees of resistance to the passage of a needle, and the anaesthetist should use this feature to try to identify the different layers as the needle is inserted. The increasing resistance of the ligamentum flavum is usually recognized, as is a loss of resistance as the needle enters the epidural space. Insertion of the needle should be gentle and unhurried at all times, but especially so once the epidural space has been entered. At this point, the anaesthetist should ease the needle forward a millimetre at a time, rather than actively pushing it. It is almost a case of allowing the patient to 'breathe' him- or herself on to the needle. After each small advance of the needle the stylet is removed so that CSF is identified as soon as the dura and arachnoid have been penetrated. A further loss of resistance, more often appreciated as a slight 'pop' or 'click', is usually noticed as the tip of the needle enters the subarachnoid space.

If bone is contacted, this is likely to be the lamina of the vertebra. The anaesthetist should check first that the spine is not rotated and remains fully flexed, and then that the needle direction is correct. If these checks do not produce success the needle should be withdrawn and reinserted, usually in a more cephalad direction.

Use of 22-g needles

Many practitioners have now abandoned the use of the relatively large 22-g needle, but it has a place in the more difficult punctures, especially in the elderly. It is relatively rigid and an introducer is not required. However, a cutting needle should be used to puncture the skin first, and care should be taken that the needle does not bend or deviate from the midline. The needle, if it has a Quincke tip, should pierce the dura with the bevel facing laterally to reduce the incidence of PDPH (Mihic 1985, Norris et al. 1989). The advantage of the Quincke tip is that CSF is identified as soon as it enters the subarachnoid space and multicompartment injection, paraesthesiae, and neural trauma are less likely.

Confirmation of dural puncture

The correct position of the needle is confirmed by free flow of CSF when the stylet is withdrawn. It will be slow with fine needles and occasionally slight rotation of the spinal needle may be required to ensure free flow. If the fluid is blood stained, time must be allowed for it to clear before injecting the solution. If it does not clear quickly, another puncture should be made. Once there is a free flow of clear CSF, the syringe containing the spinal solution is attached carefully, the hub of the spinal needle being gripped firmly (Figure 13.3) to prevent subsequent displacement. A small quantity of CSF is aspirated to ensure that the needle tip is still in the sub-arachnoid space and the solution injected at a rate of about 1 ml 5 s^{-1}. Some anaesthetists perform a further aspiration halfway through the injection and a final aspiration at the end, to confirm that all the solution has been deposited into the subarachnoid space, although neither of these practices has been shown to influence the outcome of the block (Tarkkila 1991). This final aspirate must be reinjected because it contains a high concentration of local anaes-thetic. The needles are withdrawn carefully, an adhesive plaster or plastic spray is applied to the puncture site, and the patient placed in the desired position to ensure appropriate spread of solution.

Ultrasound and lumbar puncture

While ultrasound equipment has not reached the stage where it can be used to identify the contents of the vertebral canal, and thus confirm that the level used is below the termination of the spinal cord, it can already be used in two important ways:

1. To confirm the accuracy of the intended level of needle insertion by 'counting up' from the sacrum and overcome the variability in level of Tuffier's line; and

2. To assess the orientation and 'patency' of the intended interver-tebral space and thus determine the best space and angle for needle insertion, especially in those patients with scoliosis.

Ultrasound of the vertebral canal is considered further in Chapter 14.

Factors affecting intrathecal drug spread

Spinal anaesthesia has the advantage of producing a profound nerve block in a large part of the body with a relatively simple injec-tion of a small amount of local anaesthetic. However, the greatest challenge of the technique is to produce sufficient spread of local anaesthetic through the CSF to provide an adequate block for the proposed surgery without excessive spread increasing the incidence of complications. Unfortunately, there is considerable variation between patients in the spread achieved by a particular technique, and achieving reliable results requires a detailed knowledge of the factors influencing intrathecal drug spread.

As local anaesthetic is injected, it will spread by displacement of CSF and by the effects of any currents created within the CSF. Then, and most crucially, there will be interplay, determined by gravity, between the densities of CSF and local anaesthetic solution. Gravity will be 'applied' through patient position and, in the horizontal subject, by the influence of the curves of the vertebral canal (Barker 1907). Once the injectate has spread physically, the active drug(s) will diffuse through the CSF and into the nervous tissue. Many fac-tors (Table 13.1) have been found to influence the final outcome of these processes, but the key ones are the relative physical character-istics of CSF and the solution injected, the clinical technique, and the patient's general features (Hocking & Wildsmith 2004).

Characteristics of CSF and injected solution

Three terms are used, often loosely and interchangeably, to describe the solutions used for spinal anaesthesia, but it is vital to define them precisely:

Table 13.1 Factors influencing intrathecal drug spread. (Reproduced, with permission, from Hocking & Wildsmith 2004.)

Characteristics of the injected solution	
Baricity	Volume/dose/concentration
Temperature of injectate	Viscosity
Additives	
Clinical technique	
Patient position	Level of injection
Needle type/alignment	Intrathecal catheters
Fluid currents	Epidural injection
Patient characteristics	
Age	Height
Weight	Sex
Intra-abdominal pressure	Spinal anatomy
Lumbosacral CSF volume	Pregnancy

- *Density* of a liquid is its weight per unit volume;

- *Specific gravity* (SG) of a liquid is the ratio of its density relative to that of water;

  Both density and specific gravity are temperature dependent, so the figure(s) at which the measurements are made must be quoted. The SG of a local anaesthetic is usually defined by relat-ing its density at 20°C to water at 4°C. Because it is a ratio, SG has no units.

- *Baricity* is analogous to SG, but the ratio is of the density of local anaesthetic to that of CSF, both measured at 37°C.

The mean density of CSF at 37°C is 1.0003 g l^{-1} (range 1.0000–1.0006); it is lower in women than in men, in pregnant than in non-pregnant women, and in premenopausal women than in post-menopausal women and men. These group differences are small, and probably unimportant clinically, although with all the physio-logical variation occurring at the fourth decimal place, which is often unmeasured, it is difficult to interpret the results of many studies. Given the normal range, a solution must have a baricity below 0.9990 to be hypobaric in all patients, or above 1.0010 to be hyperbaric. To be truly isobaric a solution must have a density within the normal range for CSF, but most commercially available glucose-free solutions are marginally hypobaric at 37°C, and are best referred to as 'plain'. A concentration of glucose greater than 10 mg ml^{-1} will make a solution definitively hyperbaric (McLeod 2004).

Influence of baricity

The usual choice for the clinician is between a hyperbaric solution and one with a baricity at, or just below that of, CSF. Because of the interplay between them, posture and baricity need to be considered together (see 'Patient position' section), but some general points can be made first. Hyperbaric solutions are more predictable, with greater spread in the direction of gravity and less interpatient vari-ability, a point noted by Barker (1907) over a hundred years ago. Commercially available solutions contain glucose up to 80 mg ml^{-1}, but most evidence shows that any concentration in excess of 8 mg ml^{-1} will produce a solution which behaves in a hyperbaric

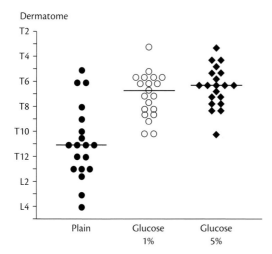

Figure 13.6 Comparison of variation in spread with plain bupivacaine and two hyperbaric solutions of ropivacaine. (Reproduced from J.B. Whiteside et al., 'Spinal anaesthesia with ropivacaine 5 mg ml^{-1} in glucose 10mg ml^{-1} or 50 mg ml^{-1}', *British Journal of Anaesthesia*, 2001, 86, 2, pp. 241–4, by permission of Oxford University Press and the *British Journal of Anaesthesia*.)

'manner' (Bannister et al. 1990, Sanderson et al. 1994). In contrast, most plain solutions produce greater variability in effect (Figure 13.6) and are less predictable so that the block may be too low, and therefore inadequate for surgery, or excessively high, causing side effects (Whiteside et al. 2001). The use of plain (glucose-free) local anaesthetic solutions should therefore be restricted to patients having surgery below the inguinal ligament (Logan et al. 1986).

Clinical technique

Having chosen the type of solution to be used, the clinician can further influence its intrathecal spread in a relatively small number of ways.

Patient position

Barker (1907) was the first to use glass models of the spinal canal and coloured solutions to demonstrate that gravity and the curves of the vertebral column (Chapter 12) influence the spread of solutions according to their densities. Gravity causes hyperbaric solutions to 'sink', and hypobaric ones to 'float', so that the degree of caudad or cephalad spread depends on the interplay between baricity and patient position. This interplay is the major determinant of the final extent of block with most techniques, but that does not mean that patient position can be used to 'control' spread as reliably as some descriptions imply.

Posture, obviously, has no influence on the spread of a truly isobaric solution.

Plain (glucose-free) bupivacaine behaves, as noted earlier, as a borderline hypobaric solution and injections made in the sitting position will spread to a higher level than those made in the lateral position. However, the patient must remain sitting for at least 2 minutes to produce any effect (2–3 segments), and for an even longer time if greater spread is needed (Kalso et al. 1982). Unfortunately, while this effect is consistent in its effect on mean spread, the interpatient variability of such solutions remains an issue, and postural hypotension is a real risk in the sitting patient with an increasing level of sympathetic block.

Hyperbaric solutions will be limited in spread if the patient is kept in the sitting or lateral position, but once placed supine the

curves of the vertebral canal will then be the primary factor 'directing' the solution, and the block will spread cephalad and or to the other side (Wildsmith et al. 1981). Such secondary extension of block due to physical movement of a hyperbaric solution after a change in posture may occur as late as 30 minutes after injection. Thus reliable production of a deliberately limited (e.g. unilateral) block will involve some delay.

Although not immediately relevant to the initial spread of solution, it should be noted that late (up to 2 hours after injection), but marked changes in patient posture can lead to significant changes in the extent of block. The effect is independent of solution baricity (Niemi et al. 1993), and probably reflects bulk movements of CSF still containing significant concentrations of local anaesthetic. All patient movements should be very gentle until the block has regressed completely.

Level of injection

The level of injection plays some role in determining the height of block achieved by a given solution in an individual patient. Moving above or below the standard level (L_3/L_4) will result in more extensive or more restricted blocks respectively, but the predictability of this effect must be considered in the light of the difficulty of identifying accurately the level of injection (Broadbent et al. 2000). Further, using a higher level risks puncture of the conus medullaris; and lumbar puncture can be more difficult at lower levels, especially in the elderly.

Effect of dose, volume, and speed of injection

Dose, rather than the volume or concentration of the solution, is a major determinant of the quality and duration of a spinal anaesthetic, but it has minimal effect on spread, and thus the extent of block. Clearly, there is a critical dose below which no block is achieved, and the accidental subarachnoid injection of a 'full' epidural dose will produce a total spinal block, but there is no correlation, within the range normally used for spinal anaesthesia, between the dose administered and the final level of block.

Slow injections (1 ml 10 s^{-1} or less) tend to produce more predictable spread, while more rapid injections act like barbotage (repeated aspiration and injection of CSF with the local anaesthetic) and decrease predictability (McClure et al. 1982).

Factors affecting the duration of spinal anaesthesia

After injection the block produced ascends progressively to its maximal spread over 20–30 minutes. Regression then proceeds from above downwards and the rate of regression depends on the individual drug's properties, the dose injected, its total spread, the use of adjuvants, and the general condition of the patient.

Individual drug properties

Ideally, a range of drugs with different durations should be available, but commercial factors and licensing regulations limit choice. For many years only hyperbaric bupivacaine was licensed for intrathecal use in the UK, although the plain solutions (0.5% and 0.75%) have been used widely. The duration of surgical anaesthesia produced ranges from 1–3 hours, depending on other related factors (see below). A shorter duration of action may be achieved using lidocaine in either plain or hyperbaric solution, but its use has declined due to the association with TNS (see 'Complications' section). Recently, a hyperbaric preparation of prilocaine 2% (Prilotekal) has become available in the UK. It requires wider evaluation, but would be expected to provide a shorter duration of action than an equivalent dose of bupivacaine. In other countries, 2-chloroprocaine, mepivacaine (intermediate duration) and tetracaine (long duration) are also used.

Of the newer drugs, ropivacaine is not licensed for intrathecal use, although clinical study has shown that it behaves very like bupivacaine, but with a shorter duration of action (Whiteside et al. 2001, Whiteside & Wildsmith 2005). The glucose free solution of levobupivacaine is licensed and, being a single isomer of bupivacaine, would be expected to have the same duration, but it is slightly longer acting. This relates to it being subject to a European Union directive which states that concentrations of hydrates and salts must be expressed in terms of milligrams of active moiety. Thus, an ampoule of 0.5% levobupivacaine contains 5 mg ml^{-1} of free base, whereas the same concentration of racemic bupivacaine, which predates the directive, contains 5 mg ml^{-1} of the hydrochloride salt. This means that a unit volume of levobupivacaine contains 11% more molecules of local anaesthetic than does racemic bupivacaine of nominally the same percentage concentration. This greater molecular concentration may explain why both the 5 mg ml^{-1} and the 7.5 mg ml^{-1} preparations of levobupivacaine are isobaric, bordering on hyperbaric, at 37°C (McLeod 2004).

Dose

Larger doses will increase the duration of action—an effect which is useful for long operations. Increasing the dose by 50% will extend the duration at T_{12} by about 50% (Wildsmith & Rocco 1985).

Spread

The greater the spread achieved with a given dose of drug, the shorter will be the duration of action. A drug limited to a small segmental area will last longer because the concentration in each of the nerves which it has reached will be higher.

Adjuvants

Opioids

Opioids inhibit pain transmission in the dorsal horn. A small dose of fentanyl (12.5–25 mcg), sufentanil (2.5–5 mcg) or morphine (0.1–0.2 mg) added to local anaesthetic exerts a synergistic action and prolongs duration of analgesia (Dahlgren et al. 1997, Kalso 1983). The effect is also seen when opioids are administered (in larger doses) intravenously (Henderson & Jones 1995).

There may also be more rapid onset and more profound block when an opioid is added to a local anaesthetic, but the combination increases the risk of respiratory depression in the postoperative period so appropriate monitoring will be required.

Clonidine

Clonidine is a selective α_2-adrenergic agonist which acts on receptors in the dorsal horn and also affects neural transmission. Doses of 75–150 mcg will prolong the block (Fogarty et al. 1993, Racle et al. 1987), but marked haemodynamic changes and sedation may limit usefulness (Elia et al. 2008).

Vasoconstrictors

Both adrenaline (0.1–0.2 mg ≡ 0.1–0.2 ml of 1:1000 solution) and phenylephrine (1 mg) constrict dural and spinal cord blood vessels, and inhibit nociception (Concepcion et al. 1984). These actions may increase duration, but the effects are neither consistent nor reliable (Chambers et al. 1981, Moore et al. 1998, Sumi et al. 1996).

Alkalinization

The addition of sodium bicarbonate to bupivacaine does not increase spread, but does prolong duration (Racle et al. 1988). However, raising the pH of bupivacaine solutions increases the risk of the drug precipitating out of solution.

Patient's physical condition

It is likely that spread will be greater and duration of action prolonged in patients in poor physical condition. In addition, the cardiovascular effects may be greater. Neither the age of the patient (Pitkanen et al. 1984, Veering et al. 1988) nor the physical state of the patient seems to affect duration.

Achieving the desired block

> The anaesthetist should never forget the capricious nature of spinal analgesia. (Lee 1984.)

Although the factors which affect *mean* spread and duration of spinal block have been identified in studies of groups of patients, there is still considerable variation in the effect obtained in individuals. Thus, the minimum and maximum effects are more important than the mean when choosing a particular technique. The minimum effect will determine the clinical utility of the technique, while the maximum effect will determine the risk of complications, especially hypotension. Therefore a technique should be chosen to give the best chance of achieving adequate block for the proposed surgery, without the risk of unnecessary spread to the upper thoracic sympathetic outflow.

Mid-thoracic block

For all lower abdominal surgery, including herniorrhaphy, a block to the mid-thoracic level is desirable, and a hyperbaric solution is preferred. Hyperbaric (glucose 5–8%) bupivacaine, ropivacaine, or levobupivacaine (2.5–3 ml of 0.5% solution) may be injected in the lateral position and the patient turned supine immediately afterwards, although this often results in a block which is more extensive than is needed. Use of lower concentrations of glucose (0.8–1%) will result in blocks which are adequate for lower abdominal surgery, but do not have the same risk of spreading to the upper thoracic sympathetic outflow (Bannister et al. 1990, Sanderson et al. 1994, Whiteside et al. 2001).

Upper lumbar block

For blocks up to L_1, 3–4 ml of glucose-free solution is usually sufficient whichever posture is used. This is particularly advantageous if patients have a painful condition such as fractured neck of femur, because they do not have to lie on the painful side during administration of the spinal. However, glucose-free solutions are unpredictable, and on occasion the block may not reach L_1. Injection at L_2/L_3 will reduce this risk, but will increase the possibility of spread to the cervical region (Logan et al. 1986). A truly isobaric solution is not associated with these risks, but is difficult to source. Early work suggested that plain levobupivacaine is as unpredictable as plain bupivacaine (Burke et al. 1999), but this has been challenged (Glaser et al. 2002), so the solution may require further study.

Saddle (perineal) block

When the maximum height of block required is S_1, 1–2 ml of hyperbaric solution may be injected in the sitting position, which should be maintained for at least 5 minutes. A risk of the sitting position is venous pooling with decreases in venous return, cardiac output, and blood pressure. In addition, the hip joint will not be blocked and this may lead to discomfort if the patient is placed in the lithotomy position. Alternatively, 2–3 ml of plain solution may be administered to the supine patient, but this can produce a much higher level of block than is required for perineal surgery.

Unilateral block

The suggested aims of producing a limited, unilateral block are twofold: first, to avoid the cardiovascular side effects of extensive spread; second, to achieve earlier patient mobilization. Because of the proximity within the theca of the nerve roots for the two sides a truly unilateral block is probably impossible to achieve, but a predominantly one-sided block may be possible. This does require that a relatively small dose of local anaesthetic (circa 1.5 ml) is used and that the patient is maintained in the lateral position for up to 30 minutes (Pittoni et al. 1995). Some spread to the other side may still occur and the delay may not be worth the minimal advantage, especially as the low dose used will limit total duration.

Overview

The aim of any spinal anaesthetic technique is to produce a block which is adequate in extent and duration for the proposed surgery with minimal risk of complications due to excessive spread, particularly hypotension. The factors which influence intrathecal drug spread may be manipulated in many ways, but the essential aim just noted may be most simply achieved by the slow injection of a hyperbaric solution containing a lower concentration of glucose (1%) than is traditional (Hocking & Wildsmith 2004). The solution spreads to almost the same level as one with a greater concentration of glucose (see Figure 13.6), but less rapidly, allowing cardiovascular adaption to increasing sympathetic block to take place more readily. Such a glucose concentration is easily achieved by mixing plain and hyperbaric solutions of local anaesthetic in appropriate proportions, but it should be noted that this is an unlicensed application.

However, any technique of spinal anaesthesia may result in hypotension so measures for its prevention, recognition, and treatment must always be available (Chapter 11). A contingency plan of management in the event of the rare partial or total failure should also be made. In essence, the options are to repeat the spinal anaesthetic (probably at an adjacent space in case some local factor has limited spread), or to give a general anaesthetic instead. The choice will depend very much on the circumstances of the case (Fettes et al. 2009).

Special techniques

Continuous spinal anaesthesia (CSA)

The problems of variability in extent and duration of block make catheter-based spinal anaesthesia an attractive concept. It allows the repeated injection of small doses of local anaesthetic to be titrated to the desired effect, but use of the method has been inhibited by fears of a high incidence of paraesthesiae, neurological complications, and PDPH.

Interest was rekindled in the 1980s with the advent of 28- and 32-g microcatheters (Hurley & Lambert 1990), but reports of CES (Rigler et al. 1991), possibly associated with pooling of highly concentrated, hyperbaric local anaesthetic in the sacral segments, inhibited the initial enthusiasm and led to the banning of catheters finer than 24 g in the USA. Further, these catheters are difficult to use, the direction taken in the subarachnoid space is unpredictable, and the inevitable slow injection prevents turbulence and decreases mixing of the local anaesthetic with CSF. As a result, inadequate blocks were common, although it has been argued that careful, considered use of the technique can avoid the complications (Denny & Selander 1998).

Currently, most systems for CSA use a 'catheter-through-needle' technique with passage of a 20–24-g catheter through a 19-g Tuohy needle placed in the subarachnoid space. Such devices are used by enthusiasts who feel that they have a place in elderly and poor-risk patients in whom slow titration of local anaesthetic is desirable, but reported failure rates still average 2.5%. As an alternative, 'catheter-over-wire' devices have become available (Burnell & Byrne 2001). A Tuohy needle is first placed in the epidural space, and the catheter/wire assembly used to penetrate the dura. Once the catheter is *in situ*, the wire and the Tuohy needle are removed, this method being said to reduce the incidence of difficulties and complications.

The safety and efficacy of CSA may be enhanced by using the larger sized systems by the paramedian approach to ensure the cephalad direction of the minimal length of catheter. Some suggest that only plain solutions should be used because of the initial association between hyperbaric solutions and CES, but it is now accepted that the problem was really due to repeated injections of concentrated local anaesthetics in the mistaken belief that more drug would extend a restricted block. The use of larger diameter systems might be expected to cause PDPH although rates of less than 1% have been claimed in very experienced hands (Denny et al. 1987, Mahisekar et al. 1991). Other complications such as sepsis, catheter breakage, and intrathecal bleeding are rare, but the practitioner must be very aware of them. CSA is a technique which should be reserved for the clinician with extensive experience of both single-dose spinal anaesthesia and other catheter techniques.

Combined spinal epidural block

Recognition of the potential advantages of CSA, but with concerns about its efficacy and safety remaining, led to the development of systems combining spinal and epidural block. It is used most widely in obstetric practice (Chapter 21), but also in orthopaedic and vascular anaesthesia. However, the overall incidence of major complications has been found to be double that of standard spinal anaesthesia (Cook et al. 2009).

Thoracic spinal anaesthesia

Although spinal anaesthesia is usually performed at the lumbar level there have been some descriptions of its use by thoracic puncture (van Zundert et al. 2007). Clearly, this is another technique which must be reserved for the very experienced practitioner.

'Selective' spinal anaesthesia

As noted earlier, spinal anaesthesia was once considered to be contraindicated in day-care patients, but changes in practice have altered the balance of risks. However, rapid mobilization and early recovery are essential so techniques, sometimes described as *selective*, have evolved, especially where suitable short-acting local anaesthetic preparations are unavailable. The method uses low doses of hyperbaric bupivacaine (5–10 mg) and fentanyl (15–25 mcg), combined with the lateral position if needed to concentrate the effects on the operative side. Considerable skill and experience are needed to achieve success with such doses and, even so, most reports mention a failure rate of at least 1%. The recent availability of a hyperbaric preparation of prilocaine, an inherently shorter acting drug, may overcome this difficulty.

Full information on spinal anaesthesia in day surgery is available in an electronic handbook (British Association of Day Surgery: see 'On-line resources').

Side effects

The technique of spinal anaesthesia is so simple that it might lead to complacency. A complete understanding of the relevant physiology and complete clinical training are essential to ensure safe management.

Cardiovascular system

The prevention and treatment of hypotension have been discussed in Chapter 11, but the benefits of maintaining venous return by keeping the patient in a slight head-down tilt should not be forgotten. This does *not* result in a significant cephalad extension of block height.

A problem perhaps specific to spinal anaesthesia is, in the event of decreased venous return or marked parasympathetic overactivity, the development of sudden bradycardia, a decrease in cardiac output, hypotension, and even asystole (see 'Complications' section). This can occur with relatively restricted blocks and is more likely in patients who are awake, or those who are hypovolaemic, have aortocaval compression, or are excessively sedated (Caplan et al. 1988). Unlike epidural block, the mass of local anaesthetic or vasoconstrictor absorbed is too small to modify the cardiovascular changes.

Respiratory system

Spinal anaesthesia is unlikely to affect resting ventilation or produce changes in blood gases. However, if the block is very high, there may be a 20% decrease in inspiratory capacity, and a marked reduction in expiratory reserve volume. Cough strength may also be impaired (Egbert et al. 1961, Freund 1969). The patient may have difficulty in taking a deep breath and may even feel dyspnoeic. Apnoea, in the absence of opioids, is rare and is usually secondary to hypotension and brainstem ischaemia, but if the block reaches the upper cervical level, it may be caused by bilateral phrenic nerve root involvement. Management of the total spinal is discussed in Chapter 21.

Gastrointestinal and genitourinary systems

The intestine becomes contracted, peristalsis continues, and the sphincters relax. Upper abdominal and intraperitoneal visceral stimuli, probably transmitted by unblocked vagal afferent fibres, may be perceived as pain, and provoke nausea and vomiting (Ratra et al. 1972). Nausea and vomiting may also be an early sign of hypotension. Hepatic and renal blood flow seem to be blood pressure dependent.

Urinary retention may be a problem in males because sacral autonomic fibre function, and thus detrusor muscle contraction, are among the last functions to recover (Axellson et al. 1974). It is difficult to micturate while lying supine, and the patient must stay in bed until the risk of postural hypotension has passed. Excessive fluid preload is a potential cause of overdistension of the bladder and should be avoided unless a urinary catheter is to be inserted.

Other effects

Blood loss is reduced and the stress response, while often incompletely blocked, may be delayed (Webster et al. 1991). It is likely that the incidence of deep venous thrombosis is also reduced, and early morbidity and mortality decreased as compared to general anaesthesia (Rodgers et al. 2000).

Complications

Postdural puncture headache

The diagnosis of PDPH is usually clear from the history of dural puncture and the postural nature of symptoms, but headache is very common postoperatively and should not be assumed to be due to the spinal anaesthetic. Aseptic and bacterial meningitis should be considered in the differential diagnosis, and a condition known as spontaneous intracranial hypotension, with similar symptoms and signs to PDPH, has been described (Weitz & Drasner 1996).

PDPH is probably due to CSF leak from the subarachnoid to the epidural space. Low CSF pressure allows descent of the brain and this stretches the dura, tentorium, venous sinuses, and dural and cerebral blood vessels, and thus the nerve endings they contain. PDPH is occipito-frontal, appears within a few days of the event, and severely incapacitates the patient. It should be mild or absent in the supine position and be aggravated by sitting up. It may be accompanied by photophobia, nausea and vomiting, neck stiffness, or cranial nerve palsies, and occasionally these may be dominant features. The key feature is that they are posturally related.

The incidence may be reduced to less than 1% by using fine, pencil-point needles (Halpern & Preston 1994) and avoiding multiple dural punctures (Seeberger et al. 1996). The bevel of a 'cutting' needle should be aligned longitudinally rather than transversely to separate rather than cut dural fibres (Mihic 1985, Norris et al. 1989). Although atraumatic needles reduce the incidence of PDPH, they have been shown to increase the likelihood of neurological deficit due to contact with either the spinal cord or the nerve roots of the cauda equina. It has been suggested that extreme flexion of the spine tenses the dura and increases the size of the puncture hole. Extension of the head on the neck may lessen this tension.

Age decreases the incidence of PDPH possibly because decreased elasticity of the tissues allows less stretching of intracranial structures. Dehydration from any cause results in low CSF pressure, which increases the severity of the headache. The headache usually resolves spontaneously within a few days, but may persist for long periods. It may be dangerous because rupture of a bridging vein as the brain moves away from the dura may lead to a subdural haematoma (Newrick & Read 1982). Thus effective treatment for the established case is essential.

Management of dural puncture headache

PDPH is a complication which should not be treated lightly because of its potential for considerable morbidity, and even mortality.

All patients who have had a spinal anaesthetic must be kept well hydrated and should avoid straining. Maintenance of the supine position after lumbar puncture does not decrease the incidence, although it reduces the symptoms (Kang et al. 1992) and may prevent complications.

Patients who develop PDPH should be encouraged to drink freely and to use mild, non-opioid analgesics. Many treatments have been proposed although studies often involve small numbers of patients and fail to recognize that, without treatment, over 85% of headaches will resolve within 6 weeks (Turnbull & Shepherd 2003). Caffeine 300–500 mg, intravenously or orally once or twice daily, may relieve the symptoms (Camann et al. 1990). If a medicinal preparation is unavailable, coffee (50–100 mg caffeine per cup) and certain soft drinks (35–50 mg per cup) may be used instead, but therapeutic doses of caffeine have been associated with central nervous system toxicity and atrial fibrillation. The serotonin receptor agonist sumatriptan, 6 mg subcutaneously, has also been recommended (Carp et al. 1994).

If the headache does not resolve within 1 or 2 days, or is incapacitating, an epidural blood patch must be considered (Chapter 21).

Backache

This is a common symptom and may be due to stretching of anaesthetized ligaments and joints during surgery. It is more common when the patient has been placed in the lithotomy position. The patient should be positioned carefully, and extreme postures should not be allowed while the block is effective because the protective effect of pain will have been removed.

Neurological complications

Neurological complications are extremely rare (Cook et al. 2009, Dripps & Vandam 1954), but can be catastrophically severe so every effort must be made to prevent them.

Local neurotoxicity

When a needle has been inserted into the subarachnoid space all of the protection afforded to the spinal cord and nerve roots has been bypassed, and these structures are very vulnerable to chemical and physical damage (see Chapter 4). Drugs and substances which are innocuous when administered intravenously or even epidurally may be harmful, so only drugs, or combinations of drugs, which have been proven to be safe should be injected, and every effort must be made to avoid contamination of the injectate with antiseptic. Equally important is the need to minimize the risk of needle trauma (Fettes & Wildsmith 2002, Reynolds 2000).

All neurological complications should be identified and investigated early by a competent neurologist with knowledge of the specific subject. The vast majority will be found to be incidental to the technique (Marinacci 1960), but they may result from the injection of inappropriate chemicals, preservatives, or drugs, or from the introduction of infection. This may result in adhesive or proliferative arachnoiditis, or transverse myelitis, usually affecting the cauda equina first, but often spreading higher. There may be low back pain, sphincter disturbances, sacral analgesia, and perhaps some numbness and weakness of the legs. The onset is variable, and the clinical course is unpredictable with recovery uncertain.

Space-occupying lesions

If neurological features produce any suspicion of a space-occupying lesion such as a haematoma, abscess, or tumour mass, a neurological opinion must be sought urgently because surgical decompression must be performed within hours (the use of central neural block in the presence of anticoagulant therapy is discussed in Chapter 9). Epidural abscesses are more often due to haematogenous spread than to the local introduction of infection.

Anterior spinal artery syndrome

Interference with the vascular supply to nerves or the spinal cord may be devastating in its consequences. The classical condition is the 'anterior spinal artery syndrome', which manifests itself as a painless paralysis of the legs and sphincters due to infarction of the anterior segments of the spinal cord. The syndrome may follow periods of hypotension especially in older patients, but may also be associated with surgical interruption of the blood supply to the cord.

Cerebral damage

Brain damage can occur due to cardiac arrest (see 'Cardiac arrest' section) or a prolonged period of hypotension. While this is more likely with a total spinal during an intended epidural, it can occur with deliberate spinal anaesthesia (Caplan et al. 1988).

Transient neurological symptoms

First described in 1993, TNS, are self-limiting pain and dysaesthesia in the buttocks and/or lower extremities after apparently uncomplicated spinal anaesthesia (Hampl et al. 1995). It is most common after day-surgery performed in the lithotomy position with lidocaine used for the spinal anaesthetic, although it has been described less commonly after other drugs. There is no evidence that TNS are due to drug toxicity, the clinical picture being of a myofascial pain condition (Selander 1999) unrelated to the CES seen after repeated injection through spinal catheters (see 'Continuous spinal anaesthesia' section). The explanation is thought to be stretching of ligaments, fasciae, and muscles when muscle relaxation leads to flattening of the lumbar lordosis, even in the supine patient. Such stretching is more widespread in the lithotomy position, and the very profound effect of lidocaine 'allows' it to happen to a greater degree than with other drugs.

Cardiac arrest

The issue of sudden, unexpected cardiac arrest, primarily in young healthy individuals undergoing relatively minor surgery was first raised in an account of 'closed' insurance claims cases by Caplan and colleagues (1988). Consideration of the details suggests that excessive sedation, coupled with elements of poor patient observation, may have been other relevant factors, but a comprehensive review of such other reports suggest that cardiovascular, rather then respiratory factors are often more relevant (Pollard 2001). Case reports do not always make for easy interpretation, but it would seem that failure of venous return and vagal overactivity are often involved so management (prevention and treatment) should be directed at both. These issues are also discussed in Chapter 11.

Key references

Fettes PDW, Jansson JR, Wildsmith JAW (2009) Failed spinal anaesthesia: mechanisms, management, and prevention. *British Journal of Anaesthesia* 102: 739–48.

Hocking G, Wildsmith JAW (2004) Intrathecal drug spread. *British Journal of Anaesthesia* 93: 568–78.

On-line resources

http://www.daysurgeryuk.net/bads/joomla/files/Handbooks/
SpinalAnaesthesia.pdf Spinal anaesthesia in day surgery.

http://www.backtobackguidetospinalanaesthesia.com Overview of spinal
anaesthesia.

References

Axellson KH, Mollefors K, Ollson JO, et al. (1974) Bladder function
in spinal anaesthesia. *Linkoping University Medical Dissertation*
184: v3–v21.

Bannister J, McClure JH, Wildsmith JAW (1990) Effect of glucose
concentration on the intrathecal spread of 0.5% bupivacaine.
British Journal of Anaesthesia 64: 232–4.

Barker AE (1907) A report on clinical experiences with spinal analgesia in
100 cases. *British Medical Journal* i: 665–74.

Broadbent CR, Maxwell WB, Ferrie R, et al. (2000) Ability of anaesthetists
to identify a marked lumbar interspace. *Anaesthesia* 55: 1122–6.

Burke D, Kennedy S, Bannister J (1999) Spinal anesthesia with 0.5% S(-)
bupivacaine for elective lower limb surgery. *Regional Anaesthesia and
Pain Medicine* 24: 519–28.

Burnell S, Byrne AJ (2001) Continuous spinal anaesthesia. *Continuing
Education in Anaesthesia, Critical Care & Pain* 1: 134–7.

Camann WR, Murray RS, Mushlin PS, Lambert DH (1990) Effects of
oral caffeine on postdural puncture headache. A double-blind,
placebo-controlled trial. *Anesthesia & Analgesia* 70: 181–4.

Caplan RA, Ward RJ, Posner K, Cheney FW (1988) Unexpected cardiac
arrest during spinal anesthesia: a closed claims analysis of predisposing
factors. *Anesthesiology* 68: 5–11.

Carp H, Singh PJ, Vadhera R, Jayaran A (1994) Effects of the serotonin
receptor agonist sumatriptan on the post dural puncture headache:
report of six cases. *Anesthesia & Analgesia* 79: 180–2.

Chamberlain DP, Chamberlain BD (1986) Changes in the skin temperature
of the trunk and their relationship to sympathetic blockade during
spinal anesthesia. *Anesthesiology* 65: 139–43.

Chambers WA, Littlewood DG, Logan MR, Scott DB (1981) Effect of
added epinephrine on spinal anesthesia with lidocaine. *Anesthesia &
Analgesia* 60: 417–20.

Concepcion MA (1989) Spinal anesthetic agents. *International
Anesthesiology Clinics* 27: 21–5.

Concepcion MA, Maddi R, Francis D, et al. (1984) Vasoconstrictors in
spinal anesthesia with tetracaine—a comparison of epinephrine and
phenylephrine. *Anesthesia & Analgesia* 63: 134–8.

Cook TM, Counsell D, Wildsmith JAW (2009) Major complications
of central neuraxial block: report of the Third National Audit
Project of the Royal College of Anaesthetists. *British Journal of
Anaesthesia* 102: 179–90.

Cope RW (1954) The Woolley and Roe case: Woolley and Roe versus
Ministry of Health and others. *Anaesthesia* 9: 249–70.

Crone LL, Vogel W (1991) Failed spinal anaesthesia with the Sprotte
needle. *Anesthesiology* 75: 717–18.

Dahlgren G, Hulstrand C, Jakobsson J, et al. (1997) Intrathecal sufentanil,
fentanyl, or placebo added to bupivacaine for Cesarean section.
Anesthesia & Analgesia 85: 1288–93.

Denny NM, Selander DE (1998) Continuous spinal anaesthesia.
British Journal of Anaesthesia 81: 590–7.

Denny N, Masters R, Pearson D, et al. (1987) Postdural puncture headache
after continuous spinal anesthesia. *Anesthesia & Analgesia* 66: 791–4.

Dripps RD, Vandam LD (1954) Longterm follow-up of patients who
received 10,098 spinal anesthetics. I: failure to discover major
neurological sequelae. *Journal of the American Medical Association*,
156: 1486–91.

Egbert LD, Tamersoy K, Deas TC (1961) Pulmonary function during
spinal anesthesia: the mechanism of cough depression.
Anesthesiology 22: 882–5.

Elia N, Culebras X, Mazza C, et al. (2008) Clonidine as an adjuvant to
intrathecal local anesthetics for surgery: systematic review of
randomized trials. *Regional Anesthesia and Pain Medicine* 33: 159–67.

Fettes PDW, Wildsmith JAW (2002) Editorial: Somebody else's nervous
system. *British Journal of Anaesthesia* 102: 760–3.

Fettes PDW, Jansson JR, Wildsmith JAW (2009) Failed spinal anaesthesia:
mechanisms, management, and prevention. *British Journal of
Anaesthesia* 102: 739–48.

Fogarty DJ, Carabine UA, Milligan KR (1993) Comparison of the analgesic
effects of intrathecal clonidine and intrathecal morphine after spinal
anaesthesia in patients undergoing total hip replacement. *British
Journal of Anaesthesia* 71: 661–4.

Freund FG (1969) Respiratory effects of subarachnoid and epidural
block. In Bonica JJ (Ed) *Clinical anesthesia 2. Regional anesthesia:
recent advances and current status*, pp. 98–107. Philadelphia,
PA: FA Davis.

Freund FG, Bonica JJ, Ward RJ, et al (1967) Ventilatory reserve and
level of motor block during high spinal and epidural anesthesia.
Anesthesiology 28: 834–7.

Gautier PE, De Kock M, Van Steenberge A, et al. (1999)
Intrathecal ropivacaine for ambulatory surgery.
Anesthesiology 91: 1239–45.

Glaser C, Marhofer P, Zimpfer G, et al. (2002) Levobupivacaine versus
racemic bupivacaine for spinal anesthesia. *Anesthesia &
Analgesia* 94: 194–8.

Greene NM, Brull SJ (1993) *Physiology of spinal anesthesia*, 4th edn.
Baltimore, MD: Williams and Wilkins.

Halpern S, Preston R (1994) Postdural puncture headache and spinal
needle design. Metanalyses. *Anesthesiology* 81: 1376–83.

Hampl KF, Schneider MC, Ummenhofer W, Drewe J (1995) Transient
neurological symptoms after spinal anaesthesia. *Anesthesia &
Analgesia* 81: 1148–53.

Henderson DJ, Jones G (1995) Effect of i.v. diamorphine on the regression
of spinal block. *British Journal of Anaesthesia* 74: 610–11.

Hocking G, Wildsmith JAW (2004) Intrathecal drug spread.
British Journal of Anaesthesia 93: 568–78.

Hoskin MF (1998) Spinal anaesthesia—the current trends towards narrow
gauge atraumatic (pencil point) needles. Case reports and review.
Anaesthesia and Intensive Care 26: 96–106.

Hurley RJ, Lambert DH (1990) Continuous spinal anesthesia with a
microcatheter technique: preliminary experience. *Anesthesia &
Analgesia* 70: 97–102.

Hutter CDD (1990) The Woolley and Roe case. A reassessment.
Anaesthesia 45: 859–64.

Kalso E (1983) Effects of intrathecal morphine, injected with
bupivacaine, on pain after orthopaedic surgery. *British Journal of
Anaesthesia* 55: 415–22.

Kalso E, Tuominen M, Rosenberg PH (1982) Effect of posture and some
c.s.f. characteristics on spinal anaesthesia with isobaric 0.5%
bupivacaine. *British Journal of Anaesthesia* 54: 1179–84.

Kang SB, Goodnough DE, Lee YK, et al. (1992) Comparison of 26- and
27-g needles for spinal anesthesia for ambulatory surgery patients.
Anesthesiology 76: 734–8.

Lee JA (1984) Personal communication.

Lee A, Ray D, Littlewood DG, Wildsmith JAW (1988) Effect of dextrose
concentration on the intrathecal spread of amethocaine. *British
Journal of Anaesthesia* 61: 135–8.

Logan ML, McClure JH, Wildsmith JAW (1986) Plain bupivacaine—an
unpredictable agent. *British Journal of Anaesthesia* 58: 292–6.

Mahisekar UL, Winnie AP, Vasireddy AR, Masters RW (1991)
Continuous spinal anesthesia and post dural puncture headache.
A retrospective study. *Regional Anesthesia* 16: 107–11.

Marinacci AA (1960) Neurological aspects of complications of spinal
anesthesia with medico-legal implications. *Bulletin of the Los
Angeles Neurological Society* 24: 170–92.

McLeod G (2004) Density of spinal anaesthetic solutions of bupivacaine, levobupivacaine and ropivacaine with and without dextrose. *British Journal of Anaesthesia* 92: 547–51.

McClure JH, Brown DT, Wildsmith JAW (1982) Effect of injected volume and speed of injection on the spread of spinal anaesthesia with isobaric amethocaine. *British Journal of Anaesthesia* 54: 917–20.

Mihic DN (1985) Postspinal headache and relationship of needle bevel to longitudinal dural fibres. *Regional Anesthesia* 10: 76–81.

Moore JM, Liu SS, Pollock JE, et al. (1998) The effect of epinephrine on small-dose hyperbaric bupivacaine spinal anesthesia: Clinical implications for ambulatory surgery. *Anesthesia & Analgesia* 86: 973–7.

Mulroy MF, Wills RP (1995) Spinal anesthesia for outpatients: Appropriate agents and techniques. *Journal of Clinical Anesthesia* 7: 622–7.

Newrick P, Read D (1982) Subdural haematoma as a complication of spinal anaesthetic. *British Medical Journal* 285: 341–2.

Niemi L, Tuominen M, Pitkanen M, Rosenberg PH (1993) Effect of late posture change on the level of spinal anaesthesia with plain bupivacaine. *British Journal of Anaesthesia* 71: 807–9.

Norris MC, Leighton BL, DeSimone CA (1989) Needle bevel direction and headache after inadvertent dural puncture. *Anesthesiology* 70: 729–31.

Pitkanen M, Haapaniemi L, Tuominen M, Rosenberg PH (1984) Influence of age on spinal anaesthesia with isobaric 0.5% bupivacaine. *British Journal of Anaesthesia* 56: 279–84.

Pittoni G, Toffoletto F, Cacarella G, et al. (1995) Spinal anesthesia in outpatient knee surgery: 22-gauge versus 25-gauge Sprotte needle. *Anesthesia & Analgesia* 81: 73–9.

Pollard JB (2001) Cardiac arrest during spinal anesthesia: common mechanisms and strategies for prevention. *Anesthesia & Analgesia* 92: 252–6.

Racle JP, Benkhadra A, Poy JY, Gleizal B (1987) Prolongation of isobaric bupivacaine spinal anesthesia with epinephrine and clonidine for hip surgery in the elderly. *Anesthesia & Analgesia* 66: 442–6.

Racle JP, Jourdren L, Benkhadra A, et al. (1988) Effect of adding sodium bicarbonate to bupivacaine for spinal anesthesia in elderly patients. *Anesthesia & Analgesia* 67: 570–3.

Ratra CK, Badola RP, Bhargrave KP (1972) A study of factors concerned in emesis during spinal anaesthesia. *British Journal of Anaesthesia* 44: 1208–11.

Rawal N, Holmstrom B, Crowhurst JA, Van Zundert A (2000) The combined spinal-epidural technique. *Anesthesiology Clinics of North America* 18: 267–95.

Rawal N (2001) Analgesia for day-case surgery. *British Journal of Anaesthesia* 87: 73–87.

Reynolds F (2000) Logic in the safe practice of spinal anaesthesia. *Anaesthesia* 55: 1045–6.

Reynolds F (2001) Damage to the conus medullaris following spinal anaesthesia. *Anaesthesia* 56: 238–49.

Rigler ML, Drasner K, Krejcie TC, et al. (1991) Cauda equina syndrome after continuous spinal anesthesia. *Anesthesia & Analgesia* 72: 275–81.

Rodgers A, Walker A, Schug S, et al (2000) Reduction of postoperative mortality and morbidity with epidural or spinal anaesthesia: results from overview of randomised trials. *British Medical Journal* 321: 1493–7.

Sanderson P, Read J, Littlewood DG, et al. (1994) Interaction between baricity (glucose concentration) and other factors influencing intrathecal drug spread. *British Journal of Anaesthesia* 73: 744–6.

Seeberger MD, Kaufmann M, Staender S, et al. (1996) Repeated dural punctures increase the incidence of post dural puncture headache. *Anesthesia & Analgesia* 82: 302–5.

Selander DE (1999) Transient lumbar pain (TLP) after lidocaine spinal anaesthesia is not neurotoxic. In Zundert A (Ed) *Highlights in Regional Anaesthesia and Pain Therapy VIII*, pp. 315–21. Cyprus: Hadjigeorgiou Printings Ltd.

Sumi M, Sakura S, Sakaguchi Y, et al. (1996) Comparison of glucose 7.5% and 0.75% with or without phenylephrine for tetracaine spinal anaesthesia. *Canadian Journal of Anaesthesia* 43: 1138–43.

Tarkkila PJ (1991) Incidence and causes of failed spinal anesthetics in a university hospital: A prospective study. *Regional Anesthesia and Pain Medicine* 16: 48–51.

Tarkkila P, Huhtala J, Tuominen M (1997) Home-readiness after spinal anaesthesia with small doses of hyperbaric 0.5% bupivacaine. *Anaesthesia* 52: 1157–60.

Turner MA, Shaw M (1993) Correspondence: Atraumatic spinal needles. *Anaesthesia* 48: 452.

Tuominen M, Taivainen T, Rosenberg PT (1989) Spread of spinal anaesthesia with plain 0.5% bupivacaine: Influence of vertebral interspace used for injection. *British Journal of Anaesthesia* 62: 358–61.

Turnbull DK, Shepherd DB (2003) Post-dural puncture headache: pathogenesis, prevention and treatment. *British Journal of Anaesthesia* 91: 718–29.

Vallejo MC, Mandell GL, Sabo DP, Ramanathan S (2000) Postdural puncture headache: a randomised comparison of five spinal needles i n obstetric patients. *Anesthesia &Analgesia* 91: 916–20.

van Zundert AAJ, Stultiens G, Jakimowicz JJ, et al. (2007) Laparoscopic cholecystectomy under segmental thoracic spinal anaesthesia: a feasibility study. *British Journal of Anaesthesia*, 98: 682–6.

Veering BT, Burm AGL, Spierduk J (1988) Spinal anaesthesia with hyperbaric bupivacaine: Effects of age on neural blockade and pharmacokinetics. *British Journal of Anaesthesia* 60: 187–94.

Webster J, Barnard M, Carli F (1991) Metabolic response to colonic surgery: extradural vs. continuous spinal. *British Journal of Anaesthesia* 67: 467–9.

Weitz SR, Drasner K (1996) Spontaneous intracranial hypotension: a series. *Anesthesiology* 85: 923–5.

Whiteside JB, Wildsmith JAW (2005) Spinal anaesthesia: an update. *Continuing Education in Anaesthesia, Critical Care & Pain* 5: 37–40.

Whiteside JB, Burke D, Wildsmith JAW (2001) Spinal anaesthesia with ropivacaine 5 mg ml^{-1} in glucose 10 mg ml^{-1} or 50 mg ml-1. *British Journal of Anaesthesia* 86: 241–4.

Whiteside JB, Burke D, Wildsmith JAW (2003) Comparison of ropivacaine 0.5% (in glucose 5%) with bupivacaine 0.5% (in glucose 8%) for spinal anaesthesia for elective surgery. *British Journal of Anaesthesia* 90: 304–8.

Wildsmith JAW, Rocco AG (1985) Current concepts in spinal anesthesia. *Regional Anesthesia* 10: 117–21.

Wildsmith JAW, McClure JH, Brown DT, Scott DB (1981) Effects of posture on the spread of isobaric and hyperbaric amethocaine. *British Journal of Anaesthesia* 53: 273–8.

Wiles MD, Nathanson MH (2010) Local anaesthetics and adjuvants—future developments. *Anaesthesia* 65 (Suppl 1): 22–37.

CHAPTER 14

Epidural block

Graeme McLeod

General considerations

Epidural block has now become well established as an adjunct to general anaesthesia and is regarded as the most effective means of providing pain relief after surgery and during labour (Dolin et al. 2002). Regardless of the type of surgery and means of assessing pain, epidural block provides better pain relief than parenteral opioids (Block et al. 2003). Several factors have contributed to this:

1. Placement of a catheter in the epidural space is a relatively straightforward procedure;

2. Epidural block may be extended for several days into the postoperative period if needed;

3. Quality pain relief allows effective coughing and early mobilization; and

4. Acute pain teams are available to provide continuity of management.

There are, however, disadvantages:

1. Visceral sensation remains intact and general anaesthesia is needed as a supplement for major surgery of the thorax and abdomen;

2. Surgery to the trunk requires thoracic epidural block, but inexperienced anaesthetists tend to insert catheters several dermatomes below the ideal, 'mid-incisional' level, resulting in inadequate pain relief *and* lower limb motor block;

3. Performance of the block adds to anaesthesia time; and

4. Pre-existing neurological conditions, coagulation disorders, and pharmacological thromboprophylaxis are weightier contraindications to epidural block than to other regional techniques because bleeding into the epidural space is not always immediately apparent, cannot be controlled directly, and may only be revealed when it causes symptoms.

Safety issues

Unfortunately the widespread use of continuous epidural block during both labour and the postoperative period has been associated with rare, but significant, complications such as neurological sequelae, pyogenic abscess and injection errors (Chapter 4). Most neurological sequelae occur in elderly postoperative rather than obstetric patients, but injection errors have been reported in both areas. Avoidable factors are often identified and some points merit further mention here.

General technique

Advice on safe practice is given in Chapters 9 and 11, but the importance of the following cannot be overemphasized:

1. Antiseptic solution such as chlorhexidine must not contaminate the epidural equipment;

2. Drugs should not be drawn up until the antiseptic has been used and removed from the sterile field;

3. The antiseptic should be given time to dry and become effective;

4. Preservative-free, single-use local anaesthetic solutions should be used, and any remnant discarded;

5. Catheters and injection ports should not be swabbed with alcohol which may be carried into the epidural space; and

6. Many hospital patients are immunocompromised and 'sensitive' to even a minor failure in aseptic technique.

Injection errors

Between 1 January 2005 and 31 May 2006, 346 epidural related drug errors were reported to the UK National Patient Safety Agency (now the National Reporting and Learning Service—NRLS), with many examples of non-epidural drug error during epidural infusion (n = 81), documentation error (n = 49), wrong epidural drug (n = 36), error with programming or operating the infusion pump (n = 31), wrong dose of drug (n = 23), accidental infusion of drug into epidural (n = 12), and inadvertent injection of local anaesthetic into a vein (n = 8) (Report 2007). Most of these errors were of little consequence, but the same report notes that between 2000 and 2004 three patients died in the UK after inadvertent intravenous infusion of bupivacaine so there is no room for complacency.

These incidents highlight the care needed with epidural injections and infusions, particularly in regard to how the medicines and devices are labelled, stored, and administered, and the report included wide.- ranging recommendations for safer practice (Table 14.1). The dispensing of epidural infusion bags by the Pharmacy, and their receipt on the wards, should be strictly regulated; and epidural pumps and tubing should be easily distinguishable from those for arterial and venous lines. Colour coding (red—arterial; blue—venous; yellow—epidural) has much to recommend it, these safeguards being in addition to the move towards entirely different connection systems for neuraxial needles and catheters.

However, accidents to surgical patients occur across a much broader front. In 2007, 129,419 incidents relating to surgical procedures were reported in England and Wales (Report 2009). Six per cent described moderate, and 1% severe, harm to patients, including 271 deaths. In response to the worldwide nature of such incidents, the World Health Organization (WHO) launched a Surgical Safety Checklist which has been adapted for England and Wales by the NRLS (Report 2009). The WHO defines a surgical procedure as 'the excision of a patient's tissue, penetration of the patient's skin or the closure of a previously sustained wound/ intervention in a "sterile" environment e.g. operating theatre or procedure room' so, by inference, the checklist should be completed for every patient undergoing a regional block.

Equipment

Trays

Commercially prepared disposable epidural trays are now readily available and manufacturers will customize the contents to suit the needs of departments. The new long-acting local anaesthetics levobupivacaine and ropivacaine are provided in sterile plastic vials, but bupivacaine and lidocaine are still produced in glass ampoules. When opening these, care should be taken not to shower the working area with glass fragments, and a filter needle should always be used to draw up the local anaesthetic.

Epidural needles

Epidural needle provision should be standardized in each department of anaesthetics in order to avoid confusion. Changing from one type of epidural needle to another is remarkably difficult, and the potential exists, with changed 'feel', for serious side effects such as accidental dural puncture.

The *Tuohy* needle (Figure 14.1) is the acknowledged standard. The shaft is 8 cm long, graduated in centimetres and available in 16-, 17-, and 18-g sizes. An 11-cm shaft is available (from Portex) for use in the obese. A stylet prevents coring of the superficial tissues and increases the rigidity of the needle. The needle point is relatively blunt and is contoured so that a catheter emerges at an angle of about 20° (the Huber tip), but this design does have the important disadvantage that the catheter cannot be withdrawn through the needle without the risk of it being transected (Figure 14.2). If it is necessary to withdraw the catheter, the needle must be withdrawn simultaneously. The choice of gauge is individual, although most trainees prefer the 16-g needle, and then graduate to the 18 g.

Combined spinal–epidural (CSE) needles

The CSE technique was introduced in an attempt to combine the reliability of spinal anaesthesia with the flexibility of continuous epidural block. The now definitive needle-through-needle technique was first used by Coates and colleagues (1982) for orthopaedics, but the technique's major application is in obstetrics so it is described in Chapter 21.

Catheters

The design and manufacture of catheters represents a compromise. The internal diameter of the catheter should be as large as possible to minimize the resistance to injection along its 90-cm length, but the wall must not be so thin that it buckles or kinks where it enters the epidural space, emerges from the skin or is caught in folds of

Table 14.1 Recommended actions for safer epidural infusion practice (Report 2007).

1	Rationalize range of epidural products
2	Rationalize procedures for preparing and administering epidural infusions to minimize the risk of confusion over different types and strengths of epidural injections and infusions
3	Ensure all staff involved in using epidural therapy have received adequate training and have the necessary work competences to undertake their duties safely
4	Clearly label infusion bags and syringes for epidural therapy (whether purchased commercially, manufactured by the hospital pharmacy service or prepared in clinical areas) with **'For Epidural Use Only'** in large font, and make judicious use of colour and design to differentiate these products from those for administration by intravenous and other routes
5	Maximize the use of ready-to-administer epidural infusions
6	Store epidural infusions in separate cupboards or refrigerators from intravenous and other types of infusions to reduce the risk of the wrong medicine being selected
7	Label all epidural administration sets with **'Epidural'** when in use
8	Use clearly identified epidural infusion devices exclusively for epidural therapy or, if not, the device should be marked clearly and unambiguously that it is **'For Epidural Use Only'** when it is being used for that purpose

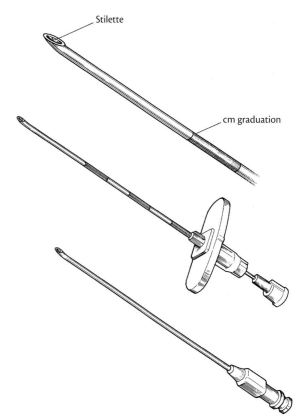

Figure 14.1 Features of a Tuohy needle.

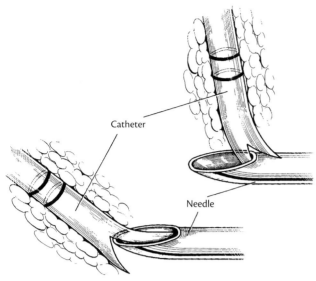

Figure 14.2 Possible mechanisms of catheter damage if one is withdrawn through a Tuohy needle.

cutaneous fat. Catheters are marked at 5-cm intervals from the tip, have a detachable connector at the proximal end (Figure 14.3), and are detectable radiologically.

Two types of catheter tip are available. The original, *open ended* version tended to puncture blood vessels and, occasionally, the dura. It was associated with a higher incidence of unilateral block, and poorer pain relief during epidural infusion. Multiport catheters, with a *closed, rounded tip* and two or more side holes within 2 cm of it, have replaced those with open ends.

Filters

The function of a filter is to exclude bacteria and microscopic debris, and several makes are capable of excluding particles as small as 0.22 micrometres. The passage of small fragments of ampoule glass is also prevented, but they will impair function so a specific filter needle should be used to draw up solutions from glass ampoules before injection.

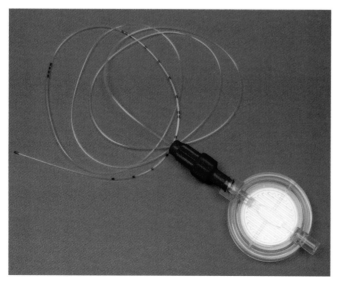

Figure 14.3 Typical markings on an epidural catheter.

Testing of equipment

Before starting, the anaesthetist should check that:

♦ The syringe plunger runs freely and evenly in the barrel;

♦ The syringe fits the hubs of both the needle and the catheter tightly enough to prevent leakage on injection;

♦ The tip of the stylet is flush with the bevel of the needle;

♦ The catheter passes easily through the needle; and

♦ The catheter and filter are patent (verified by injecting saline).

Needle and catheter insertion

Identification of the epidural space requires:

♦ A sound knowledge of the relevant anatomy (Chapter 12);

♦ An appreciation of the feel of the different tissues;

♦ A sense of where the needle tip is at every stage of the procedure;

♦ A technique which enables the anaesthetist to exert, at all times, perfect control over the movement of the needle;

♦ A constant awareness of the potentially serious clinical, social, and legal consequences which may follow an incautious approach;

♦ A willingness to seek more experienced help if any of these requirements are lacking.

♦ There are no technical 'tricks' which can obviate the need for this fundamental set of principles.

The basic technique, which should be mastered before any other, is the midline approach in the lumbar region using loss of resistance to saline.

Midline approach

Position of the patient

Either the lateral or sitting position may be chosen for fully conscious patients. Sedated patients should be placed in the lateral position, with knees bent and spine flexed. Obese and bronchitic patients may find the flexed, lateral position intolerable and prefer to be sitting. In the obstetric patient, the sitting position may seem attractive, but the risk of bloody tap is greater than with the lateral position (Harney et al. 2005). The following detailed description assumes that the patient is lying on the left side.

Identification of vertebral level

A line drawn between the iliac crests usually crosses the fourth lumbar spine when the patient is in the lateral position (Tuffier's line). The vertebral level can be checked by using ultrasound to identify the sacrum in the longitudinal plane. For a thoracic block, it is sometimes easier to count down from the prominent seventh cervical vertebral spine which in patients with a low body mass index (BMI) can be reliably identified. Inability to palpate spines is the best predictor of difficult epidural block rather than obesity.

Ultrasound

The use of ultrasound in neuraxial block is not yet well established because structures greater than 5 cm from the skin can be difficult to visualize, but both transverse and longitudinal paramedian views can provide useful information. In the transverse view, the spinous process, facet joints, and transverse processes can be identified whereas in the longitudinal paramedian view the laminae, ligamentum flavum, dura mater, and vertebral body are seen (Figure 14.4). Such images allow the pre-procedure identification of the correct vertebral level by scanning 'up' from the readily identifiable sacrum,

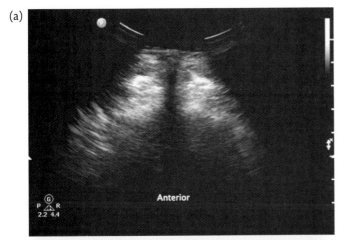

(a)

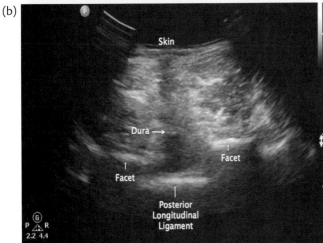

(b)

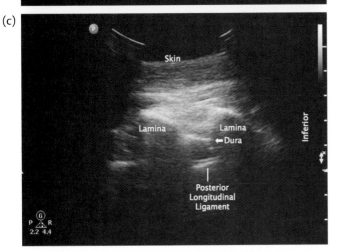

(c)

Figure 14.4 Sonograms of the lumbar spine demonstrating: (a) transverse view at the level of a lumbar spinous process with bony 'shadow' and no view of the thecal sac; (b) transverse lumbar view at the interspinous ligament demonstrating dura, facets and posterior longitudinal ligament; and (c) paramedian view at the lumbar level indicating typical view of the laminae and acoustic 'window' through to the posterior longitudinal ligament.

and calculation of the distance to the ligamentum flavum, even in the obese (Balki et al. 2009). Real-time, ultrasound-guided epidural block is not clinically feasible at present because the epidural needle is inserted out of the plane of the ultrasound beam, and is difficult to 'see', so many anaesthetists still feel that ultrasound contributes little to the outcome of the actual procedure.

However, ultrasound prior to the procedure has been shown to reduce the number of needle passes and interspaces necessary for successful epidural block (Grau et al. 2004), and further support for its use comes from a postnatal study (Schlotterbeck et al. 2008). Ninety-nine patients who had received lumbar neuraxial block for delivery were followed-up after delivery, and ultrasound showed that the recorded level of insertion was accurate in just over one-third of patients only, the actual level being more cephalad in almost 50% and more caudal in 15%. Given the risk of serious, permanent injury to the conus medullaris associated with needle insertion above L_3 (Reynolds 2001), these examples of ultrasound's utility question the continued use of Tuffier's line as the primary indicator of level.

Needle insertion

For lumbar epidural block, the appropriate space is chosen, and straddled by the second and third fingers of the left hand (Figure 14.5). This gives valuable tactile information about the underlying landmarks. The midline tissues are infiltrated with local anaesthetic and the skin pierced with a 19-g needle. The Tuohy needle is introduced through the skin puncture with the bevel facing lateral or cephalad in line with the longitudinal fibres of the ligamentum flavum. The fingers of the left hand can therefore continue to define the landmarks as the other hand advances the needle at right angles to the patient in both skin planes (Figure 14.6).

With the needle partially inserted, it is useful to test its 'feel' in the tissues by manipulating the needle slightly. While the tip is in the superficial tissues, the hub is very mobile (Figure 14.7), but when it enters the interspinous ligament, the freedom of movement is significantly restricted, and once engaged in the ligamentum flavum, the 'feel' is different again. Because the needle is now fixed at two points along its length, it behaves like a springboard

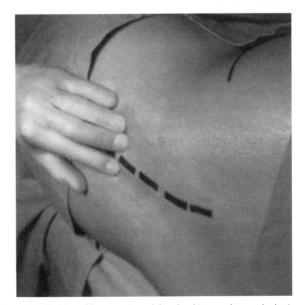

Figure 14.5 Position of fingers to immobilize the skin over the vertebral spines.

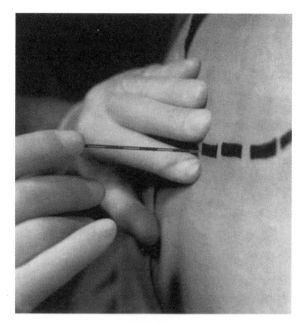

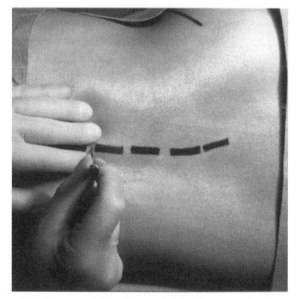

Figure 14.6 Correct angulation of the needle for midline insertion in the lumbar region.

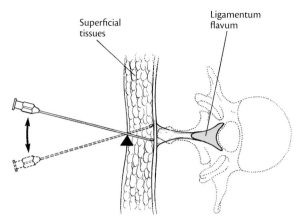

Figure 14.7 Needle mobility while the tip is in the superficial tissues. It behaves like a 'see-saw'.

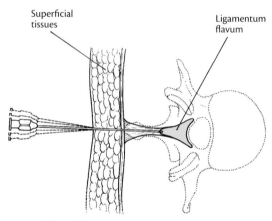

Figure 14.8 Needle mobility once the tip is firmly embedded in the ligamentum flavum. It behaves like a 'springboard'.

(Figure 14.8). When this sign has been elicited, it is worth checking again that the correct angles have been maintained during the deeper insertion of the needle. Only when the needle tip has engaged in the ligamentum flavum should the left hand alter its position.

The stylet is then withdrawn and a syringe containing saline is attached to the needle. In order to avoid accidentally advancing the needle at this stage, the hub is held firmly between the thumb and first finger of the left hand while the dorsum of the hand is steadied against the patient's back. The whole needle–syringe assembly is advanced slowly, its movement being controlled by the left hand, the dorsum of which presses firmly against the patient's back while the thumb and first finger grip the needle *hub*. Gripping the needle *shaft* provides insufficient control and does not guard against a sudden forward movement. As the assembly is advanced, steady pressure is applied to the plunger with the right thumb, and it is essential that the anaesthetist is properly balanced during this manoeuvre. This is best achieved by standing with one foot ahead of the other, as though walking in the direction of needle movement (Figure 14.9).

Location of the epidural space

Identification of the space depends on the fact that saline, being incompressible, cannot be injected if the needle tip is in the dense ligamentum flavum. When the epidural space is entered, there is a sudden loss of resistance as saline is injected.

Paramedian approach

In the paramedian approach the needle is inserted lateral to the midline, but with a cephalad angulation so it is slightly more complex than the midline route. The method has a number of advantages:

1. Calcified interspinous ligaments in the elderly are avoided;

2. Deliberate location of the lamina confirms needle position *before* it enters the ligamentum flavum;

3. The path for the needle is wider, avoiding the sometimes narrow space between the posterior spines;

4. The needle is less likely to puncture the dura because it crosses the epidural space obliquely (Figure 14.10); and

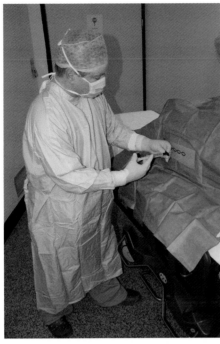

Figure 14.9 Position during needle insertion. The left hand, pressed against the patient, steadies the needle and controls its angulation and forward movement while the right provides the pressure on the syringe plunger. Balance is maintained by the forward position of the left foot.

5. The catheter is directed along the long axis of the epidural space and is more likely to thread easily.

Technique

The skin level with the lower border of a thoracic spine, and 1 cm from the midline, is immobilized with the second and third fingers of the left hand. The skin and subcutaneous tissues are infiltrated

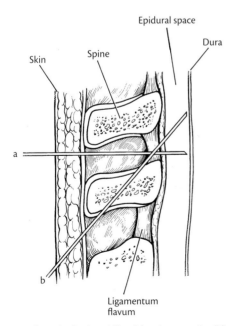

Figure 14.10 Needle angles for the midline (a) and paramedian (b) approaches. Note that the distance from the ligamentum flavum to the dura with the paramedian approach is almost twice that with the midline.

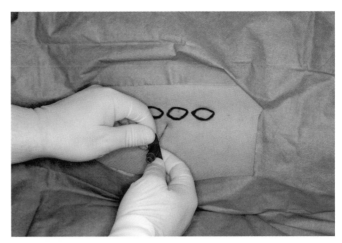

Figure 14.11 Initial needle position for the paramedian approach, about 1 cm from the midline.

with local anaesthetic (lidocaine 1%) before the needle is inserted *perpendicular* to the skin until it strikes the lamina. The depth is noted and 2–3 ml of local anaesthetic is injected to block the nerves supplying the lamina. The Tuohy needle is then inserted along the same path until it contacts the lamina (Figure 14.11), when it is necessary to redirect it in both cephalad and medial directions so that the tip enters the epidural space in the midline (Figure 14.12).

Cephalad angulation: the needle tip must be 'walked' over the lamina in a cephalad direction until it enters the ligamentum flavum above. When performing this manoeuvre, two important points of technique must be borne in mind. First, it is essential that the needle is withdrawn about 1 cm before each cephalad probe of the lamina; attempts to realign the needle without withdrawal will cause it to bend. Second, the change of angle between each probing must not be more than about 15°. It will be apparent that the more caudad the initial insertion of the needle, the greater will be the cephalad angulation when it clears the lamina, and the smaller will be the acute angle between needle and skin

Medial angulation: the second objective is to redirect the needle so that its tip enters the epidural space in the midline. The angulation will be greatest in lean patients in whom the distance between

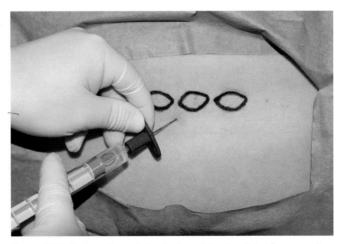

Figure 14.12 Final needle angulation, both medial and cephalad, for paramedian approach.

the skin and epidural space is short, and be smallest in obese patients in whom the 1-cm correction is made over a large distance.

Experience is needed in judging both of these angles, and the beginner will find it helpful to concentrate on one at a time, but as confidence grows it is possible to create them simultaneously to minimize the 'probing' of the lamina. In straightforward cases, the experienced anaesthetist can correctly angle the needle into the ligamentum flavum immediately after the initial location of the lamina. Once the ligament is identified the procedure is as for the midline approach.

Alternative components

Loss of resistance to air

Advocates of this method argue that any clear fluid appearing after needle or catheter insertion must be cerebrospinal fluid (CSF) so avoiding the doubt which can occur with saline (see 'Catheter insertion' section). However, air, unlike saline, is compressible and, because it is possible to 'spring' the plunger in the barrel even when the needle tip is in the ligamentum flavum, the loss of resistance sign may be inconclusive. Also, those who use air tend to spring the plunger intermittently so that advance of the needle–syringe assembly is not a smooth, steady movement. Further, a randomized comparison of liquid and air for the loss of resistance technique found that use of air was associated with four times the incidence of difficulty with catheter threading and double the frequency of 'unblocked' segments in an obstetric population (Evron 2004).

Epidural indicators

Various devices (e.g. balloons, hanging drop) have been described to help identify entry of the needle tip into the epidural space. Most were based on the premise that pressure in the epidural space is 'negative' because of transmission of intrathoracic pressure through the intervertebral foramina, but it is now recognized that other factors affect the pressure as well (Chapter 12). Thus such methods are inherently unreliable and only of historical interest now.

Catheter insertion

The catheter almost always meets some resistance on reaching the epidural space, but this can usually be overcome by threading it a little at a time. However, if the catheter does not seem to be passing beyond the end of the needle it may that the proximal part of the bevel may still be in the ligamentum flavum so it should be carefully advanced another millimetre (Figure 14.13). A second injection of 5 ml of saline or deep breathing by the patient may also help to 'open' the epidural space. Insertion of 5 cm of catheter into the space is associated with the highest incidence of satisfactory analgesia, although this does not necessarily correlate with optimal placement of the tip. Once positioned, catheters tend to be drawn inward over time with the greatest change seen in patients with a BMI greater than 30 (Choi et al. 2006).

Misplacement

If frank blood or freely flowing clear fluid (i.e. CSF) appears the procedure should be abandoned at that interspace and another one selected. This should also be the case if dural puncture occurs during needle insertion because the catheter may enter the subarachnoid space through the puncture hole. If the fluid in the catheter is only stained with blood the catheter should be flushed with saline and aspirated gently or held below the level of the patient to

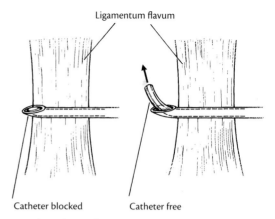

Ligamentum flavum

Catheter blocked　　　　Catheter free

Figure 14.13 The catheter will not pass into the space until the entire needle bevel is through the ligamentum flavum.

see if blood siphons along it. Clear fluid tracking along the catheter may be either injected saline or CSF. The latter usually flows briskly and can be aspirated easily. Nevertheless, if there is any doubt in either of these circumstances, another interspace should be chosen in preference to persisting with a 'difficult' epidural because inadvertent intravascular injection or total spinal anaesthesia may be life threatening.

Fixation

When the catheter has been suitably positioned, a small amount of saline or local anaesthetic should be injected to ensure that it is still patent and has not kinked in the epidural space. The catheter must be fixed firmly so that it cannot be accidentally dislodged on the operating table or during nursing procedures on the ward. However, fixing the catheter too tightly may cause it to kink at the skin, something which may be avoided by curving it around a rolled up swab or using a special fixation device (Figure 14.14). The whole area should then be covered with a transparent adhesive dressing to allow early detection of inflammation at the puncture site or dislodgement of the catheter. The remaining length of catheter is led

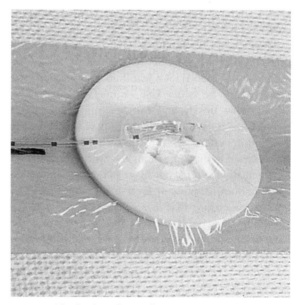

Figure 14.14 Epidural catheter fixation device in position.

up the back to the shoulder under a narrow strip of adhesive tape, and it may reduce the risk of dislodgement to ask the patient to straighten out before applying this tape. Once the patient has been turned supine, the patency of the catheter should be tested again to make sure that it has not kinked in prominent skin folds.

The test dose

The object of a test dose is to exclude intrathecal or intravascular misplacement of a needle or catheter. Various aspects have been discussed in Chapters 8 and 11, but it is worth re-emphasizing here that:

- The 'test' effect should be easily and rapidly observable (true positive);
- The drug and the dose must be *incapable* of producing the 'test' effect when injected into the correct place (true negative); and
- False positives (test positive, but actually negative effect) and false negatives (test negative, but actually positive effect) should be minimized.

In essence, this means that the test dose should produce obvious features of intravascular or intrathecal placement within a minute should the injection not have been into the epidural space. Equally though, the effects of any misplacement should not be such as to put the patient at any risk. There has been no formal study of what constitutes an appropriate test dose, but consideration of the dynamics of the onset of spinal anaesthesia with bupivacaine and other long-acting local anaesthetics suggests that they are too slow for the current purpose, even with as much as 4 ml of a 0.5% solution. The equivalent amount of lidocaine (4 ml of 2%) will usually produce clear evidence (i.e. 'heavy' legs) within a minute of intrathecal injection, as will the other shorter acting drugs (e.g. prilocaine and mepivacaine), but their rapid clearance means that a 'spinal' dose may not produce overt systemic effects. However, use of intravenous lidocaine in chronic pain states has shown that a dose of 40–50 mg injected over 5 seconds does usually produce the early features of systemic administration.

Thus the recommended test dose for epidural use is 4–5 ml of lidocaine 2%, but experience has shown that there is no absolute guarantee that even this will reveal a misplacement, especially an intravascular one, if only because the patient may not understand what symptoms to report. Test doses containing adrenaline 1:200,000 are recommended as overcoming this communication issue, causing a transient increase in heart rate and blood pressure if injected intravenously. However, there are considerable background variations in these parameters in both the preoperative and obstetric patient so that even interpretation of such 'objective' changes can be difficult. It is very easy for the test dose to become part of the 'ritual', rather than a useful preventive measure, but its careful use and sensible interpretation can help avoid major complications.

Factors affecting epidural drug spread

As with spinal anaesthesia, many factors (Table 14.2) have been shown to have some affect on the spread of drug solution through the epidural space, but most of them simply contribute to the variation in block seen between patients so that even when there is a mathematical correlation the information is of little predictive value. However, Dogliotti (1933), in his original description of the epidural technique, noted that one of its key advantages over spinal anaesthesia is that level of injection can be used to 'match' the block to the surgical site. Modern research has done nothing other than to confirm this, although the pattern of cephalad/caudad spread is dependant on the actual level used, with the mass of drug injected being the other major factor involved. The many factors involved have been reviewed comprehensively by Visser and colleagues (2008), and are summarized in the following sections.

Level of injection

Spread of solution through the epidural space has been assessed using two methods: radiological study of contrast material and clinical observation of the sensory block which develops after local anaesthetic injection. The latter depends on subjective assessment of nerve block (e.g. using pin prick) and contrast material, having different physical characteristics (e.g. viscosity), may not spread exactly like local anaesthetic, but the evidence is reasonably consistent. The extent of physical spread (i.e. number of segments reached) is much the same no matter what the level of injection, but the patterns of spread are very different. High thoracic injection produces less cranial, but more caudad spread. Spread is equal in both directions after mid thoracic placement, but is more caudad than cranial after low thoracic injection.

These differences are attributable to variation in the shape, volume, and contents of the epidural space (Chapter 12), and its narrowing at the levels of the cervical and lumbar enlargements of the spinal cord. Significant thoracic spread will only occur after lumbar injection if a relatively large volume is used. This may provide intraoperative analgesia for an abdominal procedure, but attempts to extend the duration by postoperative infusion will only result in block of the lumbar nerves leading to failed analgesia and complications due to lower limb numbness and paralysis. Epidural injections should always be 'centred' on the dermatomes involved in the surgical incision, remembering that the spinal nerves run increasingly obliquely at the lower levels.

Dose/volume/concentration

The dose (i.e. mass) of drug injected is the product of the solution's volume and concentration, so identifying the role of each factor is

Table 14.2 Factors which may influence distribution of block after epidural injection.*

Injection technique		
Major factors:	Level of injection	Mass of drug injected
Minor factors:	Speed of injection	Volume/concentration of solution
	Needle vs. catheter injection	Fractional vs. bolus injection
Patient factors		
Major factors:	Pregnancy	Age
Minor factors:	Height	Weight
	Posture	

*Influence of some factors is different during infusion.

difficult because changing one is bound to change at least one other. The traditional view is that it is the total amount of any particular drug used, not its volume or concentration, which determines onset, quality, and duration of both sensory and motor block after bolus injection at both lumbar and thoracic levels (Visser et al. 1998, 2008). However, studies using newer methods of block assessment have challenged this view. For example, surgical epidural block was produced with 200 mg lidocaine in either 1% or 2% solution and quantitative sensory analysis showed that the sensory block was more intense with the greater concentration (Sakura et al. 1999). Further, a sequential allocation method showed that there was a minimum concentration of a fixed dose of chloroprocaine which would provide good pain relief in 50% of women in labour (Columb et al. 1997).

Mass of drug is also the most important factor in continuous techniques, high-volume, low-concentration and low-volume, high-concentration solutions containing the same dose having the same analgesic effect when delivered by continuous infusion or by patient control (Dernedde et al. 2006). However, there is some evidence that the low-volume, high-concentration combination produces less motor block and better haemodynamic stability (Dernedde et al. 2003).

An overview interpretation of this evidence is that total mass *is* the key determinant, but that the effects can be fine tuned by adjusting volume/concentration.

Injection factors

Needle or catheter injection

Many experienced practitioners feel that 'better' spread results after epidural injection through a needle than a catheter, and it has been shown to result in better quality block and fewer adverse events such as paraesthesiae and venous catheterization (Cesur et al. 2005). Thus administering the first dose through the needle before catheter insertion may be advantageous, but a cautious incremental technique is still required because accidental intrathecal and intravenous injection both remain possible.

Direction of needle bevel

In young patients there is no difference, but in those over 40 years there is a tendency for spread to be in the direction in which the needle bevel is facing, but the effect is small (Visser et al. 2008). The alignment of the needle bevel does not reliably predict the final position of the catheter tip after insertion so no more than 5 cm of catheter should be inserted to ensure that the tip stays close to the intended level.

Rate of injection

Rate of injection has no effect on spread, but rapid injections can be uncomfortable for the patient and will increase the severity of any systemic reaction if placement is accidentally intravascular.

Single bolus versus fractionation

The incremental injection of a specified dose of local anaesthetic to reduce the risk of systemic toxicity will not affect the resulting block. For example, the low-thoracic injection of two 5-ml increments as much as 5 minutes apart produces the same epidural block as a single injection of 10 ml, although fewer segments are blocked when the time interval is extended to 10 minutes (Okutomi et al. 2001).

Patient factors

Age

Local anaesthetic spread through the epidural space correlates well with age, although the mean difference between young and old adults is only 2–3 dermatomes (Simon et al. 2004). It was thought that occlusion of intervertebral foramina was the explanation, but recent work suggests otherwise (Saitoh et al. 1995). The epiduroscopic observation that the amount of epidural fat decreases with age (Igarashi et al. 1997) suggests that this allows easier spread of solution through the space although changes in neuronal sensitivity to local anaesthetics may also be involved (Olofsen et al. 2008).

Posture

Generally the interaction between posture and gravity has little impact on epidural drug spread, keeping the patient in the lateral position only producing minor improvements in onset, total, spread and duration in the dependent side (Visser et al. 2008) However, posture may occasionally be used to encourage solution to spread towards the nerve root supplying a 'missed segment' or to improve perineal analgesia in labour.

Height and weight

Physical stature has little effect on epidural spread. Tall patients need slightly more solution to achieve a certain degree of spread, but the correlation is poor (Visser et al. 2008). Obesity, while making identification of the epidural space more difficult, also has little effect on spread although some evidence indicates how different factors can interact. Height of block was the same when injection was made in the horizontal or sitting position in lean patients awaiting Caesarean section, but was lower after injection in the sitting position in an obese group (Hodgkinson & Husain 1981).

Pregnancy

Pregnant patients require less local anaesthetic for a given extent of lumbar epidural block. This may be related to transmission of intraabdominal pressure to distended epidural veins and an increased sensitivity to local anaesthetics (see Chapter 21).

Vertebral canal dimensions

Modern imaging methods allow measurement of novel aspects of the physical dimensions of the vertebral canal, and the evaluation of how these relate to epidural spread. For example, dural surface area correlates inversely with peak sensory block; posterior epidural fat volume correlates inversely, with regression to L_5–S_3 and determines duration of block (Higuchi et al. 2004). Such measurements may not be of any practical clinical value, but they may lead to better understanding of the processes involved.

Clinical profile of block

The previous main section describes the factors which influence the spread of local anaesthetic solution throughout the epidural space, but this knowledge is only the first component of developing a clinical technique. Even with local anaesthetics the *pattern of spread*, and thus the clinical effect, which develops with different levels of injection needs to be understood as well, and the same applies to the other classes of drug which are used epidurally. The physical properties of these drug solutions are very similar to those of local anaesthetics so it is assumed that their spread is governed by the same factors, but methods are needed to assess their clinical impact. Thus consideration of the clinical effectiveness of different classes of drugs, and of different drugs of the same class, requires an understanding of how they are assessed clinically.

Pattern of local anaesthetic effect

Judging the clinical effect of an injection of local anaesthetic is an inexact art (Hocking & Wildsmith 2004), but the most widely used method is pin-prick: inability to appreciate 'sharpness' being defined as 'analgesia', and inability to appreciate touch as 'anaesthesia'. Other modalities of sensation can be used, especially temperature ('cold'), but pin-prick perhaps has more clinical relevance although it should not be applied over-vigorously! Figure 14.15 shows the segmental block with time profile after a single lumbar epidural injection assessed in this way. At this injection level matters are complicated by the thickness of the lumbosacral nerve roots, this slowing drug penetration, delaying onset, and shortening duration. The diagram also shows that onset is delayed, and duration shorter, at the limits of spread because less drug solution has spread to these segments. That pattern, slower onset and shorter duration at the limits of spread, is seen with higher injection levels where the nerve roots are of more consistent thickness.

Onset and duration of sensory block

Obviously, defining time intervals is, given the factors noted earlier, less than straightforward and many figures have been used. If surgery to the lower limb is be performed then the time to complete block of all segments below T_{10} is probably the most clinically relevant, as is time to block of all the relevant dermatomes for surgery at a higher level. For more objective, comparative purposes time to block of a specific dermatome or the average time to block of all affected dermatomes, the *mean segmental latency profile*, can be used.

Determination of the time to complete regression in all blocked segments will provide the *mean segmental latency profile*, but obtaining this may be complicated by surgical dressings. The time taken for block to regress by two (or four) segments from its maximum spread—the *two or four segmental regression time*—is more straightforward, but even that may be difficult if the patient has

also received general anaesthesia or sedation. Time to request for first postoperative analgesia is a pragmatic solution to the difficulty, but requires standardization of the surgical procedure. In addition, in the era of the pro-active, multimodal approach to postoperative analgesia time to first request for analgesia is going to be a judgement of the overall technique, not just local anaesthetic duration.

In spite of these difficulties (which are compounded by the interpatient variation noted in the previous section) it is possible to obtain an overview of the block profiles of the different local anaesthetics used epidurally, and use this information to incorporate the appropriate drug into the technique to be used in a particular clinical situation (Visser et al. 1998)

Assessment of motor block

A block with the distribution shown in Figure 14.15 will, if sufficient drug is injected, block the motor nerves to the lower abdomen and legs. Lower limb motor block is usually assessed using the 'Bromage' method (Table 14.3), a scale which indicates a mixture of both the degree and extent of motor block. A more quantitative assessment of power, certainly at hip and knee joints, can be obtained with the Medical Research Council rating system for nerve injury, but it is used rarely in anaesthetic practice.

Assessing the degree of abdominal (or even thoracic) wall motor block is even more difficult. The rectus abdominis muscle score (Table 14.3) is based on the ability to sit up from the supine position, a score greater than 3 being sufficient to permit abdominal surgery (Kopacz et al. 2000). Given that the anterior abdominal wall is the major 'muscle' of active expiration, measurement of forced expiratory lung volume probably gives the most quantitative assessment.

Information on motor block is needed for two very different reasons. When an epidural is used for surgery it gives an indication of the likely adequacy of 'relaxation' just as a nerve stimulator

Table 14.3 Methods of assessing muscle weakness during epidural block.

Lower limb		Abdomen
Bromage	**Medical Research Council**	**Rectus abdominis muscle**
0 = No motor block	5 = Normal strength	0 = Can sit up from supine with arms behind head
1 = Inability to straight leg raise	4 = Reduced power, but moves against resistance and gravity	1 = Can sit up only with arms extended
2 = Additional inability to extend the knee	3 = Moves against gravity, but not resistance	2 = Can lift head and shoulders off bed
3 = Additional inability to flex the ankle (indicates total paralysis)	2 = Active only with gravity eliminated	3 = Can raise shoulders only
	1 = Flicker of contraction, but no movement	4 = Abdominal muscles tense, but no shoulder movement
	0 = No movement or contraction	5 = Cannot even tense muscles

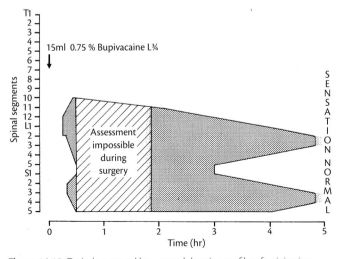

Figure 14.15 Typical segmental latency and duration profiles after injection of 15 ml of 0.75% bupivacaine.

would during neuromuscular block. In the context of continuous block for pain relief during labour or after surgery, muscle weakness is a 'side effect', indicating that either the degree of block or its spread is excessive and requires adjustment.

Assessment of pain relief

While local anaesthetic action can be assessed in terms of the effects on sensory and motor nerve conduction, much of their epidural use is for the production of analgesia. However, the methods described previously are of little direct relevance to, and are of no use at all in judging, the actions of other drugs. Epidural analgesia is, of course, amenable to assessment by exactly the same methods, such as visual analogue scales (VAS), as systemic drugs, but these were developed for comparing individual drugs and performing dose response studies. Most epidural regimens now combine two or more drugs and traditional methods of assessment would require many groups of patients, each group receiving a different dose or concentration of drug to establish the optimum combination.

Overcoming this problem was the prime reason for the development of the *sequential analysis technique* (Lyons et al. 1998), often referred to as the 'up/down' method. Cutaneous numbness and muscle weakness are, in essence, side effects of epidural local anaesthetics when used solely for analgesia so the effectiveness of combination with other agents is assessed by the reduction in the amount required. The initial concentration is based on clinical experience and, assuming that the epidural bolus produces a defined effect (e.g. VAS (visual analogue score) equal or less than 1/10 within 30 minutes), the next patient in the series receives an injection with a defined reduction in the concentration of local anaesthetic. Depending on whether that injection is effective or not, the third patient will receive a decreased or increased concentration, the sequence continuing until the variation between patients is small. Statistical analysis allows calculation of the *minimum local anaesthetic concentration* (MLAC), the concentration which will produce the desired effect in 50% of subjects.

This elegant method is very suitable for its original intended purpose, comparison of the *local anaesthetic sparing effect* of other classes of analgesic drugs given by the epidural route in labour. However, its simplicity and 'efficient' use of patient numbers has meant that it has been adapted for other purposes, notably direct comparisons of the potency of different local anaesthetic drugs. MLAC defines the mid-point of the dose response curve, but the sequential method does not provide any information about its slope, and thus the concentration which is effective in 95% of patients, although attempts are being made to rectify this (Panni et al. 2010).

This is an important issue because sequential studies have claimed differences in potency between local anaesthetics which are not apparent when equal concentration are compared using more traditional methods (Wildsmith 2000). Thus caution should be exercised in the interpretation of any data obtained with this method in any situation other than the one noted previously.

Drugs in the epidural space

Local anaesthetics

Short-acting drugs

Lidocaine 2% (15–20 ml) produces very profound sensory and motor block after lumbar injection. Onset is short, pin-prick analgesia appearing in the dermatomes close to the point of injection after 5–6 minutes, but duration is also short, two segment regression appearing after about an hour. Adrenaline 1:200,000 will prolong this time by 50–100% (and also reduce systemic concentrations). The 2% solution is arguably the local anaesthetic of choice if an epidural is used in an emergency situation. Lidocaine 2% can also be used to induce thoracic epidural block, but in lower volumes (5–10 ml). Lower concentrations produce less block of longer onset and shorter duration unless very large volumes are used, but can be used to produce an 'analgesic' block (e.g. 10 ml of 1%).

Prilocaine and *mepivacaine* have similar profiles to lidocaine, but the plain solutions have durations of the same order as lidocaine with adrenaline. Plasma concentrations are also lower, especially with prilocaine.

Chloroprocaine, especially in 3% concentration, is even faster in onset, although shorter in duration, than lidocaine, but it is not available in the UK.

Long-acting drugs

All of the listed short-acting drugs will require frequent repeat administration if a continuous block is required, and this is likely to lead to cumulative toxicity. The longer acting drugs, being more lipid soluble, are absorbed more by adipose tissue which 'buffers' the increase in systemic concentration.

Bupivacaine is the standard long-acting agent for both surgical and analgesic use. A dose of 100–110 mg will produce profound sensory and motor block within 20–30 minutes after lumbar injection, regression occurring after 4–6 hours. Adrenaline shortens onset and prolongs duration. Increments of 25–50 mg are used for thoracic block.

An interesting feature of bupivacaine is that, after lumbar injection of a 'surgical' dose, motor block develops more slowly than sensory, and regresses sooner. This *motor-sensory separation* is even more obvious when lower concentrations/doses are used and is another reason why bupivacaine first became very popular in obstetric practice.

Unfortunately, wider use of greater concentrations of bupivacaine led to identification of its potential to cause primary cardiotoxicity and thus a search for alternative drugs (see Chapters 6 and 7), this resulting in the introduction of *levobupivacaine* and *ropivacaine*. Differences in their systemic toxicity are considered in earlier chapters, but at the concentrations needed to produce surgical anaesthesia by the epidural route there is little between them in the degree of sensory block which is produced. However, the newer drugs produce even greater degrees of motor-sensory separation, the rank order for the degree of motor block produced being bupivacaine > levobupivacaine > ropivacaine. One early study showed that ropivacaine 0.2% and 0.3%, while producing effective analgesia, were both associated with less motor block than bupivacaine 0.25% although regression of block was slower with the latter when the infusions were discontinued (Zaric et al. 1996).

All three drugs can be used for continuous epidural block, usually in concentrations in the 0.1–0.2% range, but hypotension and lower limb weakness are common when any local anaesthetic is used alone in effective doses. Thus analgesic techniques usually feature combinations of drugs (see 'Local anaesthetic and opioid combinations' section).

Epidural opioids

After local anaesthetics, the commonest drugs used by the epidural route are the opioids although none is licensed for this route of administration in the UK. However, good safety data are available for a few drugs so routine practice should be limited to those already in widespread clinical use.

All drugs administered by the epidural route have to traverse both lipid and aqueous environments to reach the receptors in the dorsal horn of the spinal cord so, as with local anaesthetics, the ideal drug is one with intermediate lipid and water solubility. Morphine has poor lipid solubility and a long half-life in CSF, this accounting for its slow onset, long duration, and propensity for respiratory depression (Bernards et al. 2003). In contrast, the highly lipid soluble drugs (e.g. fentanyl and sufentanil) diffuse rapidly into nervous tissue (and then into the circulation) so that they have rapid onset and short duration, but less risk of respiratory depression.

In many ways the ideal drug is diamorphine (diacetylmorphine), although it is only clinically available in the UK. It is highly water soluble, but after administration it is metabolized to the more lipid soluble monoacetyl morphine, which has a profound effect (McLeod et al. 2005). Compared to morphine it is faster in onset, but shorter in duration and with much less risk of respiratory depression. Hydromorphone has not dissimilar properties and is used commonly in North America.

Opioids have been used as the sole epidural analgesic agent by both bolus injection and continuous infusion, but (as with their systemic use) there is little relief of pain on movement, and side effects (especially pruritus, nausea, and respiratory depression) are common.

Liposomal opioid preparation

A slow release, liposomal preparation of morphine (Depodur) has become available for epidural use in the USA and Europe. It is effective for up to 48 hours and patients have less need for additional medication compared to standard epidural morphine (Gambling et al. 2005), but there are two significant side effects. Respiratory depression has occurred in clinical trials (Hartrick et al. 2006) of larger doses (20–30 mg) so prescribing recommendations are to use only 5–15 mg depending on age and health. Secondly, systemic release of morphine and side effects are enhanced if the preparation is combined with a local anaesthetic so at least 30 minutes should elapse after administration before any local anaesthetic is injected (Viscusi et al. 2005).

Local anaesthetic and opioid combinations

Arguably the single most important fact to emerge from attempts to improve pain relief over the last 30 or more years is that by the time an effective dose of one drug has been administered by a single route the patient is on the threshold of complications. This applies fully to the epidural route, and is the reason why most regimens combine a local anaesthetic with an opioid. Their interaction is synergistic (Robinson et al. 2001) so that effectiveness is improved, lower doses are needed, and the risk of side effects (of both drugs) is reduced considerably.

Many different combinations of local anaesthetic and opioid are possible, even before variations in the rate of administration of each drug are factored in, and this has perhaps inhibited formal study to define which regimen is optimum. One study did attempt this, and found, using a stepwise optimization technique, that the best balance between analgesia and side effects was obtained using either bupivacaine 8 mg h^{-1} and fentanyl 30 mcg h^{-1} or bupivacaine 13 mg h^{-1} and fentanyl 25 mcg h^{-1}, both given in an infusion of 9 ml h^{-1} (Curatolo et al. 2000). Unfortunately, 190 patients were required to reach this conclusion, and this number provides another reason why no other combination has been so studied.

Many different 'mixtures' are used, this suggesting that the exact details are not crucial, it perhaps being more important that each hospital department agrees a specific technique which all involved can become familiar with. Efficacy and side effects should be audited, and compared with experience elsewhere to see if any improvement can be made.

Other epidural analgesics

A number of other drugs have been used to produce analgesia by the epidural route, this reflecting the many transmitter substances which are involved in the pain pathway at spinal level (see Chapter 2). Many are effective, especially at reducing the amount of local anaesthetic required, but the clinician should recognize that epidural injection is an unlicensed use, and that there are not even formal stability data available to indicate whether it is safe to mix them with other drugs in solution.

Adrenaline

The effect of adrenaline on local anaesthetic action is well known, but it may also act on adrenergic components of the pain pathway, pain relief being improved by its addition to a thoracic infusion containing fentanyl and either ropivacaine or bupivacaine (Niemi & Breivik 2002).

Clonidine

Clonidine (an α2 adrenergic agonist with some α1 activity) is increasingly added to solutions of local anaesthetics and opioids to enhance pain relief and spare local anaesthetic use after knee arthroplasty. The addition of clonidine to patient-controlled epidural analgesia (PCEA) with ropivacaine and morphine after laparotomy, and lower limb arthroplasty improved analgesia without the characteristic side effects of sedation or hypotension (Huang et al 2007).

Neostigmine

Neostigmine stimulates muscarinic cholinergic activity within the descending inhibitory pathways, and offers the potential for pain relief without respiratory depression. Side effects such as nausea and vomiting are common (Walker et al 2002).

Ketamine

N-methyl-D-aspartate receptors in the spinal cord are activated by severe postoperative pain and this may lead to central sensitization, hyperalgesia, allodynia, and (potentially) the development of chronic pain. Ketamine blocks these receptors and may have a role in the treatment of patients on long-term opioids and those with neuropathic, cancer, or opioid-resistant pain (De Kock et al. 2001). Although ketamine did not affect early pain scores a reduction in secondary hyperalgesia was found 6 months after surgery (Lavand'homme et al. 2005).

Management of epidural anaesthesia and analgesia

Careful selection of patients and a knowledge of the principles, practice, and limitations of epidural block are essential for satisfactory and consistent results, but supplementary sedation, systemic opioids, and even light general anaesthesia may still be required at some stage. Their use, far from implying that the block has failed, acknowledges that there are sources of discomfort which an epidural is incapable of relieving (see Chapter 11).

The operative period

Epidural block in the conscious patient

For operations on conscious patients, profound block is required and 15–20 ml lidocaine or prilocaine (other than in obstetrics) 2% is suitable when either rapid onset or short duration is required. Prolonged duration can be produced by bupivacaine 0.75% or ropivacaine 1%, but great care is needed with such large doses and it may be wiser (assuming that a catheter can be inserted) to start with lidocaine and then extend the block with increments of a longer acting agent. Injection should be at the appropriate vertebral level, so that the extent of anaesthesia 'matches' the operation, taking into account not only innervation of the incision, but also of structures handled during surgery. For example, 10 ml injected at L_1/L_2 is adequate for inguinal herniorrhaphy, but more is needed to ensure that the sacral nerves are blocked during abdominal hysterectomy.

'Balanced' epidural anaesthesia

The combination of epidural block with general anaesthesia can provide superb conditions for even the most extensive surgery, the epidural providing most of the analgesic component. However, it requires training and experience in all aspects of managing both anaesthetic and major surgery, particularly in regard to maintaining circulatory balance, if complications are to be avoided. Even then, an extensive epidural may cause profound hypotension, but usually the object is to provide analgesia only so a fairly limited block is all that is required if the correct level of insertion has been chosen. Small increments of drugs (4–5 ml) are all that are required to institute the block, with the postoperative infusion being started thereafter.

For upper abdominal and thoracic procedures, control of ventilation is essential to provide a 'quiet' surgical field, so neuromuscular block is needed as well as general anaesthesia, but this has several advantages. The airway is secured, lung ventilation is adequate, and each aspect of the technique has a synergistic effect on the others, reducing drug requirements. The method is particularly suitable in situations where respiration is impeded by obesity, severe respiratory disease, posture, or the nature of the surgery although overventilation may contribute to circulatory depression.

The postoperative period

If the full potential of an epidural is to be realized after major surgery, it should be continued into the postoperative period, either alone or in conjunction with other analgesic methods, the object being to prevent pain rather than to relieve it. Prevention is more effective at controlling acute pain than treatment after it has occurred (Kissin 2000), it being argued that continued use of the term 'pain relief' probably does more than anything to retard progress in this field (Armitage 1989). The epidural should be continued for as long as the patient needs it (Kehlet 1994), and there should be no arbitrary time after which all epidurals are discontinued routinely.

Mode of solution delivery

The advantage of starting the postoperative regimen whilst the surgery is in progress, as noted earlier, is that it should be fairly stable when the patient recovers consciousness, and its adequacy (or otherwise) can be judged at an early stage. A number of ways of delivering the solution have been described, the earliest being continuous, gravity-fed drip infusion (Dawkins 1966), but, as with the intravenous route, this is unreliable. *Intermittent bolus administration* was used more widely, but repeat injections were usually triggered by return of pain which could be severe if there was delay in obtaining a qualified individual. The level of block also varied and, as a result, so did the blood pressure and the degree of leg weakness. Developments in infusion technology led to better delivery, the earliest pumps allowing *constant volume infusion* after the block had been established by bolus injection. This avoided many of the problems, but the block often regresses down to a few dermatomes close to the catheter tip after more than a few hours so occasional bolus injections were still needed. Many variations, ranging from low-volume/high-drug concentration to high-volume/low-drug concentration, were tried, but it was the introduction of combination regimens that produced more consistent analgesia.

Further technical development allowed the introduction of *PCEA*, which reduces the requirement for 'rescue' injections and is associated with better patient satisfaction (Nightingale et al. 2007). The problems associated with changing level of block after each injection still occur, but this can be minimized by combining constant infusion with PCEA. This technique is now widely used: postoperatively, a local anaesthetic and opioid mixture is infused at a low rate (4–8 ml h^{-1}) and supplemented by patient-controlled boluses (2–5 ml every 20–30 minutes).

However, some (the elderly especially) have difficulty understanding patient-controlled systems and this led to the utilization of pumps which can deliver *regular bolus injections*. Appropriate choice of bolus volume and time interval can result in almost static level of block and have been shown to produce equivalent analgesia with less need for rescue medication than the same amount given as constant infusion, both postoperatively (Duncan et al. 1998) and in labour (Fettes et al. 2006).

Personnel and organization

After surgery, the patient is moved to an adjacent *recovery area* where the anaesthetist hands over to the nursing staff. This involves a brief description of the type and course of the anaesthetic, a review of the record chart (with particular reference to the patient's response to the epidural infusion), the setting of limits for physiological variables beyond which corrective action must be taken, and any other suggestions for management. When patients are conscious, stable, and pain free they should be transferred, either to Ward or High Dependency Unit, but (irrespective of what it is called) the staff should have experience and training in the management of epidural analgesia. Patient care should be protocol driven, with those protocols advising nursing and junior medical staff how the patient should be monitored and what action should be taken if readings and observations stray beyond pre-set limits. Pain management should be supervised by a named anaesthetist or a member of the Acute Pain Team, contact information for the responsible individual being readily available.

Attention is re-drawn to the safety issues surrounding confusion of epidural and venous lines noted at the start of the chapter.

Monitoring and side effects

If a continuous epidural is to provide safe, effective analgesia both delivery system and patient will require close monitoring. Sudden failure of delivery of the solution to the epidural space will result in the patient rapidly developing severe pain and this must be avoided by the early identification of any equipment malfunction or disconnection.

Patient observations should assess the adequacy of analgesia and warn of the development of excessive block or the onset of other side effects so that they can be dealt with before they are severe enough to be classified as complications.

Increasing block: with the routine use of low concentrations of local anaesthetic, increasing numbness or leg weakness are usually due to the infusion rate being greater than is needed. Unless the rate is reduced patients can suffer injury to skin or joints, but the same features also warn of two major complications: catheter migration into the subarachnoid space (leading to total spinal anaesthesia) or development of a vertebral canal haematoma. Both are dealt with later, but staff should have clear instructions on their actions in the event of any increase in epidural block, with a low threshold for obtaining senior anaesthetic advice if this does not result in regression in effect.

The patient in pain: deciding whether a patient in pain requires supplementary medication or an increase in epidural dosage can be difficult, but if the pain is unilateral or associated with evidence of regression of block, it is likely that the epidural needs reinforcing. Any action must recognize that there is still a significant amount of drug in the epidural space, even though the block is inadequate, and a 5-ml bolus of the infusion solution is usually sufficient. If the pain is unilateral, the patient should lie on the unblocked side for 15 minutes after injection.

Hypotension: it is common for the blood pressure of a patient receiving epidural analgesia to be lower than one receiving conventional analgesia, but often because inadequate analgesia increases the pressure of the latter! A 'hypotensive' patient who is comfortable, rational, well perfused, producing urine, and able to move the lower limbs is unlikely to be in any danger, but it is vital that hypovolaemia is avoided because it is tolerated badly by the patient with a sympathetic block. More detailed aspects of hypotension occurring in association with regional block are considered in Chapter 11.

Respiratory depression: the incidence of respiratory depression with epidural analgesia depends on the criteria used to define it (e.g. increased somnolence, respiratory rate <10 bpm, raised $PaCO_2$ or hypoxaemia), but a large survey of the literature found that the incidence is much the same (around 1%) no matter what route of opioid administration is used (Cashman & Dolin 2004). However, patients who have received neuraxial opioids require close monitoring and the most comprehensive guidelines are from North America (Table 14.4, Horlocker et al. 2009), these suggesting that increased monitoring (e.g. frequency, duration, or method) may be warranted in patients at increased risk of respiratory depression

(e.g. unstable medical condition, obesity, obstructive sleep apnoea, concomitant administration of opioid analgesics or hypnotics by other routes, extremes of age).

Retention of urine: bladder catheterization will be needed during continuous epidural block, often because the overall management of the patient demands close monitoring of urine output. Some concern has been expressed that insertion of the catheter will cause a bacteraemia which may increase the risk of infection after arthroplasty, but this is not the case if the antibiotic prophylaxis is administered first.

Hypothermia: sympathetic block causes vasodilation and increased heat loss so temperature should be monitored and standard preventive measures used to avoid hypothermia.

Failure of epidural analgesia

Postoperative epidural analgesia may 'fail' in as many as one in every seven patients (Ballantyne et al. 2003, Mcleod et al. 2001) and for a wide range of reasons:

1. Misplacement of the catheter ($\approx$1%);

2. Technical problems during infusion (13–14%, e.g. pump malfunction, solution leakage, catheter migration, etc.); and

3. True failure of analgesia despite a correctly functioning delivery system (3–8%, inadequate solution or spread thereof).

The median time to failure in this large series was 27 (range 14–46) hours, indicating that maintenance of effective epidural analgesia requires constant vigilance and attention to detail. *Such problems are better prevented* and a few key points bear emphasis:

1. Continuous epidural block for major surgery should be instituted by, or under the immediate supervision of, an experienced practitioner;

2. The catheter must be placed at the correct level relative to the site of surgery;

3. The catheter level should be adjusted in the light of both the method of solution administration intended and the patient's likely posture. In a classic paper Dawkins (1966) showed that local anaesthetic infused into the epidural space of semi-recumbent patients spreads caudally, but in both directions in those placed horizontally (Figure 14.16);

4. Combined drug regimens are more effective and less prone to problems such as unilateral block;

5. Patients may have sources of discomfort arising from outside the distribution of the epidural block and these may require small doses of systemic drugs to deal with them.

Table 14.4 Recommendations for the respiratory monitoring of patients who have received neuraxial opioid drugs (derived from Horlocker et al. 2009).

Method of administration	Duration of monitoring	Frequency
Single-injection lipophilic drug (e.g. fentanyl)	Minimum of 2 hours	Regularly for 20 minutes then hourly for 2 hours
Single-injection hydrophilic drug (e.g. morphine)	Minimum of 24 hours	Hourly for the first 12 hours; two-hourly for the next 12 hours
Continuous infusion or PCEA with any drug	Duration of administration	Hourly for first 12 hours; two-hourly for next 12 hours; four-hourly thereafter
Sustained- or extended-release drug	Minimum of 48 hours	Hourly for first 12 hours; two-hourly for next 12 hours; four-hourly thereafter

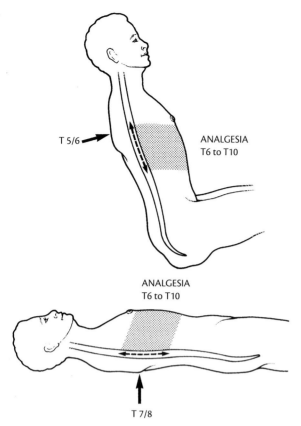

T 5/6

ANALGESIA
T6 to T10

ANALGESIA
T6 to T10

T 7/8

Figure 14.16 Distribution of analgesia during continuous epidural infusion in sitting and supine positions.

Discontinuing the epidural

Patients who have undergone major surgery usually require at least 48 hours of effective analgesia, and after thoraco-abdominal procedures the epidural should continue for as long as intensive chest physiotherapy is required and until the chest drains have been removed. Because the sudden withdrawal of effective analgesia can cause the patient much anxiety, and even lead to myocardial ischaemia, the infusion should be reduced gradually while other methods become effective, the catheter being removed only when the patient agrees. Instituting an epidural catheter for surgery and removing it immediately afterwards, but before the patient's analgesic requirements are established, is a practice with questionable risk/benefit balance.

Complications

The more routine side effects of epidural block have been considered earlier, and most aspects of neurological sequelae, local anaesthetic toxicity, and physiological consequences are considered in earlier chapters. This section will focus on the more specific complications of epidural needle and catheter insertion.

Accidental dural puncture

The incidence varies with the skill and experience of the anaesthetist, but if the technique is taught according to sound anatomical principles and is carefully performed, dural puncture should not occur in more than 1% of cases. Puncture by the needle is usually obvious, resulting in a brisk flow of warm liquid, but it is harder to

identify with a catheter because flow is comparatively slow and CSF may be mistaken for saline or local anaesthetic if these have been injected previously. If dural puncture is obvious, it is usual for the procedure to be abandoned and re-started at an adjacent interspace although an alternative, suitable in some situations, is to place the catheter in the subarachnoid space and convert to a continuous spinal technique.

However, dural puncture may not be obvious or the catheter may enter the CSF through the original dural puncture hole when using an adjacent space, and this is one reason why 'test' doses are so important (see 'The test dose' section). Further, an accurately positioned catheter can later migrate through the dura so that the injections or infusion become intrathecal, this being why regular monitoring of sensory and motor block is so vital.

Total spinal

If dural puncture is not recognized and a full epidural dose is injected into the CSF, profound and extensive block with circulatory collapse and apnoea will develop, an emergency requiring full cardiorespiratory resuscitation until the block regresses (see Chapter 21).

Postdural puncture headache

Headache is common after accidental dural puncture, occurring in up to 40% of obstetric patients when a Tuohy needle is used (Norris et al. 1989). Its features and treatment are exactly the same as when it occurs after spinal anaesthesia (Chapter 13) although the size of the needle means that the headache is more likely to be severe and an epidural blood patch (Chapter 21) is more likely to be needed.

Accidental venous puncture

Accidental puncture of an epidural vein is rare with the needle because the venous plexuses are laterally placed, but occurs in about 10% of obstetric cases when the catheter is inserted, the incidence being reduced to about 3% by prior injection of 10 ml of liquid (Verniquet 1980). Definitive venous cannulation is obvious, but the situation is more difficult if clear, but blood stained fluid is obtained during insertion or at a later stage. The catheter should be flushed with saline, held below the patient, and watched carefully to see if any blood 'siphons' back through it. A test dose should be administered, but if there is any doubt the catheter should be removed and a new one inserted.

Epidural haematoma

Bleeding into the epidural space is concealed and impossible to control. Some minor degree of bleeding must be inevitable during epidural catheterization, but a frank haematoma is a rare event. The various issues are discussed in Chapters 4 and 9, but it is worth repeating here that:

1. Clear policies on managing patients with 'disorders' of coagulation must be available; and

2. A careful, gentle technique will minimize the degree of 'trauma' to the space and, hopefully, the risk of a haematoma developing.

Catheter problems

Measures for preventing *kinking* of a catheter were discussed earlier, but if this should occur a change in patient posture may help. Otherwise the dressings should be carefully removed and replaced looking for the obstruction, but if it is deep to the skin the catheter may be withdrawn very slightly. Occasionally, *bacterial filter disconnection* from the catheter will break the sterility of the system, and the safest response is to replace the whole system, but there are situations where this can be difficult. Rarely, a catheter may form a loop if an excessive length is introduced, and a *knot* can form when it is withdrawn. A knotted catheter, or one that is otherwise *difficult to remove*, may be freed by placing the patient in the fully flexed position and pulling firmly. Changes in posture may help, but if this fails, or the *catheter breaks*, surgical removal may be considered. However, finding small fragments of material in the epidural space can be difficult, and leaving well alone is an option which has been pursued previously (Dawkins 1969).

Key references

Armitage EN (1989) Postoperative pain—prevention or relief? *British Journal of Anaesthesia* 63: 136–8.

Curatolo M, Schnider TW, Petersen-Felix S, et al. (2000) A direct search procedure to optimize combinations of epidural bupivacaine, fentanyl, and clonidine for postoperative analgesia *Anesthesiology* 92: 325–37.

Visser WA, Lee RA, Gielen MJ (2008) Factors affecting the distribution of neural blockade by local anesthetics in epidural anesthesia anaesthesia and a comparison of lumbar versus thoracic epidural anesthesia. *Anesthesia & Analgesia* 107: 708–21.

On-line resource

http://www.britishpainsociety.org/pub_professional.htm#epidural_analgesia
The British Pain Society. Best practice in the management of epidural analgesia in the hospital setting (2010).

References

Apfel CC, Saxena A, Cakmakkaya OS, et al. (2010) Prevention of postdural puncture headache after accidental dural puncture: a quantitative systematic review. *British Journal of Anaesthesia* 105: 255–63.

Armitage EN (1989) Postoperative pain—prevention or relief? *British Journal of Anaesthesia* 63: 136–8.

Balki M, Lee Y, Halpern S, Carvalho JC (2009) Ultrasound imaging of the lumbar spine in the transverse plane: the correlation between estimated and actual depth to the epidural space in obese parturients. *Anesthesia & Analgesia* 108: 1876–81.

Ballantyne JC, McKenna JM, Ryder E (2003) Epidural analgesia—experience of 5628 patients in a large teaching hospital derived through audit. *Acute Pain* 4: 89–97.

Bernards CM, Shen DD, Sterling ES, et al. (2003) Epidural, cerebrospinal fluid, and plasma pharmacokinetics of epidural opioids (part 1): differences among opioids. *Anesthesiology* 99: 455–65.

Block BM, Liu SS, Rowlingson AJ, et al. (2003) Efficacy of postoperative epidural analgesia: a meta-analysis. *Journal of the American Medical Association* 290: 2455–63.

Cashman JN, Dolin SJ (2004) Respiratory and haemodynamic effects of acute postoperative pain management: evidence from published data. *British Journal of Anaesthesia* 93: 212–23.

Cesur M, Alici HA, Erdem AF, et al. (2005) Administration of local anesthetic through the epidural needle before catheter insertion improves the quality of anesthesia and reduces catheter-related complications. *Anesthesia & Analgesia* 101: 1501–5.

Choi DH, Lee SM, Cho HS, Ahn HJ (2006) Relationship between the bevel of the Tuohy needle and catheter direction in thoracic epidural anesthesia. *Regional Anesthesia and Pain Medicine* 31: 105–12.

Coates MB, Mumtaz MH, Daz M, Kuz M (1982) Combined subarachnoid and epidural techniques. *Anaesthesia* 37: 89–90.

Columb MO, Lyons G, Naughton NN, Becton WW (1997) Determination of the minimum local analgesic concentration of epidural

chloroprocaine hydrochloride in labor. *International Journal of Obstetric Anaesthesia* 6: 39–42.

Curatolo M, Schnider TW, Petersen-Felix S, et al. (2000) A direct search procedure to optimize combinations of epidural bupivacaine, fentanyl, and clonidine for postoperative analgesia *Anesthesiology* 92: 325–37.

Dawkins CJM (1966) Postoperative pain relief by means of continuous epidural block. *Acta Anaesthesiologica Scandinavica* 23(Supplement): 438–41.

Dawkins CJM (1969) An analysis of the complications of extradural and caudal block. *Anaesthesia* 24: 554–63.

De Kock M, Lavand'homme P, Waterloos H (2001) Balanced analgesia in the perioperative period: is there a place for ketamine? *Pain* 92: 373–80.

Dernedde M, Stadler M, Bardiau F, Boogaerts JG (2003) Continuous epidural infusion of large concentration/small volume versus small concentration/large volume of levobupivacaine for postoperative analgesia *Anesthesia & Analgesia* 96: 796–801.

Dernedde M, Stadler M, Bardiau F, et al. (2006) Low vs. *high concentration of levobupivacaine for post-operative* epidural analgesia: influence of mode of delivery. *Acta Anaesthesiologica Scandinavica* 50: 613–21.

Dolin SJ, Cashman JN, Bland JM (2002) Effectiveness of acute postoperative pain management: I. Evidence from published data. *British Journal of Anaesthesia* 89: 409–23.

Dogliotti AM (1933) A new method of block anesthesia. Segmental peridural spinal anesthesia. *American Journal of Surgery* 20: 107.

Duncan LA, Fried MJ, Lee A, Wildsmith JAW (1998) Comparison of continuous and intermittent administration of extradural bupivacaine for analgesia after lower abdominal surgery. *British Journal of Anaesthesia* 80: 7–10.

Evron S, Sessler D, Sadan O, et al. (2004) Identification of the epidural space: loss of resistance with air, lidocaine, or the combination of air and lidocaine. *Anesthesia & Analgesia* 99: 245–50.

Fettes PD, Moore CS, Whiteside JB, et al. (2006) Intermittent vs continuous administration of epidural ropivacaine with fentanyl for analgesia during labour. *British Journal of Anaesthesia* 97: 359–64.

Gambling D, Hughes T, Martin G, et al. (2005) A comparison of Depodur, a novel, single-dose extended-release epidural morphine, with standard epidural morphine for pain relief after lower abdominal surgery. *Anesthesia & Analgesia* 100: 1065–74.

Grau T, Leipold RW, Fatehi S, et al. (2004) Real-time ultrasonic observation of combined spinal-epidural anaesthesia. *European Journal of Anaesthesiology* 21: 25–31.

Halpern SH, Carvalho B (2009) Patient-controlled epidural analgesia for labor. *Anesthesia & Analgesia* 108: 921–8.

Harney D, Moran CA, Whitty R, et al. (2005) Influence of posture on the incidence of vein cannulation during epidural catheter placement. *European Journal of Anaesthesiology* 22: 103–6.

Hartrick CT, Martin G, Kantor G, et al. (2006) Evaluation of a single-dose, extended-release epidural morphine formulation for pain after knee arthroplasty. *Journal of Bone and Joint Surgery of America* 88: 273–81.

Higuchi H, Adachi Y, Kazama T (2004) Factors affecting the spread and duration of epidural anesthesia with ropivacaine. *Anesthesiology* 101: 451–60.

Hodgkinson R, Husain FJ (1981) Obesity, gravity, and spread of epidural anesthesia. *Anesthesia & Analgesia* 60: 421–4.

Hocking G, Wildsmith JA (2004) Intrathecal drug spread. *British Journal of Anaesthesia* 93: 568–78.

Horlocker TT, Burton AW, Connis RT, et al. (2009) Practice guidelines for the prevention, detection, and management of respiratory depression associated with neuraxial opioid administration. *Anesthesiology* 110: 218–30.

Huang YS, Lin LC, Huh BK, et al. (2007) Epidural clonidine for postoperative pain after total knee arthroplasty: a dose-response study. *Anesthesia & Analgesia* 104: 1230–5.

Igarashi T, Hirabayashi Y, Shimizu R, et al. (1997) The lumbar extradural structure changes with increasing age. *British Journal of Anaesthesia* 78: 149–52.

Jorgensen H, Wetterslev J, Moiniche S, Dahl JB (2000) Epidural local anaesthetics versus opioid-based analgesic regimens on postoperative gastrointestinal paralysis, PONV and pain after abdominal surgery. *Cochrane Database of Systematic Reviews* 4: CD001893.

Karmakar MK, Li X, Ho AM, et al. (2009) Real-time ultrasound-guided paramedian epidural access: evaluation of a novel in-plane technique. *British Journal of Anaesthesia* 102: 845–54.

Kissin I (2000) Preemptive analgesia. *Anesthesiology* 93:1138–43.

Kehlet H (1994) Postoperative pain relief—what is the issue? *British Journal of Anaesthesia* 72: 375–8.

Kopacz DJ, Allen HW, Thompson GE (2000) A comparison of epidural levobupivacaine 0.75% with racemic bupivacaine for lower abdominal surgery. *Anesthesia & Analgesia* 90: 642–8.

Lavand'homme P, De Kock M Waterloos H (2005) Intraoperative epidural analgesia combined with ketamine provides effective preventive analgesia in patients undergoing major digestive surgery. *Anesthesiology* 103: 813–20.

Liu SS, Wu CL (2007) The effect of analgesic technique on postoperative patient-reported outcomes including analgesia: a systematic review. *Anesthesia & Analgesia* 105: 789–808.

Liu SS, Wu CL (2007) Effect of postoperative analgesia on major postoperative complications: a systematic update of the evidence. *Anesthesia & Analgesia* 104: 689–702.

Lyons G, Columb M, Wilson RC, Johnson RV (1998) Epidural pain relief in labour: potencies of levobupivacaine and racemic bupivacaine. *British Journal of Anaesthesia* 81: 899–901.

McLeod G, Davies H, Munnoch N, et al. (2001) Postoperative pain relief using thoracic epidural analgesia: outstanding success and disappointing failures. *Anaesthesia* 56: 75–81.

McLeod GA, Munishankar B, Columb MO (2005) Is the clinical efficacy of epidural diamorphine concentration-dependent when used as analgesia for labour? *British Journal of Anaesthesia* 94: 229–33.

McLeod GA, Dell K, Smith C, Wildsmith JAW (2006) Measuring the quality of continuous epidural block for abdominal surgery. *British Journal of Anaesthesia* 96: 633–9.

McLeod GA, Munishankar B, Columb M (2007) An isobolographic analysis of diamorphine and levobupivacaine for epidural analgesia in early labour. *British Journal of Anaesthesia* 98: 497–502.

Niemi G, Breivik H (2002) Epinephrine markedly improves thoracic epidural analgesia produced by a small-dose infusion of ropivacaine, fentanyl, and epinephrine after major thoracic or abdominal surgery: a randomized, double-blinded crossover study with and without epinephrine. *Anesthesia & Analgesia* 94: 1598–605.

Nightingale JJ, Knight MV, Higgins B, Dean T (2007) Randomized, double-blind comparison of patient-controlled epidural infusion vs nurse-administered epidural infusion for postoperative analgesia in patients undergoing colonic resection. *British Journal of Anaesthesia* 98: 380–4.

Nishimori M, Ballantyne JC, Low JH (2006) Epidural pain relief versus systemic opioid-based pain relief for abdominal aortic surgery. *Cochrane Database of Systematic Reviews* 3: CD005059.

Norris MC, Leighton BL, DeSimone CA (1989) Needle bevel direction and headache after inadvertent dural puncture. *Anesthesiology* 70: 729–31.

Okutomi T, Hashiba MM, Hashiba S, et al. (2001) The effects of single and fractionated doses of mepivacaine on the extent of thoracic epidural block. *Regional Anesthesia and Pain Medicine* 26: 450–5.

Olofsen E, Burm AG, Simon MJ, et al. (2008) Population pharmacokinetic-pharmacodynamic modeling of epidural anesthesia. *Anesthesiology* 109: 664–74.

Panni MK, George RB, Allen TK, et al. (2010) Minimum effective dose of spinal ropivacaine with and without fentanyl for postpartum tubal ligation. *International Journal of Obstetric Anesthesia* 19: 390–4.

Report (2007) *Safer practice with epidural injections and infusions.* National Reporting and Learning Service: http://www.nrls.npsa.nhs.uk/resources/?entryid45 = 59807

Report (2009) *WHO Surgical Safety Checklist.* National Reporting and Learning Service: http://www.nrls.npsa.nhs.uk/resources/clinical-specialty/surgery/?entryid45 = 59860

Reynolds F (2001) Damage to the conus medullaris following spinal anaesthesia. *Anaesthesia* 56: 238–47.

Robinson AP, Lyons GR, Wilson RC (2001) Levobupivacaine for epidural analgesia in labor: the sparing effect of epidural fentanyl. *Anesthesia & Analgesia* 92: 410–14.

Saitoh K, Hirabayashi Y, Shimizu R (1995) Extensive extradural spread in the elderly may not relate to decreased leakage through intervertebral foramina. *British Journal of Anaesthesia* 75: 688–91.

Sakura S, Sumi M, Kushizaki H, et al. (1999) Concentration of lidocaine affects intensity of sensory block during lumbar epidural anesthesia. *Anesthesia & Analgesia* 88: 123–7.

Schlotterbeck H, Schaeffer R, Dow WA, et al. (2008) Ultrasonographic control of the puncture level for lumbar neuraxial block in obstetric anaesthesia. *British Journal of Anaesthesia* 100: 230–4.

Simon MJ, Veering BT, Stienstra R, et al. (2004) Effect of age on the clinical profile and systemic absorption and disposition of levobupivacaine after epidural administration. *British Journal of Anaesthesia* 93: 512–20.

Verniquet AJ (1980) Vessel puncture with epidural catheters. Experience in obstetric patients. *Anaesthesia* 35: 660–2.

Viscusi ER, Martin G, Hartrick CT, et al. (2005) Forty-eight hours of postoperative pain relief after total hip arthroplasty with a novel, extended-release epidural morphine formulation *Anesthesiology* 102: 1014–22.

Visser WA, Liem TH, van Egmond J, Gielen MJ (1998) Extension of sensory blockade after thoracic epidural administration of a test dose of lidocaine at three different levels. *Anesthesia & Analgesia* 86: 332–5.

Visser WA, Lee RA, Gielen MJ (2008) Factors affecting the distribution of neural blockade by local anesthetics in epidural anesthesia anaesthesia and a comparison of lumbar versus thoracic epidural anesthesia. *Anesthesia & Analgesia* 107: 708–21.

Walker SM, Goudas LC, Cousins MJ, Carr DB (2002) Combination spinal analgesic chemotherapy: a systematic review. *Anesthesia & Analgesia* 95: 674–715.

Wildsmith JAW (2000) Relative potencies of ropivacaine and bupivacaine. *Anesthesiology 2000* 92: 283–4.

Zaric D, Nydahl PA, Philipson L, et al. (1996) The effect of continuous lumbar epidural infusion of ropivacaine (0.1%, 0.2%, and 0.3%) and 0.25% bupivacaine on sensory and motor block in volunteers: a double-blind study. *Regional Anesthesia* 21: 14–25.

CHAPTER 15

Sacral epidural (caudal) block

Edward Doyle and Jon McCormack

The sacral approach to the epidural space provides a reliable and effective block for operations which involve low lumbar and sacral dermatomes. The technique of using a single injection of local anaesthetic via the caudal approach combines the advantages of simplicity with a high success rate and a low incidence of side effects. It can be combined with general anaesthesia to reduce the requirement for anaesthetic agent and systemic opioid, allowing rapid pain-free recovery with minimal postoperative vomiting and an early resumption of oral intake. Over 50,000 such blocks are performed annually in the UK (Cook et al. 2008), with satisfactory analgesia being achieved in 95–97% of them (Mercan et al. 2009). The benefits are multifaceted, the technique producing better patient satisfaction and less analgesic requirement than infiltration of local anaesthetic solution for surgery (Siddiqui et al. 2007), and being as effective as lumbar epidural block for total hip arthroplasty (Kita et al. 2007). Caudal analgesia also has a place in the management of chronic pain, with evidence accumulating to support the injection of caudal steroids for low back pain (Conn et al. 2009).

Success depends upon accurate localization of the sacral hiatus for access to the sacral epidural space, but there are considerable anatomical differences in its size and shape. These variations may make identification difficult and needle insertion impossible in some cases.

Anatomical variations

Interest in the anatomy of the sacrum was aroused in the 1940s with the development of continuous caudal block for analgesia during childbirth. Reviews of large collections of skeletons documented the wide range of normal measurements and the variations which may occur (Trotter 1947, Trotter & Lanier 1945, Trotter & Letterman 1944) (Figure 15.1). The sacrum is formed from five distinct semicartilagenous sacral vertebrae which ossify and fuse to differing degrees, so that many variations of 'normal' may occur. The sacral hiatus which is roughly triangular in shape, results from failure of fusion of the laminae of the fifth sacral vertebra, and is covered by the sacrococcygeal ligament. The 'classical' position of the superior apex is level with the lower third of the body of S_4, although this is the case in only 35% of subjects. The mean distance between the apex and a line joining the cornua is 20 mm (range 0–66 mm), although the cornua may be impalpable in up to 24% of adults (Aggarwal et al. 2009). The upper sacral vertebrae may fail to

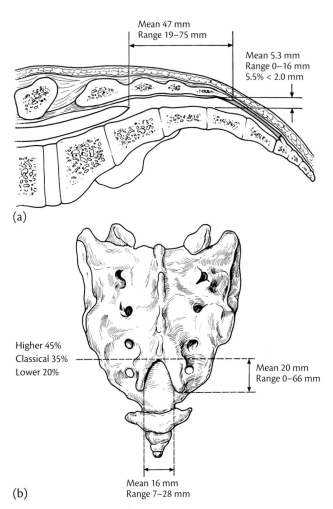

Figure 15.1 Variations in sacral anatomy.

fuse in about 5%, leaving defects through which local anaesthetic solution may escape and result in block failure. The base of the hiatus (the line joining the sacral cornua) is subject to some variation also, having a mean length of 16 mm (range 7–28 mm). The mean anteroposterior diameter of the sacral canal is 5–6 mm (range 0–16 mm) (Sekiguchi et al. 2004), with similar variation in the position of the inferior extremity of the dura (Lanier et al. 1944). The mean position was S_2, but it was caudad to this in 46% of subjects and cephalad in 38%. The mean distance from the apex of the sacral hiatus to the dura was 47 mm (range 19–75 mm).

Magnetic resonance imaging (MRI) has been used increasingly to study sacral anatomy (Crighton et al. 1997) and shown differences in comparison to the older cadaver studies. The median position of the apex of the sacral hiatus was found to be lower, level with the body of S_5, and the sacrococcygeal ligament was absent in 11%. The anteroposterior dimensions of the canal were similar, with its maximal diameter adjacent to the upper third of the sacrococcygeal ligament. The position of the inferior extremity of the dura was confirmed at the middle third of S_2, but the mean distance from the apex of the hiatus to the dura was greater at 60 mm (range 34–80 mm).

Technique of sacral epidural block

Explanation of the procedure, including the likelihood of some postoperative lower limb motor block, and consent from the patient are required preoperatively. Some patients are concerned at the thought of an epidural technique being performed for what they may regard as minor surgery and a simple explanation of the procedure and its benefits is often reassuring.

Indications and contraindications

Caudal epidural block has a defined place in surgery on the anus, rectum, penis, prostate, urethra, vagina, and cervix, but local infection and bleeding disorders contraindicate its use. Anatomical abnormalities of the sacrum or overlying skin, which may lead to difficulty in identifying the sacral hiatus, and neurological abnormalities are relative contraindications.

Position of patient

Caudal injections are usually carried out with the patient in the *lateral position* with the back flexed and the knees drawn in front of the abdomen, although alternatives are possible. The patient usually lies on the left side for the right-handed anaesthetist, such that the natural movement of the wrist facilitates the needle insertion.

The *prone position* is easier for the operator, but less comfortable for the patient, particularly if there is any respiratory impairment. The patient's head and shoulders should be supported by a suitable pillow or padding, and another pillow should be placed under the pelvis to tilt it and bring the sacral hiatus into greater prominence. The ankles should also be supported on a pillow with the lower limbs slightly abducted and the feet internally rotated to prevent tightening of the gluteal muscles.

Caudal injection with the patient in the lithotomy position has been described (Berstock 1979).

Location of sacral hiatus

The approximate position of the sacral hiatus can be identified in two ways. First, an equilateral triangle with its base on the line joining the two posterior superior iliac spines will have its apex over the sacral hiatus (Figure 15.2). Second, if the index finger is laid in the natal cleft with the distal end at the tip of the coccyx, the sacral hiatus will be level with the proximal interphalangeal joint. The exact position is confirmed by palpation of the cornua and the depression over the hiatus.

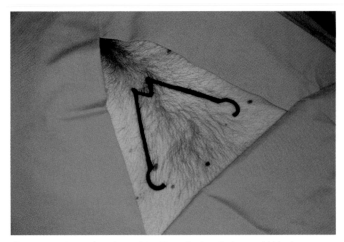
Figure 15.2 Triangular relationship of bony landmarks for caudal block.

Choice of needle

Ordinary disposable hypodermic needles may be used for injection, but their length may be inadequate in obese patients. It is more satisfactory to use a longer, more substantial needle, preferably with a trocar *in situ*, which may reduce the possibility of introducing a core of skin into the epidural space. Spinal needles of 18 or 19 g can be used, as can epidural needles with a straight point. Huber pointed needles are more difficult to insert through the sacrococcygeal ligament. A short bevelled needle will also reveal an appreciable loss of resistance as the sacrococcygeal ligament is pierced.

Needle insertion

The skin should be prepared with an appropriate antiseptic solution. A skin wheal is raised over the hiatus and the subcutaneous tissue infiltrated with a small quantity of local anaesthetic solution. The sacrococcygeal ligament and the adjacent periosteum should also be infiltrated, but large volumes should be avoided because the landmarks are easily obscured.

The caudal needle should then be inserted close to the apex of the sacral hiatus (Figure 15.3), keeping it in the midline throughout. Ultrasound studies indicate that an angle of 20° to the skin is optimal if an adequate depth of insertion is to be achieved without

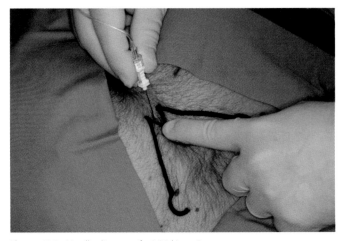
Figure 15.3 Needle alignment for initial insertion.

risking intraosseous injection. (Park et al. 2006). Once a loss of resistance has been felt as the sacrococcygeal ligament is pierced, the needle hub is 'depressed' through 55–60° to bring the shaft into alignment with the sacral canal (Figure 15.4). The needle should be held firmly by the ligament at this stage and should only be advanced far enough to establish its position in the sacral canal, bearing in mind the variations in distance to the dural space detailed earlier to minimize the risk of dural puncture.

Incorrect insertion

The needle may be inserted superficial to the canal (Figure 15.5a), so that the injection is made into the subcutaneous tissue. A swelling will usually be visible or palpable if this occurs, but in cases of doubt the injection of a few millilitres of air will produce localized surgical emphysema which will confirm the misplacement. Alternatively, the needle may enter the canal, but become embedded in the periosteal lining. Attempts at injection will then meet with considerable resistance. It is also possible for the needle to enter the canal, but leave it through a superior defect so that the injection will again be subcutaneous.

A more serious malposition may occur if the needle is inserted too vigorously and too far. It will pass through the sacrococcygeal joint into the pelvic cavity (Figure 15.5b). In this case both the rectum and birth canal may be punctured and the needle will become contaminated. Subsequent withdrawal and reinsertion into

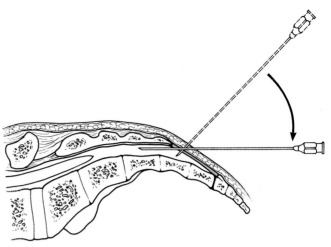

Figure 15.4 Change of alignment needed to advance needle along sacral canal.

the sacral canal will carry with it the danger of infection. If this malposition is suspected the procedure should be abandoned. It is also possible to force the point of the needle into the marrow cavity of a sacral vertebra and any local anaesthetic injected will be absorbed rapidly. Misplacement, as opposed to malposition, may occur if the needle enters an epidural vein, or is advanced too far and punctures the dura.

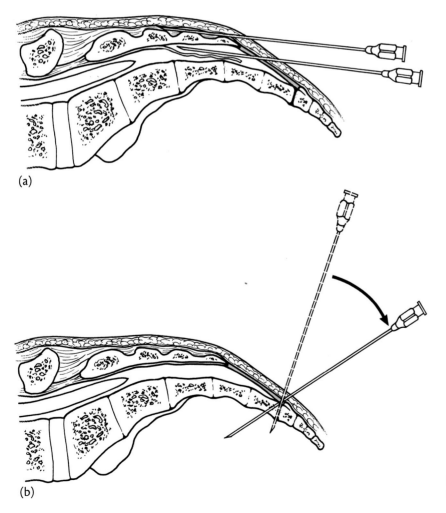

(a)

(b)

Figure 15.5 Some possible misplacements of the needle during caudal block.

Injection

When the needle is satisfactorily positioned it should be left 'open' for 10–20 seconds to help detect blood or CSF in case of accidental venous or dural puncture. This is the ideal time to draw up the local anaesthetic solution. The syringe with local anaesthetic should then be attached and a gentle aspiration test performed. A dural 'tap' is, in fact, very rare, but should it occur it is wise to abandon the procedure and consider an alternative technique. A 'bloody tap' is more common and is usually due to bleeding from veins damaged during needle insertion, rather than to venous placement. The needle should be withdrawn slightly and, if the aspiration test is negative, a small quantity of local anaesthetic may be injected. The patient is questioned and observed for any signs of systemic toxicity and, if none appear, the full dose of anaesthetic is injected slowly, in small increments. It should be remembered that aspiration from small epidural veins may be negative, yet intravenous injection can still occur. If the needle is correctly placed in the sacral canal there will be only slight resistance to injection similar to that experienced with an epidural or venous injection. If any force is required malposition should be suspected, but the needle should be rotated to see whether that helps before it is repositioned.

Many techniques have been described to confirm correct placement of the needle tip. The anaesthetist may inject 1–2 ml of air through it while listening with a stethoscope placed over the lower lumbar vertebrae. If the needle is within the sacral canal a loud bruit will be heard (Lewis et al. 1992). This procedure, known as the 'whoosh test', has been the subject of some controversy regarding both its usefulness (Eastwood et al. 1998) and the (in)advisability of injecting air into the epidural space (Sethna & Berde 1993). When a clear bruit is heard, it is a useful confirmatory sign of correct placement. When there is no bruit, or there is some doubt about it, the position of the needle should be reviewed. Similarly, correct needle placement may be checked by injection of 1 ml of saline whilst auscultating for a bruit. This has a 96% positive predictive rate, which compares with a 93% positive predictive rate following injection of 1 ml of air, but without the risk of air embolism or pneumocephalus (Talwar et al. 2006).

Volume of solution

The spread of solution in the sacral canal is dependent on the volume injected. The early anatomical studies suggested that the mean volume of the sacral canal in adults is about 30 ml (range 12–65 ml), but these figures were obtained from 'dry' bones, devoid of any contents. MRI studies have shown the mean volume to be 14.4 ml (range 9.5–26.6 ml) although variable and unpredictable leakage through the sacral foramina may reduce cephalad spread.

The maximal block height is not dependent on the rate of injection. Cousins and Bromage (1971) found wide variation in the upper level of block after injection of 20 ml of 2% lidocaine, there being no correlation with age, height, or weight of the patient. However, 20 ml of solution can be relied upon to produce analgesia of the sacral nerves, so this is recommended as the standard volume for adults irrespective of the drug used (for dose recommendations in children see Chapter 22).

Continuous caudal analgesia

It is possible to insert an epidural catheter in the sacral region. Because the size of the canal may limit the diameter of the needle, the smallest available system should be used. Provided that the needle tip is lying freely in the canal, no difficulty should be experienced in threading the catheter, about 5 cm being advanced beyond the needle. An ordinary venous cannula is simpler to insert, but difficult to secure and it may be uncomfortable for the patient. The use of caudal catheters in children is considered in Chapter 22.

Suitable local anaesthetics

Bupivacaine 0.25% is the most commonly used agent for postoperative analgesia, but is occasionally associated with motor block which may delay discharge in outpatients where lidocaine or prilocaine may be preferred. Given that the consequences of the venous injection of bupivacaine are among the most serious complications of caudal epidural block, ropivacaine or levobupivacaine may offer a safety advantage and less lower limb motor block.

An effective caudal block may be followed by severe pain when it wears off. This must be anticipated and sequential analgesia provided. Inpatients should have adequate systemic or oral analgesia prescribed, and day-patients should be discharged with a supply of appropriate analgesic drugs and instructions for home use. In either case, the first dose should be given in advance of complete block regression.

Additives

Adrenaline 1:200,000 may prolong the action of the local anaesthetic drug, but there is wide and unpredictable variation in its effect. The caudal route has also been used for epidural opioid administration alone and with local anaesthetic, but the results have been variable (Farad & Naguib 1985). The use of other additives for caudal injection is considered in Chapter 22.

Ultrasound-guided techniques

Ultrasound has been used to assess the feasibility of caudal block (Chen et al. 2010) and to guide both needle insertion (Chen et al. 2004) and subsequent injection (Yoon et al. 2005). No randomized study has as yet compared ultrasound with traditional techniques for successfully placing caudal anaesthetics in adults.

Complications

The incidence of serious adverse events directly attributable to caudal anaesthetic or adjuvant agent injection is low. The most acute and potentially serious complication is intravenous injection of local anaesthetic, occurring in 5.6% of caudal injections in children (Fisher et al. 1997). Neurological complications are rare (Chapter 4).

Further reading

Hadzic A (2007) *Textbook of Regional Anesthesia and Acute Pain Management*. New York: McGraw-Hill Professional.

On-line resource

www.nysora.com/regional_anesthesia/neuraxial_techniques/3010-caudal_anesthesia.html New York School of Regional Anesthesia

References

Aggarwal A, Kaur H, Batra YK, et al. (2009) Anatomic consideration of caudal epidural space: a cadaver study. *Clinical Anatomy* 22: 730–7.

Berstock DA (1979) Haemorrhoidectomy without tears. *Annals of the Royal College of Surgeons of England* 61: 51–4.

Conn A, Buenaventura RM, Datta S, et al. (2009) Systematic review of caudal epidural injections in the management of chronic low back pain. *Pain Physician* 12: 109–35.

Chen CP, Tang SF, Hsu TC, et al. (2004) Ultrasound guidance in caudal epidural needle placement. *Anesthesiology* 101: 181–4.

Chen CP, Wong AM, Hsu CC, et al. (2010) Ultrasound as a screening tool for proceeding with caudal epidural injections. *Archives of Physical Medicine and Rehabilitation* 91: 358–63.

Cook TM, Mihai R, Wildsmith JA (2008) Royal College of Anaesthetists Third National Audit Project Working Group. A national census of central neuraxial block in the UK: results of the snapshot phase of the Third National Audit Project of the Royal College of Anaesthetists. *Anaesthesia* 63: 143–6.

Cousins MJ, Bromage PR (1971) A comparison of the hydrochloride and carbonated salts of lignocaine for caudal anaesthesia in out-patients. *British Journal of Anaesthesia* 43: 1149–55.

Crighton IM, Barry BP, Hobbs GJ (1997) A study of the anatomy of the caudal space using magnetic resonance imaging. *British Journal of Anaesthesia* 78: 391–5.

Eastwood D, Williams C, Buchan I (1998) Caudal epidurals: the whoosh test. *Anaesthesia* 53: 305–7.

Farad H, Naguib M (1985) Caudal morphine for pain relief following anal surgery. *Annals of the Royal College of Surgeons of England* 67: 257–8.

Fisher QA, Shaffner DH, Yaster M (1997) Detection of intravascular injection of regional anaesthetics in children. *Canadian Journal of Anaesthesia* 44: 592–8.

Kita T, Maki N, Song YS, et al. (2007) Caudal epidural anesthesia administered intraoperatively provides for effective postoperative analgesia after total hip arthroplasty. *Journal of Clinical Anesthesia* 19: 204–8.

Lanier VA, McKnight HE, Trotter M (1944) Caudal analgesia: an experimental and anatomical study. *American Journal of Obstetrics and Gynecology* 47: 633–41.

Lewis MPN, Thomas P, Wilson LF, Mulholland C (1992) The 'whoosh' test. *Anaesthesia* 47: 57–8.

Mercan A, Ture H, Sayin MM, et al (2009) Comparison of the effect of sevoflurane and halothane anesthesia on the fall in heart rate as a predictor of successful single shot caudal epidural in children. *Saudi Medical Journal* 30: 72–6.

Park JH, Koo BN, Kim JY, et al. (2006) Determination of the optimal angle for needle insertion during caudal block in children using ultrasound imaging. *Anaesthesia* 61: 946–9.

Sekiguchi M, Yabuki S, Satoh K, Kikuchi S (2004) An anatomic study of the sacral hiatus: a basis for successful caudal epidural block. *Clinical Journal of Pain* 20: 51–4.

Sethna NF, Berde CB (1993) Venous air embolism during identification of the epidural space in children. *Anesthesia & Analgesia* 76: 925–7.

Siddiqui ZI, Denman WT, Schumann R, et al. (2007) Local anesthetic infiltration versus caudal epidural block for anorectal surgery: a randomized controlled trial. *Journal of Clinical Anesthesia*, 19: 269–73.

Talwar V, Tyagi R, Mullick P, Gogia AR (2006) Comparison of 'whoosh' and modified 'swoosh' test for identification of the caudal epidural space in children. *Paediatric Anaesthesia* 16: 134–9.

Trotter M (1947) Variations of the sacral canal: their significance in the administration of caudal analgesia. *Current Researches in Anesthesia and Analgesia* 26: 192–202.

Trotter M, Lanier PF (1945) Hiatus canalis sacralis in American whites and negroes. *Human Biology* 17: 368–81.

Trotter M, Letterman GS (1944) Variations of the female sacrum. *Surgery, Gynecology and Obstetrics* 78: 419–24.

Yoon JS, Sim KH, Kim SJ, et al. (2005) The feasibility of color doppler ultrasonography for caudal epidural steroid injection. *Pain* 118: 210–14.

CHAPTER 16

Regional anaesthesia of the trunk

John McDonnell and Dominic Harmon

The use of peripheral nerve blocks in the trunk has been an area of significant development and expansion in recent years even though most methods were first described long ago. Two factors, other than the general increase in interest in regional anaesthesia, have been relevant:

1. Concerns about the systemic effects and complications of epidural analgesia coupled with a desire to deliver equally high-quality postoperative analgesia;

2. The availability of ultrasound scanning to identify the target tissue planes, a more definitive method than the elicitation of a fascial 'pop' as the needle is advanced. This should increase both efficacy and safety.

Innervation of the trunk

The somatic supply

The thoracic and first lumbar spinal cord segments supply the major part of the innervation of the trunk (see Figure 2.3). The course, branches, and relations of the first 11 thoracic nerves are sufficiently similar to allow them to be described as 'typical' segmental nerves (Figure 16.1). Each has a ventral and a dorsal ramus, the latter passing posteriorly to supply the muscles and skin of the paravertebral region. Close to its origin the ventral ramus communicates with the associated sympathetic ganglion through the white and grey rami communicantes. It then continues as the intercostal nerve which has three main branches:

1. The *lateral cutaneous branch* arises approximately in the mid-axillary line and pierces the internal and external intercostal muscles obliquely before dividing into anterior and posterior branches. The anterior branch runs forward to supply skin over the pectoral region (T_1–T_6) or that of the anterior abdominal wall (T_7–T_{12}). The posterior branch supplies skin over the scapula and latissimus dorsi;

2. The *anterior cutaneous branches* pierce the external intercostal and pectoralis major muscles to supply the skin of the anterior part of the thorax near the midline (T_1–T_6), or pierce the posterior rectus sheath to supply the rectus muscle and the overlying skin (T_7–T_{12});

3. A *collateral branch* arises from most nerves in the posterior intercostal space and runs forward in the inferior part of

the space. It lies parallel to the main nerve and may rejoin it anteriorly or end as a separate anterior cutaneous nerve.

Other branches exist, but are less easily defined. Numerous slender filaments supply the intercostal muscles and parietal pleura and these branches may cross to adjoining intercostal spaces.

Exceptions to this pattern occur at either end of the thoracic outflow. Most of the fibres from T_1 join those from C_8 to form the inferior trunk of the brachial plexus. Some fibres from T_2 and T_3 join to form the intercostobrachial nerve which supplies the medial aspect of the upper arm. The lower six nerves extend beyond the costal margin to innervate the anterior abdominal wall,

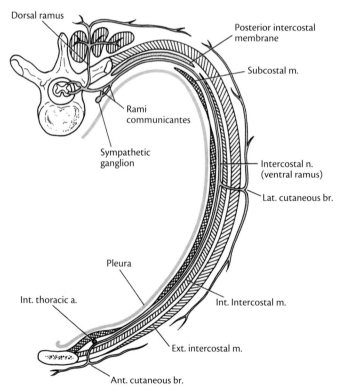

Figure 16.1 Anatomy of a typical intercostal nerve showing also the boundaries of the paravertebral space. The recurrent nerve and smaller branches have been omitted for clarity.

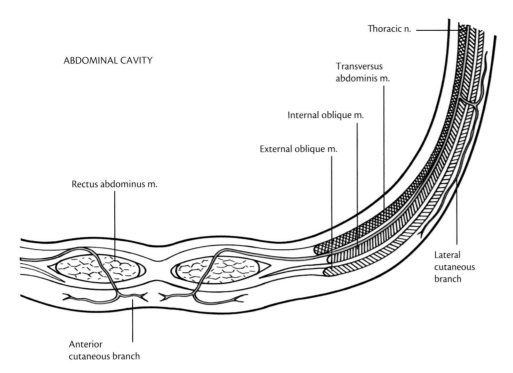

ABDOMINAL CAVITY

Thoracic n.

Transversus
abdominis m.

Internal oblique m.

External oblique m.

Rectus abdominus m.

Lateral
cutaneous
branch

Anterior
cutaneous branch

Figure 16.2 Section through anterior
abdominal wall

creating a plexus of nerves between the internal oblique and transversus abdominis muscles, with terminal anterior branches penetrating the rectus abdominis muscle (Figure 16.2). The ventral ramus of T_{12} is larger than the others, and its smaller anterior branch follows the lower border of the twelfth rib to continue (in the same plane as the other nerves) as the *subcostal nerve*. However, the larger portion joins L_1 to form the *iliohypogastric*, *ilio-inguinal*, and *genitofemoral* nerves (Figure 16.3).

Initially, the iliohypogastric and ilio-inguinal nerves lie within the upper part of psoas major, emerging from its latter border to lie between the kidney and quadratus lumborum (see Figure 23.4). They then pierce the lumbar fascia at the lateral border of quadratus lumborum to run, like the lower five intercostals and the subcostal nerves, between the internal oblique and transversus muscles. About 2 cm medial to the anterior iliac spine the iliohypogastric nerve pierces the internal oblique to lie between it and the external oblique. More medially, and some 3 cm above the

superficial inguinal ring it pierces the external oblique aponeurosis (Figure 16.4) to supply the skin above the pubis and medial end of the inguinal ligament. The ilio-inguinal nerve pierces the internal oblique muscle further inferomedially than the iliohypogastric nerve and then enters the inguinal canal to lie below the spermatic cord. It supplies the skin over the root of the penis and scrotum as well as structures within the canal. The genitofemoral nerve also pierces psoas major (see Figure 23.4), and then runs down its anterior surface before the genital branch enters the inguinal canal (Figure 16.4). It may supply skin in the medial part of the groin.

Key points

The course and relations, particularly the deeper ones, of the thoracic nerves must be understood if safe, effective blocks are to be produced. Initially, the nerve crosses the *paravertebral space* (Figure 16.1), a triangular compartment lying anterior to the transverse process and formed:

1. *Medially* by the vertebra and intervertebral foramina and discs;

2. *Posteriorly* by the intercostal membrane and the superior costo-transverse ligament; and

3. *Anterolaterally* by the parietal pleura.

Each space communicates with the adjacent two vertically, the vertebral canal medially, and the intercostal space laterally, so solution can spread in all directions when injected from any point medial to the angle of the rib. Significant epidural spread is not unknown.

Medial to the angle of the rib, the nerve is deep to the posterior intercostal membrane with very little tissue separating it from the pleura and lung. Beyond the angle of the rib the nerve lies in the subcostal groove, running between the subcostal and internal intercostal muscles. The nerve lies below the intercostal artery with

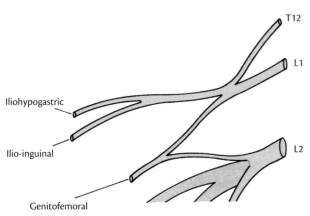

T12

L1

L2

Iliohypogastric

Ilio-inguinal

Genitofemoral

Figure 16.3 Formation of the nerves supplying the inguinal region.

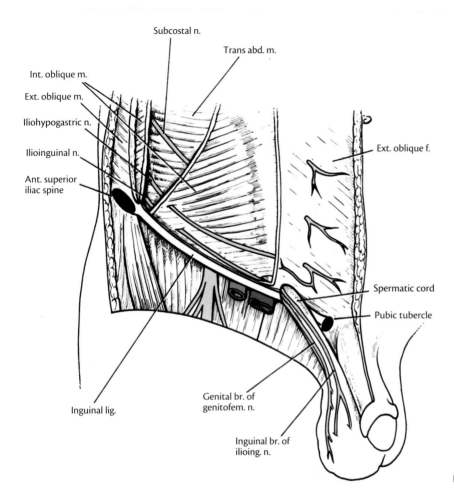

Figure 16.4 Nerves in the inguinal region.

the vein above that, a relationship which is constant to the anterior end of the space, but is less so medial to the angle of the rib. Beyond the costal margin the lower six nerves are separated from the peritoneum and abdominal contents by extraperitoneal fat, the transversus muscle, and the posterior rectus sheath medially.

However, this latter description has to be qualified. The medial extension of the fascial sheath of the internal oblique muscle splits about the rectus muscle, blending with that of external oblique anteriorly and transversus abdominis muscle posteriorly. The sheaths from either side fuse and meet medial to the rectus muscles to form the linea alba, but in the lower third of the abdomen (below the arcuate line) the fascial extensions of *all* three abdominal muscles pass *anterior* to the rectus. This means that the fascia transversalis and peritoneum are immediately deep to the posterior surface of that muscle. Further, the anterior rectus sheath is attached to the muscle by horizontal bands of tissue meaning that local anaesthetic injected into the anterior sheath does not spread vertically very widely.

The autonomic supply

The *sympathetic* supply is from the 12 thoracic and the first (and occasionally second) lumbar segments. The preganglionic fibres pass from the segmental nerves through the white rami communicantes to form the chain of sympathetic ganglia in the paravertebral space, and lying on the necks of the ribs in the thoracic region. Here, the fibres either synapse diffusely, returning to the segmental

nerves in grey rami communicantes, or continue uninterrupted to more peripheral sites such as the coeliac plexus and adrenal glands (Figure 16.5).

The largest sympathetic ganglion, the stellate, receives fibres from the first three thoracic segments and lies in the thoracic inlet at the level of first rib and the transverse process of the C_7 vertebra (see Figure 23.1). The heart is innervated by a diffuse system of nerves from the third to fifth rami, but below this level fibres form the more discrete greater, lesser and least splanchnic ganglia and nerves. Initially, they are closely applied to the vertebral bodies of T_{11} and T_{12}, but below the diaphragm they coalesce to form the more diffuse coeliac plexus overlying the aorta at the level of L_1 (see Figure 23.3). From there, fibres run with the blood vessels to supply the abdominal organs. The supply to the pelvic viscera is from the lowest outflow (T_{10}–L_1), then through the lumbar sympathetic chain and the ill-defined hypogastric plexus.

The *parasympathetic* supply to the trunk is through branches of the vagus nerves except for the pelvic viscera where it is from the second to fourth sacral nerves.

Implications of block

Spinal and epidural block involving the lumbar and sacral segments will thus totally denervate the pelvic structures, but the parasympathetic innervation of other viscera will be unaffected, even by very extensive block, and can lead to discomfort in conscious patients.

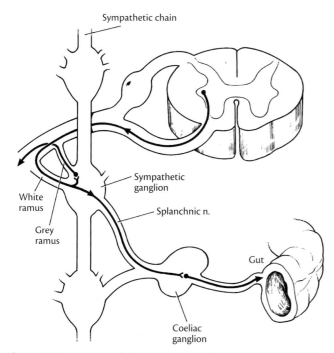

Figure 16.5 Synaptic sites of efferent sympathetic fibres.

lateral, or prone. It can be performed at any point from high thoracic to mid lumbar, although the psoas muscle complicates matters at the lower levels.

The tip of the relevant vertebral spine is identified and a point 2–3 cm lateral to it marked as the site of needle insertion. With full aseptic precautions, the skin and superficial tissues are infiltrated with local anaesthetic solution, and an 18-g Tuohy needle is inserted at right angles to the skin and advanced until the transverse process is encountered (Figure 16.6a), usually at a depth of 2–4 cm. The needle is then angled slightly cephalad (Figure 16.6b), 'walked off' the superior margin of the process, and a loss of resistance technique is used to identify passage through the costo-transverse ligament. If no such loss of resistance is identified the needle should not be advanced more than 1–1.5 cm beyond the transverse process so that it remains in the paravertebral space (Figure 16.1). An aspiration test is performed and the procedure abandoned without injection if air, blood, or cerebrospinal fluid are obtained. A test dose of local anaesthetic is injected to eliminate vascular and intrathecal (into a dural cuff) placement, and usually causes the patient to complain of some chest pain or tightness.

Significant sympathetic block will accompany spinal, epidural, and paravertebral block of thoracic segments, and can be associated with haemodynamic compromise. With the more peripheral techniques both somatic and sympathetic nerves will be blocked, but in a fairly limited distribution so that the cardiovascular consequences are minimal.

Paravertebral block

A number of blocks are performed very close to the vertebral column (e.g. interscalene), but the term 'paravertebral' is reserved for the thoracic or high lumbar approaches to the space. The technique was first described over a century ago, but only started to become popular after reappraisal by Eason and Wyatt (1979). Recent studies have shown that it can produce high-quality analgesia, even after thoracotomy (Davies et al. 2006). It is also used widely in the management of chronic pain.

It is very suited to use after mastectomy, decreasing chronic as well as acute pain (Iohom et al. 2006, Kairaluoma et al. 2006), and has been used after a wide range of abdominal surgery (Naja et al. 2002, Shine et al. 2004). Retrospective work has even shown that paravertebral analgesia is associated with a tendency towards lower incidence of tumour recurrence after breast and prostatic cancer surgery managed with opioid analgesia alone (Exadaktylos et al. 2006). Confirmation of the effect, and establishment of the mechanism, could require major changes in practice (Sessler 2008).

Standard technique

Injection into the paravertebral space can be very uncomfortable so the procedure should be preceded by administration of a moderate dose of opioid (e.g. fentanyl 50–75 mcg intravenously) combined with the intravenous anxiolytic (midazolam 1–3 mg). The technique is the same whether a single injection or catheter insertion is planned, and can be performed with the patient sitting,

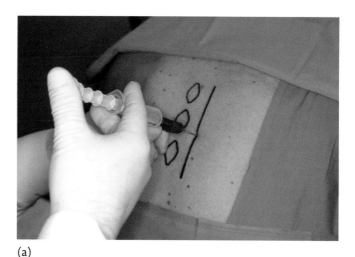

(a)

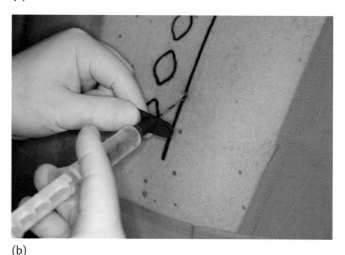

(b)

Figure 16.6 Paravertebral block: (a) needle insertion for location of transverse process. (b) Needle re-angled to pass cephalad to transverse process and pierce costotransverse ligament.

The usual bolus dose is 20 ml of long-acting local anaesthetic (e.g. bupivacaine 0.25–5%), and using adrenaline 1:200,000 may reduce peak plasma concentrations in some individuals (Snowden et al. 1994). The injection should be made slowly in 5-ml increments with repeated aspiration tests to eliminate misplacement. The patient should be asked to breathe slowly and deeply during injection, firstly to prevent breath holding which may cause a vaso-vagal reflex, secondly to encourage correct spread of solution, and thirdly to decrease epidural spread. This volume of local anaesthetic solution will spread to the two spaces above and below the injection point, a total of five segments (Richardson and Lonnqvist 1998). Once the injection is complete a catheter may be inserted before the needle is withdrawn if a prolonged block is required. An infusion of ropivacaine 0.1–0.2% at 8–10 ml h^{-1} provides good analgesia.

Alternative measures

In North America it is more common to inject 5-ml doses of local anaesthetic at several levels, but this increases the risk profile. The 'hanging drop' method can be used to confirm placement because the fluid will be sucked in when the patient breathes in if the needle tip is correctly placed, but the reverse will happen if it is in the posterior spinal muscles. Nerve stimulation has also been used to aid identification of the paravertebral space, and elicitation of paraesthesiae is a useful sign if it occurs.

In some centres during thoracic surgery a catheter has been placed under direct vision by the surgeon with good results (Davies 2006).

Complications

Despite the potential benefits of paravertebral block, there is some reluctance to use it because of concern about side effects. In expert hands the incidence of pneumothorax is 0.5%, and of epidural spread 0.05–0.14% (Naja 2001). There are no reports of cumulative toxicity with infusions.

Ultrasound techniques

The landmarks used, and other details, are as in the standard technique. First, a curvilinear 2–5-MHz ultrasound probe is placed 3–4 cm lateral to the point of needle insertion and aligned parallel to the vertebral column. The ribs above and below the target space, with the pleura between them, are identified (Figure 16.7) before the probe is moved slowly medially. The signal from the ribs will decrease as they curve anteriorly and then a 'step up' of bone, the transverse process, will appear as the rib disappears anteriorly (Figure 16.8). The pleura can still be visualized if the probe is angled laterally. The Tuohy needle is then inserted as described earlier, but in-plane with the probe (Figure 16.9) so that the tip can be followed until it has passed just deep to the transverse process where the injection will be seen to displace the pleura.

An alternative method is to place a linear array probe horizontally, between the ribs at the required level, identify the pleura as a hyperechoic structure, and move the probe medially and superiorly until the acoustic shadow of the transverse process is seen. The needle is inserted lateral to the probe and directed in-plane medially towards the paravertebral space until it lies just deep to the transverse process (Karmakar 2001). However, there is a greater risk of entering the intervertebral foramen and catheter insertion is more difficult.

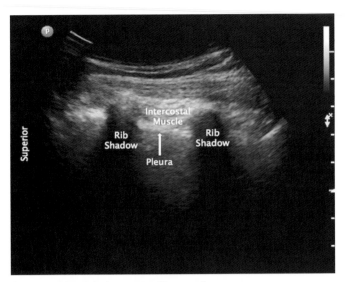

Figure 16.7 Parasagittal sonogram of intercostal space.

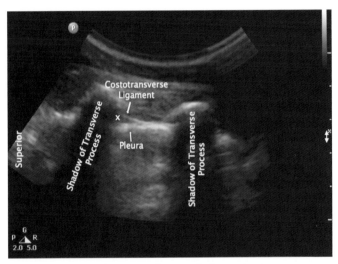

Figure 16.8 Parasagittal sonogram of paravertebral space showing transverse process of thoracic vertebra with target point (x) deep to the costotransverse ligament.

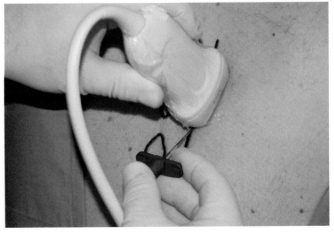

Figure 16.9 Ultrasound probe position for paravertebral block.

Intercostal nerve block

Intercostal nerve block is an extremely useful and effective technique for providing pain relief for unilateral conditions such as fractured ribs or herpes zoster. It can also be used for superficial surgical procedures on the abdomen and thorax such as insertion of drainage tubes, minor breast surgery (Atanassoff et al. 1991), and cardiac pacemaker insertion (Raza et al. 1991). The best effects are produced if the injections are performed posterior to the origin of the lateral cutaneous branch.

Standard technique

Like paravertebral block, intercostal injection can be uncomfortable, especially if multiple injections are needed, so prior administration of an opioid is advised, certainly if the patient is already in pain. For ease of performance the patient is best placed prone with the arms abducted at the shoulder so that they lie beside the head (Figure 16.10). This draws the scapulae laterally to allow access to the angles of the upper ribs. However, the sitting or lateral positions may be more comfortable for the patient, and the ribs may be more readily palpable in the posterior axillary line in obese or muscular individuals. The vertebral spines are identified and a vertical line is drawn along the along the lateral edge of the paraspinal muscles where the ribs are most superficial. The inferior edge of each rib is then marked with a horizontal line crossing the vertical line to identify the injection points for the nerves to be blocked. Most indications will only require unilateral injections, but analgesia for midline abdominal incisions will require block of the lower six nerves bilaterally.

Using full aseptic precautions, the anaesthetist stands behind the patient and starts by infiltrating each injection point with local anaesthetic using a 25-g needle. Then, the index and middle finger of one hand are placed over the angle of the rib and used to retract the skin cephalad, up and over rib (Figure 16.11a). A 23-g, 25-mm needle, attached to a syringe, is introduced between the tips of the fingers, angled 20° cephalad, and advanced until it contacts the rib. The left hand then relaxes the skin retraction (Figure 16.11b) and both hands are moved inferiorly, with the needle point being 'walked' down the rib to its inferior margin. Both hands are then steadied by being rested against the patient's back before they grip the needle's hub and shaft firmly, and gently advance it 2–4 mm

into the subcostal groove. Occasionally a 'pop' is noted as the needle penetrates the external intercostal muscle and the posterior intercostal membrane. An aspiration test is performed and, if negative, 3–5 ml of local anaesthetic is injected. The risk of pneumothorax will be reduced if the patient is asked to breath hold during advancement of the needle into the subcostal groove and during injection.

The intercostal space is one the most vascular sites into which local anaesthetics are injected, and absorption is very rapid (Chapter 7); thus the risk of systemic toxicity is high if multiple, bilateral injections, as for abdominal wound analgesia, are required. A long-acting agent is usually required, and bupivacaine 0.25% with adrenaline 1:200,000 has long been recommended; the adrenaline decreases plasma concentrations, but does not increase duration. If only a few nerves are to be blocked, the local anaesthetic concentration can be increased, but adrenaline is still advisable. Catheter techniques have been described to prolong duration and reduce the risks of multiple repeat injections (Kolvenbach et al. 1989).

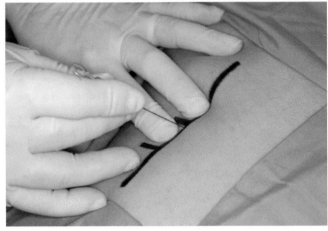

(a)

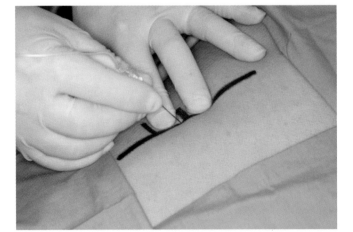

(b)

Figure 16.11 Technique of intercostal nerve block. (a) The fingers of the left hand have pushed the skin overlying the rib cephalad, and the needle tip has been advanced down to the rib. (b) The left hand then moves the skin and needle downwards so that the needle tip can slide under the rib.

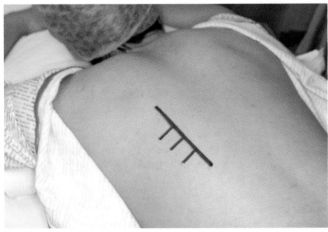

Figure 16.10 Skin marking for intercostal block.

Complications

Apart from systemic toxicity, the greatest risk is of pneumothorax, the incidence of which is said to be 0.42% (Shanti et al. 2001).

Ultrasound technique

The chest wall is best imaged in a parasagittal plane with a high-frequency linear transducer. The ribs appear above and below the space as dense dark oval structures with bright surfaces (periosteum) casting dark shadows. In between them the pleura may be visualized deep to the intercostal space (Figure 16.7), and the depth of the space identified. General aspects of the technique are as described for the standard method, but both preliminary infiltration and block needle insertion are followed under real-time, in-plane ultrasound guidance. Because one hand will be holding the transducer and the other advancing the needle, the latter is attached by a length of sterile tubing to a syringe held by an assistant. A 21-g needle is inserted from the caudad end of the transducer, parallel to the beam, and at an angle of about 45° to the skin. Once the tip is at the correct depth at the inferior aspect of the rib, the injection is made.

Interpleural block

This technique enjoyed a wave of popularity when first introduced in the 1980s (Kvalheim & Reiestad 1984), particularly for analgesia after cholecystectomy through a subcostal incision, but its use declined with the advent of laparoscopic surgery. It has also been used for a range of other unilateral surgical procedures, but it does not preserve respiratory function any better than opioid analgesia (Scott et al. 1989), possibly another reason for the decline in use.

Technique

The aim is simple: the introduction into the pleural cavity of a catheter through which local anaesthetic can be injected, repeatedly if necessary. A needle, attached to a freely moving syringe full of air, is advanced though an intercostal space until the tip penetrates the parietal pleura, at which point the air will be sucked out of the syringe. Thus the essence is detection of negative pleural pressure, so the procedure should be performed in the conscious patient before or after surgery, or during general anaesthesia with the patient breathing spontaneously. It must *not* be performed during positive pressure ventilation because pleural pressure becomes positive and lung puncture is a serious risk.

The procedure is performed under aseptic precautions and with the patient either prone or in the lateral position. It seems sensible to use the interspace at the centre of the distribution of the nerves requiring block. In the conscious patient the skin and subcutaneous tissues over the chosen interspace, and the rib below it, are infiltrated with local anaesthetic 8–10 cm lateral to the posterior midline. An 18-g Tuohy needle, with air-filled syringe attached, is then advanced down to the rib before being 'walked' off its superior aspect and advanced cautiously through the intercostal muscles, the different layers of which are usually readily appreciated. As the parietal pleura is punctured, the syringe barrel will be sucked in, at which point the syringe is removed from the needle and a catheter inserted some 5–6 cm as expeditiously as possible to minimize any further air entry. The needle is removed and the catheter secured with an occlusive dressing. The standard dose of local anaesthetic is 20 ml bupivacaine 0.5% with adrenaline 1:200,000 which will last 4–5 hours and can be followed with an infusion of 10 ml per hour of bupivacaine 0.2–0.25%. Smaller doses have been used in children (McIlvaine et al. 1988).

Mode of action

Local anaesthetics injected into the pleural cavity act by diffusing through the parietal pleura to act on nerves which run in close proximity to its external surfaces. The intercostal nerves are close relations in the chest wall, particularly posteriorly, and both phrenic and sympathetic nerves run under the mediastinal surface. The lung must be fully expanded to keep the local anaesthetic solution in contact with the parietal pleura, and efficacy is impaired if there is air, blood, or other fluid in the space.

Spread of solution in the pleural space is determined primarily by gravity, the volume injected, and the location of the catheter so the patient should be placed in a position to maximize the desired effect before injection. Gravity will cause the local anaesthetic to 'pool' at the most dependent point (Riegler et al. 1989), so solution should accumulate near the intercostal nerves if the patient is supine and perhaps tilted slightly towards the operative side. A head-up or -down tilt may further direct the solution towards the target nerves, and the position should be maintained for 20–30 minutes to give time for drug diffusion. Tilting the patient away from the injected side encourages medial spread and block of sympathetic and phrenic nerves.

Complications

Significant pneumothorax occurs in approximately 2.0% of patients (De Cosmo 2009), and phrenic nerve block occurs occasionally (Kowalski 1992). Nitrous oxide should not be used during subsequent general anaesthesia to avoid expansion of the small pneumothorax created during insertion.

Transversus abdominis plane block

This relatively new technique involves injection of local anaesthetic between the transversus abdominis and internal oblique muscles, the plane of the abdominal wall in which the lower six thoracic nerves run (Figure 16.2). Initially it was thought that this would produce a local 'field' block (Cornish and Deacon 2007), but recent work has shown spread as far back as the paravertebral space (Rafi 2001). It has been used to provide analgesia after a wide range of (mostly) lower abdominal operations, but *only* as one part of a multimodal technique. It does not seem to be very effective when used alone.

Standard technique

The landmark for this technique is the triangle of Petit at the lower end of the lateral abdominal wall (Figures 16.12 and 16.13), although the anatomy of this area is inconstant (Jankovic et al. 2009). The base of the triangle is the iliac crest, with the other two sides formed by the anterior border of latissimus dorsi, and the posterior border of the muscular component of external oblique. The latter's aponeurosis usually forms the floor of the triangle (McDonnell et al. 2007, McDonnell et al. 2008).

With the patient in the supine position, the triangle is identified by running a finger along the iliac crest until the insertion point of latissimus dorsi muscle is palpated. After superficial infiltration, a short bevel 24-g regional block needle is inserted near the apex of

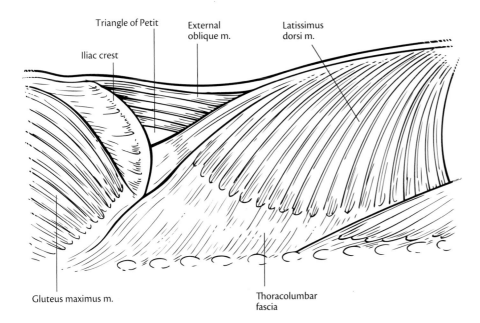

Figure 16.12 Anatomy of the triangle of Petit.

the triangle and advanced at right angles to the skin through the subcutaneous tissues until resistance is encountered. This indicates that the needle tip is abutting the external oblique aponeurosis, gentle advance resulting in a 'pop' (or loss of resistance) to indicate that the needle tip is between the external and internal oblique muscles. Further advance results in a second pop as the needle tip punctures internal oblique to lie between that muscle and transversus abdominis.

After careful aspiration to exclude vascular puncture 0.3 ml kg^{-1} of local anaesthetic is injected with repeated aspiration tests. Bilateral blocks are required for incisions which cross or involve the midline, therefore a low concentration of a long-acting agent (e.g. levobupivacaine 0.125%) should be used to reduce total dose (Griffiths et al. 2010).

Complications

Unless the various muscle layers are identified there is always the risk of entering the peritoneal cavity and puncturing bowel.

Ultrasound technique

There are a number of different approaches to the transversus abdominis plane (TAP) block described with ultrasound (Carney et al. 2008, Hebbard et al. 2007), the majority encouraging the identification of the three abdominal muscles: external and internal oblique and transversus abdominis (Figure 16.14). These muscles are identified either in the mid-axillary line or the subcostal region and, once identified, the TAP is approached using an in-plane technique. The needle is visualized as it passes through the subcutaneous tissue and the body of both internal and external oblique muscles. On passing through the deep aspect of the internal oblique muscle, the needle tip passes into the TAP. After aspiration to exclude vascular puncture, 0.2–0.3 ml kg^{-1} of local anaesthetic solution is injected with repeated aspiration, remembering at all times the maximal allowable dose. The use of ultrasound allows visualization of correct needle placement and allows the operator to observe the expansion of local anaesthetic solution within the space.

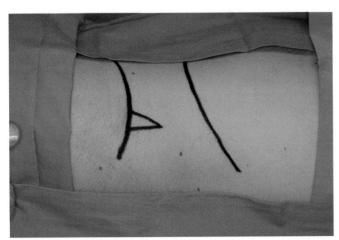

Figure 16.13 Position and landmarks of triangle of Petit.

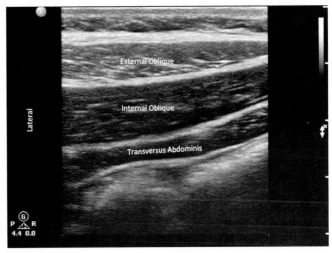

Figure 16.14 Sonogram of anterior abdominal wall indicating three muscle layers lateral to rectus abdominis.

Rectus sheath block

Originally the rectus sheath block was introduced to produce (not very effective) muscle relaxation for surgery, but now it is being used with increasing frequency to produce postoperative analgesia (Yentis et al. 1999). Bilateral blocks are needed for midline incisions, and the injection must be made into the posterior compartment of the sheath to ensure reasonably extensive spread. The block must not be performed below the arcuate line because peritoneal perforation is a significant risk.

Landmark technique

The rectus sheath block can be performed using a loss of resistance technique with the patient awake, sedated, or anaesthetized. The skin is cleaned and infiltrated with local anaesthetic as necessary. A short bevel 22-g needle is inserted at right angles to the skin, a little above the umbilicus, just medial to the lateral border of the rectus sheath and advanced through the subcutaneous tissue until resistance is encountered. Gentle pressure results in a 'pop' sensation so that the needle tip will lie deep to the anterior rectus sheath. The needle is then advanced through the muscle until the posterior rectus sheath is encountered, this best being appreciated by moving the needle from side to side until a 'scratching' sensation is felt. The needle now lies superficial to the posterior wall of the rectus sheath and an aspiration test should be performed and followed by a test dose of local anaesthetic. The full dose of local anaesthetic (a total of 20 ml for each side) is then injected incrementally with repeated aspiration tests. A long acting agent (e.g. ropivacaine 0.2%) is preferred.

The block may also be performed under direct vision by the surgeon prior to abdominal closure.

Complications

The major risk is puncture of the peritoneum with consequent bowel perforation. This is minimized by making sure that the injection is made well above the arcuate ligament.

Ultrasound technique

Ultrasound can be used to aid identification of the correct plane and to facilitate catheter placement. Abdominal wall preparation and most other aspects are as described for the landmark method, but ultrasound is used to identify the structures in the upper anterior abdominal wall, particularly the rectus muscle and its sheath. The block needle is then inserted in-plane with the probe so that it can be seen as it passes through the subcutaneous tissues, the anterior sheath and belly of the rectus muscle, and into the plane deep to the latter. Details of injection are also as described previously but the local anaesthetic should be seen to distend the posterior rectus sheath during injection. A catheter may also be inserted using the same technique and the usual precautions to avoid intravascular placement. An infusion of local anaesthetic (levobupivacaine 0.125%) can then be started depending on patient size with a typical adult having a solution running at 8 ml per hour per side.

Ilio-inguinal/iliohypogastric nerve block

These blocks are used widely for analgesia for inguinal hernia repair performed under general anaesthesia, but will require supplementation for surgery (see 'Field block for herniorrhaphy' section). The specific blocks are useful in diagnosing nerve entrapment syndromes following herniorrhaphy.

Standard technique

The patient lies supine and the skin is punctured 1 cm medial and 1cm inferior to the anterior superior iliac spine. A 35-mm, 21-g needle is advanced at right angles to the skin in all planes until a characteristic 'click' is felt as the external oblique is penetrated, at which point 6–8 ml of ropivacaine or levobupivacaine 0.5% is injected to block the iliohypogastric nerve. Further advance of the needle will result in a second 'click' as the needle penetrates the internal oblique and a further 6–8 ml is injected for the ilio-inguinal nerve. If bilateral blocks are performed for bilateral surgery under light general anaesthesia no more than 40 ml of 0.375% solution should be used.

Complications

Complications include haematoma, both subcutaneous and pelvic, and rarely femoral nerve block or bowel perforation.

Ultrasound technique

Using ultrasound, the nerves are visualized where they both still lie deep to the external oblique muscle, medial to, but slightly above the anterior superior iliac spine. The probe is placed obliquely, at right angles to the line of the nerves, which appear as hypoechoic structures with hyperechoic rims sandwiched between internal oblique and transversus abdominis (Figure 16.15). The nerves, the peritoneum, and the needle during insertion should all be visualized to help prevent nerve or visceral injury.

After preliminary superficial infiltration, a 23-g short bevel needle attached with sterile extension to a syringe containing 20 ml bupivacaine 0.5%, all flushed clear of air, is inserted at the caudad end of the probe. The needle is advanced 'in plane', its entire path to the vicinity of the nerve being observed carefully. An aspiration test is then performed before local anaesthetic injection is started, when the space between the two muscles should be seen to expand (hydro-dissection). A comparative study has found the rate of successful block to be higher with ultrasound (96% vs. 55%) than with the landmark technique (Willschke et al. 2005).

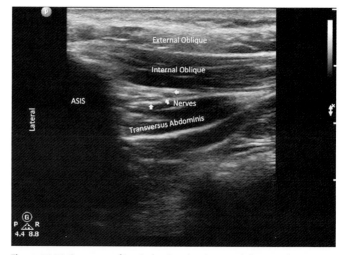

Figure 16.15 Sonogram of inguinal region showing muscle layers and nerve targets.

Complications

Complications should be rare with the ultrasound technique, but it is vital that the needle is visualized throughout if they are to be avoided.

Field block for herniorrhaphy

If herniorrhaphy is to be performed under local anaesthesia alone then further injections are needed once the iliohypogastric and ilioinguinal nerves have been blocked. The terminal cutaneous branches of the subcostal nerve are blocked by the subcutaneous injection of 3–5 ml of local anaesthetic (both superomedially and inferolaterally) from a point just anterior to the anterior superior iliac spine. The equivalent branches of the genitofemoral nerve are blocked by a similar injection over the pubic tubercle. Finally, the surgeon should inject 5 ml of solution into the coverings of the spermatic cord as soon as it is exposed to block the genitofemoral nerve, sympathetic fibres, and the peritoneal sac. A wider area than may be imagined needs to be anaesthetized to ensure patient comfort (Figure 16.16).

Drug dosage

Up to 40 ml of solution may be needed, and prilocaine 0.5–1% should be used for the poor-risk patient. For the healthy outpatient, bupivacaine 0.5% may be used for the deep injections, and 0.25% with adrenaline 1:200,000 for the skin infiltrations.

Penile block

This is a useful, simple procedure for reduction of paraphymosis and, as an adjunct to general anaesthesia, for dorsal slit, circumcision, or meatotomy. It provides excellent analgesia while avoiding the other effects of more central regional techniques such caudal or spinal block. For hypospadias surgery, blocks performed at the start and end of the repair provide better postoperative analgesia than either block alone (Chibber et al. 1997).

Anatomy

Most of the somatic supply to the penis is from the second, third, and fourth sacral nerve roots through the dorsal nerve of the penis, a terminal branch of the pudendal nerve. The dorsal nerve runs with the artery along the inferior ramus of the pubis, through the suspensory ligament of the penis and under the pubic arch. There it lies in the floor of the suprapubic space, before entering Buck's fascia, the fibrous tissue which invests the corpus cavernosum (Dalens et al. 1989) (Figure 16.17). It supplies the skin and glans. The autonomic supply is from the inferior hypogastric plexus in the pelvis, fibres either running in the pudendal nerves or with the blood vessels. The base of the penis and scrotum are innervated by cutaneous branches of the genitofemoral nerve through its genital branch.

Technique

With the patient supine a finger is placed under the pubic symphysis in the midline. A skin wheal is raised before a 23-g needle 5 cm long is inserted in the midline, vertical to the skin, to pass under the pubis into the subpubic space. There, 5 ml of local anaesthetic (0.25–0.5% plain bupivacaine) should be injected on each side of the midline without encountering any resistance. Forced injection of large volumes of solution within the non-elastic tissues of Buck's fascia, especially in children, may cause arterial compression and penile gangrene even if adrenaline has not been used (Sara & Lowry 1984). Frequent aspiration is required to avoid intravascular injection in this highly vascular area, and it is imperative that adrenaline is not used. For complete anaesthesia, another 5–10 ml of solution should be placed in a loose subcutaneous 'ring' around the base of the penis. Formal subpubic penile block provides better anaesthesia for surgery than subcutaneous ring block (Holder et al. 1997).

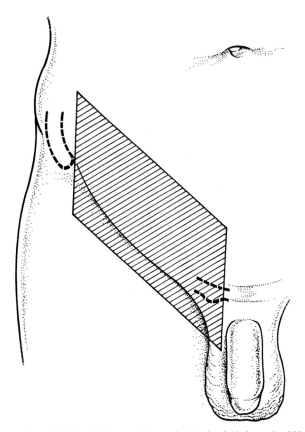

Figure 16.16 Field block for inguinal herniorrhaphy: the shaded area should be infiltrated once the primary injections have been made near the anterior superior iliac spin and pubic tubercle.

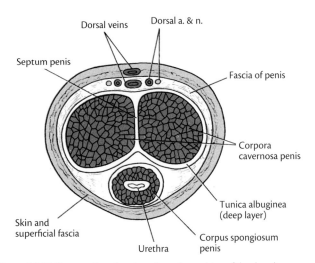

Figure 16.17 Cross section of penis to show the position of the dorsal nerves.

Choice of block for surgery to the trunk

There is no doubt that regional anaesthesia for surgery on the trunk offers many advantages, both during and after operation. Several techniques are available, each with advantages and disadvantages, so the anaesthetist must decide which is the most appropriate. Consideration must be given to several factors, including the skills and experience of the anaesthetist, the availability of adequate monitoring and supervision during and after the procedure, anatomical and physiological features of the individual patient, and the amount of time available. If there are major reasons for avoiding general anaesthesia, even mastectomy may be performed under a field block (Dennison et al. 1985).

For *thoracic surgery* the practical choice lies between intercostal, interpleural, paravertebral, and thoracic epidural block. Apart from simple procedures on the chest wall, thoracic surgery requires general anaesthesia, with intermittent positive-pressure ventilation, to allow adequate control of respiration and manipulation of the diaphragm. The latter is innervated from the cervical region, so it is unaffected by the above regional techniques. Regional anaesthesia is therefore used as a supplement to general anaesthesia, particularly to provide postoperative pain control. Intercostal block by the surgeon or the anaesthetist is the easiest technique and has a relatively low incidence of serious side effects, but it is limited in efficacy and duration of effect. Cryoanalgesia, applied from within the chest, may be used, or placement of a paravertebral or interpleural catheter considered, but close monitoring of infusions and injections is vital, particularly in the first few postoperative hours because the effects are variable. The best pain control is probably obtained with an epidural infusion, but meticulous monitoring and control of hydration are required.

For *abdominal surgery* the choice lies between subarachnoid, epidural, or intercostal block. During upper abdominal procedures, conscious patients will not tolerate large packs or stimulation of the diaphragm, so general anaesthesia with controlled ventilation is required. Regional techniques may be used as supplements to, but virtually never as replacements for, general anaesthesia. For lower abdominal and pelvic procedures, however, excellent anaesthesia and relaxation is obtained with spinal and epidural techniques, and if sedation or light general anaesthesia is required it may be considered to be the supplement. Given adequate postoperative facilities and expertise, epidural anaesthesia is superior to other methods as it is suitable for long surgical procedures, and excellent postoperative pain control can be obtained with top-ups or continuous infusion of local anaesthetic, or with the epidural injection of opioid. If this form of postoperative analgesia is not to be used, and if the surgery is sure to be completed in the available time, spinal anaesthesia is preferable because it is quicker to perform, has a more rapid onset and is more effective than epidural anaesthesia.

Intercostal block is useful in abdominal surgery in three situations: first, where spinal or epidural techniques are not possible, because of a major spinal deformity such as spina bifida or ankylosing spondylitis; second, for subcostal incision for open gall bladder surgery, where it is quick and easy to apply at the end of surgery and gives reasonable postoperative analgesia; third, and most important, where sympathetic block may result in dangerous hypotension due to the relative hypovolaemia associated with many acute conditions, such as haematemesis, peritonitis, and intestinal obstruction. Spinal and epidural anaesthesia are contraindicated in these conditions, but it should be remembered that sympathetic block, although rare, is possible after posteriorly placed intercostal injections. The final place of the transversus abdominis plane technique has yet to be determined, but early studies demonstrate promising results.

The type of regional anaesthesia applicable to *renal surgery* depends to a large extent on the patient's position during surgery. The 'renal position', with the patient on the side and with maximum operating table 'break', may impair venous return regardless of the anaesthetic technique employed, but the use of spinal or epidural anaesthesia will magnify this problem. This is a situation where unilateral intercostal blocks may offer an advantage.

Low spinal, or lumbar or caudal epidural blocks are all useful in a variety of *gynaecological*, *urological*, *perineal*, and *anal* procedures. After some of these, for example, transurethral prostatectomy, profound postoperative analgesia is not necessary and spinal anaesthesia with an agent of suitable duration is the technique of choice. For anal procedures (but only in those in which sphincter relaxation is surgically acceptable or desirable), low spinal or caudal block may be employed. A short-acting opioid such as alfentanil may be used to supplement general anaesthesia, followed by caudal injection of local anaesthetic at the end of the procedure to provide postoperative analgesia. If the patient is to remain conscious a spinal injection is less painful, quicker in onset and more effective than caudal block, which has a significant failure rate even in expert hands. The main advantage of the caudal approach is that it avoids post-spinal headache, which may be a serious disability in younger patients who would normally mobilize quickly after surgery.

Regional anaesthesia is commonly used for *inguinal hernia repair*. Peripheral nerve block has gained popularity in day-care surgery and for the very frail patient. The advantages include lack of sympathetic block and resulting hypotension, lack of accessory respiratory muscle involvement, no risk of spinal headache and no muscle paralysis of the lower limbs, the patient being able to walk from the table. However, the technique requires careful patient counselling and the cooperation of both patient and surgeon. If the block is performed after the induction of general anaesthesia the discomfort of injection is avoided, minimal general anaesthesia is required thereafter, and the advantage of good postoperative pain control is retained. For the patient undergoing penile surgery, regional techniques have much to offer.

Key references

Abrahams MS, Horn JL, Noles LM, Aziz MF (2010) Evidence-based medicine: ultrasound guidance for truncal blocks. *Regional Anesthesia and Pain Medicine* 35: S36–42.

Charlton S, Cyna AM, Middleton P, Griffiths JD (2010) Perioperative transversus abdominis plane (TAP) blocks for analgesia after abdominal surgery. *Cochrane Database of Systematic Reviews* 12: CD007705.

Finnerty O, Carney J, McDonnell JG (2010) Trunk blocks for abdominal surgery. *Anaesthesia* 65(Suppl 1): 76–83.

On-line resources

http://www.asra.com/pain-resource-center-regional-anesthesia-truncal-blocks.phphttp://www.usra.ca/ugt_sb

References

Atanassoff PG, Alon E, Pasch T, et al. (1991) Intercostal nerve block for minor breast surgery. *Regional Anesthesia and Pain Medicine* 16: 23–7.

Carney J, Lane J. Quondamatteo F, et al. (2008) Defining the limits and the spread beyond the transversus abdominis plane block—radiological and anatomical study. *Regional Anesthesia and Pain Medicine* 33(Suppl. 1): e7.

Chibber AK, Perkins FM, Rabinowitz R, et al. (1997) Penile block timing for postoperative analgesia of hypospadias repair in children. *Journal of Urology* 158: 1156–9.

Cornish P, Deacon A (2007) Rectus sheath catheters for continuous analgesia after upper abdominal surgery, Australia and New Zealand. *Journal of Surgery* 77: 84.

Dalens B, Vanneuville G, Dechelotte P (1989) Penile block via the subpubic space in 100 children. *Anesthesia & Analgesia* 69: 41–5.

Davies RG, Myles PS, Graham JM (2006) A comparison of the analgesic efficacy and side effects of paravertebral vs epidural blockade for thoracotomy – a systemic review and meta-analysis of randomized trials. *British Journal of Anaesthesia* 96: 418–26.

De Cosmo G, Aceto P, Gualtieri E, Congedo E (2009) Analgesia in thoracic surgery: review. *Minerva Anesthesiologica* 75: 393–400.

Dennison AR, Walkins RM, Ward ME, Lee ECG (1985) Simple mastectomy under local anaesthesia. *Annals of the Royal College of Surgeons of England* 67: 243–4.

Eason MJ, Wyatt R (1979) Paravertebral thoracic block—a reappraisal. *Anaesthesia* 34: 638–42.

Exadaktylos AK, Buggy DJ, Moriarty DC, et al. (2006) Can anesthetic technique for primary breast cancer surgery affect recurrence or metastasis? *Anesthesiology* 105: 660–4.

Griffiths JD, Barron FA, Grant S, et al. (2010) Plasma ropivacaine concentrations after ultrasound-guided transversus abdominis plane block. *British Journal of Anaesthesia* 105: 853–6.

Hebbard P, Fujiwara Y, Shibata Y, Royse C (2007) Ultrasound-guided transversus abdominis plane (TAP) block. *Anaesthesia and Intensive Care* 35: 616–17.

Holder KJ, Peutrell JM, Weir PM (1997) Regional anaesthesia for circumcision. Subcutaneous ring block of the penis and subpubic penile block compared. *European Journal of Anesthesia* 14: 495–8.

Iohom G, Abdalla H, O'Brien J, et al. (2006) The associations between severity of early postoperative pain, chronic postsurgical pain and plasma concentration of stable nitric products after breast surgery. *Anesthesia & Analgesia* 103: 995–1000.

Jankovic ZB, du Feu FM, McConnell P (2009) An anatomical study of the transversus abdominis plane block: location of the lumbar triangle of Petit and adjacent nerves. *Anesthesia & Analgesia* 109: 981–5.

Kairaluoma PM, Bachmann MS, Rosenberg PH, Pere PJ (2006) Preincisional paravertebral block reduces the prevalence of chronic pain after breast surgery. *Anesthesia & Analgesia* 103: 703–8.

Karmakar MK (2001) Thoracic paravertebral block. *Anesthesiology* 95: 771–80.

Kolvenbach H, Lauven PM, Schneider B, Kunath U (1989) Repetitive intercostal nerve block via catheter for postoperative pain relief after thoracotomy. *Thoracic and Cardiovascular Surgeon* 37: 273–6.

Kowalski SE, Bradley BD, Greengrass RA, et al. (1992) Effects of interpleural bupivacaine (0.5%) on canine diaphragmatic function. *Anesthesia & Analgesia* 75: 400.

Kvalheim L, Reiestad F (1984) Interpleural catheter in the management of postoperative pain. *Anesthesiology* 61: A231.

McDonnell JG, O'Donnell BD, Farrell T, et al. (2007) Transversus abdominis plane block: a cadaveric and radiological evaluation. *Regional Anesthesia and Pain Medicine* 32: 399–404.

McDonnell JG, Curley G, Carney J, et al. (2008) The analgesic efficacy of transversus abdominis plane block after cesarean delivery: a randomized controlled trial. *Anesthesia & Analgesia* 106: 186–91.

McIlvaine WB, Knox RF, Fennessey PV, Goldstein M (1988) Continuous infusion of bupivacaine via intrapleural catheter for analgesia after thoracotomy in children. *Anesthesiology* 69: 261–4.

Naja Z, Lonnqvist PA (2001) Somatic paravertebral nerve blockade. Incidence of failed block and complications. *Anaesthesia* 56: 1184–8.

Naja Z, Ziade MF, Lonnqvist PA (2002) Bilateral paravertebral somatic nerve block for ventral hernia repair. *European Journal of Anesthesia* 19: 197–202.

Rafi AN (2001) Abdominal field block: a new approach via the lumbar triangle. *Anaesthesia* 56: 1024–6.

Raza SM, Vasireddy AR, Candido KD, et al. (1991) A complete regional anesthesia technique for cardiac pacemaker insertion. *Journal of Cardiothoracic and Vascular Anesthesia* 5(1): 54–6.

Riegler FX, Vade BT, Pelligrino DA (1989) Interpleural anesthetics in the dog: Differential somatic neural blockade. *Anesthesiology* 71: 744.

Richardson J, Lonnqvist PA (1998) Thoracic paravertebral block. *British Journal of Anaesthesia* 81: 230–38.

Sara CA, Lowry CJ (1984) A complication of circumcision and dorsal nerve block of the penis. *Anaesthesia and Intensive Care* 13: 79–85.

Scott NB, Mogensen T, Bigler D, Kehlet H (1989) Comparison of the effects of continuous intrapleural vs epidural administration of 0.5% bupivacaine on pain, metabolic response and pulmonary function following cholecystectomy. *Acta Anaesthesiologica Scandinavica* 33: 535–9.

Sessler DI, Ben-Eliyahu S, Mascha EJ, et al. (2008) Can regional analgesia reduce the risk of recurrence after breast cancer? Methodology of a multicentre randomized trial. *Contemporary Clinical Trials* 29: 517–26.

Shanti CM, Carlin AM, Tyburski JG (2001) Incidence of pneumothorax from intercostal nerve block for analgesia in rib fractures. *Journal of Trauma* 51: 536–9.

Shine TSJ, Greengrass RA, Feinglass NG (2004) Use of continuous paravertebral analgesia to facilitate neurologic assessment and enhance recovery after thoracoabdominal aortic aneurysm repair. *Anesthesia & Analgesia* 98: 1640–3.

Snowden CP, Bower S, Conacher I (1994) Plasma bupivacaine levels in paravertebral blockade in adults. *Anaesthesia* 49: 546.

Willschke H, Marhofer P, Bosenberg A, et al. (2005) Ultrasonography for ilioinguinal/iliohypogastric nerve blocks in children. *British Journal of Anaesthesia* 95: 226–30.

Yentis SM, Hills-Wright P, Potparic O (1999) Development and evaluation of combined rectus sheath and ilioinguinal blocks for abdominal gynaecological surgery. *Anaesthesia* 54: 466–82.

CHAPTER 17

Upper limb blocks

David Coventry

Nerve block techniques can play a major role in the management of procedures on the upper limb, providing both anaesthesia for operative surgery and analgesia thereafter. Brachial plexus block can greatly simplify the anaesthetic management of patients with significant medical co-morbidity, particularly those with respiratory or cardiovascular disease, obesity, diabetes, altered conscious level, or a compromised or difficult airway. In addition, prolonged infusion techniques for more major surgery may facilitate earlier limb mobilization and have the potential to reduce hospital stay and improve functional outcome.

The pattern of block is partly determined by the approach used, and it is important to relate the surgical requirements to the features of the specific method because each has its limitations in regard to the extent of block and the risk of side effects (Table 17.1). Local infiltration or distal individual nerve blocks can also be used to supplement brachial plexus techniques or to produce a restricted field of block according to surgical need. This would include local anaesthesia for brief surgical procedures, those not requiring a proximal arm tourniquet, and those where additional general anaesthesia is employed for other indications such as iliac crest bone graft harvesting.

In recent years, the development of ultrasound-guided approaches has stimulated widespread interest and reappraisal of many of these techniques, leading to hopes of more successful blocks and fewer side effects (Chapter 10). Although there is a lack of well-controlled, large-scale studies comparing rates of block efficacy and complications when ultrasound or peripheral nerve stimulation is used, there is a growing volume of work in the literature to support the former's routine use for upper limb blocks (McCartney et al. 2010).

Anatomy of the brachial plexus

The brachial plexus (Figure 17.1) innervates the entire upper limb except for the skin over the shoulder which is supplied by the supraclavicular nerves of the cervical plexus. The intercostobrachial nerve (T_2) and a branch of T_3 (Figure 17.2) supply the skin of the inner aspect of the upper arm and axilla.

The plexus is formed from the anterior primary rami of the fifth cervical to the first thoracic nerve roots. Contributions occasionally arise from C_4 (prefixed) and T_2 (postfixed). The *five roots* form *three trunks*, each of which divides into an anterior and a posterior division. The *six divisions* recombine to form *three cords*, which in turn each divide into two terminal branches. The six terminal branches recombine to form the *five terminal nerves* which supply the majority of the upper limb. The proximal branches of the plexus supply the deep structures of the shoulder and thoracic wall. Although the plexus is a complex structure, there is a degree of symmetry in that the plexus originates from five roots and terminates in five peripheral nerves, while the intervening structures—the trunks, anterior and posterior divisions and cords—all occur in groups of three.

Table 17.1 Techniques of upper limb block.

Technique	Sensory block	Advantages	Disadvantages
IVRA	Hand, forearm	Simple, low failure rate	Tourniquet pain, risk of toxicity, no prolonged analgesia
Interscalene	Shoulder, humerus, elbow, lateral aspect forearm and hand	Blocks deep structures of shoulder and upper arm	C_8, T_1 often missed, phrenic nerve palsy inevitable, occasional serious complications
Supraclavicular	Whole limb except shoulder	Widest area of block	Risk of pneumothorax, phrenic nerve palsy
Infraclavicular	Hand, forearm, elbow	Ease of arm positioning. Secure site for catheter fixation	Risk of pneumothorax. Landmarks not always obvious
Axillary	Hand, forearm, elbow	Easy technique, low risk of complications	Difficult to position painful limb. Need for multiple injection technique
Peripheral nerves	Individual nerve territories	Easy techniques, long duration	Limited area of block, may need multiple injections. Tourniquet pain if utilized

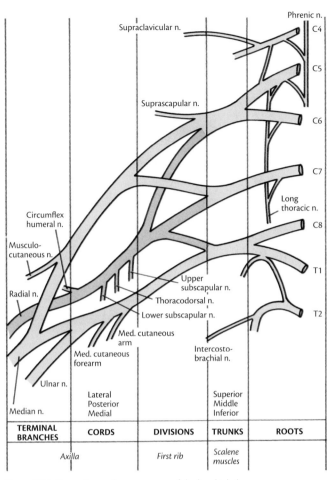

Figure 17.1 Formation and components of the brachial plexus.

Dermatomal distribution is different from the cutaneous territory of individual nerves because peripheral nerves carry fibres from several roots as a result of interconnections within the plexus. Similarly, the innervation of deep structures is different from that of the overlying skin and subcutaneous tissues (Figure 17.2). For example, the musculocutaneous nerve (C_5–C_7) supplies the biceps muscle in the upper arm, but the skin of the anterolateral aspect of the forearm.

Plexus relations

The *roots* of the brachial plexus lie between the anterior and middle scalene muscles which arise from the transverse processes of the cervical vertebrae and insert into the first rib (Figure 17.3). The vertebral artery, the stellate ganglion, and the cervical epidural space are immediately deep to the plexus. The phrenic nerve (C_3–C_5) is formed at the lateral border of scalenus anterior and descends across the body of this muscle. The recurrent laryngeal nerve also lies close to the roots, between the oesophagus and the trachea (Figure 17.4). Superficially, the external jugular vein crosses the interscalene groove, often at the level of C_6 and the cricoid cartilage.

The *trunks* form at the lateral margin of the interscalene groove and are arranged vertically (i.e. superior, middle, and inferior) above the first rib where they are superficially placed, being covered only by skin, the platysma, and deep fascia of the neck. They are crossed by the inferior belly of omohyoid, the transverse cervical artery, and the supraclavicular nerves as well as the external jugular vein. The subclavian artery lies between the inferior trunk and the anterior scalene muscle, with the subclavian vein lying anterior to this muscle. The cupola of the pleura is inferomedial to the first rib at this level. At the lateral edge of the first rib each trunk divides into *two divisions* which pass behind the clavicle to form the *three cords* around the axillary artery. At first, the medial cord lies behind the artery with the lateral and posterior cords lateral to

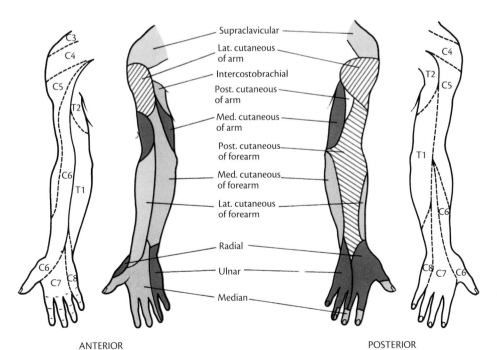

Figure 17.2 Cutaneous innervation and dermatomal maps of the upper limb. The segmental innervation of the deep structures is different from that of the skin: C_5 supplies the shoulder, C_7 the elbow, and T_1 the hand.

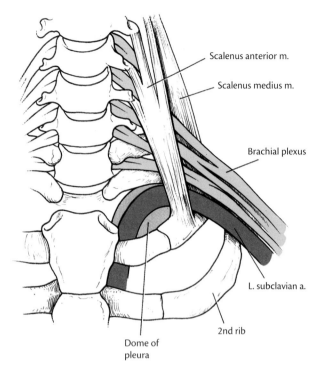

Figure 17.3 Major relations of the brachial plexus.

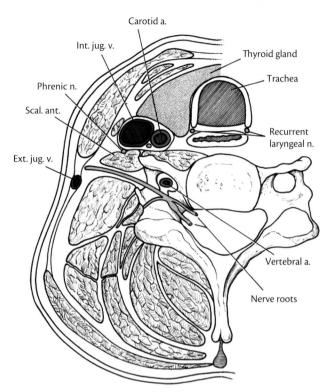

Figure 17.4 Transverse section of the neck.

this vessel, before reaching their true anatomical positions, in the pericoracoid area behind pectoralis minor. Each cord divides into two branches at the level of the lateral border of pectoralis minor and two of the branches combine so that *five terminal nerves* are formed (Table 17.2). The musculocutaneous nerve leaves the plexus high in the axilla, lying in a plane between the short-head of biceps and the coracobrachialis muscle or within the latter muscle (Figure 17.5), where it is liable to remain unblocked with the traditional single injection approach to axillary block.

The plexus sheath

The nature and relevance of those tissues which surround the brachial plexus is highly debated and incompletely understood. A fibrous sheath enveloping the neurovascular bundle is formed from the prevertebral fascia and the fascial reflections from the two scalene muscles (Winnie 1970), but its structural integrity appears variable along the course of the plexus. The sheath appears to be contiguous with that of the cervical plexus so that cervical plexus (and phrenic nerve) block can occur with proximal brachial plexus injection techniques. However, some investigators (Thompson & Rorie 1983) have also described connective tissue septae forming a multicompartmental structure, particularly in the axilla, which encourages longitudinal rather than circumferential spread of local anaesthetic relative to the axillary artery. This incomplete cross-sectional spread has also been confirmed with magnetic resonance imaging (Klaastad et al. 2002). The terminal nerves in the axilla may therefore travel independently of each other in their own connective tissue envelopes and this would correlate with the clinical observations seen with ultrasound location as well as the improved success rates of triple- versus single-injection approaches of the more distal axillary approaches.

Brachial plexus block—general issues

Nerve finding

The original descriptions of brachial plexus techniques used elicitation of paraesthesiae in the distribution of the required block to identify the point of injection. However, most modern practitioners prefer to take advantage of the more objective evidence provided by electrical stimulation or, increasingly, ultrasound scanning.

Nerve stimulation

Peripheral nerve stimulation was, until recently, the standard technique for confirming correct needle placement, without the need to elicit paraesthesiae, during brachial plexus block. Success is more likely if an appropriate motor response can be obtained with the current in the optimum range of 0.5–0.8 mA (Franco et al. 2004). Although it is often said that intraneural injection can be avoided by ensuring that there is no motor response below 0.3 mA, animal studies have shown that, occasionally, the current has to exceed 1 mA (Chan et al. 2007). Thus, this is not a fail-safe technique for preventing intraneural injection, particularly in the heavily sedated or anaesthetized patient.

Ultrasound guidance

A variety of high-quality scanning devices is now available, and vast improvements in image quality have contributed greatly to advances in these techniques. Ultrasound location is not only useful for visualizing nerve structures and local anaesthetic spread, but also allows adjustment of needle position to optimize local anaesthetic distribution and identification of other important structures such as blood vessels and pleura in order to avoid complications. This is a major consideration in brachial plexus block.

Table 17.2 The terminal nerves of the brachial plexus, and their principal branches.

Terminal nerve	Principal sensory function	Principal motor branches
Axillary (circumflex humeral)	Upper lateral cutaneous nerve of arm	Deltoid and teres minor
Radial	Lower lateral cutaneous nerve of arm	Upper arm extensors
	Posterior cutaneous nerve of forearm	Forearm extensors
	Cutaneous nerves to dorsum of hand	
Ulnar	Cutaneous nerves to medial third of hand	Forearm flexors
		Flexor carpi ulnaris
		Flexor digitorum profundus (4th & 5th digits)
		Intrinsic muscles of hand
		Medial two lumbricals
Median	Cutaneous nerves to palm of hand	Forearm flexors
		Flexor digitorum profundus (2nd & 3rd digits)
		Thenar muscles
		Lateral two lumbricals
Musculo-cutaneous	Lateral cutaneous nerve of forearm	Upper arm flexors

NB the medial cutaneous nerves of the arm and forearm are branches of the medial cord of the brachial plexus.

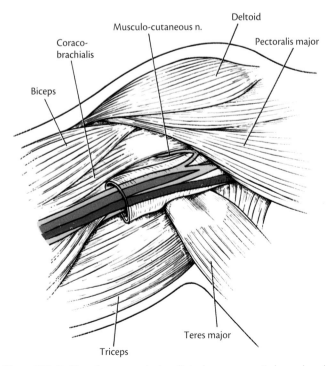

Figure 17.5 Position of neurovascular bundle in the upper arm. Both vessels and nerves are within the sheath at this level.

The brachial plexus lies superficially (depth 1–3 cm) through most of its course, allowing high-frequency linear probes to be used for best image quality. However, the infraclavicular section is relatively deeply located, lying beneath both pectoralis major and minor, and may be better visualized using a small, lower frequency (6–9 MHz) curved array probe, particularly in the more muscular or obese patient. For all ultrasound-guided blocks, a sterile field should always be prepared using antiseptic solution and the probe covered with a sterile sheath or adhesive dressing before commencing the block. It is vitally important to cover the skin with sterile conductivity gel to remove the air–skin interfaces and allow good ultrasound wave penetration and reflection.

The combination of ultrasound-guidance with peripheral nerve stimulation, although useful as a teaching aid, does not appear to improve block outcome compared to using ultrasound alone (Arcand et al. 2005, Sinha et al. 2007). The combination may lead to longer block performance time due to conflicting endpoints for injection and increase the frequency of unnecessary needle-nerve contact.

Block needles

The debate regarding the choice between a short-bevel (or pencil-point) needle and a conventional hypodermic one remains unresolved, although few anaesthetists now use the latter. Standard hypodermic needles have long been thought to increase the risk of nerve injury (Selander et al. 1977), but a short bevel may cause more damage than a longer one if the nerve sheath is penetrated (Rice & McMahon 1992). Nevertheless, the greater 'feel' for different tissue planes provided by a short-bevelled needle increases the awareness and accuracy of placement, and reduces the likelihood of nerve sheath penetration (Moore et al. 1994). Ultrasound guidance allows the needle to be placed close to the nerve, with subsequent visualization of local anaesthetic spread, without risking nerve penetration which, in theory at least, is more likely with a 'blind' or nerve stimulator based technique.

Most custom-made regional block needles, with or without insulation for nerve stimulation, provide a short, flexible, extension tube between the syringe and needle. This allows the anaesthetist to position the needle accurately, hold it firmly in position, and minimize the risk of it being displaced during aspiration and injection. Ultrasound 'bright' or echogenic needles are now available, and improve visualization of the needle shaft during the performance of in-plane techniques.

Pharmacology of plexus block

Drugs and dosage

Lidocaine and prilocaine 1–2% are both effective when a short duration is required, prilocaine being the drug of choice because of its lower potential for systemic toxicity (Wildsmith et al. 1977). However, the 2% solution is no longer available and 1% prilocaine may not produce adequate muscle relaxation so lidocaine will have to be used for more profound blocks although it should be used with adrenaline to reduce peak plasma concentrations and provide an adequate duration of action. The commercial preparation contains adrenaline 1:200,000 (5 mcg ml^{-1}), but 1:400,000 (2.5 mcg ml^{-1}) may be preferred in patients with myocardial ischaemia or those prone to nerve injury as a consequence of decreased blood flow secondary to diabetes or atherosclerosis (Neal

2003). Bupivacaine 0.5%, ropivacaine 0.75% and levobupivacaine 0.5% are all appropriate if a longer duration is required, the latter two having less risk of serious systemic toxicity and not requiring the addition of adrenaline.

Traditionally, a volume of 30–40 ml of solution has been recommended with 'blind' or nerve stimulator-guided brachial plexus block. Such a volume implies a large dose of local anaesthetic (Table 17.3), one which must be injected cautiously and incrementally, in all patients, and will need to be reduced in children and frail, elderly patients. However, the volume and concentration of solution really needed is controversial because it may be that 'supramaximal' doses are often used to ensure success, particularly when a block is used as the sole technique for surgery. Already, significant reduction in dosage, without sacrificing block quality, has been demonstrated with some, but not all, ultrasound-guided approaches (Riazi et al. 2008) so this is obviously an area for further development.

Latency of block: the core/mantle concept

The arrangement of nerves within a plexus, and fibres within a peripheral nerve, is not random (Winnie et al. 1977), those supplying the distal structures in its territory lie at the centre or 'core', whereas those supplying the proximal areas are in the outer layer or 'mantle'. Thus when local anaesthetic is deposited around a nerve it will diffuse into, and block, the fibres supplying the more proximal structures first. In most mixed peripheral nerves the proportion of sensory and motor fibres is the same in both mantle and core, but this is not the case with the brachial plexus. A large proportion of the core fibres are those providing the rich sensory innervation to the hand, and the mantle fibres are predominantly those providing motor supply to the shoulder and elbow, the skin over the shoulder being supplied by the cervical plexus. The clinical consequence is that the first sign of a successful brachial plexus block is likely to be weakness of either the shoulder or elbow joint. Weakness of joint movement usually progresses from proximal to distal joints and may precede sensory loss.

Whichever technique is used, there will be a latent period of 5–10 minutes before the first evidence of block becomes apparent because of the time it takes for drug to diffuse through the considerable coverings of the plexus. The intensity of the block will continue to increase for a further 10–20 minutes with the time taken for the block to be 'ready' for surgery depending on the accuracy of local anaesthetic placement as well as the agent and mass of local anaesthetic used. The importance of these factors has been shown

in studies of ultrasound-guidance involving precise application of local anaesthetic around individual nerves or nerve trunks and resulting in faster onset and longer duration (Kapral et al. 2008, Marhofer et al. 2004).

Duration

Lidocaine (with adrenaline) typically provides up to 120 minutes of surgical anaesthesia, and 3–4 hours of analgesia, whereas longer acting drugs may produce analgesia lasting 14–18 hours, and occasionally longer, particularly if a higher dosage is used (Liisanantti et al. 2004). However, if such prolonged duration is needed, a catheter technique should be used.

Adjuvant drugs

Opioid and α_2-adrenergic agonist drugs have been added to the local anaesthetic to try and improve the quality and duration of brachial plexus block, but properly designed studies with adequate control groups suggest that there is no clinically relevant perineural opioid effect (Murphy et al. 2000). Clonidine 0.5 mcg kg^{-1} (to a maximum of 150 mcg) may usefully prolong lidocaine block without causing significant systemic side effects (hypotension, bradycardia, sedation), but its effects are less pronounced when added to long-acting local anaesthetics (McCartney et al. 2007a). Again, significant prolongation of duration is best achieved with catheter techniques

Nerve injury and brachial plexus block

Given the functional importance of the upper limb, the avoidance of even very minor neurological sequelae is particularly important. Pre-existing neurological and vascular disease, surgical injury, limb traction and posture, inadequate limb padding and support, tourniquet pressure, and ischaemia are all important risk factors for nerve damage associated with upper limb surgery, surgical factors being responsible for 89% of such complications (Horlocker et al. 1999). Regional anaesthesia may contribute through mechanical trauma (needle injury, intraneural injection, high injection pressure), ischaemic injury (adrenaline), local anaesthetic neurotoxicity, or, most likely, a combination of factors. In addition, there appears to be a higher incidence of short-term neurological injury with the interscalene than the axillary approach (4% vs. 1% respectively) (Fanelli et al. 1999), particularly when paraesthesiae occur during placement (Candido et al. 2005). All of these issues need to be considered, and formal neurophysiological investigation undertaken, before a diagnosis of needle or injection neuritis can be made. Symptoms of nerve damage may be apparent immediately postoperatively, but can take a week or more to develop and the duration can vary from 2–3 weeks up to 1–2 years. Full recovery is usual, with permanent disability being rare.

Techniques of brachial plexus block

Numerous approaches to the plexus have been described, but most in widespread use fall into one of four categories:

1. Interscalene;

2. Supraclavicular;

3. Axillary;

4. Infraclavicular.

Table 17.3 Suggested drugs, concentrations, and volumes for brachial plexus block in the healthy adult. Doses actually used should reflect features of the individual patient.

Drug	Plain solution	With adrenaline 1:200,000
Lidocaine	Not advised; risk of toxicity too great	500 mg (33 ml 1.5%)
Prilocaine	400 mg (40 ml 1%)	Not available
Levobupivacaine	150 mg (30 ml 0.5%)	Not available
Bupivacaine	150 mg (30 ml 0.5%)	150 mg (30 ml 0.5%)
Ropivacaine	225–300 mg (30–40 ml 0.75%)	Not available

With the introduction of ultrasound guidance these approaches continue to be refined, with less dependence on specific surface landmarks, but rather greater appreciation and application of relevant cross-sectional anatomy. This allows modification of needle approaches and position with a view to reducing block latency, improving efficacy, and minimizing side effects.

The distribution of block depends on the approach used (Lanz & Theiss Djankovic 1983). Interscalene injection blocks the proximal components of the plexus, including the axillary and suprascapular nerves, as well as the supraclavicular nerves which originate from the cervical plexus, making it the block of choice for shoulder and proximal humeral surgery. However, the C_8 and T_1 dermatomes, which supply the ulnar aspect of the forearm and hand, are often unaffected. Conversely, the axillary approach produces reliable block of the medial arm, elbow, forearm, and hand, often including the intercostobrachial nerve (T_2). The supraclavicular technique may result in the most widespread block because it is performed at the level of the trunks/divisions, although the inferior trunk may be missed unless local anaesthetic is deposited close to the first rib. The infraclavicular approach has a similar distribution of block to the axillary approach, with the vertical injection approach being preferred when using nerve stimulation and the pericoracoid with ultrasound.

In experienced hands, the choice of technique is determined by the surgical requirements and the preferences of the anaesthetist. For the occasional practitioner, the axillary approach may be the best compromise between a good distribution of block and a low risk of complications, and can be used safely in the out-patient setting.

Interscalene block

Clinical indications

This, the most proximal approach to the plexus, involves injection onto the roots of the plexus, preferentially affecting C_5–C_7, and with the C_8 and T_1 roots not being blocked reliably. Thus, the skin and deep structures of the shoulder, the upper arm, the elbow, and the lateral aspects of the forearm and hand are consistently blocked (Figure 17.6), while structures in the medial aspect of the arm, forearm, and hand often need supplementary nerve block or local infiltration. It is usually possible to produce partial cervical plexus block with an interscalene approach.

Patient position

The patient lies supine with the head supported by a pillow and the head turned slightly away from the site of needle insertion. The arm should be placed by the patient's side to depress the shoulder slightly. If the posture is exaggerated the neck muscles will be too tense and obscure the interscalene groove.

Landmarks

The cricoid cartilage is palpated and, at that level, the index finger of the non-dominant hand is placed immediately posterior to the border of sternocleidomastoid. The finger tip will then lie on the belly of the anterior scalene muscle and, as the finger is moved slightly posterolaterally, the interscalene groove is felt as a depression between the two scalene muscles. If the patient is asked to 'sniff' or inhale vigorously, the scalene muscles contract and the groove is accentuated. The external jugular vein often crosses the interscalene groove at the intended point of needle insertion.

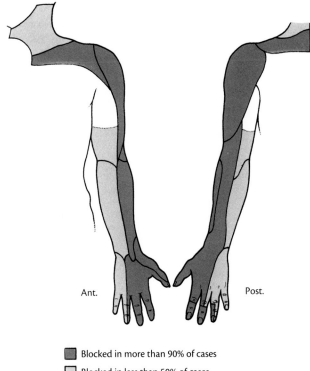

Ant.   Post.

■ Blocked in more than 90% of cases
□ Blocked in less than 50% of cases

Figure 17.6 Distribution of interscalene block.

Technique

The groove is identified and the needle inserted at the level of the cricoid cartilage, perpendicular to the skin, but at a caudad angle (Figure 17.7) to reduce the risk of it passing between adjacent transverse processes and entering the vertebral artery or the intervertebral foramen and spinal canal (Sardesai et al. 2006). An optimal nerve stimulator response distal to the acromion (deltoid/biceps) is usually considered adequate for obtaining successful block (Silverstein et al. 2000).

Ultrasound-guided technique

The patient is positioned as just described or in the lateral position if a lateral-to-medial, needle in-plane approach is preferred.

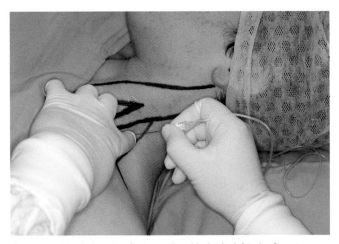

Figure 17.7 Needle insertion for interscalene block. The left index finger is palpating the interscalene groove.

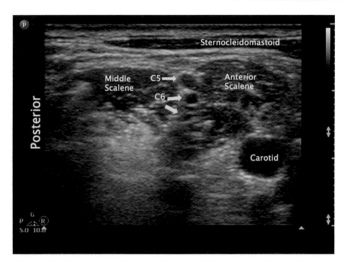

Figure 17.8 Sonogram of the roots of the brachial plexus in the interscalene groove.

The ultrasound probe is positioned in a transverse, oblique plane at or above C_7. With the ultrasound beam positioned perpendicular to the plexus, the best transverse views of the C_5 and C_6 nerve roots are obtained, these appearing as distinct round or oval, dark, hypoechoic structures (often three) lying in the plane between the scalenus anterior and medius muscles (Chan 2003) (Figure 17.8) If the roots are difficult to locate, it is often helpful to scan caudally to the supraclavicular region where they can often be seen as a hypoechoic cluster, superior and lateral to the subclavian artery. Colour flow Doppler can be used to differentiate vascular from neural structures. Once their location there is confirmed, the roots can be traced back to their interscalene location and the view optimized by tilting the probe in an anterior or posterior direction.

After local anaesthetic infiltration, a 50-mm needle is advanced from lateral to medial towards the plexus, along the axis of the probe (in-plane approach—Figure 17.9) or in a more conventional direction along the interscalene groove (out-of-plane approach). The latter may provide a more favourable angle for catheter insertion. A volume of 20–30 ml of local anaesthetic is usual to produce complete anaesthetic block (including the cervical plexus), but as

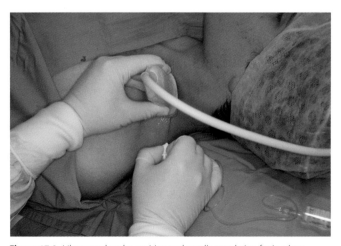

Figure 17.9 Ultrasound probe position and needle angulation for in-plane, ultrasound-guided interscalene plexus block.

little as 5 ml will produce reliable postoperative analgesia after shoulder surgery (Riazi et al. 2008).

Complications

Although relatively easy to perform, interscalene brachial plexus block is associated with rare, but serious, side effects, which should limit its use by inexperienced practitioners, especially where a less hazardous approach can be used. It is best performed in the awake patient.

Phrenic nerve block: the ipsilateral hemidiaphragm is almost always paralysed when larger volumes are used (Urmey et al. 1991), but the incidence is much lower (although not zero) when ultrasound guidance is used to inject only 5 ml for an analgesic block (Riazi et al. 2008). Phrenic nerve block rarely causes respiratory distress unless the patient has significant respiratory disease or is obese (Erickson et al. 2009), spirometric measures of pulmonary function usually being reduced by around 25%.

Recurrent laryngeal nerve block: hoarseness develops occasionally after interscalene or supraclavicular block (6–8%) and is of little consequence, although it is necessary to reassure the patient that this is the case. However, bilateral blocks should not be performed because of the potentially adverse effect on laryngeal competence. Hoarseness may also be caused by vasodilatation of the arytenoid and laryngeal mucosa.

Horner's syndrome (miosis, ptosis, enophthalmos): about 50% of interscalene and supraclavicular blocks produce this effect so patients should be warned about facial flushing and unequal pupils.

Vertebral artery injection: this is a constant risk of the interscalene approach and is potentially very hazardous because small volumes (as little as 1 ml) can cause serious cerebral toxicity.

Epidural and subarachnoid injection: serious complications from inadvertent total spinal and high epidural injection, and even direct spinal cord injury, have been reported (Benumof 2000). The minimum distance from skin to the C_6 foramen is only 23 mm (Sardesai et al. 2006) and may be significantly less if tissues are compressed with the application of an ultrasound probe. Careful placement using shorter needles, directing the needle in a slightly caudad direction and frequent aspiration are essential to avoid serious complications.

Supraclavicular block

Clinical indications

This approach involves injection onto the trunks/divisions of the plexus as they run across the surface of the first rib, immediately posterior to the subclavian artery, and within the plexus sheath (Figure 17.3). A successful block provides consistent anaesthesia of the limb beyond the shoulder joint (Figure 17.10), although the artery may occasionally prevent solution spreading to the inferior trunk so that the block is deficient in the C_8–T_1 distribution. However, this is uncommon if sufficient volume is injected or spread is visualized using ultrasound guidance. Landmarks may be difficult to determine, especially in the obese, and the risk of pneumothorax or hemidiaphragmatic paresis might detract from its use in these patients or those with significant respiratory disease.

Position

The patient position is the same as for interscalene block previously described.

Landmarks

The interscalene groove is identified (as described previously) and traced caudally towards the clavicle until the pulse of the subclavian

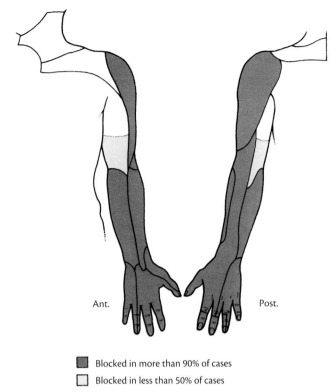

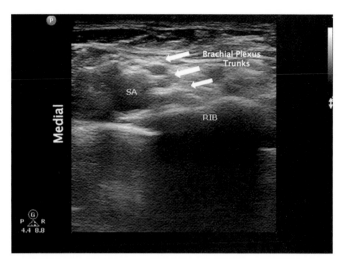

Figure 17.11 Sonogram of the brachial plexus as it crosses the first rib; SA = subclavian artery.

Ant.   Post.

■ Blocked in more than 90% of cases
□ Blocked in less than 50% of cases

Figure 17.10 Distribution of supraclavicular block.

artery is palpated, usually at a point posterior to the midpoint of the clavicle. The artery emerges from behind the insertion of scalenus anterior on the first rib and passes beneath the midpoint of the clavicle.

Standard technique

With the subclavian pulse identified at the base of the interscalene groove, the needle is inserted immediately above the palpating finger. It should be aligned parallel to the midline in the horizontal plane (in the supine patient), without any medial angulation, and advanced slowly until a distal nerve stimulator response is obtained. Even with a careful technique the risk of pleural puncture is such that many would argue against the use of this approach to the plexus *without* ultrasound guidance. Prior visualization of pleura and first rib reduces significantly the risk of pneumothorax (Perlas et al. 2009).

Ultrasound location

The probe is placed in a coronal oblique plane above the clavicle in the supraclavicular fossa scanning caudally, towards the first rib. The subclavian artery is located above the rib where the plexus can be seen as a cluster of hypoechoic structures, often likened to a 'bunch of grapes', lying superolateral to the artery (Figure 17.11). Colour Doppler imaging can be used to confirm the vascular nature of structures, such as the transverse cervical artery, which may be confused with the target nerves. The pleura should also be visualized, and is usually seen as a hyperechoic line sliding with respiration medial and deep to the first rib.

After local anaesthetic infiltration, the block needle is advanced, in-plane, towards the plexus in a lateral to medial direction (Figure 17.12) It is often easier, and safer initially, to locate the needle superficially before changing the angle to a slightly deeper

plane and advancing it, slowly and carefully, towards the plexus. Because this trajectory is also towards the pleura the needle must be kept in view throughout, and the proximity of the tip to the plexus can be confirmed with small (0.5-ml) injections of local anaesthetic, repeated if necessary, as the needle is advanced to its final position. A conventional volume of 30 ml is usually required for complete plexus block, and this does not appear to be reduced by ultrasound guidance (Duggan et al. 2009), although it does allow needle repositioning to ensure local anaesthetic spread around all elements of the plexus.

Complications

Pneumothorax: this is the most significant complication, the incidence varying widely (0.1–6%) in different studies (Neal et al. 2009), but likely to be less than 1% in experienced hands. A pneumothorax may remain small and undetected, or increase slowly in size for up to 24 hours before becoming apparent. Cough, chest pain or dyspnoea indicate the need for an erect chest X-ray to confirm the diagnosis.

Block of adjacent nerves: as with interscalene block, solution may spread to other major nerves in the neck.

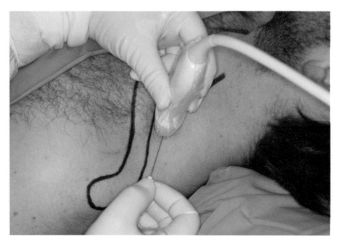

Figure 17.12 Arrangement for ultrasound-guided supraclavicular block.

Axillary block

Clinical indications

This is a relatively safe and simple method of blocking the brachial plexus, although the extent of the block is restricted with single injection approaches, even when a large volume is used. The presence of septae may limit circumferential spread in some individuals (Klaastad et al. 2002), some nerves may travel in their own connective tissue 'envelopes', and both musculocutaneous and axillary nerves leave the plexus sheath proximally so remain unblocked in the majority of patients. Finally, the radial nerve, lying inferoposterior to the axillary artery, is missed in up to 40% of cases when a single injection is made (Coventry et al. 2001). Conversely, success rates greater than 95% can be achieved with triple injection techniques (Figure 17.13), whether using nerve stimulation or ultrasound guidance (Casati et al. 2007), so this variation is preferred.

The absence of significant side effects makes the block ideal for the out-patient, and a safer block than most for the occasional practitioner. It is used mainly for surgery of the hand, forearm, and elbow, although it also provides reliable block of the medial aspect of the upper arm, making it useful for proximal superficial surgery such as brachio–basilic fistula formation and skin graft harvesting.

Position

The patient lies supine with the shoulder abducted to 90° and the elbow flexed to 90° so that the dorsum of the hand lies on the pillow. Over-abduction of the shoulder should be avoided because the arterial pulse may be more difficult to palpate. In patients with shoulder stiffness and discomfort from trauma, arthritis or muscle spasticity, the optimal position may be more difficult to achieve and selection in these situations should be made on a case by case basis after careful consideration of the alternatives.

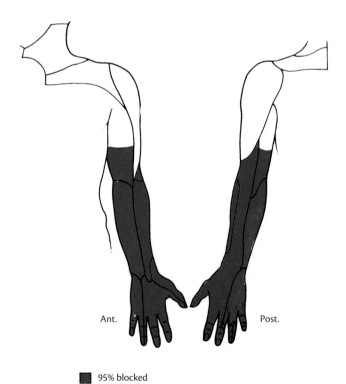

Ant.   Post.

■ 95% blocked

Figure 17.13 Distribution of triple injection axillary block.

Variations in technique

A number of methods of axillary block have been described, each involving a single injection, but utilizing a variety of methods for identifying its placement point: fascial 'pop', proximity to arterial pulsation, paraesthesiae, or deliberate arterial puncture. The transarterial approach was described originally as being highly successful (Cockings et al. 1987), but this is disputed, and routine puncture of the artery should be discouraged. Historically, the axillary arterial pulse was traced medially to enable injection high in the axilla, but most modern techniques, whether nerve stimulator or ultrasound guided, now use more distal injection, usually level with the lateral border of pectoralis major. For reasons noted earlier, a triple injection technique is preferred, specific nerves being identified where they lie in different relationship to the axillary vessels (Figure 17.14).

An initial, 2-ml subcutaneous infiltration, superficial to and below the arterial pulse, can be used to block the branches of the intercostobrachial nerve as well as the block needle insertion site.

Nerve stimulator technique

The artery is compressed gently against the humerus with the index finger of the non-dominant hand, at a point approximately level with the lateral border of the pectoralis major muscle. An insulated short-bevel needle is inserted, above the artery and perpendicular to the skin, directed towards the musculocutaneous nerve, and advanced slowly until biceps contraction is elicited. The needle is then withdrawn and angled in a slightly caudal direction towards the median nerve which lies superficially, although deep to the fascia, finger flexion usually being elicited immediately after feeling a 'pop' as the fascia is penetrated. Finally, the needle is again withdrawn to skin and angled below the artery to locate the radial nerve, ideally by obtaining finger and wrist extension because triceps contraction alone may not result in complete radial block. In each case, the stimulator current should be optimized to 0.5 mAmp before performing careful aspiration tests and injecting the local anaesthetic in 5-ml increments: totals of 5 ml for the musculocutansous, 15 ml for the median, and 10 ml for the radial. Specific location of the ulnar nerve does not appear to be necessary in the majority of cases because there is adequate spread from the other sites, although it will reduce block onset time.

Ultrasound guidance

The nerves of the plexus lie superficially in the distal axilla and are best visualized using a linear, high-frequency (8–13 MHz) probe, and a brief anatomical survey should be performed first to identify the important vascular, muscular, and neural structures. (Figure 17.15) The probe is positioned perpendicular to skin, in a transverse orientation to the humerus (Figure 17.16), so that the neurovascular bundle is visualized in a short-axis view. The needle can be advanced in-plane, allowing its shaft to be visualized, or out-of-plane in a more traditional orientation, where the needle tip or cross-section will be visualized.

Most of the nerves in this location will be seen as hyperechoic structures, with the hypoechoic fascicles giving them a 'honeycomb' appearance. Their positions relative to the axillary article are variable (Christophe et al. 2009), but the more common orientation is as illustrated (Figures 17.14 and 17.15). The musculocutaneous

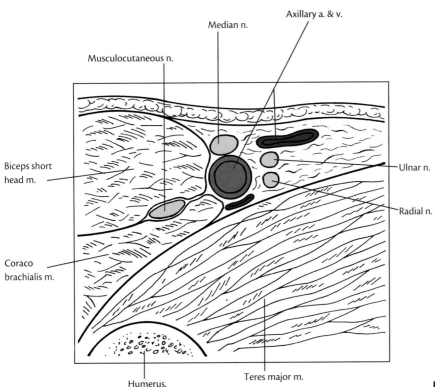

Figure 17.14 Cross section through distal axilla.

nerves lies in the plane between the short-head of biceps and cora-cobrachialis muscles, and often appears as a flat hyperechoic structure with a round hypoechoic core. The median nerve is usually located superficially, and adjacent to the artery in a 9–12 o'clock position, with the ulnar nerve located in a corresponding medial position, although usually distinct from the artery and not infrequently lying deep to the axillary vein. The radial nerve is generally regarded as the hardest to locate and tends to lie beneath the ulnar nerve. As with the nerve stimulator technique already described, a total of 20–30 ml of local anaesthetic solution is usually employed,

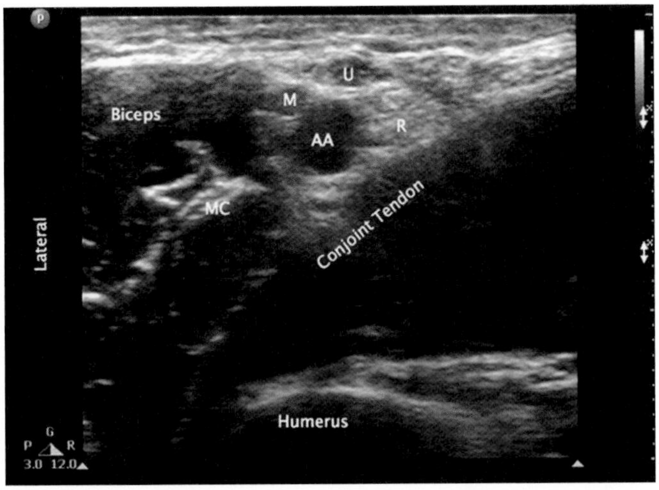

Figure 17.15 Sonogram of distal axilla; MC = musculocutaneous, M = median, U = ulnar and R = radial nerves, and AA = axillary artery.

depending on spread, but successful block with much lower volumes has been described (O'Donnell et al. 2009).

Infraclavicular block

Infraclavicular injection produces a similar block distribution to the axillary approach without the need to abduct the arm for access, and may be used for hand, forearm, and elbow surgery. An advantage over supraclavicular injection is that phrenic nerve block is unlikely.

Many variations in technique have been described, but each falls into one of two broad categories related to needle insertion site:

1. *Midclavicular* techniques, such as the vertical infraclavicular block (Kilka et al. 1995), are usually performed with nerve stimulation. Disadvantages include variable and indistinct landmarks, a high incidence of vascular puncture, pneumothorax (< 0.5%), and slow set-up time, often with the need for multiple injections to improve efficacy.

2. *Pericoracoid* techniques, such as the lateral sagittal infraclavicular block, can be performed using nerve stimulation, but are more reliable with ultrasound guidance, this allowing the limitations of the more medial techniques to be addressed and efficacy improved, usually with a single injection (Desgagnés et al. 2009).

Injection in this location is onto the cords of the plexus, deep to pectoralis minor, where they surround the axillary artery in lateral, posterior, and medial positions (Figure 17.17), the neurovascular bundle lying approximately 4–5 cm from the skin. A lower frequency (6.5–8 MHz) linear probe can be used, but a small curved array probe allows better access below the clavicle.

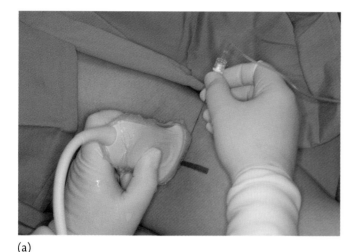

(a)

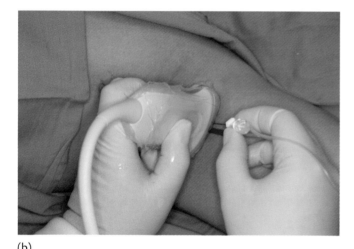

(b)

Figure 17.16 Ultrasound-guided axillary block showing in plane (a) and out of plane (b) needle angulations.

The block needle is inserted in-plane, just medial to the coracoid process, and once localized is advanced at an angle of 45–60° to the skin, (Figure 17.18) in a caudal direction to lie below and behind the axillary artery. Successful block with a single injection of around 30 ml of local anaesthetic is best achieved by placing it posterior to the artery (Figure 17.19), although this can be modified according to spread if the plexus cords are visualized.

Catheter techniques

All four approaches to the brachial plexus can be used to insert a catheter through which continuous infusions or intermittent top-up injections can be given to extend the duration of block to provide prolonged analgesia and vasodilatation. Both physiotherapy and mobilization may be facilitated in the postoperative period.

The infraclavicular approach is particularly successful because the catheter can be fixed to the anterior chest wall where catheter movement and dislodgement are less likely than with other approaches. However, after shoulder surgery an interscalene catheter is more appropriate to ensure continuing block of the upper plexus roots and the supraclavicular nerves. Maintaining the position of an indwelling catheter can be difficult because of the wide range of movement at the shoulder and neck, and the elasticity of the skin and subcutaneous tissues. 'Tunnelling' the catheter a short distance under the skin may be useful to reduce movement as well as infection risk.

A number of specialist equipment sets have been developed for continuous brachial plexus block, their catheters being connected to disposable elastomeric pumps which run at 5 or 10 ml hr^{-1}. Alternatively, a more sophisticated electronic pump will allow a range of background infusion rates to be used, with an intermittent bolus function allowing a patient controlled option. A typical infusion regimen after shoulder surgery is ropivacaine 2 mg ml^{-1} at 8 ml hr^{-1} with an additional patient controlled bolus of 2 ml every hour (Ilfeld et al. 2004).

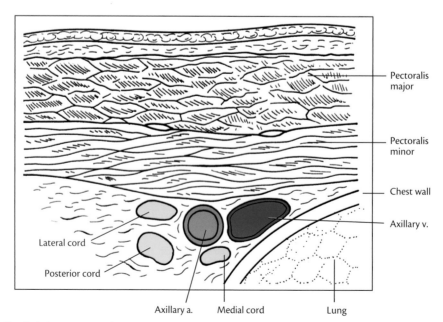

Figure 17.17 Relationship of brachial plexus to proximal axillary artery.

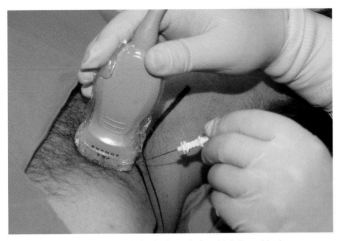

Figure 17.18 Ultrasound-guided infraclavicular brachial plexus block.

Peripheral nerve blocks

Individual peripheral nerve blocks have a limited role compared to brachial plexus block, but are useful as supplements to an incomplete brachial plexus block, and can also be used with light general anaesthesia to provide prolonged postoperative analgesia after distal surgery. The distal nerves of the arm can be blocked at almost any point in their courses (Figure 17.20), injections being performed singly or in combination at the arm, elbow, or wrist depending on clinical requirements. However, they should only be used as the sole technique when tourniquet time is short (<15 minutes) (Delaunay et al. 2001) or when a finger tourniquet is employed. Injection at or above the elbow produces motor and sensory block in both forearm and hand, whereas injection at the wrist restricts sensory loss to the hand and preserves some motor control of the digits (Table 17.2).

Peripheral blocks have traditionally been performed at the elbow or wrist where surface landmarks are readily identifiable. However, needle trauma to both nerves and related vessels is possible, and injection at the wrist may produce incomplete block because of proximal nerve division. Delaunay and colleagues (2001) reported the need for supplementary injection in 14% of patients to achieve adequate analgesia at this site.

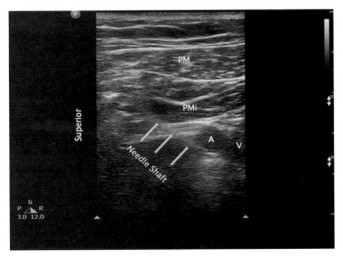

Figure 17.19 Sonogram of infraclavicular brachial plexus block.

Equipment

Block success can be improved by using either nerve stimulation or ultrasound guidance (Macaire et al. 2008). However, nerve stimulation can only be used to locate nerves which have mixed motor and sensory function, although it is especially useful for the radial and median nerves at the elbow. Ultrasound allows all nerves to be visualized, and at a variety of sites which are not landmark dependent (McCartney et al. 2007b). In addition, ultrasound guidance may be reassuring when attempting to supplement a partially blocked nerve, or when performing a specific peripheral block with a long-acting agent for postoperative analgesia in a patient who already has a functional, but short duration, brachial plexus block. Finally, by allowing nerves to be blocked at more proximal sites in the forearm, ultrasound reduces the need for subcutaneous injection of their distal branches.

Standard 22-g regional block needles are suitable for all peripheral techniques in the upper limb.

Drugs

Levobupivacaine and ropivacaine give prolonged analgesia of up to 12 hours, although lidocaine or prilocaine can be used for minor surgical procedures.

Complications

Neural damage

Injury to peripheral nerves during regional anaesthesia is extremely rare (Auroy et al. 2002), although transient symptoms of paraesthesiae may be relatively minor and go unreported. It is important to avoid direct neural contact, which is both painful and potentially traumatic, and it may be wise to avoid some blocks in the presence of existing nerve compression (e.g. median nerve block at the wrist for carpal tunnel syndrome). The ulnar nerve is particularly vulnerable to damage in the sulcus of the medial epicondyle of the humerus.

Vascular injury

There are blood vessels in close proximity to most distal nerves in the upper limb, and care must taken to avoid both intravascular injection and haematoma formation. Ultrasound minimizes these risk by allowing identification of the vessels before needle insertion.

Standard techniques

Blocks at the elbow

The skin and subcutaneous tissues of the forearm are supplied by the medial, lateral, and posterior cutaneous nerves, and those of the hand by the median, radial, and ulnar nerves; the latter also innervate the muscles of the hand and forearm (Figure 17.2). Depending on the clinical requirements, the median and medial cutaneous nerves, and the radial and lateral cutaneous nerves, are usually blocked together.

Ulnar nerve: this block can be used in isolation for procedures on the little finger and ulnar aspect of the hand or in combination with median and radial nerve blocks for more extensive analgesia. The nerve lies in the ulnar sulcus of the medial epicondyle where it is constrained by the medial ligaments of the elbow. The incidence of neuritis is high if the nerve is blocked within the sulcus so the injection should be made 2–3 cm proximal to the epicondyle if using

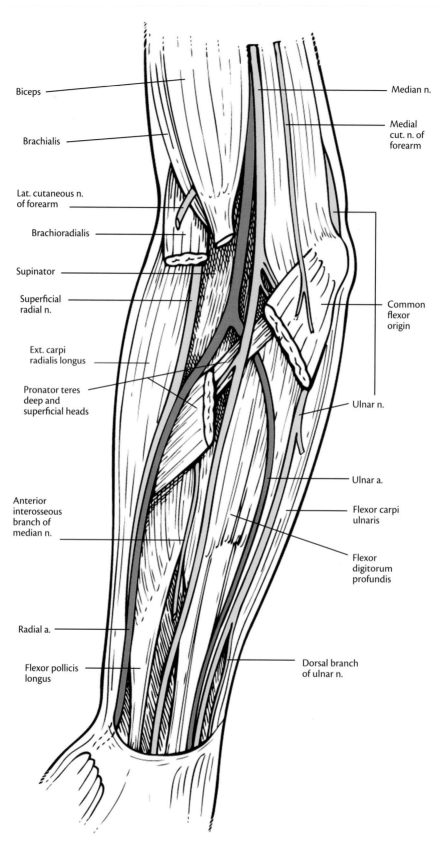

Biceps

Brachialis

Lat. cutaneous n. of forearm

Brachioradialis

Supinator

Superficial radial n.

Ext. carpi radialis longus

Pronator teres deep and superficial heads

Anterior interosseous branch of median n.

Radial a.

Flexor pollicis longus

Median n.

Medial cut. n. of forearm

Common flexor origin

Ulnar n.

Ulnar a.

Flexor carpi ulnaris

Flexor digitorum profundis

Dorsal branch of ulnar n.

Figure 17.20 Nerves of the forearm.

nerve stimulation. The needle is inserted to a depth of 0.5–1 cm and 3–4 ml of local anaesthetic injected.

Median nerve: the nerve lies medial to the brachial artery just proximal to the antecubital fossa. After the course of the artery has been identified, a short-bevel needle is inserted just medial to the pulsation (Figure 17.21) until it penetrates the deep fascia, often with a distinct 'pop' approximately 0.5–1 cm beneath the skin. Paraesthesiae may occur, but should not be sought, and 4–5ml of local anaesthetic is injected. Nerve stimulation can be used to confirm needle location.

Medial cutaneous nerve of forearm: once the median nerve injection is complete, the needle is withdrawn until it is superficial to the deep fascia and then redirected proximally (Figure 17.21), parallel to the medial border of the biceps tendon. As the needle is advanced, 5 ml of local anaesthetic is injected subcutaneously. The combination of these two injections provides sensory block of the medial aspect of the forearm and the lateral aspect of the palm, and motor block of the forearm flexors and intrinsic muscles of the hand.

Radial nerve: the radial nerve is blocked 2 cm proximal to the elbow crease where it lies in the groove between brachioradialis and biceps tendon, at a depth of 1–2 cm (Figure 17.22). If a peripheral nerve stimulator is used, extension of the fingers and abduction of the thumb indicate successful location, and 5–10 ml of local anaesthetic is injected.

Lateral cutaneous nerve of forearm: this, the sensory continuation of the musculocutaneous nerve, is usually blocked with the radial nerve to provide anaesthesia of the lateral aspect of the forearm and hand (dorsal surface). After completing the radial injection, the needle is redirected proximally, parallel to the lateral border of the biceps tendon (Figure 17.22), and 5 ml of local anaesthetic deposited as the needle advanced.

Blocks at the wrist

Ulnar nerve: the nerve is blocked at the wrist by injecting 3–4 ml of local anaesthetic beneath the tendon of flexor carpi ulnaris, 1 cm medial to the ulnar artery. Efficacy can be improved with nerve stimulation.

Median nerve: the nerve enters the hand deep to the flexor retinaculum, lateral to the tendon of palmaris longus and medial to flexor carpi radialis. The needle is inserted about 1 cm medial to flexor carpi radialis and 1 cm proximal to the flexor skin crease of the wrist to a depth of about 1cm. The retinaculum may offer some resistance to needle advancement. Nerve stimulation will confirm the nerve's position, and 2–3 ml of local anaesthetic is injected, with a further 1ml subcutaneously as the needle is withdrawn to block the superficial palmar branch.

Radial nerve: a subcutaneous injection of 5–7 ml of local anaesthetic across the dorsal surface of the wrist at the level of the ulnar styloid process blocks the terminal dorsal branches of the nerve which supply the radial two-thirds of the hand up to the distal phalanges (Figure 17.2).

Ultrasound-guided forearm blocks

Ultrasound guidance allows the peripheral nerves of the forearm (Figure 17.20) to be located and blocked at convenient sites which are potentially safer in terms of avoiding neurological or vascular injury.

The *median and ulnar nerves* are readily visualized in the midforearm where they can be blocked from a single needle insertion

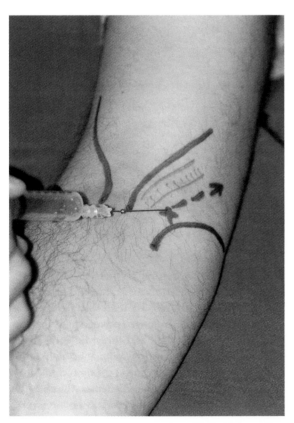

Figure 17.21 Injection for median nerve block at the elbow. The arrow indicates the direction of the subcutaneous injection for the medial cutaneous nerve.

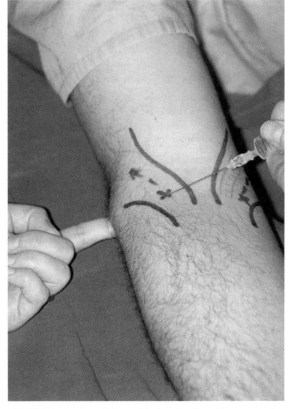

Figure 17.22 Injection for radial nerve block at the elbow. The arrow indicates the direction of the subcutaneous injection for the lateral cutaneous nerve.

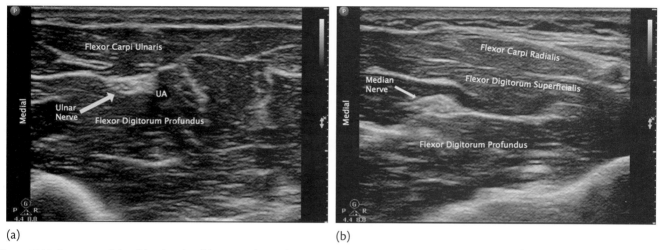

(a)   (b)

Figure 17.23 Sonograms of ulnar (a) and median (b) nerves in the mid-forearm; UA = ulnar artery.

point, and at a level which should facilitate block of their distal branches (palmar branch of the median and dorsal branch of the ulnar). First, the ulnar artery and nerve are identified at the wrist where they lie side by side, the nerve medial to the artery, before they are traced proximally until they diverge, the artery moving laterally away from the nerve (Figure 17.23a). At this point, the block needle can be introduced in-plane (Figure 17.24) without concern about vascular puncture. The median nerve is then be located by moving the probe laterally until the median nerve is seen lying in the plane between flexor digitorum superficialis and flexor digitorum profundus (Figure 17.23b). Each nerve can be blocked by injecting 3–5 ml of local anaesthetic.

The *radial nerve* is readily visualized in the lateral aspect of the lower arm where it emerges from the spiral groove behind the humerus; it can then be traced distally to where it divides into superficial and deep branches approximately 2–3 cm proximal to the elbow. It is usually accompanied by the recurrent radial artery which is usefully highlighted with colour flow Doppler if it is less obvious or difficult to distinguish from the nerve. The nerve can be blocked at either the traditional location in front of the elbow, where it lies in fascia deep to brachioradialis (Figure 17.25), or on the lateral aspect of the distal humerus where it lies close to the bone.

Digital nerve block

This block somewhat inaccurately referred to as a 'ring' block, is very effective for minor surgery to the fingers. Each digit is innervated by two dorsal and two palmar nerves which are blocked by injecting 2–3ml of local anaesthetic into the web space either side of the digit (Figure 17.26). The injection is made in the vertical plane, advancing the needle from the dorsal skin surface towards the palmar aspect of the hand. Local anaesthetics containing vasoconstrictor (e.g. adrenaline) must not be used because of the risk of prolonged ischaemia. Furthermore, excessive volumes of local anaesthetic may cause vascular compression, and should be avoided.

Intravenous regional anaesthesia (IVRA)

Bier originally described the intravenous injection of local anaesthetic into an exsanguinated limb in 1908, but his method has been modified over the years and the technique currently used is based on the method described by Holmes (1963). IVRA is a reliable and

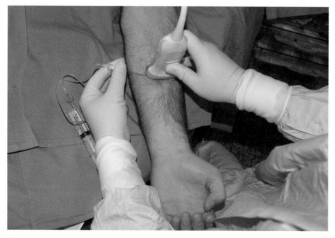

Figure 17.24 Arrangement for ultrasound-guided block of ulnar and median nerves in the forearm.

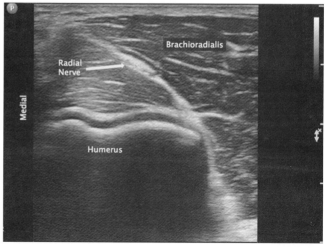

Figure 17.25 Sonogram of radial nerve at the level of the elbow joint.

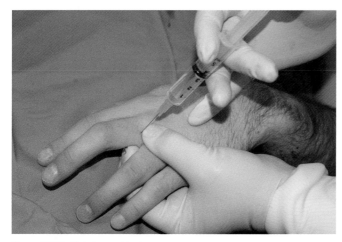

Figure 17.26 Digital nerve block.

successful method of upper limb anaesthesia, but its success depends on the intravenous injection of a large dose of local anaesthetic. The use of bupivacaine by inexperienced clinicians in combination with unreliable equipment resulted in fatal complications (Heath 1982). The use of bupivacaine is now contraindicated in IVRA.

Clinical indications

IVRA provides sensory and motor block in the forearm and hand with up to 98% success and is suitable for surgery distal to the elbow with a tourniquet time of about 1 hour. Tourniquet pain is difficult to prevent and limits the duration of surgery, although prolonged use of IVRA has been reported. The simplicity, high success rate, and speed of recovery of limb function following tourniquet deflation mean that the technique is suited to use in the day-surgery unit and accident and emergency department in experienced hands. A major limitation of IVRA is the lack of any analgesia once the tourniquet is deflated, but this can be overcome by supplementation with peripheral nerve blocks.

Contraindications

IVRA is contraindicated for patients in whom ischaemia would cause significant problems—sickle cell trait, Raynaud's disease, and significant soft tissue injury or infection—because tissue necrosis may occur. Severe cardiac disease (cardiac failure, heart block, severe hypertension) is also a contraindication.

Tourniquet equipment

A variety of tourniquet designs are available with either manual or automatic inflation and single or double cuffs. For simplicity and safety, a manual pump with high-pressure tubing and accurate pressure gauge leading to a single orthopaedic tourniquet is recommended (Figure 17.27), and this equipment must be maintained properly and calibrated regularly. Double cuffs have been recommended as a means of avoiding pain from the tourniquet, but this is often not achieved and there is a risk of confusion when inflating and deflating the cuffs in the correct sequence. Sphygmomanometer cuffs, of any design, must *never* be used.

Drugs and doses

A fit adult usually requires 40 ml, with smaller volumes being administered for elderly patients or children. Preservative-free

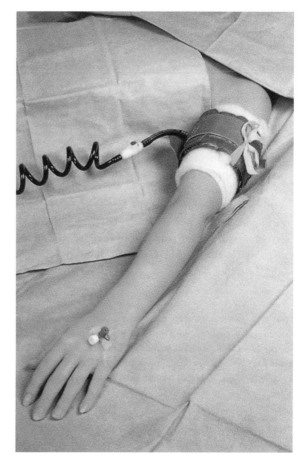

Figure 17.27 Arrangement for intravenous regional anaesthesia.

prilocaine 0.5% has long been considered the agent of choice, but unfortunately this preparation is no longer commercially available in the UK. The clinician is left with the option of using preservative-free lidocaine 0.5%, or carefully diluting the 1% solution of prilocaine.

Opioid drugs such as morphine, pethidine, and fentanyl have been used as adjuvants, but do not improve analgesia, and result in drowsiness and nausea after tourniquet release.

Technique

Despite the apparent simplicity of the technique, the usual precautions for managing the potentially serious complications of regional anaesthesia must be observed:

♦ Venous access established in the other arm;

♦ A full range of resuscitation equipment and drugs immediately available;

♦ The patient fasted prior to the block;

♦ The tourniquet checked beforehand and the inflation pressure monitored during use;

♦ The block performed by an experienced clinician who is responsible for monitoring the patient during the procedure.

The intravenous cannula in the opposite arm is checked for patency before a 20-g cannula is inserted into a vein on the dorsum of the hand or the distal part of the forearm of the limb to be blocked. Scalp vein or other infusion needles are not recommended because of the increased risk of vessel wall puncture and displacement. The tourniquet is placed securely on the upper arm and is adequately padded to prevent damage to the skin.

The patient's blood pressure is measured, and then the limb is exsanguinated by applying an Esmarch bandage firmly from fingers to tourniquet, care being taken not to displace the cannula. If the limb has been traumatized and the patient cannot tolerate application of the bandage, the limb should be elevated and the brachial artery compressed for 2 minutes, just distal to the tourniquet, before the tourniquet is inflated to 100 mmHg above the patient's systolic pressure. The Esmarch bandage is removed, and the limb should appear pallid with no evidence of arterial pulsation or venous congestion. Adequate exsanguination is essential because patchy sensory block and inadequate muscle relaxation may be a problem, especially with large muscular arms, and venous bleeding can interfere with the surgery. If necessary, the process should be repeated with a slightly higher tourniquet inflation pressure.

Once satisfactory exsanguination is achieved, the local anaesthetic is injected slowly over 2–3 minutes through the intravenous cannula. There will be rapid onset of paraesthesiae and a blotchy appearance to the skin, with full sensory block occurring within 10 minutes, although motor block may take a further 10 minutes to develop. Rapid or forceful injection must be avoided because it can generate high intravenous pressure and force the drug beyond the tourniquet into the systemic circulation. The tourniquet inflation pressure should be monitored continuously throughout the duration of the block, and the tourniquet should remain inflated for a minimum of 20 minutes after the injection, even if surgery is completed sooner. Circumoral tingling, tinnitus, and drowsiness may occur after tourniquet deflation, and occasionally bradycardia and hypotension may be observed, indicating that minor systemic toxicity can occur even with 0.5% prilocaine. The patient must be kept under close supervision for 30 minutes after tourniquet deflation.

Complications

Systemic toxicity

Serious sequelae have not been reported when the technique is performed correctly using prilocaine, but the risk of systemic toxicity due to failure of equipment or a faulty technique is always present. Local anaesthetic can be forced beneath the tourniquet into the systemic circulation if the cannula is placed in a proximal forearm or antecubital fossa vein, or if the injection is made rapidly or with force (Haasio et al. 1989). Inadvertent tourniquet deflation can occur with inadequate supervision of the equipment or inexperienced personnel. This technique should not be used by inexperienced doctors, unfamiliar with the hazards of regional anaesthesia and untrained in its management. It is not suitable for single operator-anaesthetist use, and the patient should always be attended by a trained doctor, experienced in the technique and solely responsible for the patient's care.

Tourniquet compression injury

Nerve damage due to inappropriate tourniquet application is uncommon, but it is important to pad the arm before applying the tourniquet and to position the cuff carefully over the mid-part of the upper limb, avoiding the epicondyles of the humerus. Duration of tourniquet time is not directly related to the risk of nerve damage, but the pain from direct pressure of the cuff as well as from ischaemia usually limits duration to about 1 hour.

Key references

McCartney CJL, Lin L, Shastri U (2010) Evidence basis for the use of ultrasound for upper-extremity blocks. *Regional Anesthesia & Pain Medicine* 35(Suppl 1): 10–15.

Neal JM, Gerancher JC, Hebl JR, et al. (2009) Upper extremity regional anesthesia: essentials of our current understanding 2008. *Regional Anesthesia and Pain Medicine* 34: 134–70.

On-line resources

http://www.usra.ca/
http://www.nysora.com

References

Arcand G, Williams SR, Chouinard P, et al. (2005) Ultrasound-guided infraclavicular versus supraclavicular block. *Anesthesia & Analgesia* 101: 886–90.

Auroy Y, Benhamou D, Bargues L, et al. (2002) Major complications of regional anesthesia in France: The SOS Regional Anesthesia Hotline Service. *Anesthesiology* 97: 1274–80.

Benumof JL (2000) Permanent loss of cervical spinal cord function associated with interscalene block performed under general anesthesia. *Anesthesiology* 93: 1541–4.

Candido KD, Sukhani R, Doty R, et al. (2005) Neurologic sequelae after interscalene brachial plexus block for shoulder/upper arm surgery: the association of patient, anaesthetic and surgical factors to the incidence and clinical course. *Anesthesia & Analgesia* 100: 1489–95.

Casati A, Danelli G, Baciarello M, et al. (2007) A prospective, randomized comparison between ultrasound and nerve stimulation guidance for multiple injection axillary brachial plexus block. *Anesthesiology* 106: 992–6.

Chan VWS (2003) Applying ultrasound imaging to interscalene brachial plexus block. *Regional Anesthesia and Pain Medicine* 28: 340–3.

Chan VW, Brull R, McCartney CJ, et al. (2007) An ultrasonic and histologic study of intraneural injection and electrical stimulation in pigs. *Anesthesia & Analgesia* 104: 1281–4.

Christophe JL, Berthier F, Boillot A, et al. (2009) Assessment of topographic brachial plexus nerves variations at the axilla using ultrasonography. *British Journal of Anaesthesia* 103: 606–12.

Cockings E, Moore PL, Lewis RC (1987) Transarterial brachial plexus blockade using high doses of 1.5% mepivacaine. *Regional Anesthesia and Pain Medicine* 12: 159–64.

Coventry DM, Barker KF, Thomson M (2001) Comparison of two neurostimulation techniques for brachial plexus block. *British Journal of Anaesthesia* 86: 80–3.

Delaunay L, Chelly JE (2001) Blocks at the wrist provide effective anaesthesia for carpal tunnel release. *Canadian Journal of Anaesthesia* 48: 656–60.

Desgagnés MC, Lévesque S, Dion N, et al. (2009) A comparison of a single or triple injection technique for ultrasound-guided infraclavicular block: a prospective randomized controlled study. *Anesthesia & Analgesia* 109: 668–72.

Duggan E, El Beheiry H, Perlas A, et al. (2009) Minimum effective volume of local anesthetic for ultrasound-guided supraclavicular brachial plexus block. *Regional Anesthesia and Pain Medicine* 34: 215–18.

Eisenach JC, De Kock M, Klimscha W (1996) Alpha2 agonists for regional anesthesia. *Anesthesiology* 85: 655–74.

Erickson JM, Louis DS, Naughton NN (2009) Symptomatic phrenic nerve palsy after supraclavicular block in an obese man. *Orthopedics* 32: 368.

Fanelli G, Casati A, Garancini P, Torri G (1999) Nerve stimulator and multiple injection technique for upper and lower limb blockade: failure rate, patient acceptance and neurological complications. Study Group on Regional Anaesthesia. *Anesthesia & Analgesia* 88: 847–52.

Franco CD, Domashevich V, Voronov G, et al. (2004) The supraclavicular block with a nerve stimulator: to decrease or not to decrease, that is the question. *Anesthesia & Analgesia* 98: 1167–71.

Haasio J, Hiippala S, Rosenberg PH (1989) Intravenous regional anaesthesia of the arm: effect of the technique of exsanguination on the quality of anaesthesia and prilocaine plasma concentrations. *Anaesthesia* 44: 19–21.

Heath ML (1982) Deaths after intravenous regional anaesthesia [Editorial]. *British Medical Journal* 285: 913–14.

Holmes C McK (1963) Intravenous regional anaesthesia: a useful method of producing analgesia of the limbs. *Lancet* 1: 245–7.

Horlocker TT, Kufner RP, Bishop AT, et al. (1999) The risk of persistent paraesthesia is not increased with repeated axillary blocks. *Anesthesia & Analgesia* 88: 382–7.

Ilfeld BM, Morey TE, Wright TW, et al. (2004) Interscalene perineural ropivacaine infusion: a comparison of two dosing regimens for postoperative analgesia. *Regional Anesthesia and Pain Medicine* 29: 9–16.

Kapral S, Greher M, Huber G, et al. (2008) Ultrasonic guidance improves success rate of interscalene brachial plexus block. *Regional Anaesthesia and Pain Medicine* 33: 253–8.

Kilka HG, Geiger P, Mehrkens HH (1995) Infraclavicular vertical brachial plexus blockade. A new method for anesthesia of the upper extremity. An anatomical and clinical study. *Anaesthesist* 44: 339–44.

Klaastad Ø, Smedby O, Thompson GE, et al. (2002) Distribution of local anesthetic in axillary brachial plexus block: a clinical and magnetic resonance imaging study. *Anesthesiology* 96: 1315–24.

Lanz E, Theiss Djankovic D (1983) The extent of blockade following various techniques of brachial plexus block. *Anesthesia & Analgesia* 62: 55–8.

Liisanantti O, Luukkonen J, Rosenberg PH (2004) High dose bupivacaine, levobupivacaine and ropivacaine in axillary brachial plexus block. *Acta Anaesthesiologica Scandinavica* 48: 601–6.

Macaire P, Singelyn F, Narchi P, Paqueron X (2008) Ultrasound or nerve stimulation guided wrist blocks for carpal tunnel release: a randomized prospective comparative study. *Regional Anesthesia and Pain Medicine* 33: 363–8.

Marhofer P, Sitzwohl C, Greher M, Kapral S (2004) Ultrasound guidance for infraclavicular brachial plexus anaesthesia in children. *Anaesthesia* 59: 642–6.

McCartney CJL, Duggan E, Apatu E (2007a) Should we add clonidine to local anaesthetics for peripheral nerve blockade? A qualitative systematic review of the literature. *Regional Anesthesia and Pain Medicine* 32: 330–8.

McCartney CJL, Xu D, Constantinescu C, et al. (2007b) Ultrasound examination of peripheral nerves in the forearm. *Regional Anesthesia and Pain Medicine* 32: 434–9.

McCartney CJL, Lin L, Shastri U (2010) Evidence basis for the use of ultrasound for upper-extremity blocks. *Regional Anesthesia & Pain Medicine* 35(Suppl 1): 10–15.

Moore DC, Mulroy MF, Thompson GE (1994) Peripheral nerve damage and regional anaesthesia. *British Journal of Anaesthesia* 73: 435–6.

Murphy DB, McCartney CJL, Chan VWS (2000) Novel analgesic adjuncts for brachial plexus block: a systematic review. *Anesthesia & Analgesia* 90: 1122–8.

Neal JM (2003) Effects of epinephrine in local anesthetics on the central and peripheral nervous systems: neurotoxicity and neural blood flow. *Regional Anesthesia and Pain Medicine* 28: 124–34.

Neal JM, Gerancher JC, Hebl JR, et al. (2009) Upper extremity regional anesthesia: essentials of our current understanding 2008. *Regional Anesthesia and Pain Medicine* 34: 134–70.

O'Donnell BD, Iohom G (2009) An estimation of the minimum effective anaesthetic volume of 2% lidocaine in ultrasound-guided axillary brachial plexus block. *Anesthesiology* 111: 25–9.

Perlas A, Lobo G, Lo N, et al. (2009) Ultrasound-guided supraclavicular block. *Regional Anesthesia and Pain Medicine* 34: 171–6.

Riazi S, Carmichael N, Awad I, et al. (2008) Effect of local anaesthetic volume (20ml vs 5 ml) on the efficacy and respiratory consequences of ultrasound-guided interscalene brachial plexus block. *British Journal of Anaesthesia* 101: 549–56.

Rice ASC, McMahon SB (1992) Peripheral nerve injury caused by injection needles used in regional anaesthesia: influence of bevel configuration, studied in a rat model. *British Journal of Anaesthesia* 69: 433–8.

Sardesai AM, Patel R, Denny NM, et al. (2006) Interscalene brachial plexus block: can the risk of entering the spinal cord be reduced? A study of needle angles in volunteers undergoing magnetic resonance imaging. *Anesthesiology* 105: 9–13.

Selander D, Dhuner KG, Lundborg G (1977) Peripheral nerve injury due to injection needles used for regional anaesthesia. An experimental study of the acute affects of needle point trauma. *Acta Anaesthesiologica Scandinavica* 21: 182–8.

Silverstein WB, Saiyed MU, Brown AR (2000) Interscalene block with a nerve stimulator: a deltoid motor response is a satisfactory endpoint for successful block. *Regional Anesthesia and Pain Medicine* 25: 356–9.

Sinha SK, Abrams JH, Weller RS (2007) Ultrasound-guided interscalene needle placement produces successful anaesthesia regardless of motor stimulation above or below 0.5 mA. *Anesthesia & Analgesia* 105: 848–52.

Thompson G, Rorie D (1983) Functional anatomy of the brachial plexus sheath. *Anesthesiology* 59: 117–22.

Urmey WF, Talts KH, Sharrock NE (1991) One hundred percent incidence of hemidiaphragmatic paresis associated with interscalene brachial plexus anesthesia as diagnosed by ultrasonography. *Anesthesia & Analgesia* 72: 498–503.

Wildsmith JAW, Tucker GT, Cooper S, et al. (1977) Plasma concentrations after interscalene brachial plexus block. *British Journal of Anaesthesia* 49: 461–6.

Winnie AP (1970) Interscalene brachial plexus block. *Anesthesia & Analgesia* 49: 455–66.

Winnie AP, Tay CH, Patel KP, et al. (1977) Pharmacokinetics of local anesthetics during plexus blocks. *Anesthesia & Analgesia* 56: 852–61.

CHAPTER 18

Lower limb blocks

Colin McCartney

Peripheral nerve blocks of the lower limb can provide profound intraoperative anaesthesia and postoperative analgesia without many of the side effects of central techniques. However, spinal and lumbar epidural anaesthesia and analgesia remain the most commonly performed regional techniques for lower limb surgery, and all anaesthetists should be competent in these methods. Central blocks have several disadvantages, especially when used for postoperative analgesia, and in the last decade the use of peripheral nerve blocks has become more common. This is related to a number of factors including the association of continuous epidural analgesia with increased side effects such as urinary retention and pruritis compared to peripheral (especially continuous) techniques, fear of epidural haematoma with newer more potent anticoagulants, and the significant incidence of failure of continuous epidural analgesia (up to 20% in some studies). In addition, the emergence of better techniques for localizing nerves and the availability of improved equipment have increased the popularity of blocks of the lumbar and sacral plexus.

Lower limb peripheral nerve block techniques can be challenging, especially in obese individuals, but the view that all nerve blocks of the lower limb are difficult and unreliable is incorrect. The aim of this chapter is to present simple techniques which give consistent results and may be used routinely. The use of ultrasound has, in a number of cases, increased our ability to locate lower limb nerves and appropriate techniques have been included. Only brief reference will be made to techniques which have not been found useful in routine clinical practice.

General considerations

Anatomy

Knowledge of anatomy is essential for the performance of nerve blocks in the lower limb, but no attempt will be made to describe the complete course of each nerve or to describe its anatomical relations because only comparatively small areas need to be understood in detail. The anatomy described is sufficient to permit reliable identification of each nerve.

Lumbosacral plexus

The nerve supply of the lower limb is from the lumbosacral plexus, which is formed from the anterior primary rami of the second lumbar to the third sacral roots (Figure 18.1). Each root divides

into an anterior and posterior division, and these divisions then join and branch to form the individual nerves.

Cutaneous innervation

Whereas knowledge of *dermatomal* distribution in the lower limb is needed for the proper use of spinal and epidural blocks, it is the *cutaneous* distribution of the various nerves (Figure 18.2) which determines the practical application of peripheral nerve block. This cutaneous distribution varies. For example, the junction between

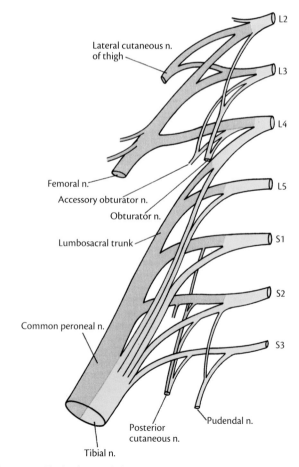

Figure 18.1 The lumbo-sacral plexus.

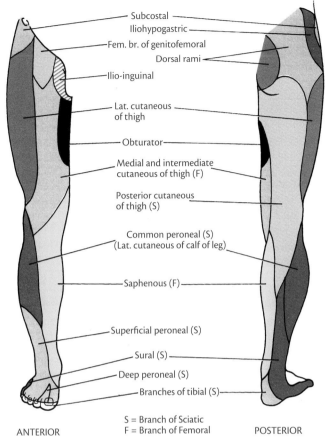

Figure 18.2 Distribution of cutaneous nerves in the lower limb.

Labels on figure:
Subcostal
Iliohypogastric
Fem. br. of genitofemoral
Dorsal rami
Ilio-inguinal
Lat. cutaneous of thigh
Obturator
Medial and intermediate cutaneous of thigh (F)
Posterior cutaneous of thigh (S)
Common peroneal (S) (Lat. cutaneous of calf of leg)
Saphenous (F)
Superficial peroneal (S)
Sural (S)
Deep peroneal (S)
Branches of tibial (S)
ANTERIOR
S = Branch of Sciatic
F = Branch of Femoral
POSTERIOR

the areas supplied by the saphenous (femoral) and the superficial peroneal (sciatic) nerves can be anywhere between the upper edge of the medial malleolus and the big toe. Such variation must be borne in mind if an operation is to be performed near the edge of the distribution of a nerve. It is essential to test carefully and block the nerve supplying the adjacent area if necessary. Most common mistakes relate to failure to block the saphenous, in addition to the popliteal nerve, for foot and ankle surgery (especially great toe surgery) or failure to block the nerves at a more proximal level if a thigh tourniquet is to be used for any duration during the operation.

Innervation of deep structures

The sensory nerve supply to deep tissues has not been as well elucidated as that of the skin. It is generally safe to assume that muscles and bones are supplied by the same peripheral nerves as the skin overlying them, but joints generally have a more complex nerve supply and receive innervation from all the nerves supplying structures around them. For example, the hip and knee joints are supplied by femoral, sciatic, and obturator nerves, and the ankle is supplied by branches of both femoral and sciatic nerves. As in the upper limb, the dermatomal innervation of *deep* structures is quite different from that of the skin. The foot is supplied by the lower roots (S_3–S_4) and the upper parts of the limb by the upper roots (L_1–L_2). However, analgesia provided by certain lower limb blocks may also relate to the musculature surrounding traumatized joints. For example, femoral nerve block after hip surgery provides

effective analgesia not only because of block of articular branches, but also relief of quadriceps muscle spasm related to the surgery (Singelyn et al. 2001).

Factors influencing choice of technique

The art of anaesthesia lies in giving each patient the most suitable anaesthetic for each operation. The choice of technique depends on the variables considered in the first part of this book, but a few points apply particularly to the use of local anaesthesia in the lower limb.

The patient

Peripheral nerve blocks have advantages in patients with cardiovascular disease because the extensive sympathetic block which may be associated with spinal or epidural anaesthesia is avoided (Fanelli et al. 1998). Spinal and epidural anaesthesia may also be contraindicated or complicated by spinal disease associated with the lower limb condition requiring surgery, or by the position of the patient who may, for example, be in fixed traction and cannot be moved until anaesthesia has been induced. Conversely, a peripheral nerve block will be impossible to perform if a plaster of Paris cast covers the injection site. Many lower limb nerves are blocked at points where they lie close to arteries. If the latter are affected by peripheral vascular disease it is important to avoid needle trauma to them and the use of ultrasound guidance can reduce this risk.

A relatively large volume of local anaesthetic is required for major lower limb blocks. If bilateral femoral and sciatic nerve blocks were to be performed at the hip, as much as 80 ml of local anaesthetic could be required, and this, in standard concentrations, could amount to a potentially toxic dose. It must be stressed that systemic concentrations after these blocks tend to be low (Connolly et al. 2001, Misra et al. 1991, Robison et al. 1991), and that toxicity is not a common problem. However, if factors are present which make such large doses particularly undesirable, a technique requiring a smaller dose of drug, such as a spinal, may be preferable. Recent studies in the literature indicate that with suitable expertise the use of ultrasound can permit effective lower limb peripheral nerve blocks with lower volumes of local anaesthetic (Casati et al. 2007).

The patient's wishes must be taken into account. Most patients will accept regional anaesthesia if it is properly explained to them, and if it is accepted practice in the unit. Generally, patients are most concerned about being awake during both block performance and surgery, but are usually much more willing to undergo these procedures if reassured that they will be adequately sedated.

The operation

Obviously, the operation dictates what sort of block is appropriate. For most orthopaedic operations on the leg, a tourniquet is used and the block must eliminate pain from the tourniquet as well as from the operative site. If tourniquet discomfort does develop, it must be dealt with promptly and effectively before the patient's response disrupts the operation. Sedation, even with an opioid analgesic, may not be adequate and recourse to a light general anaesthetic may well be necessary.

The time factor

Sciatic and femoral nerve blocks take a relatively long time because the patient has to be positioned twice and two separate injections are required. The blocks take between 15 and 30 minutes to become effective so, if speed is important, a spinal anaesthetic is a better choice. When lower limb blocks are being performed it is particularly important to organize the operating list to take this time factor into account, otherwise delay will occur and the anaesthetist will become unpopular. This is especially so if continuous catheter techniques are being performed. Having the support and cooperation of colleagues is as important as knowing where to put the needle.

Broad recommendations

Choice of block for operations on the lower limb in the average patient is not difficult: epidural and spinal blocks are undoubtedly the most useful for intraoperative anaesthesia. They are adaptable to almost all operations on the lower limb, and are so easy to perform and so reliable that they are an essential part of every anaesthetist's repertoire. They are the methods of choice for hip and knee surgery and operations involving the femoral shaft, and are also useful for bilateral operations below the knee.

However, peripheral blocks have their place especially for postoperative analgesia where their profound site specific effects produce equivalent pain control, but fewer adverse effects, than central techniques (Singelyn et al. 1998). For skin grafts from the thigh, blocks of the femoral and lateral cutaneous nerves are useful. For unilateral varicose veins, femoral nerve block, together with local infiltration to the groin, is often adequate (Vloka et al. 1997). For unilateral operations below the knee, femoral and sciatic nerve blocks are, in the opinion of many, the methods of choice. More recently the use of continuous techniques has become common, especially for hip and knee arthroplasty, where a continuous block of the lumbar plexus can reduce pain and side effects related to opioid analgesics, and facilitate rehabilitation (Singelyn et al. 1998). Major foot and ankle surgery can be extremely painful postoperatively and the use of a peripheral technique in addition to either a spinal anaesthetic or light general anaesthetic can be very beneficial (Ilfeld et al. 2002).

Individual nerve blocks are also useful in the diagnosis and treatment of chronic pain, and every anaesthetist involved in such work should be familiar with the commoner lower limb nerve blocks.

Technical aspects

The general principles of technique for blocks of the major nerves of the lower limb (factors such as choice of equipment, aseptic technique, and the dosage, latency, and duration of drugs) are much the same as for the brachial plexus (see Chapter 17). Lidocaine 1.5% and bupivacaine 0.5%, with or without adrenaline, are suitable for most lower limb blocks, but ropivacaine or levobupivacaine 0.5–0.75% may be safer alternatives to bupivacaine when prolonged block is required (see Chapters 7 and 8). Ultrasound is useful for locating the femoral nerve in the groin and sciatic nerve in the popliteal fossa, but nerve stimulation may still be preferred for location of the sciatic nerve in the thigh because it is so deeply situated, especially in obese patients.

The *siting of the tourniquet* should also be considered. For operations on the knee, it must be applied to the thigh, but, it may be applied to the calf for operations on the ankle and foot. This position is widely used in some Scandinavian countries and has been used for many years without any problems, although the precise position is important. If it is placed too high there may be pressure on the common peroneal nerve as it winds around the neck of the fibula or on the saphenous nerve where it lies on the anteromedial surface of the tibia just below the knee. If the tourniquet is too low, it will be in the surgeon's way. The advantage of placing the tourniquet on the middle of the calf (as in Figure 18.15) for operations on the ankle and foot is that nerve block at the knee will provide anaesthesia for both the tourniquet and the operation (Figure 18.2).

Lumbar plexus blocks

A number of approaches, both anterior and posterior, to the lumbar plexus have been described (Hanna et al. 1993), all with the essential aim of blocking both femoral and obturator nerves with a single injection. However, the evidence is that the posterior approaches are the most effective (Parkinson et al. 1989), there being little to choose (in terms of efficacy) between block at the L_2–L_3 (Hanna et al. 1993) or the L_4–L_5 levels (Chayen et al. 1976). The latter is also known as the '*psoas compartment*' block and has two potential advantages: the components of the plexus are somewhat closer together at that level; and the landmarks are rather better defined. The caveat to the use of the psoas compartment block is that it has the highest incidence of complications (including epidural spread) of all peripheral blocks (Gadsden et al. 2008). It also produces a high incidence of haematoma and therefore any coagulopathy should be regarded as a contraindication to its use (Horlocker et al. 2010).

Psoas compartment block

Anatomy

The lumbar plexus is formed by the ventral rami of the first three and major part of the fourth lumbar nerves (Figure 18.1). After emerging from the lateral foramina of the vertebral column, the nerves run inferolaterally and are first located within the posterior part of the psoas major muscle (see Figure 23.9). This muscle is enclosed in a fascial sheath limited medially by the bodies of the lumbar vertebrae, and posteriorly by the lumbar transverse processes, ligaments, and quadratus lumborum. The femoral and lateral cutaneous nerves emerge from the lateral, and the obturator nerve from the medial aspects of psoas, respectively. After emerging from psoas, the nerves lie in a fascial compartment between it and quadratus lumborum. Local anaesthetic injected into psoas, or into the potential space between psoas and quadratus lumborum, should block all three nerves.

Clinical application

Lumbar plexus block is frequently combined with sciatic nerve block to provide analgesia of the whole lower limb in situations when central nerve block is contraindicated. It may be used as the sole technique for femoral neck surgery or be combined with a general anaesthetic to provide postoperative analgesia. This combination is particularly useful for prolonged revision hip surgery. Although there is usually good cardiovascular stability, epidural spread can occur and appears more common with the psoas compartment approach (Parkinson et al. 1989), particularly in children (Dalens et al. 1988) and when high injection pressures are used (Gadsden et al. 2008). Parkinson and colleagues (1989) recorded a block as high as T_6, but this may have been related to the relatively large dose of local anaesthetic used (0.5 ml kg^{-1}). Hanna and colleagues (1993) believe that as little as 10 ml will block the lumbar plexus without the risk of epidural spread, but volumes of 25–30 ml are used more commonly.

Technique

The patient is positioned in the lateral decubitus position with the operative side uppermost. Initially, the fourth lumbar spine is identified from its relationship to the iliac crests. A point 3 cm caudad to this, and 5 cm lateral to the midline, is marked and the skin and subcutaneous tissue infiltrated with local anaesthetic. A 21-g, 100-mm short-bevelled insulated needle is attached to a nerve stimulator and advanced perpendicular to all planes until the transverse process of L_5 is located at a depth of approximately 5 cm. Usually the paraspinal muscles can be seen to contract before the needle reaches the transverse process. The needle is then withdrawn and advanced with progressively increased cephalad angulation until it 'glides' above the transverse process. As the needle is advanced further, contractions of the quadriceps femoris muscle are elicited, usually when the needle tip is 1–2 cm deeper than the transverse process. When the stimulating current can be decreased to 0.5 mA whilst maintaining quadriceps contractions 25–30 ml of local anaesthetic is injected incrementally and slowly, and will usually produce complete block within 15 minutes.

Ultrasound guidance can be used both to judge vertebral level (Chapter 14) and to guide needle placement toward the space above the transverse process (Karmakar et al. 2008) and the lumbar plexus. Nerve stimulation is very helpful in assisting with correct placement of the needle tip when combined with ultrasound. A catheter can be inserted, and is usually placed after the initial bolus of local anaesthetic (Capdevila et al. 2005).

Nerve block at the hip

Block of the lumbar plexus

The sheath concept and the 3-in-1 block

Winnie and colleagues (1973) noted that the femoral, lateral cutaneous, and obturator nerves, all branches of the lumbar plexus, lie in the same myofascial plane, and theorized that injection of a large volume of local anaesthetic into that plane would result in spread to affect all three nerves. Their original description (Winnie et al. 1973) demonstrated such spread radiographically, but subsequent studies have failed to confirm satisfactory spread to all three nerves. Local anaesthetic appears to spread under the fascia iliaca, between the iliacus and psoas muscles, but only rarely reaches the lumbar plexus (Capdevila et al. 1998). In practice, injection of sufficient local anaesthetic under the fascia iliaca at most points along the inguinal ligament will block the femoral and lateral cutaneous nerves, but obturator block is rare (20%) with this method, and only achieved with large (> 20 ml) volumes of local anaesthetic.

Femoral nerve block

Anatomy

The femoral nerve (L_2–L_4) runs down the posterolateral wall of the pelvis behind the fascia iliaca, lying on the psoas and iliacus muscles. The femoral artery and vein lie anterior to the fascia iliaca, which sweeps downwards and forwards from the posterior and lateral walls of the pelvis and blends with the inguinal ligament. As the vessels pass behind the inguinal ligament they become invested in a fascial sheath. The femoral nerve lies *behind and lateral* to this sheath and, unlike the vessels, is not within it. All three are deep to the fascia lata. Just below the inguinal ligament the nerve divides into several branches (Figure 18.3). Because of these factors, femoral nerve block is not as easy as may be thought. Moore (1965), states that when sciatic and femoral nerve blocks are combined, and found to be inadequate, it is usually the femoral nerve which has been missed. The location of the nerve is more consistent closer to the inguinal ligament where the nerve is almost always seen at the anteromedial border of the iliopsoas muscle (see Figure 18.5b) just lateral to the common femoral artery. Below this level the origin of the profunda femoris artery does lead to greater variability in the location of the nerve.

Clinical application

It is important to stress that, although femoral nerve block is not always easy, it is a useful technique, and well worth mastering. The majority of incisions for varicose vein surgery are made within its distribution and it may be used alone or in combination with block of the lateral cutaneous nerve for the taking of skin grafts from the thigh. It is suitable for many orthopaedic operations on the leg and foot, and can provide analgesia for a fracture of the upper part of the femoral shaft. Femoral nerve catheter techniques are very useful for providing continuous pain relief after major knee surgery, reducing opioid consumption and facilitating postoperative rehabilitation (Carli et al. 2010).

Technique

A line drawn between the anterior superior iliac spine and the pubic tubercle marks the position of the inguinal ligament. The femoral artery is palpated where it passes behind the midpoint of the ligament, and the needle is inserted just below the ligament and

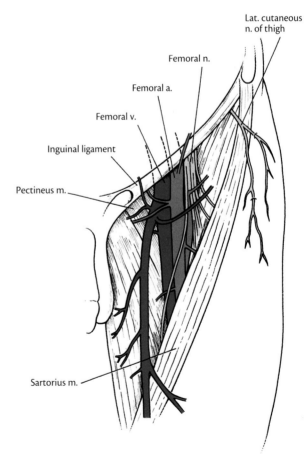

Figure 18.3 Positions of the femoral and lateral cutaneous nerves.

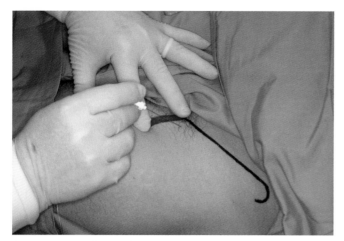

Figure 18.4 Femoral nerve block.

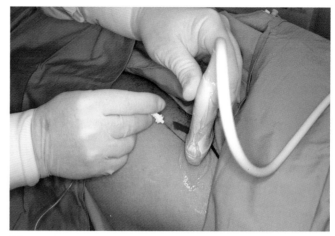

(a)

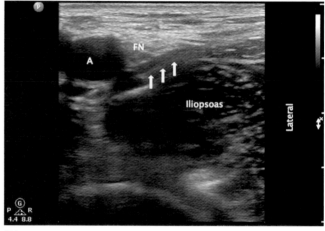

(b)

Figure 18.5 Technique of ultrasound-guided femoral nerve block (a) and sonographic anatomy (b). (FN = femoral nerve, A = artery, arrows indicate needle shaft passing from anterolateral to posteromedial.)

1 cm lateral to the artery (Figure 18.4). With the nerve stimulator set at 1.5 mA, the needle is advanced towards the nerve at an angle of about 45°. A 'click' is felt as the needle passes through the fascia lata and, after advancing with a gentle probing motion, a second 'click' is noted as the needle penetrates the fascia iliaca. The needle is advanced further until quadriceps contractions are seen to move the patella ('patellar tap') before the current is reduced and the needle manipulated until contractions are maintained at 0.5 mA. If the needle has been inserted to a depth of 3 or 4 cm without finding the nerve, it should be withdrawn and the direction changed slightly, either medially or laterally. Once the nerve is located, the needle is immobilized and an aspiration test performed before 15–20 ml of local anaesthetic solution is injected.

Using ultrasound a very similar (out-of-plane) technique can be used, the nerve being visualized just lateral to the femoral artery at the level of the inguinal ligament (see Figure 18.5). A linear, high-frequency probe is used because of the superficial position of the nerve, and prepared for a sterile procedure in the usual manner. Often, the fasciae are not visible, but the needle tip can be seen 'popping' through the individual layers prior to reaching its final position, with stimulation being a useful (but not essential) adjunct for confirming correct placement. An in-plane technique can also be used to place the needle tip (or catheter) either lateral to the nerve (just under the fascia iliaca) or deep to it prior to injection.

Lateral cutaneous nerve of thigh

Anatomy

The lateral cutaneous nerve of the thigh (lateral femoral cutaneous nerve) (L_2–L_3) runs forward in a curve on the iliacus muscle outside the pelvic viscera and fascia iliaca. Anteriorly, it passes behind the inguinal ligament to enter the thigh deep to the fascia lata, 1–2 cm medial to the anterior superior iliac spine (Figure 18.3). In the thigh, it divides into two branches, anterior and posterior, which pierce the fascia lata about 10 cm below the anterior superior iliac spine and supply the skin of the lateral aspect of the thigh.

Clinical application

The block is usually combined with others to provide anaesthesia of the lower limb. Because the lateral aspect of the thigh is used frequently as a skin graft donor site, this block is a useful adjunct to general anaesthesia for skin harvesting, providing excellent postoperative analgesia. However, it should only be used as the sole anaesthetic technique if the donor site is small and lies well within the distribution of the nerve.

Technique

The nerve is blocked where it emerges below the inguinal ligament. The patient lies supine and the anterior superior iliac spine is palpated and marked. The needle is introduced perpendicularly through the skin 1 cm medial to, and 2 cm below, the anterior superior iliac spine. After passing through skin and subcutaneous tissue, slight resistance to needle advancement is felt and then a 'click' as the needle passes through the fascia lata. After aspiration, 2 ml local anaesthetic solution is injected. The needle tip is then withdrawn into the subcutaneous tissues, redirected laterally and advanced deep to the fascia lata where it will be approximately 1 cm from the original injection site. A further 2 ml of local anaesthetic is then injected. This process is repeated medial to the original injection site.

This is a fairly easy block with a high success rate although, like many blocks, it can be difficult in obese patients because the correct tissue plane is hard to identify. However, the following procedure may overcome this. Once the needle tip is in the subcutaneous tissues, a finger is placed either side of the needle shaft and moved from side to side. Initially, the needle will move with the subcutaneous tissues, but once it has penetrated the fascia lata it will be anchored in place.

Using ultrasound the lateral femoral cutaneous nerve can be identified just below the level of the inguinal ligament, deep to the fascia lata and superficial to sartorius. A needle is inserted in-plane towards the nerve, and a single injection of 5 ml of local anaesthetic is usually sufficient to block the nerve at this level.

Obturator nerve block

The obturator nerve (L$_2$–L$_4$) slants down the side wall of the pelvis to the upper part of the obturator foramen where it divides into anterior and posterior branches and passes into the thigh. It sends branches to the hip and knee joints and supplies the adductor muscles as well as a variable area of skin on the inside of the thigh. Although obturator nerve block is a relatively simple technique (Choquet et al. 2005), its clinical usefulness is limited because the contribution to the innervation of the knee is both variable and relatively small. However, an occasional patient may complain of medial pain after knee surgery and benefit from an obturator block once the more common cause of pain in the distribution of the femoral and sciatic nerves has been excluded.

Sciatic nerve block

Anatomy

The sciatic, the largest nerve in the body, starts in the pelvis as the continuation of the sacral plexus (Figure 18.1) and passes from the pelvis into the buttock through the greater sciatic foramen. At this point, it is accompanied by the posterior cutaneous nerve of the thigh which can be thought of as a branch of the sciatic.

After emerging from the greater sciatic foramen, the nerve is just posterior to the acetabulum and the head of the femur (Figure 18.6), lying on the muscles around the hip joint (piriformis then quadratus femoris) and covered by gluteus maximus. It then runs vertically downwards in the hamstring compartment (deep to biceps femoris) to reach the popliteal fossa, where it divides into common peroneal and tibial branches (see Figure 18.10). Occasionally, this division occurs much higher up. The tibial nerve passes vertically downwards through the calf to supply the heel and sole of the foot. The common peroneal nerve winds diagonally across the popliteal fossa to the lateral aspect of the calf before descending to the foot where its branches innervate the dorsal structures. The sural nerve is formed from branches of these two nerves and supplies the lateral border of the foot (see Figure 18.14).

Clinical application

Block of the sciatic in the buttock is easy and reliable, producing anaesthesia of the back of the thigh (because of the close relationship to the posterior cutaneous nerve), the anterolateral part of the leg, and most of the foot. In combination with femoral or saphenous nerve block, it provides anaesthesia for the whole of the leg below the knee. It causes motor block of the hamstrings as well as of the muscles of the lower leg.

Techniques

Several landmark-based methods have been described for blocking the sciatic nerve at the level of the hip joint including the posterior (Labat 1922), anterior (Beck 1963), superficial (Raj et al. 1975),

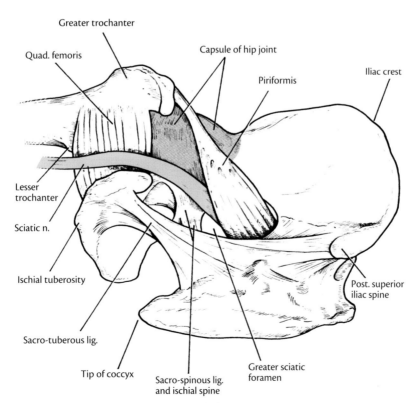

Figure 18.6 The position of the sciatic nerve relative to the major structures near the hip joint.

lateral (Guardini et al. 1985), and parasacral (Mansour 1993) approaches. A modification of the 'Raj' technique is preferred because it is undoubtedly the easiest and it has the highest success rate, although the anterior approach may be useful if the patient is in pain and cannot be moved. Ultrasound can be used (Chan et al. 2006), but the sciatic can be a challenging nerve to locate, especially in the obese individual.

Modified Raj approach

Correct positioning is vital if this block is to be carried out effectively. The patient lies with the side to be blocked uppermost, the lower leg straight, and both hip and knee joints flexed so that the thigh is at right angles to the body. The greater trochanter and ischial tuberosity are palpated and their greatest prominences marked so that the midpoint between the two can be identified and also marked as the point for needle insertion (Figure 18.7). The nerve is just lateral to the ischial tuberosity and if the fingers are 'rolled' off it in a lateral direction a groove may be felt between the two bony prominences. This is where the nerve lies, just deep to gluteus maximus.

Under aseptic conditions, local anaesthetic is infiltrated into the skin and muscle. A 100-mm needle, connected to a nerve stimulator set to deliver 2 mA, is inserted at right angles to the skin and advanced until dorsiflexion or plantar flexion of the foot is elicited. Hamstring muscle contraction usually indicates that the needle tip is too deep and medial to the nerve. If bone is encountered without muscle contraction, the needle is withdrawn, its direction reassessed, and it is reinserted more medially or laterally. With the correct motor response, the needle is manipulated until the contractions are maintained with the current reduced to about 0.5 mA. The needle is then held firmly in position and 20 ml of local anaesthetic is injected.

The utrasound technique (Chan et al. 2006) visualizes the nerve deep in the gluteus maximus muscle between the bony landmarks of the greater trochanter and ischial tuberosity (Figure 18.8). A low-frequency, curved array probe is used to enable a wider field of view and visualization of deeper structures. Usually the bony landmarks are identified first, then the muscles, and finally the nerve is seen as a 'lozenge'-shaped structure just lateral to the ischial tuberosity. A common error is to mistake the conjoint tendon (common tendon of the hamstrings) for the nerve at this level so it is good practice to trace the nerve, once identified, up and down the thigh to confirm the anatomy. A needle can then be inserted either in or out of plane to reach the sciatic nerve. Nerve stimulation can be used for secondary confirmation, but a motor response is not always obtained despite proximity of needle tip to nerve (see Chapter 10). After careful injection of local anaesthetic spread around the nerve can be confirmed by ultrasound visualization.

Anterior approach

The patient lies supine. The anterior superior iliac spine and the pubic tubercle are palpated and marked, and a line is drawn between them to represent the inguinal ligament (Figure 18.9). This line is divided into three equal parts and a perpendicular dropped from the junction of the medial and middle thirds. A line is then drawn from the top of the greater trochanter parallel to the line of the inguinal ligament and the point where it meets the perpendicular is the point of needle insertion. This overlies the lesser trochanter on the inner aspect of the femur and, at this level, the sciatic nerve lies close behind the acetabulum and the head of the femur.

After skin cleansing, a wheal of local anaesthetic is raised, a fairly long (e.g. 150-mm, 21-g) insulated needle is inserted and directed slightly laterally so that it strikes the medial surface of the femur. It is then withdrawn and 'walked' off the femur so that it passes medial to the femoral head. Some anaesthetists believe that if the needle is inserted 5 cm deeper than its point of contact with the femur it will lie very close to the nerve, and that a good block will result if the local anaesthetic can be injected easily and without resistance. However, this is not always the case so it is better to use a nerve stimulator and elicit plantar flexion of the foot. After careful aspiration, 20 ml of local anaesthetic is injected.

Computed tomography (Charlton et al. 1987) has shown that the sciatic nerve often lies more laterally behind the femur than was previously appreciated so that it is impossible to insert the needle close to the nerve when using the landmarks already described. Use of a more medial insertion point, with more lateral direction of the needle may lead to a higher success rate, but recent cadaver and volunteer studies have suggested that *internal* rotation of the hip may be more helpful (Moore et al. 2004, Vloka et al. 2001).

An ultrasound-guided technique has been described (Ota et al. 2009).

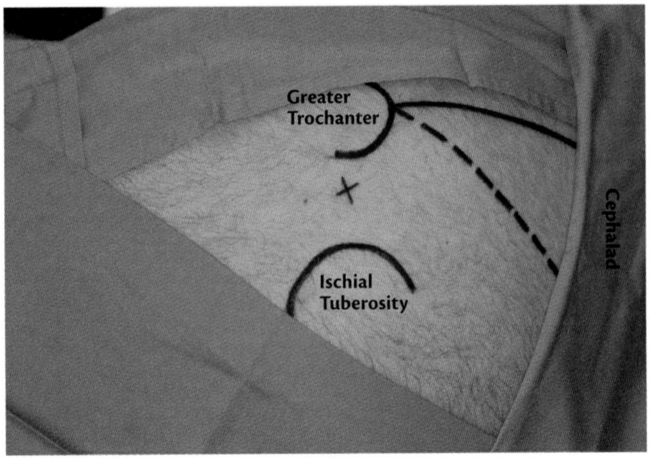

Figure 18.7 Landmarks for modified Raj approach to the sciatic nerve with the point of needle insertion marked.

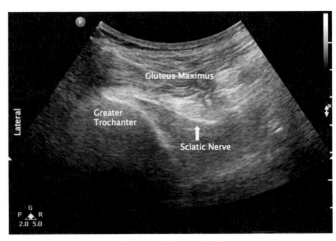

Figure 18.8 Ultrasound-guided sciatic block at the hip.

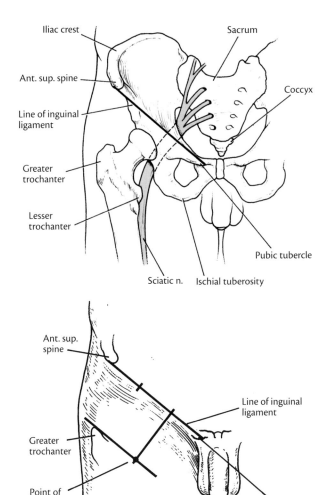

Figure 18.9 Landmarks for the anterior approach to the sciatic nerve.

Nerve block at the knee

Sciatic nerve (popliteal fossa) block

Block of the sciatic nerve in the popliteal fossa anaesthetizes the foot and most of the leg, although complete block of the two major terminal nerves may be less consistent than with the posterior approach at the hip (Kilpatrick et al. 1992). Its advantage is that widespread motor block above the knee is avoided making it more suitable for many patients and for day surgery. When positioning is a problem, a lateral approach can be considered, but will not be described further here (Hadzic & Vloka 1998).

Technique

The patient lies prone and the leg is gently lifted to flex the knee joint so that the tendons of the biceps femoris (laterally) and semi-membranosus with semitendinosus (medially) stand out. A line is drawn in the flexion crease between these tendons and, from its middle, a perpendicular is drawn upwards for 10–15 cm to the apex of the fossa (Figure 18.10). The point of needle insertion is 1 cm lateral to the top of this perpendicular, the sciatic nerve lying slightly to the side, not in the middle, of the fossa. A 50-mm, 22-g insulated needle, attached to a nerve stimulator, is inserted parallel to the perpendicular, but angled 30–45° cephalad, and advanced gently until a motor response in the foot is elicited. The nerve is normally 3–5 cm deep to the skin. If no response is obtained the needle is withdrawn almost to the skin and redirected laterally or medially, but with only small changes in direction or the nerve may be missed. The most complete block of both terminal nerves appears to be obtained by eliciting either dorsiflexion, inversion, or a combination of inversion and plantar flexion with the current at or below 0.5 mA (Benzon et al. 1997).

The ultrasound-guided block (Figure 18.11) can be performed either in or out of plane. It is easiest to start by visualizing the tibial nerve just lateral and posterior to the popliteal artery at the popliteal crease, and then to trace it superiorly until it joins the

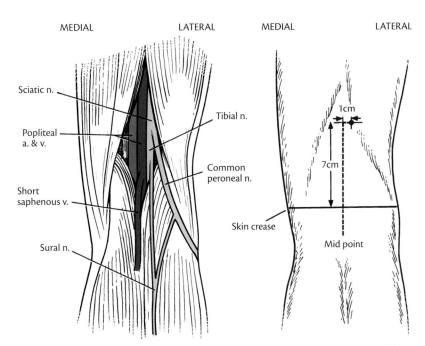

Figure 18.10 Sciatic nerve block in the popliteal fossa. The perpendicular from the skin crease is extended to overlie the apex of the fossa.

peroneal at the apex of the fossa (Figure 18.10) (Tsui & Finucane 2006). The nerve can be accentuated by asking the patient to dorsiflex and plantarflex the ankle causing the nerve to rotate (the 'see-saw' sign: Shafhalter-Zoppoth et al. 2004).

Popliteal block is performed with 20–30 ml of local anaesthetic, but the onset time can be at least 40 minutes. Recent studies have shown that onset is fastest when the block is performed just distal to the bifurcation of tibial and peroneal nerves (Buys et al. 2010).

Saphenous nerve block

The saphenous nerve (Figure 18.12) is the terminal branch of the femoral nerve and supplies the skin of the anteromedial aspect of the leg although the lower border of this area is variable. Because most operations on the ankle and foot require a tourniquet, saphenous nerve block can be used to provide complete analgesia for a mid-calf tourniquet.

The nerve runs down through the thigh in the adductor canal under the sartorius muscle. It pierces the fascia lata between the tendons of sartorius and gracilis on the inner aspect of the knee joint and becomes subcutaneous. In thin people, the nerve can often be rolled under the fingers where it lies on the medial aspect

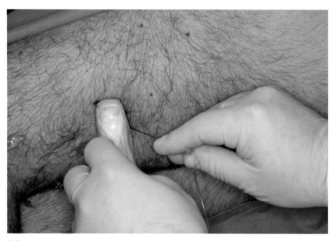

(a)

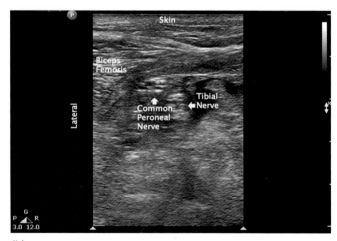

(b)

Figure 18.11 Technique of ultrasound-guided popliteal block (a) and related sonographic anatomy (b).

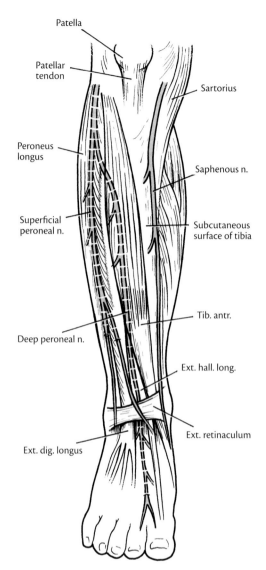

Figure 18.12 Nerves on the anterior aspect of the leg and foot.

of the head of the tibia, about 2 cm below the lower border of the patella. The long saphenous vein is a close relation here and is a useful landmark. The nerve is blocked by infiltrating 10 ml of local anaesthetic into the subcutaneous tissues at this point, the proximity of the vein making aspiration particularly important.

The most practical ultrasound technique (Figure 18.13) blocks the nerve as it lies just superficial to the femoral artery under sartorius in the adductor canal 10–15 cm proximal to the knee joint (Manickam 2009). Five to 10 ml of local anaesthetic will block the nerve at this level.

Distal blocks of the lower limb

Ankle block

In order to anaesthetize the foot by injecting at the level of the ankle, it is necessary to block five nerves: the saphenous (terminal branch of the femoral) and four (tibial, sural, superficial peroneal, and deep peroneal) derived from the sciatic. Although technically straightforward, ankle block has limited use because multiple injections are uncomfortable for the patient (anatomical knowledge may

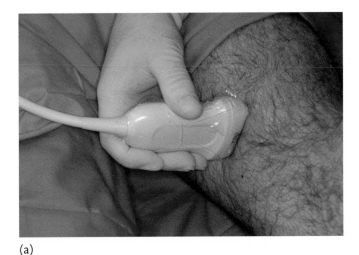

(a)

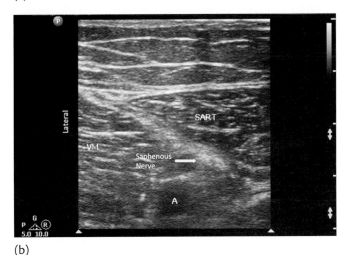

(b)

Figure 18.13 Ultrasound-guided saphenous nerve block (a) and sonographic anatomy (b). (VM = vastus medialis, A = artery, SART = sartorius.)

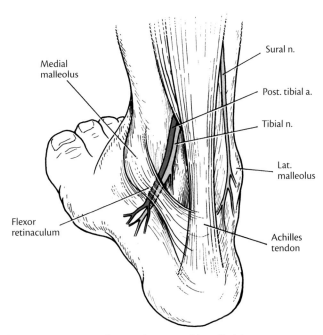

Figure 18.14 Nerves on the posterior aspect of the ankle joint.

help reduce the number, but most procedures will require tibial nerve block with at least one other) and incomplete blocks occur with depressing regularity. Further, most procedures on the foot require a tourniquet so ankle block is only really appropriate for supplementing incomplete proximal blocks or to provide postoperative analgesia.

The saphenous nerve is blocked just above, and slightly anterior to, the medial malleolus by infiltrating subcutaneously from the midline to the medial malleolus (Figure 18.12); the tibial nerve immediately behind the medial malleolus and posterior to the posterior tibial artery (Figure 18.14); the sural behind the lateral malleolus (Figure 18.14); the deep peroneal between the tendons of tibialis anterior and extensor digitorum longus on the anterior aspect of the ankle (or on either side of the dorsalis pedis if palpable) (Figure 18.12); and the superficial peroneal nerve by infiltrating subcutaneously across the anterior aspect of the ankle joint (Figure 18.12).

The important landmark of the tibial artery may be absent and a more distal structure, the sustentaculum tali, felt as a bony ridge 1–2 cm distal to the medial malleolus, provides a much more useful landmark for accurate tibial nerve block (Wassef 1991). The needle is inserted perpendicularly at a point inferior and posterior to this

ridge, and 5–8 ml of local anaesthetic injected. There should be no resistance to injection.

Ultrasound can be useful for identifying and infiltrating around the tibial nerve posterior to the medial malleolus where it lies posterior to the tendon of tibialis posterior and the tibial artery (TAN: tendon, artery, nerve).

Digital nerve block

Digital nerve block is a simple, safe, effective, and extremely useful technique and is probably underused, especially as a means of postoperative analgesia. After operations on the toes in which periosteum is damaged (e.g. osteotomy or nail-bed ablation), postoperative pain can be severe and out of all proportion to the scale of the procedure. Even if a general anaesthetic is used for the operation itself, a digital nerve block with 0.5% *plain* bupivacaine can provide analgesia for more than 12 hours. The technique is essentially the same as described for the upper limb (see Chapter 17).

Intravenous regional anaesthesia (IVRA)

IVRA (Figure 18.15) is not used as widely for lower limb as for upper limb procedures. Although this may be because procedures for which it is suited are seen less often in the lower limb, it is more probably because the technique is not considered to be practical. The large dose of local anaesthetic required if the tourniquet is placed on the thigh can result in a significant incidence of problems due to systemic toxicity, yet operative and tourniquet pain are very frequent (Valli et al. 1987). If the tourniquet is placed at mid-calf level the dose of drug used is the same as in the upper limb and the technique is identical in every respect (see Chapter 17). However, tourniquet discomfort can still be a problem and some workers find that anaesthesia is not as reliable as in the upper limb (Fagg 1987, Valli & Rosenberg 1986). This suggests that case selection is very important.

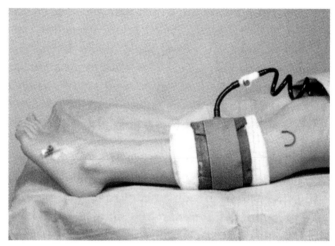

Figure 18.15 IVRA in the lower limb. The head of the fibula has been marked to show that the tourniquet is well below the lateral popliteal nerve.

Continuous infusion techniques

One of the great advantages of peripheral block techniques is the ability to extend the excellent analgesia into the postoperative period. With bupivacaine and ropivacaine, even a single injection will last in excess of 14, and sometimes as long as 24, hours, but many procedures, such as knee replacement or amputation, are associated with considerable pain for at least the first 48 hours. Continuation of the block using a catheter technique will allow for this and, in some situations, may also facilitate active rehabilitation and physiotherapy, and encourage earlier mobilization and restoration of limb function. The effectiveness of continuous blocks will depend on the innervation of the area involved, but careful selection of the key nerve as the site of infusion will provide excellent analgesia, particularly if combined initially with single block of other relevant nerves. The effect may be enhanced further, if necessary, by incorporation in a multimodal approach to reduce the need for opioids and minimize their well-recognized side effects.

Two recent advances have facilitated the use of continuous peripheral blocks. First, the stimulating catheter has increased the ability to place the tip adjacent to the nerve and reduce the incidence of secondary failure of analgesia (failure after the effect of the primary bolus has receded) (Morin et al. 2010). Secondly, ultrasound guidance not only facilitates accurate placement of both needle and catheter, but also allows identification of appropriate spread of local anaesthetic from the catheter and around the nerve (Koscielniak-Nielsen et al. 2008).

Continuous sciatic block

Continuous sciatic nerve block, possible at a number of sites, is the most useful single nerve infusion technique in the lower limb, with the modified Raj approach being very effective for procedures carried out below the knee, particularly amputation (Connolly & Coventry 1998). A 110-mm, 18-g needle is placed as described earlier, and catheter insertion can be facilitated by creating space with an initial injection of 20 ml of local anaesthetic solution through the needle. Some 5–10 cm of catheter can usually be inserted before the needle is removed and the catheter carefully secured to skin with a clear adhesive dressing and tape. A femoral nerve block is added to complete surgical anaesthesia, and the sciatic block continued postoperatively by infusing ropivacaine 0.2% at about 6 ml h^{-1}.

Continuous parasacral block by infusion of bupivacaine 0.1% at 8 ml h^{-1} has also been described for similar cases, an insulated Tuohy needle being used for catheter placement (Morris & Lang 1997). For surgery around the foot and ankle, the sciatic nerve catheter can be placed in the popliteal fossa (Singelyn et al. 1997).

Continuous lumbar plexus or femoral block

The applicability of a single infusion for analgesia after most surgery of the hip or knee is less clear because of the multiple innervation of these joints, the issue being further complicated by debate over exactly which nerves are blocked by the various approaches to the lumbar plexus. In addition, the incision for hip arthroplasty may extend into the lower thoracic (T$_{12}$) dermatome or curve into the sacral innervation of the buttock so it is unlikely that a single infusion will provide complete pain control after most hip and knee procedures. However, such techniques can make a highly significant contribution to improving the quality of analgesia and reducing opioid requirements.

Continuous femoral nerve block is very useful for minimizing pain and adverse effects after knee surgery, and allowing more effective rehabilitation compared to both intravenous and epidural approaches (Singelyn et al. 1998). For complete immediate postoperative analgesia, an additional sciatic nerve block is needed, although longer-term pain control can be achieved by continuous lumbar plexus block alone performed using the femoral approach (Mansour & Bennetts 1996). It is probable that many patients will do well without sciatic nerve block after knee surgery, but it is difficult to predict who they are so many practitioners combine a continuous femoral block with a single bolus sciatic technique for that reason.

Providing continuous analgesia after major hip surgery is more contentious, with few appropriate, controlled studies available. Often, obturator nerve block is used to relieve hip pain, but the anterior capsule is innervated by branches of the femoral nerve, and the posterior capsule by branches of sciatic and superior gluteal nerves (Birnbaum et al. 1997). In addition, the majority of incisions are within the lateral cutaneous nerve's territory, and often extend into sacral and lower thoracic dermatomes. All of these nerves need to be blocked to provide complete surgical anaesthesia, although the posterior approaches to the lumbar plexus can be used to provide postoperative analgesia. More reliable block of the principal lumbar plexus nerves is produced, particularly the obturator nerve which is not blocked consistently by the femoral approach (Capdevila et al. 1998, Parkinson et al. 1989). In the majority of cases the plexus can be reached using a 110-mm, 18-g cannula and catheter by the posterior approach described earlier. The initial injection of 30 ml ropivacaine 0.75% through the needle should create space to facilitate catheter insertion. Subsequent infusion of ropivacaine 0.2% at a rate of about 6 ml h^{-1} is then used to prolong the analgesia. Given the dose of local anaesthetic used, it would be inappropriate to combine this block with others if subsequent infusion is contemplated.

Local infiltration analgesia (LIA)

The injection of local anaesthetics and other, adjuvant drugs into the tissues around the surgical site is increasing in popularity partly because of its simplicity, and partly because of the improved analgesia reported in comparison to placebo techniques after both hip

(Kerr & Kohan 2008) and knee arthroplasty (Essving et al. 2009). Typical mixtures include ropivacaine (200–400 mg), ketorolac 30 mg, and adrenaline 0.5 mg injected into the joint capsule in a total volume of 100–150 ml once the prosthesis is inserted. It is also possible to place a periarticular catheter on completion of surgery for the injection of further doses in the postoperative period (Toftdahl et al. 2007). Current evidence suggests that LIA lacks benefit after hip arthroplasty, but does provide short duration (6–12 hours) pain relief after knee arthroplasty (Kehlet & Andersen 2011). It may be a useful technique, but only in the absence of expertise at performing effective continuous femoral nerve block (Carli et al. 2010), and is possibly better than epidural analgesia (Spreng et al. 2010). A recent randomized study also demonstrated the benefit of the use of a low dose of intrathecal morphine (100 mcg) in comparison with single injection femoral block for total knee arthroplasty (Frassanito et al. 2010). However, continuous femoral nerve block remains the peripheral block of choice both for improved pain control and rehabilitation after total knee arthroplasty (Carli et al. 2010, McCartney & McLeod 2011).

Key reading

Enneking FK, Chan V, Greger J, et al. (2005) Lower-extremity peripheral nerve blockade: essentials of our current understanding. *Regional Anesthesia & Pain Medicine* 30: 4–35.

On-line resources

http://asra.com/pain-resource-center-regional-anesthesia-lower-extremity-blocks.php
http://www.usra.ca/ugt_sb
http://www.nysora.com

References

Beck GP (1963) Anterior approach to sciatic nerve block. *Anesthesiology* 24: 222.

Benzon HT, Kim C, Benzon H, et al. (1997) Correlation between evoked motor responses of the sciatic nerve and sensory blockade. *Anesthesiology* 87: 547–52.

Birnbaum K, Prescher A, Hessler S, Heller KD (1997) The sensory innervation of the hip joint—an anatomical study. *Surgical and Radiologic Anatomy* 19: 371–5.

Buckley JR, Hood GM, Macrae W (1989) Arthroscopy under local anaesthesia. *Journal of Bone and Joint Surgery* 71B: 126–7.

Buys MJ, Arndt CD, Vagh F, et al. (2010) Ultrasound-guided sciatic nerve block in the popliteal fossa using a lateral approach: onset time comparing separate tibial and common peroneal nerve injections versus injecting proximal to the bifurcation. *Anesthesia & Analgesia* 110: 635–7.

Capdevila X, Biboulet P, Bouregba M, et al. (1998) Comparison of the 3-in-1 and fascia iliaca compartment blocks in adults: clinical and radiographic analysis. *Anesthesia & Analgesia* 86: 1039–44.

Capdevila X, Coimbra C, Choquet O (2005) Approaches to the lumbar plexus: success, risks and outcome *Regional Anesthesia & Pain Medicine* 30: 150–62.

Carli F, Clemente A, Asenjo JF, et al. (2010) Analgesia and functional outcome after total knee arthroplasty: periarticular infiltration vs continuous femoral nerve block. *British Journal of Anaesthesia* 105: 185–95.

Casati A, Baciarello M, Di Cianni S, et al. (2007) Effects of ultrasound guidance on the minimum effective anaesthetic volume required to block the femoral nerve. *British Journal of Anaesthesia* 98: 823–7.

Chan VW, Nova H, Abbas S, et al. (2006) Utrasound examination and localization of the sciatic nerve: a volunteer study *Anesthesiology* 104: 309–14.

Charlton JE, Nicholls BJ, White E (1987) Anterior and lateral approaches to the sciatic nerve: a study using computerized tomography. *British Journal of Anaesthesia* 59: 127P.

Chayen D, Nathan H, Chayen M (1976) The psoas compartment block. *Anesthesiology* 45: 95–9.

Choquet O, Capdevila X, Bennourine K, et al. (2005) A new inguinal approach for the obturator nerve block: anatomical and randomized clinical studies. *Anesthesiology* 103: 1238–45.

Connolly C, Coventry DM (1998) Combined sciatic/femoral block followed by sciatic infusion of ropivacaine 2mg/ml for below knee amputation; a feasibility study. *Regional Anesthesia* 23 (Suppl): 81.

Connolly C, Coventry D, Wildsmith JAW (2001) A double-blind comparison of ropivacaine 7.5mg/ml with bupivacaine 5mg/ml for sciatic nerve block. *British Journal of Anaesthesia* 86: 674–7.

Dalens B, Tanguy A, Vanneuville G (1988) Lumbar plexus block in children. A comparison of two procedures in 50 patients. *Anesthesia & Analgesia* 67: 750–8.

Essving P, Axelsson K, Kjellberg J, et al. (2009) Reduced hospital stay, morphine consumption, and pain intensity with local infiltration analgesia after unicompartmental knee arthroplasty. *Acta Orthopaedica* 80: 213–19.

Fagg P (1987) Intravenous regional anaesthesia for lower limb orthopaedic surgery. *Annals of the Royal College of Surgeons of England* 69: 274–5.

Fanelli G, Casati A, Aldegheri G, et al. (1998) Cardiovascular effects of two different regional anaesthetic techniques for unilateral leg surgery. *Acta Anaesthesiologica Scandinavica* 42: 80–4.

Frassanito L, Vergari A, Zanghi F, et al. (2010) Post-operative analgesia following total knee arthroplasty: comparison of low-dose intrathecal morphine and single-shot ultrasound-guided femoral nerve block: a randomized, single blinded, controlled study. *European Review of Medical and Pharmacological Science* 14: 589–96.

Gadsden JC, Lindenmuth DM, Hadzic A, et al. (2008) Lumbar plexus block using high-pressure injection leads to contralateral and epidural spread. *Anesthesiology* 109: 683–8.

Greengrass RA, Klein SM, D'Ercole FJ, et al. (1998) Lumbar plexus and sciatic nerve block for knee arthroplasty: comparison of ropivacaine and bupivacaine. *Canadian Journal of Anaesthesia* 45: 1094–6.

Guardini R, Waldron BA, Wallace WA (1985) Sciatic nerve block: a new lateral approach. *Acta Anaesthesiologica Scandinavica* 29: 515–19.

Hadzic A, Vloka JD (1998) A comparison of the posterior versus lateral approaches to block of the sciatic nerve in the popliteal fossa. *Anesthesiology* 88: 1480–6.

Hanna MH, Peat SJ, D'Costa F (1993) Lumbar plexus block: an anatomical study. *Anaesthesia* 48: 675–8.

Horlocker TT, Wedel DJ, Rowlingson JC, et al. (2010) Executive summary: regional anesthesia in the patient receiving antithrombotic or thrombolytic therapy (Third edition). *Regional Anesthesia & Pain Medicine* 35: 102–5.

Ilfeld BM, Morey TE, Wang RD, Enneking FK (2002) Continuous popliteal sciatic nerve block for postoperative pain control at home: a randomised, double-blinded, placebo-controlled study. *Anesthesiology* 97: 959–65.

Karmakar MK, Ho AM, Li X, et al. (2008) Ultrasound-guided lumbar plexus block through the acoustic window of the lumbar ultrasound trident. *British Journal of Anaesthesia* 100: 533–7.

Kehlet H, Andersen L (2011) Local infiltration analgesia in joint replacement: the evidence and recommendations for clinical practice. *Acta Anaesthesiologica Scandinavica* 55: 778–84.

Kerr DR, Kohan L (2008) Local infiltration analgesia: a technique for the control of acute postoperative pain following knee and hip surgery: a case study of 325 patients. *Acta Orthopaedica* 79: 174–83.

Kilpatrick A, Coventry DM, Todd JG (1992) A comparison of two approaches to sciatic nerve block. *Anaesthesia* 47: 155–7.

Koscielniak-Nielsen Z, Rasmussen H, Hesselbjerg L (2008) Long-axis ultrasound imaging of the nerves and advancement of perineural catheters under direct vision: a preliminary report of four cases *Regional Anesthesia and Pain Medicine* 33: 477–82.

Labat G (1922) *Regional Anesthesia: Its Technic and Clinical Application.* Philadelphia, PA: WB Saunders Co.

Lang SA, Yip RW, Chang PC, Gerard MA (1993) The femoral 3-in-1 block revisited. *Journal of Clinical Anesthesiology* 5: 292–6.

Manickam B, Perlas A, Duggan E, et al. (2009) Feasibility and efficacy of ultrasound-guided block of the saphenous nerve in the adductor canal. *Regional Anesthesia and Pain Medicine* 34: 578–80.

Mansour NY, Bennetts FE (1996) An observational study of combined continuous lumbar plexus and single-shot sciatic nerve blocks for post-knee surgery analgesia. *Regional Anesthesia* 21: 287–91.

McCartney CJL, McLeod GA (2011) Local infiltration analgesia for total knee arthroplasty. *British Journal of Anaesthesia* 107: 487–9.

Misra U, Priddie AK, McClymont C, Bower S (1991) Plasma concentrations of bupivacaine following combined sciatic and femoral 3-in-1 nerve block in open knee surgery. *British Journal of Anaesthesia* 66: 310–13.

Moore C, Sheppard D, Wildsmith JAW (2004) Thigh rotation and the anterior approach to the sciatic nerve: a magnetic resonance imaging study. *Regional Anesthesia and Pain Medicine* 29: 32–5.

Moore DC (1965) *Regional block* (4th edn). Springfield: CC Thomas.

Morin AM, Kranke P, Wulf H, et al. (2010) The effect of stimulating versus nonstimulating catheter techniques for continuous regional anesthesia: a semiquantitative systematic review *Regional Anesthesia and Pain Medicine* 35: 194–9.

Morris GF, Lang SA (1997) Continuous parasacral sciatic nerve block: two case reports. *Regional Anesthesia* 22: 469–72.

Morris GF, Lang SA, Dust WN, Van der Wal M (1997) The parasacral sciatic nerve block. *Regional Anesthesia* 22: 223–8.

Ota J, Sakura S, Hara K, Saito Y (2009) Ultrasound-guided anterior approach to sciatic nerve block: a comparison with the posterior approach *Anesthesia & Analgesia* 108: 660–5.

Parkinson SK, Mueller JB, Little WL, Bailey SL (1989) Extent of blockade with various approaches to the lumbar plexus. *Anesthesia & Analgesia* 68: 243–8.

Raj PP, Parks RI, Watson TD, Jenkins MT (1975) New single position supine approach to sciatic–femoral nerve block. *Anesthesia & Analgesia* 54: 489.

Robison C, Ray DC, McKeown DW, Buchan AS (1991) Effect of adrenaline on plasma concentrations of bupivacaine following lower limb nerve block. *British Journal of Anaesthesia* 66: 228–31.

Schafhalter-Zoppoth I, Younger SJ, Collins AB, Gray AT (2004) The 'seesaw' sign: improved sonographic identification of the sciatic nerve. *Anesthesiology* 101: 808–9.

Serpell MG, Millar FA, Thomson MF (1991) Comparison of lumbar plexus block versus conventional opioid analgesia after total knee replacement. *Anaesthesia* 46: 275–7.

Singelyn FJ, Aye F, Gouverneur JM (1997) Continuous popliteal- sciatic nerve block: an original technique to provide postoperative analgesia after foot surgery. *Anesthesia & Analgesia* 84: 383–6.

Singelyn FJ, Deyaert M, Joris D, et al. (1998) Effects of intravenous patient-controlled analgesia with morphine, continuous epidural analgesia, and continuous three-in-one block on postoperative pain and knee rehabilitation after unilateral total knee arthroplasty. *Anesthesia & Analgesia* 87: 88–92.

Singelyn FJ, Vanderelst PE, Gouverneur JM (2001) Extended femoral nerve sheath block after total hip arthroplasty: continuous versu patient-controlled techniques. *Anesthesia & Analgesia* 92: 455–9.

Spreng UJ, Dahl V, Hjall A, et al. (2010) High volume local infiltration analgesia combined with intravenous or local ketorolac + morphine compared with epidural analgesia after total knee arthroplasty. *British Journal of Anaesthesia* 105: 675–82.

Toftdahl K, Nikolajsen L, Haraldsted V, et al. (2007) Comparison of peri- and intraarticular analgesia with femoral nerve block after total knee arthroplasty *Acta Orthopaesica* 78: 172–9.

Tsui BC, Finucane BT (2006) The importance of ultrasound landmarks: a 'traceback' approach using the popliteal blood vessels for identification of the sciatic nerve. *Regional Anesthesia and Pain Medicine* 31: 481–2.

Valli H, Rosenberg PH (1986) Intravenous regional anesthesia below the knee. *Anaesthesia* 41: 1196–201.

Valli H, Rosenberg PH, Hekali R (1987) Comparison of lidocaine and prilocaine for intravenous regional anesthesia of the whole lower extremity. *Regional Anesthesia* 12: 128–34.

Vloka JD, Hadzic A, Mulcare R, et al. (1997) Femoral nerve block versus spinal anesthesia for outpatients undergoing long saphenous vein stripping surgery. *Anesthesia & Analgesia* 84: 749–52.

Vloka JD, Hadzic A, April E, Thys DM (2001) Anterior approach to the sciatic nerve: the effects of leg rotation. *Anesthesia & Analgesia* 92: 460–2.

Wassef MR (1991) Posterior tibial nerve block. A new approach using the bony landmark of the sustentaculum tali. *Anaesthesia* 46: 841–4.

Winnie A P, Ramamurthy S, Durrani Z (1973) The inguinal paravascular technic of lumbar plexus anesthesia: the '3 in 1 block'. *Anesthesia & Analgesia* 52: 989–96.

CHAPTER 19

Head, neck, and airway blocks

Neil Smart, Stephen Hickey, and Alistair Nimmo

Nerve blocks in the head and neck were, for long, the preserve of the surgeons (dental, maxillofacial, ophthalmic, and ear, nose & throat) specializing in that region of the body. In dentistry the size of the workload means that this is still the case, but developments in other areas have meant that anaesthetists are now using these methods in all of the other areas. Simple nerve block techniques can provide all that is needed for minor surgery and contribute much to patient comfort after major procedures. More recently, regional anaesthesia has found a place in the management of carotid endarterectomy to allow monitoring of consciousness and provide an indication of the adequacy of cerebral blood flow during arterial cross clamping. Finally, these methods have a place in the diagnosis of both acute and chronic pain syndromes.

Innervation of the head and neck

For the purposes of nerve block for surgery the most important nerves are those which supply the skin (Figure 19.1) and the structures of the airway, so their anatomy will be described in detail. Fortunately, sensory and motor innervation in the head and neck is often quite distinct: thus sensory block can be produced without motor paralysis. This is a distinct advantage with intraoral blocks because the muscles maintaining and controlling the airway remain unaffected.

Trigeminal nerve

This, the fifth and largest of the cranial nerves, supplies the muscles of mastication and is also the principle sensory nerve of the head (Figures 19.2 and 19.3), supplying:

1. The skin of the face and the anterior half of the head (the mask area);

2. The mucous membranes of the nose, sinuses, mouth, and anterior two-thirds of the tongue;

3. The teeth and the temporomandibular joint;

4. The contents of the orbit (except the retina); and

5. Part of the dura.

The *trigeminal* (also known as the *semilunar* or *Gasserian*) *ganglion* lies in the middle cranial fossa in a recess near the apex of the petrous temporal bone. At the ganglion the sensory component of the nerve divides into three, each with a discrete area of distribution (Figure 19.1).

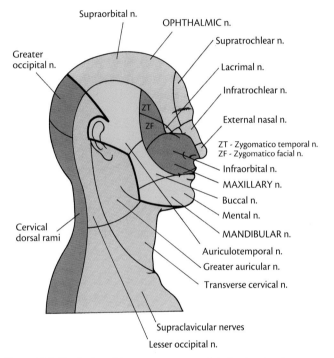

Figure 19.1 Distribution of the cutaneous nerves of the head and neck.

Ophthalmic nerve

The ophthalmic nerve enters the orbit through the superior orbital fissure and divides into three main branches:

1. The *frontal nerve*, which has two terminal cutaneous branches. The *supraorbital nerve* emerges from the supraorbital foramen, turns upwards and supplies the upper eyelid, the forehead, and upper anterior part of the scalp as far as the vertex. The *supratrochlear nerve* emerges at the supraorbital margin, a finger's breadth from the midline, to supply the paramedian part of the forehead and the medial part of the upper eyelid.

2. The *nasociliary nerve*, which also has two terminal branches. The *infratrochlear nerve* emerges from the orbit just above the medial palpebral ligament to supply the medial parts of the eyelids and the root of the nose. The *anterior ethmoidal nerve* leaves the orbit through the anterior ethmoidal foramen. It gives

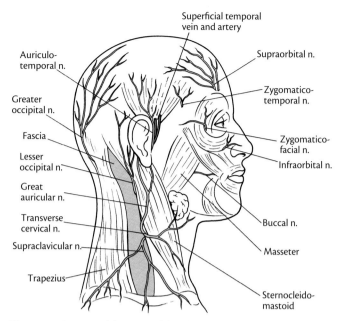

Figure 19.2 Positions of the nerves of the right side of the scalp, face, and neck. Note that the superficial branches of the cervical plexus emerge together from the midpoint of the posterior border of sternocleidomastoid, and that the branches of the facial nerve have been omitted from the area in front of the ear for clarity.

off *internal nasal branches* to the mucous membrane of the adjacent lateral and septal nasal walls, and then emerges between the nasal bone and the lateral nasal cartilage as the *external nasal nerve* to supply the skin of the lower half of the dorsum of the nose.

3. The *lacrimal nerve*, the terminal component of which is the *palpebral branch*. It pierces and supplies the lateral part of the upper eyelid.

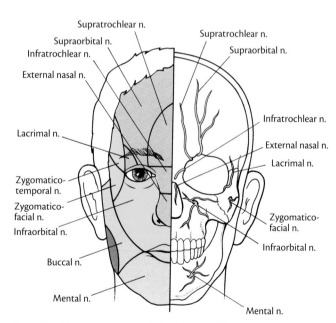

Figure 19.3 Cutaneous branches of the divisions of the trigeminal nerve. The territory supplied by each nerve is shown on the left while the positions of the major nerves are on the right. Note the straight-line relationship between the supraorbital, infraorbital, and mental foramina.

Maxillary nerve

The maxillary nerve leaves the cranium through the foramen rotundum, crosses the pterygopalatine fossa anterior to the lateral pterygoid plate, and enters the orbit through the inferior orbital fissure. The relevant terminal cutaneous branches are:

1. The *infraorbital nerve* which emerges from the infraorbital foramen beneath the orbicularis oculi muscle and supplies the skin and mucous membrane of the upper lip, the lower eyelid, the skin between them and that on the side of the nose.

2. The *zygomaticofacial nerve* which leaves the orbit through the zygomaticofacial foramen and supplies skin over the bony part of the cheek.

3. The *zygomaticotemporal nerve* which emerges from the temporal surface of the zygomatic bone to supply the skin over the anterior part of the temple.

Mandibular nerve

The mandibular nerve leaves the skull through the foramen ovale accompanied by the motor root of the *trigeminal nerve*, and crosses the pterygopalatine fossa posterior to the lateral pterygoid plate, but anterior to the neck of the mandible. There it divides into a small anterior (mostly motor) and a large posterior (mostly sensory) division. An important sensory branch of the anterior division is the *buccal nerve* which supplies the skin over, and the mucous membrane deep to, the buccinator muscle. The posterior division trunk has three main branches:

1. The *auriculotemporal nerve* which hooks round the posterior surface of the neck of the mandible, lying close to the superficial temporal vessels and the parotid gland. It supplies the skin of the temple and the superior two-thirds of the anterior aspect of the ear.

2. The *inferior dental nerve* which enters the mandibular foramen on the medial surface of the ramus of the mandible. Within the mandible it gives off branches to the teeth and gums, and finally exits through the mental foramen as the *mental nerve* supplying the skin of the chin, and the skin and mucous membrane of the lower lip.

3. The *lingual nerve* which runs between the medial pterygoid muscle and the ramus of the mandible, and is covered only by mucous membrane at the level of the third molar. It supplies the mucous membrane of the anterior two-thirds of the tongue and the adjacent parts of the floor of the mouth and gum.

Thus the trigeminal nerve supplies all of the skin of the face except for the area over the parotid gland and the angle of the mandible which is supplied by the great auricular nerve (see 'Cervical nerves' section). It is important to note that the landmarks identifying the three main terminal cutaneous branches of the trigeminal nerve, the supraorbital foramen, the infraorbital foramen, and the mental foramen, all lie in a straight line (Figure 19.3).

Facial nerve

As it traverses the parotid gland in front of the ear, the facial (seventh) nerve divides into five main branches—temporal, zygomatic, buccal, mandibular, and cervical—which radiate out to supply the muscles of expression in the respective parts of the face. The mandibular branch runs forward below the angle of the mandible before turning upwards and forwards to supply the angle of the mouth.

Glossopharyngeal nerve

The glossopharyngeal (ninth) nerve supplies sensation to the posterior third of the tongue, the pharynx, palatine tonsil, part of the soft palate, and the anterior surface of the epiglottis. It emerges from the skull through the jugular foramen and descends between the internal carotid artery and the internal jugular vein. It curves round the lateral surface of the stylopharyngeus muscle and passes with it into the pharynx between the superior and middle constrictor muscles. Here it lies deep to the mucous membrane of the lower part of the tonsillar fossa, and then passes forwards into the tongue.

Vagus nerve

The vagus (tenth) nerve also emerges from the skull through the jugular foramen. The *pharyngeal branch* arises immediately below the skull and runs between the internal and external carotid arteries to form, with the glossopharyngeal nerve, a large part of the pharyngeal plexus innervating the pharyngeal wall. There are two other branches of particular interest:

1. The *superior laryngeal nerve* arises from the inferior ganglion of the vagus and runs downwards, forwards and medially to cross in front of the greater horn of the hyoid bone where it divides into two. The *internal branch* pierces the thyrohyoid membrane to supply the mucous membrane of the larynx (including the posterior surface of the epiglottis) down to the level of the vocal cords. The *external branch* is the motor nerve to the cricothyroid muscle.

2. The *recurrent laryngeal nerve* loops under the aorta on the right, and the subclavian artery on the left, ascends in the groove between the trachea and the oesophagus and enters the larynx posteriorly, deep to the inferior border of the inferior constrictor muscle. It supplies the mucous membrane of the larynx below the vocal cords and all the muscles of the larynx except cricothyroid.

Hypoglossal nerve

The hypoglossal (twelfth) nerve is the motor nerve to the tongue. From the base of the skull, where it is closely related to the glossopharyngeal and vagus nerves, it passes between the internal jugular vein and the internal carotid artery, and curves downwards and forwards to the base of the tongue

Cervical nerves

Branches of the cervical nerves supply the neck and the back of the head (Figures 19.1 and 19.2).

The dorsal rami of C_2–C_4 supply the skin of the back of the neck and, through the medial branch of the dorsal ramus of C_2 (the *greater occipital nerve*), the scalp. This, the thickest cutaneous nerve in the body, crosses the suboccipital triangle and pierces semispinalis capitis. It supplies the scalp as far as the vertex.

The ventral rami of C_1–C_4 form the *cervical plexus* which may be divided into two parts. The *deep* cervical plexus lies posterior to the internal jugular vein and the prevertebral fascia, and extends inferiorly from the root of the auricle to the superior border of the thyroid cartilage. It gives rise to the *phrenic nerve* and smaller branches which innervate the muscles and other deep structures of the neck.

The *superficial* cervical plexus has a number of cutaneous branches and these emerge from behind the mid-portion of the sternomastoid muscle, from where they are distributed widely. The *lesser occipital nerve* supplies the skin over the mastoid process, and the *great auricular nerve* the skin on both surfaces of the ear and over the angle of the mandible. The *transverse cervical nerve* passes forwards across the superficial surface of sternomastoid and supplies most of the skin on the side and front of the neck. Finally, the *supraclavicular nerves* radiate out to supply skin of the chest and shoulder down to the level of the second rib—the 'cape' area.

Clinical application

Techniques for blocking the main trunks and branches of all the cranial nerves, not just those mentioned already, have been described. However, many of these methods involve injection near the base of the skull, require very detailed knowledge of anatomy, and are technically difficult. These issues, together with lack of clearly defined clinical need and concerns about safety, mean that major cranial nerve blocks are used rarely. Even with the more distal blocks, where the target nerves are more accessible and associated risks are lower, it is important that these points are kept clearly in mind, especially the safety issue.

Safety

The close proximity of the major nerves to other important structures in the area below the base of the skull means that major complications can be produced by intravascular or local spread all too easily. Accidental injection of as little as 1 ml of local anaesthetic into the carotid or vertebral arteries, or one of their branches, will produce major central nervous system toxicity, and even if arterial puncture is identified it may lead to significant haematoma. Subarachnoid spread of local anaesthetic from injection into the dural cuff around a cranial nerve will also produce consequences out of proportion to the dose involved. The more proximal the injection, the more likely it is that both sensory and motor nerves to the airway will be affected, with consequent risk of obstruction or aspiration. Thus essential prerequisites are intravenous access for all but the most peripheral of these methods, use of appropriate monitoring equipment, and the ready availability of resuscitation equipment. Small volumes of local anaesthetic also minimize the risk of unintended spread.

Similar concerns apply to the classic technique of deep cervical plexus block. Diaphragmatic paralysis is inevitable, and careful needle angulation is needed to avoid injection into the vertebral artery, or the epidural or subarachnoid spaces. Both cervical epidural and high spinal blocks have been used for head and neck surgery, but the potential problems and the availability of alternative methods mean that such techniques are employed rarely.

Nerve damage from needle trauma may be influenced by bevel configuration (Chapter 4), but other factors can influence choice. Short bevel needles are useful for some blocks because they allow better appreciation of passage through tissue planes, but they offer little advantage in the mouth, and their relative bluntness makes them more painful. The American Dental Association recommends long bevel needles for intraoral and circumoral blocks. Intraoral blocks can be performed using standard hypodermic syringes and needles, but it is worth the regular user becoming proficient with the dental cartridge system because this is very suited to these methods (Rosenburg et al. 2009).

Postinjection infection is a rare complication in the head and neck with few case reports, even with blocks which involve penetration of the mucous membranes of the mouth.

Indications

Head and neck blocks, used alone or in combination with general anaesthesia, can benefit patients in a range of clinical situations:

◆ *Postoperative pain control.* The longer acting agents can produce prolonged analgesia, reducing the need for opioids (which may be relatively contraindicated in surgery in close proximity to the airway), improving patient comfort, and facilitating early discharge.

◆ *Sole anaesthetic technique.* Many elderly patients presenting for excision of basal or squamous cell carcinomas of the face have significant comorbidities and are poor risks for general anaesthesia. Infiltration techniques tend to distend the skin and distort the local anatomy, making surgery difficult. Peripheral nerve blocks offer an effective, simple, and safe alternative. Major resections and reconstruction under regional block have also been reported (Neill 1996).

◆ *Awake intubation.* Regional block allows instrumentation of the airway and endotracheal intubation prior to induction of general anaesthesia.

◆ *Chronic pain management.* Head and neck nerve blocks have an important role in the diagnosis and treatment of conditions such as trigeminal neuralgia, postherpetic pain, and intractable pain associated with malignancy.

◆ *Carotid artery surgery.* This is discussed in the 'Regional anaesthesia for carotid endarterectomy' section.

Suggested techniques

The trigeminal nerve and its branches

The trigeminal nerve system can be blocked at several points along its course, but the distal blocks have more favourable risk/benefit profiles. The terminal branches are more easily identified (Figure 19.3) and so can be blocked more consistently, while their greater separation from the major subcranial structures means that accidental misplacement of the injectate has less serious consequences.

Trigeminal ganglion block

Trigeminal ganglion block is technically difficult and requires radiographic control. Its use is largely confined to specialist units dealing with intractable trigeminal neuralgia and cancer pain. The reader is referred to more specialized texts for a description (Bonica 1990, Suresh & Jagannathan 2009).

Branches of the ophthalmic nerve

Block of the *supraorbital* and *supratrochlear nerves* is useful for surgery of the forehead and the scalp as far as the vertex. The important bony landmark is the supraorbital foramen which is palpable on the superior orbital rim at a point immediately above the pupil when the patient gazes straight ahead. A single subcutaneous injection of 3–4 ml of local anaesthetic, starting in the midline at the root of the nose and directed laterally above the eyebrow as far as the supraorbital foramen, will block both nerves.

The landmark for *external nasal nerve* block is the junction of the lateral nasal cartilage and nasal bone. Injection of 2 ml of local anaesthetic immediately lateral to the midline anaesthetizes the apex and vestibule of the nose. The *infratrochlear nerve* can be blocked by infiltration of 1–2 ml of solution, starting at the superomedial border of the orbit and moving towards, but stopping just short of, the medial palpebral ligament. This results in anaesthesia of the nose around the medial angle of the eye. When bilateral external nasal and infratrochlear nerve blocks are combined with bilateral infraorbital nerve blocks (see 'Maxillary nerve and its branches' section), superficial surgery on the nose can be performed. However, if the surgery involves the skeleton or mucosa, anaesthesia of the nasal cavity (see next section) is required also.

An infiltration starting at the zygomatic foramen and directed upwards along the lateral margin of the orbit anaesthetizes the lateral part of the upper eyelid supplied by the *lacrimal nerve*. When this is combined with supraorbital and supratrochlear nerve block, surgery on the entire upper eyelid is possible.

The nasal cavity

Topical analgesia is simple to perform and quite safe provided that it is remembered that local anaesthetic uptake from mucosal surfaces is rapid and extensive. Total uptake can be reduced if the local anaesthetic is confined to the intended site of action by applying it with soaked cotton pledgets, but it is essential that the *total* dose is kept under review, particularly when several blocks are combined. Cocaine 10%, to a maximum 1.5 mg kg^{-1} (but see the discussion in Chapters 7 and 8 on weight-related doses), has long been the traditional drug for this method because its local anaesthetic action is accompanied by intense vasoconstriction which improves the surgical field. However, large doses of cocaine are associated with severe hypertension and arrhythmia, and lidocaine 5% with phenylephrine 0.5% (Co-phenylcaine Forte) is a less toxic and more readily available option.

The *anterior ethmoidal nerve* is blocked by inserting a pledget parallel to the bridge of the nose, backwards and upwards as far as the superior border of the nasal cavity. Similarly, the *sphenopalatine ganglion and nerves* are blocked by inserting a pledget at an angle of about 20° to the floor of the nose so that it passes along the upper border of the inferior turbinate to a depth of about 6–7 cm until bone is felt at the posterior pharyngeal wall. The pledgets should be left in place for 10 minutes.

The maxillary nerve and its branches

It is possible to block the main trunk of the maxillary nerve in the pterygopalatine fossa, using a lateral approach (Figure 19.4). The superficial landmarks are the midpoint of the zygomatic arch and the notch between the condyle and the coronoid process of the mandible. The notch is accentuated as the mouth is opened and closed. A 22-g, 9-cm short bevelled needle is inserted perpendicular to the skin, through the notch below the midpoint of the zygomatic arch. The needle is advanced through the masseter and temporalis muscles until the tip contacts the lateral pterygoid plate, usually at a depth of about 4 cm. It is then redirected superiorly and anteriorly until bony resistance is lost, when it is advanced a further 1 cm. The tip will then lie in the pterygopalatine fossa and in close proximity to the mandibular nerve. Injection of 4 ml of solution, without eliciting paraesthesia and after very careful aspiration tests, will produce anaesthesia of the whole maxilla.

However, the potential complications (as outlined above) of such a proximal technique make this an unwise method for the inexperienced, particularly when much of the same area can be blocked using simpler and safer distal procedures.

The *infraorbital nerve* can be approached either extraorally or, preferably, from within the mouth. Not only is the intraoral route considered to be more reliable (Hanke 2001, Lynch et al. 1994), but accidental entry to the infraorbital foramen, with the attendant hazards of damage to the artery, nerve, or floor of the orbit, is less likely. A 27-g dental needle is inserted just lateral to the lateral incisor tooth, and advanced upwards through the upper buccal sulcus towards the infraorbital foramen which is located just below the orbital rim, approximately 2 cm from the lateral surface of the nose. Care should be taken to ensure that the needle stops short of the orbital rim (to avoid damage to the eye) and does not enter the canal (to avoid nerve damage). One millilitre of local anaesthetic is injected in the vicinity of the foramen with gentle massage of the skin over the injection point to promote spread of local anaesthetic into the foramen. Widespread anaesthesia (of the lower eyelid, cheek, lateral nose, ala, and upper lip) results. This technically simple and relatively safe nerve block is a valuable and commonly used method for superficial plastic surgery.

The zygomatic foramen, 1–2 cm lateral to the lower lateral margin of the orbit, is the landmark for block of both *the zygomaticofacial* and *zygomaticotemporal nerves*. The zygomaticofacial nerve emerges from the foramen itself (Figure 19.3) while the zygomaticotemporal nerve pierces the temporal fascia approximately 2 cm above this point. Infiltration of 2 ml of local anaesthetic at each site produces anaesthesia in the distribution shown in Figure 19.1.

The mandibular nerve and its branches

Extensive analgesia (the temple, auricle, external auditory meatus, cheek, lower lip, tongue, gums, and mandible) results from block of

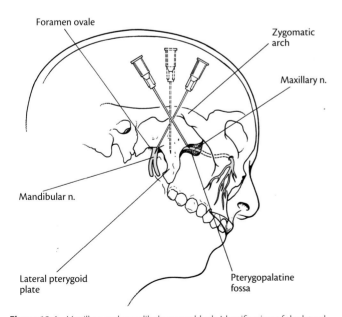

Figure 19.4 Maxillary and mandibular nerve block. Identification of the lateral pterygoid plate is necessary for both blocks, but subsequent angulation of the needle is different: the maxillary nerve is found anterosuperiorly and the mandibular posteriorly (Reproduced from Murphy TM, 'Somatic block of the head and neck', in: Cousins MJ, Bridenbaugh PO (eds) *Neural Blockade in clinical anaesthesia and management of pain*, Second edition, pp. 537–58. Copyright Wolters Kluwer, 1988.)

the main trunk of the mandibular nerve where it lies in the infratemporal fossa (Figure 19.4). As with the maxillary nerve, the clinical value of mandibular nerve block is limited by complications, but it is undoubtedly useful in patients with widespread pain associated with intraoral malignancy. However, the occasional user will be able to achieve much, and with a greater margin of safety, by blocking the more distal branches of the nerve (see later in this section).

The landmarks, and the needle insertion point, are the same as for maxillary nerve block, but once the needle contacts the lateral pterygoid plate it is redirected posteriorly until bony contact is lost. At this point paraesthesiae in the distribution of the nerve confirm correct needle position, but the needle should not be advanced much beyond the depth of the lateral pterygoid plate because of the risk of pharyngeal puncture. Fortunately, paraesthesiae are not essential because local anaesthetic injected just beyond the lateral pterygoid plate will reach the nerve by diffusion.

Inferior dental and lingual nerves: the inferior dental foramen lies in the centre of the medial aspect of the vertical ramus of the mandible. It may be located by palpating the concavity of the retromolar trigone with the index finger, the nail identifying the medial ridge. With the barrel of the syringe resting on the contralateral premolar, the needle is inserted parallel to the occlusal surface just beyond the midpoint of the palpating finger. As the injection (2 ml) is made, the syringe is swung across to allow the needle to be inserted a further 2 cm parallel to the horizontal ramus of the mandible. The injection will anaesthetize both nerves.

The *buccal nerve* is also blocked using an intraoral approach. A 27-g dental needle is inserted into the mucous membrane of the cheek, level with the occlusive plane of the first mandibular molar, and advanced posteriorly towards the external oblique ridge of the mandibular ramus. Infiltration of 2 ml of local anaesthetic between the needle entry point and the ridge will block the nerve.

Mental nerve block provides soft tissue anaesthesia of the lower lip, its underlying mucosa, and the chin, and requires identification of the mental foramen, the position of which varies with age and dentition. In the young adult it is situated below the first premolar tooth halfway between the gum margin and the lower border of the body of the mandible, but with advancing age the foramen 'moves' superiorly and posteriorly. The opening is often difficult to palpate, but its position may be confirmed using the straight-line relationship with the other foramina (Figure 19.3). A 25-g needle is introduced through the skin of the lower lip, below and in front of the second premolar tooth. It is directed towards the foramen, around which 1–2 ml of local anaesthetic should be infiltrated. It is neither necessary nor desirable for the needle to enter the foramen.

The *auriculotemporal nerve* is associated closely with the superficial temporal artery and vein in front of the ear. Using the pulsation of the artery just above the temporomandibular joint as a landmark, the nerve can be blocked by infiltration of 2–3 ml of local anaesthetic around the vessels. Branches of the facial nerve lie close by and facial paresis may result also.

Cervical nerves

Deep cervical plexus block

Deep cervical plexus block is a paravertebral block of C_2–C_4 in which local anaesthetic is injected into the deep cervical space. With the patient lying supine, and the head turned to the opposite side, the tip of the mastoid process and Chassaignac's tubercle (the anterior tubercle on the transverse process of the sixth cervical vertebra) are marked (Figure 19.5). A line is drawn from the posterior

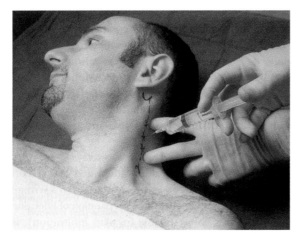

Figure 19.5 Deep cervical plexus block. The crosses mark the tips of the transverse processes of the cervical vertebrae. The needle has been inserted at C_3.

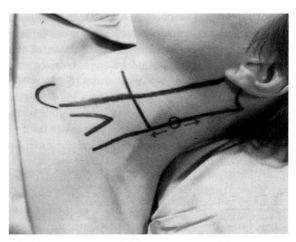

Figure 19.6 Landmarks for superficial cervical plexus block. The circle marks the point of needle insertion, and the arrows mark the direction in which solution should spread.

margin of the mastoid process to Chassaignac's tubercle. The transverse processes of C_2, C_3, and C_4 all lie on this line and can usually be palpated, with that of C_2 located approximately 1.5 cm below the tip of the mastoid process and those of C_3 (needle position in Figure 19.5) and C_4 found at further 1.5-cm intervals. The needle should be inserted in a caudal direction towards each transverse process to ensure that the epidural or subarachnoid spaces or the vertebral artery are not entered accidentally.

Originally, deep cervical plexus block was described using three separate injections, one at the level of each of the three relevant vertebrae (Moore 1979). However, a single injection at C_4 is equally effective because the cervical nerve roots are contained in a continuous sheath between the scalenus anterior and scalenus medius muscles (Winnie et al. 1975), this allowing the local anaesthetic to spread to all components of the plexus. A 22-g needle is inserted through the skin at the C_4 level on the line noted earleir, and then directed slightly caudad. Usually, the transverse process of C_4 is contacted at a depth of 1.5–3 cm, and paraesthesiae are obtained. Careful aspiration is essential to exclude vascular puncture or entry to the subarachnoid space before the injection of 10–15 ml of local anaesthetic. Accidental injection of local anaesthetic into the vertebral artery (which lies close by in the transverse foramen) results in immediate convulsions, while spread to the epidural or subarachnoid spaces produces cardiorespiratory collapse of slower onset. Paralysis of the diaphragm is a consequence of phrenic nerve block, so bilateral blocks are contraindicated. Although, the overall incidence of block related complications is low, the superficial approach (see next section) causes even fewer problems (Pandit et al. 2007).

Ultrasound has been used recently to facilitate deep cervical plexus block (Sandeman et al. 2006).

Superficial cervical plexus block

Block of the superficial branches of the cervical plexus anaesthetizes the skin, but not the deeper structures, of the anterolateral aspect of the neck from the mandible to the clavicle and below. Technically easy to perform, there is little risk of blocking the phrenic or recurrent laryngeal nerves, so bilateral blocks are not contraindicated. The main landmark is the sternocleidomastoid muscle which can be accentuated if the supine patient is asked to lift the head from the pillow. All four branches of the plexus emerge

from behind the midpoint of the muscle (approximately 1–2 cm above the point at which the external jugular vein crosses it). With the head turned to the opposite side a total of 20–30 ml of local anaesthetic is injected subcutaneously along the posterior border of the muscle in cranial and caudal directions from the midpoint of the muscle (Figure 19.6). If combined deep and superficial or bilateral blocks are to be performed the volume or concentration should be reduced to ensure that a safe dose of local anaesthetic is not exceeded.

Great auricular nerve block

The great auricular nerve can be blocked selectively by injecting 2–3 ml of local anaesthetic in a straight line running anteriorly and posteriorly from the tip of the mastoid process. Its area of distribution to the ear is also included as part of superficial cervical plexus block.

Greater occipital nerve block

The simplest technique for blocking this nerve is to infiltrate 10 ml of local anaesthetic superficially on a line running between the mastoid process and the greater occipital protuberance. The lesser occipital nerve is blocked simultaneously. Greater occipital nerve block is useful in the diagnosis and treatment of occipital neuralgia and can be combined with lesser occipital, auriculotemporal, supraorbital, and supratrochlear nerve blocks to produce surgical anaesthesia of the scalp in a 'skull cap' distribution.

Regional anaesthesia of the ear

The posterior surface of the ear and the lower third of the anterior surface are supplied by the great auricular nerve and, often, the lesser occipital nerve, both branches of the cervical plexus. The superior two-thirds of the anterior surface are supplied by the auriculotemporal nerve, a branch of the mandibular nerve. Block of these nerves allows extensive surgery from otoplasty and wedge resection to amputation. Anaesthesia of the concha may be inadequate, but it can be reinforced by subcutaneous infiltration of 2–3 ml of local anaesthetic posteriorly through the conchal cartilage. In children, postoperative nausea and vomiting may be reduced by block of the auricular branch of the vagus. This requires infiltration of 2 ml of local anaesthetic at the bony-cartilaginous junction of the external auditory meatus over its lower aspect.

The tympanic membrane can be anaesthetized with 10% lidocaine spray. This is best applied by directing it at the roof of the auditory canal rather than at the tympanic membrane itself.

Awake intubation

A technique which depends on blocking the individual nerves which supply the upper airway is not practical, and most practitioners use a technique which is predominantly topical. This will require separate applications to anaesthetize the nose, pharynx, and larynx, and close monitoring is needed of the amount of drug used and the early signs of systemic toxicity. Antisialogogue pre-medication (e.g. glycopyrrolate 0.4 mg intravenously) will improve both the effect of topically applied local anaesthetic and the view through the fibreoptic endoscope. The use of sedative and or analgesic drugs to make the procedure more acceptable to the patient is well described, but no general recommendations can be made. Each case must be considered on its own merits and the choice of drug made according to the experience of the practitioner and the clinical scenario, bearing in mind the risk to airway maintenance and aspiration of stomach contents, blood or pus. The preliminary administration of nebulized lidocaine (6 mg kg^{-1} of 10% solution) from a facemask results in acceptable plasma concentrations, but has limited effect as the sole technique (Parkes et al. 1997).

The *nasal cavity* (assuming that this route is used) can be blocked by using the technique described earlier or by using an atomizer to produce topical anaesthesia with the same lidocaine/phenylephrine mixture mentioned for that technique. A soft nasopharyngeal airway coated in 5% lidocaine gel will supplement these while also time dilating the airway before insertion of the endotracheal tube.

The *posterior pharyngeal wall* is anaesthetized with an atomizer administering lidocaine 10 mg per spray. The patient is asked to gargle with the spray before swallowing or expectorating it.

The *larynx* can be anaesthetized in a number of ways, all of which render the patient at risk of aspiration. The endoscope can be used to direct a spray of lidocaine 4% onto, and then below, the vocal cords (2 ml per spray). Injection down an epidural catheter passed through the suction channel of the endoscope to protrude about 1 cm from the end may help direct the spray onto the vocal cords.

Alternatively the superior laryngeal nerve is blocked specifically using a cotton wool ball soaked in lidocaine 4% topical applied to each piriform fossa using Krause's forceps, or an external approach can be used. A needle is passed in a posteromedial direction to make contact with the greater cornu of the hyoid and then 'walked off' caudally. A loss of resistance may be felt as the needle penetrates the thyrohyoid membrane: 3 ml of lidocaine 2% is then injected.

Finally, transtracheal injection through a cricothyroid cannula can be used, this having the advantage that it will provide a route for emergency oxygenation if required. The cricoid cartilage is usually easily palpable, but ultrasound has been used to identify the trachea in patients with abnormal anatomy (Orr et al. 2007). A skin bleb is raised with injectable lidocaine and a 20-g cannula is inserted through the cricothyroid membrane in the midline (Figure 19.7), its correct position being confirmed by the free aspiration of air. The needle is removed to prevent damage to the wall of the trachea during injection and a syringe containing 2 ml of topical lidocaine 4% is attached to the cannula. The patient is told to exhale maximally at which point the lidocaine is injected. This causes the patient to breathe in deeply and then cough, so ensuring that the larynx and trachea are well coated. A second injection is performed as a routine.

Regional anaesthesia for carotid endarterectomy

Carotid endarterectomy (CEA) may be undertaken under regional or general anaesthesia, or the combination of a regional block and a light general anaesthetic. Regional anaesthesia in an awake or lightly sedated patient has the advantage of permitting clinical assessment of the adequacy of cerebral perfusion when the carotid artery is clamped. The GALA trial, a mulicentre randomized trial of general against local anaesthesia for CEA, found no significant difference in the incidence of stroke, myocardial infarction, and death, but that surgery under local anaesthesia was more cost-effective (GALA Trial Collaborative Group 2008, Gomes et al. 2010).

The operation is performed in the territory of the cervical plexus, and three regional anaesthetic techniques may be used: cervical epidural anaesthesia, cervical plexus block. or local infiltration alone. Local infiltration is less likely to produce satisfactory anaesthesia than the other techniques and cervical plexus block is used most frequently. Both superficial and deep approaches (or a combination of the two) as described earleir are appropriate using levo-bupivacaine or ropivacaine 0.375%.

During superficial cervical plexus block the local anaesthetic may be injected subcutaneously or a little deeper, below an apparent fascial layer, the 'intermediate cervical plexus block' (Telford & Stoneham 2004). These techniques provide equivalent anaesthesia to deep cervical plexus block (Stoneham et al. 1998) or combined deep and superficial block (Pandit et al. 2000). However, superficial and intermediate blocks are associated with a lower risk of serious complications than deep or combined block (Pandit et al. 2007). With any technique of cervical plexus block, local anaesthetic may spread to the roots of the ipsilateral brachial plexus so any temporary weakness in the arm, particularly the shoulder, should be distinguished from that due to a cerebrovascular cause.

Cervical plexus block usually provides good anaesthesia for the skin incision and initial dissection, but it may not block the whole surgical field. Discomfort may occur at the upper and lower ends of the wound and require supplementary infiltration by the surgeon. Retractor pressure on the mandible, dissection within the carotid

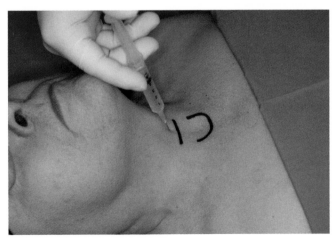

Figure 19.7 Cricothyroid puncture.

sheath, and cross clamping of the artery can all produce pain, often referred to the teeth, Carotid pain may be prevented or reduced if the surgeon injects 1 ml of local anaesthetic into the sheath at an early stage. This should be done very cautiously with repeated aspiration to reduce the risk of inadvertent intra-arterial injection. Topical application of local anaesthetic to the artery has also been used. Using prilocaine rather than lidocaine for the supplementary local anaesthesia will reduce the risk of toxicity.

Some anaesthetists avoid supplementary analgesia or sedation because they may mask a change in conscious level or make the patient uncooperative. However, the block does not always provide complete pain relief, and both anxiety and discomfort from lying still with the neck extended for a long period are common. Heavy premedication, and long-acting sedative and analgesic drugs, should be avoided, but careful titration of short-acting agents can improve the patient's comfort without impairing assessment. Low-dose target-controlled infusions of propofol (0–1 mcg ml^{-1}) and or remifentanil (0–1 ng ml^{-1}) may be started before the block is performed and adjusted to ensure that the patient is appropriately sedated before surgery starts. The level of sedation should be light enough to allow identification of changes in conscious level or power in the contralateral arm, and detection of dysphasia or dysarthria.

Other measures which improve patient comfort during surgery include use of a transparent surgical drape to prevent claustrophobia, placing a pillow under the knees to prevent back pain, the use of a fan to cool the face, wetting the lips with water, and restricting administration of intravenous fluids to avoid a full bladder.

Key references

GALA Trial Collaborative Group (2008) General anaesthesia versus local anaesthesia for carotid surgery (GALA): a multicentre, randomised controlled trial. *Lancet* 372: 2132–42.

Neill RS (1996) Regional anaesthesia in ophthalmology and otorhinolaryngology. In Brown DL (Ed) *Regional anaesthesia and analgesia*, pp. 487–94. Philadelphia, PA: WB Saunders.

References

Bonica JJ (1990) Neurolytic blockade and hypophysectomy. In Bonica JJ (Ed) *Managment of Pain*, 2nd edn, pp. 1980–2039. Philadelphia, PA: Lea and Febiger.

GALA Trial Collaborative Group (2008) General anaesthesia versus local anaesthesia for carotid surgery (GALA): a multicentre, randomised controlled trial. *Lancet* 372: 2132–42.

Gomes M, Soares MO, Dumville JC, et al. (2010) GALA Collaborative Group. Cost-effectiveness analysis of general anaesthesia versus local anaesthesia for carotid surgery (GALA Trial). *British Journal of Surgery* 97: 1218–25.

Hanke CW (2001) The tumescent facial block: Tumescent local anaesthesia and nerve block anaesthesia for full face laser resurfacing. *Dermatologic Surgery* 27: 1003–5.

Lynch MT, Syverud SA, Schwab RA, et al. (1994) Comparison of intraoral and percutaneous approaches for infraorbital nerve block. *Academic Emergency Medicine* 1: 514–19.

Moore DC (1979) *Regional Block: A Handbook for Use in Clinical Practice of Medicine and Surgery*, 4th edn. Springfield, IL: Charles C Thomas.

Murphy TM (1988) Somatic block of head and neck. In Cousins MJ, Bridenbaugh PO (Eds) *Neural Blockade in Clinical Anesthesia and Management of Pain*, 2nd edn, pp. 537–58. Philadelphia, PA: JB Lippincott.

Neill RS (1996) Regional anaesthesia in ophthalmology and otorhinolaryngology. In Brown DL(Ed) *Regional Anaesthesia and Analgesia*, pp. 487–94. Philadelphia, PA: WB Saunders.

Orr JA, Stephens RS, Mitchell VM (2007) Ultrasound-guided location of the trachea. *Anaesthesia* 62: 972.

Pandit JJ, Bree S, Dillon P, et al. (2000) A comparison of superficial versus combined (superficial and deep) cervical plexus block for carotid endarterectomy: a prospective, randomized study. *Anesthesia & Analgesia* 91: 781–6.

Pandit JJ, Satya-Krishna R, Gration P (2007) Superficial or deep cervical plexus block for carotid endarterectomy: a systematic review of complications. *British Journal of Anaesthesia* 99: 159–69.

Parkes SB, Butler CS Muller R (1997) Plasma lignocaine concentration following nubulization for awake intubation. *Anaesthesia & Intensive Care* 25: 369–71.

Rice ASC, McMahon SB (1992) Peripheral nerve injury caused by injection needles used in anaesthesia; influence of bevel configuration studied in a rat model. *British Journal of Anaesthesia* 69: 433–8.

Rosenberg MB, Giovannitti JA, Phero JC (2009) Neural blockade of oral and circumoral structures. In Cousins MJ, Carr DB, Horlocker TT, Bridenbaugh PO (Eds) *Neural Blockade in Clinical Anaesthesia and Pain Medicine*, 4th edn, pp. 426–42. Philadelphia, PA: Lippincott Williams & Wilkins.

Sandeman DJ, Griffiths MJ, Lennox AF (2006) Ultrasound guided deep cervical plexus block. *Anaesthesia & Intensive Care* 34: 240–4.

Stoneham MD, Doyle AR, Knighton JD, et al. (1998) Prospective, randomized comparison of deep or superficial cervical plexus block for carotid endarterectomy surgery. *Anesthesiology* 89: 907–12.

Suresh S, Jagannathan N (2009) Somatic blockade of the head and neck In Cousins MJ, Carr DB, Horlocker TT, Bridenbaugh PO (Eds) *Neural Blockade in Clinical Anaesthesia and Pain Medicine*, 4th edn, pp. 405–25. Philadelphia, PA: Lippincott Williams & Wilkins.

Telford RJ, Stoneham MD (2004) Correct nomenclature of superficial cervical plexus blocks. *British Journal of Anaesthesia* 92: 775.

Winnie AP, Ramamurthy S, Durrani Z, Radonjic R (1975) Interscalene cervical plexus block: a single injection technique. *Anesthesia & Analgesia* 54: 370–5.

CHAPTER 20

Ophthalmic regional anaesthesia

Hamish McLure

Regional anaesthesia provides excellent conditions for virtually all types of ophthalmic surgery. The ideal block provides a painless, hypotonic, still eye, with rapid return of function once the surgery has been completed. Techniques vary from simple application of local anaesthetic drops to semi-surgical techniques involving incision and dissection of the orbital tissues. All techniques have side effects, and the clinician needs to have a comprehensive knowledge of orbital anatomy and physiology, pharmacology, the techniques and their side effects, as well as practical experience of resuscitation.

History

All of modern regional anaesthesia stems from the 1884 work of Carl Koller, a young Viennese surgeon, who wished to become an ophthalmologist and who had sought an alternative to the early techniques of general anaesthesia (Chapter 1). Postoperative vomiting with both chloroform and ether could lead to an increase in intraocular pressure sufficient to cause extrusion of the contents of the globe through the incision, so destroying any possible benefit from the surgery. Koller's introduction of topical anaesthesia produced by the instillation of cocaine solution was a major advance, and within a year Knapp (1884) had developed the technique by injecting cocaine behind the eye to perform an enucleation.

The uptake of this new method was limited by the inherent toxicity of cocaine, but the development of a safer agent, procaine, led to renewed interest. In 1934 Atkinson (1934) described retrobulbar block in which local anaesthetic is injected deep within the orbit. Despite the significant risks of perforation, haemorrhage, and brainstem spread, it remained the standard technique until Davis and Mandel (1986) described the peribulbar technique in which injections are made more anteriorly. The final step in the evolution of ophthalmic regional anaesthesia was the description of injection beneath Tenon's fascia by Stevens (1992), a technique which requires basic surgical skills and insertion of a blunt cannula rather than a sharp needle.

As anaesthetic techniques developed, there was a similar evolution in surgical practice. Cataract extraction changed from a 10-day in-patient procedure involving an open eye and multiple sutures, to a self-sealing incision, phacoemulsification method which allows the procedure to be performed during a brief day-stay visit. This rapid, minimally invasive technique made fewer demands on both patient and anaesthesia, with surgeons soon realizing that topical anaesthesia alone can be used in a significant proportion of cases. The result is that ophthalmic local anaesthesia has almost come full circle back to topical techniques. However, topical anaesthesia is not suitable for all patients, surgeons, or procedures, and the clinician must retain the skills to perform a variety of techniques.

Orbital anatomy

The orbit is a four-sided pyramid with its apex pointing postero-medially (Figure 20.1) and its base, formed by the orbital margins (Figure 20.2), facing anteriorly. Of the four walls, the medial is parallel to the sagittal plane, the lateral is angled 45° backwards, the inferior slopes 10° upwards towards the apex, and the roof is horizontal. The globe sits slightly medially and superiorly in the anterior half of the orbit (Figure 20.3), suspended by a framework of muscles and fascia. It is 2.3–2.5 cm long (the axial length), with the 'equator' about half-way back. Myopic eyes may be longer with thinner sclera, and thus be at greater risk of needle perforation.

The six extraocular muscles comprise the four rectus (medial, lateral, superior, and inferior) and two oblique (superior and inferior) muscles, these rotating the globe in various planes within the orbit. The rectus muscles arise from the annulus of Zinn at the back of the orbit (Figures 20.2 and 20.4), sweep forward to be inserted into the globe just anterior to the equator and thus form an incomplete cone behind the eye. This cone divides the orbit into *retrobulbar* and *peribulbar* spaces, with many key structures (optic nerve, ophthalmic artery, ciliary ganglion, and the nerves to the muscles) running within the cone. Anterior to the globe are the eyelids which are closed by the circumferential orbicularis orbis, with the upper lid being opened by levator palpebrae superioris.

Numerous fascial sheets enclose and support the tissues within the orbit, and subdivide it into compartments containing nerves, muscles, blood vessels, and adipose tissue. However, these compartments are rarely complete, and fluid in one may flow readily into others (Ripart et al. 2001). Of particular anaesthetic interest is Tenon's fascia which surrounds the rectus muscles and provides a smooth, shiny capsule within which the globe can rotate. Posteriorly, it fuses with fibres of the dura where the optic nerve enters the orbit, and anteriorly it fuses with the conjunctiva, 2–3 mm from the limbus of the eye.

The blood supply is by the ophthalmic artery which runs with the optic nerve through the optic canal and into the rear of the

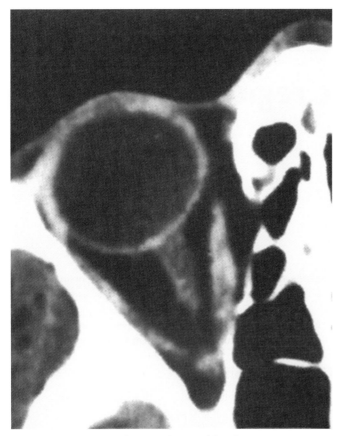

Figure 20.1 Axial computed tomography scan of the orbit.

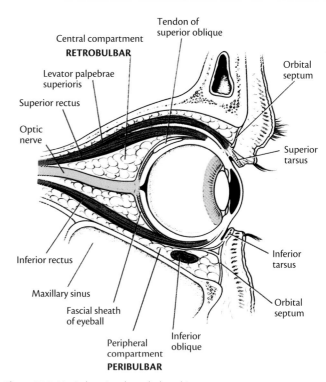

Figure 20.3 Vertical section through the orbit.

orbit. It divides into many branches, but the main vessel winds forwards, superiorly and medially, into the superonasal quadrant.

Innervation

The oculomotor (third cranial) nerve supplies the superior, inferior, and medial rectus muscles, the inferior oblique, and levator palpebrae superioris; the trochlear (fourth) nerve supplies the superior oblique, the abducent (sixth) nerve the lateral rectus, and the facial (seventh) nerve the orbicularis oculi through its temporal and zygomatic branches (see Chapter 19). Autonomic fibres run from the ciliary ganglion which lies within the cone, near the apex of the orbit.

The retina is innervated by the optic (second cranial) nerve, but all other sensory supply is by branches of the trigeminal (fifth).

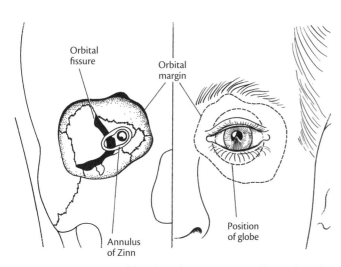

Figure 20.2 Anterior view of the orbit and its contents. Dotted lines indicate the positions of the orbital margin and globe.

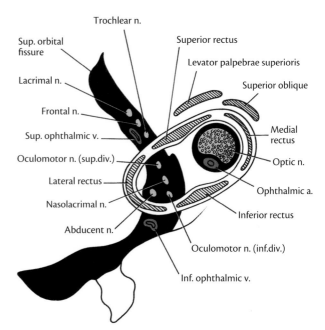

Figure 20.4 Structures at the apex of the orbit.

The lower eyelids are supplied by the maxillary division, and all of the other structures by the ophthalmic: the cornea, sclera, iris, and ciliary body by the nasociliary branch, the conjunctiva by the lacrimal.

The branches of the trigeminal nerve are the main targets for regional anaesthesia, but assessment of efficacy prior to surgery usually involves tests of function of the muscles supplied by oculomotor, trochlear, and abducent nerves. Fortunately, they are closely related anatomically to the trigeminal branches so assessment of their function provides a good marker of effect.

Pharmacology

Local anaesthetics

The general pharmacology of the local anaesthetics has been described in Chapters 6–8, and most aspects apply, but a few specific points may be made here.

Mixing of local anaesthetics is common in ophthalmic regional anaesthesia. Modest alterations in efficacy can be achieved, although any benefit will be lost by poor placement of the solution. Virtually all of the currently available local anaesthetic agents may be used in high concentrations.

Lidocaine

Lidocaine is used widely in ophthalmic anaesthesia because of its admirable toxicity profile and low cost. The 2% solution provides rapid onset and duration of action of up to an hour. Lower concentrations may be used, but do not provide sufficient anaesthesia for most procedures.

Prilocaine

The higher concentrations (3% and 4%) of prilocaine were popular with ophthalmic anaesthetists, but cases of retinal and optic nerve damage after orbital injection led to withdrawal of the licence for this application. The lower concentrations are still available for ophthalmic use, but they do not provide reliable anaesthesia for ocular procedures.

Articaine

Structurally similar to prilocaine (Chapter 6), articaine is used widely for dentistry and has recently been applied to ophthalmic practice, although without a great deal of formal study. The 3% and 4% solutions provide rapid onset and intermediate duration of block although the offset may be abrupt compared to other local anaesthetics. As long as the surgical procedure is comfortably within the duration of action, this rapid offset is advantageous because postoperative pain is rarely severe and return of nerve function allows the patient to resume normal activities.

Bupivacaine

In larger volumes, bupivacaine (0.5% or 0.75%) can provide 2 or more hours of block after orbital injection, but it also has a relatively slow onset, adequate anaesthesia, and orbital akinesia requiring about 5 minutes after retrobulbar placement and up to 25 minutes with peribulbar techniques.

Improvements in onset have been sought by co-administration with lidocaine or a variety of adjuvants. Equal volumes of lidocaine and bupivacaine are often mixed in the hope of combining the rapid onset of lidocaine with the prolonged duration of bupivacaine, but the actual outcome is a solution with onset and duration intermediate between the two agents used alone.

Levobupivacaine

The lower toxicity of levobupivacaine may be useful for peribulbar block in elderly patients with significant cardiovascular co-morbidity, allowing a large volume of a high concentration of local anaesthetic to be administered.

Ropivacaine

While the lower toxicity of ropivacaine might also be appealing in high-risk patients, it also produces either less motor block than other long acting agents, or motor block of shorter duration. This makes it unappealing in ophthalmic practice given that akinesia can be very important.

Topical local anaesthetics

Oxybuprocaine 0.4%, proxymetacaine 1%, and tetracaine 0.5–1% are all used commonly in the UK, but the former two are preferred for initial instillation because they cause much less discomfort than tetracaine. However, it has a longer duration and is used commonly with intracameral lidocaine to provide anaesthesia without injection.

Adjuvants

Vasoconstrictors

Vasoconstrictors may be added to local anaesthetic solutions for ophthalmic use for the usual reasons of minimizing bleeding and slowing absorption of the drug, although the practice has declined. Commercial preparations containing adrenaline also include a stabilizer (e.g. metabisulphite) which may cause local tissue toxicity or allergic reactions, and they have a low pH which increases discomfort on injection. Adding the adrenaline immediately prior to injection overcomes these concerns, but affords the opportunity of inadvertently concocting a dangerous mixture. In addition, the longer acting drugs provide sufficient duration without vasoconstrictor although some use lidocaine or prilocaine with adrenaline to provide a medium duration and less need for postoperative eye protection. However, the concentration of adrenaline should not exceed 1:200,000. The impact of intense vasoconstriction of the ophthalmic artery is unknown, but it is likely to compromise retinal circulation.

Hyaluronidase

Hyaluronidase temporarily hydrolyses the hyaluronic acid component of ground substance, improving local anaesthetic spread through tissues. It is believed to improve the speed of onset and quality of block after retrobulbar and sub-Tenon's fascia injections, but the evidence is equivocal for peribulbar block. Hyaluronidase appears to have a beneficial effect after peribulbar injection of less than 9 ml of solution, but the effect is lost with larger volumes which may flood the orbit and mask any effect. The optimal concentration and volume of hyaluronidase is not known, but addition of 7.5 IU ml^{-1} to the injectate is usual (Thomson 1988).

General management

Patient selection

Virtually all ophthalmic procedures in adults can be performed in the awake patient, and absolute contraindications to regional anaesthesia are rare, but include patient refusal, coagulopathy, local infection, inability to communicate (severe deafness, confusion, dementia, language barrier), and difficulty keeping still (involuntary movement, cough). Other conditions such as anxiety, dizziness, mild tremors, claustrophobia, obstructive sleep apnoea, severe reflux, restless leg syndrome, and difficulty lying flat (scoliosis, kyphosis, heart failure) are challenging, but do not preclude the use of local anaesthesia.

The widespread success of local anaesthesia reduced the use of general anaesthesia for cataract extraction surgery from 24.2% in 1996 to 4.1% in 2003 (Eke & Thomson 1999, 2007). Increasing confidence with local anaesthesia for cataract surgery has extended its use to longer, more complex surgery, including a significant proportion of vitreo-retinal surgery.

Patient preparation

Patient selection for local anaesthesia is usually determined by the surgeon with preassessment in nurse-led clinics, but high-risk patients should be referred for an anaesthetic opinion. With the exception of clotting tests in patients taking warfarin, routine investigations are unnecessary, but may be required if the patient has developed new symptoms or familiar symptoms have worsened (Report 2001). An outline of the procedure, as well as the risks involved, should be given to patients in a format which can be taken home from the clinic. In particular, they should be told that, even with a functioning block, they may experience visual 'sensations', including colours and movements, during surgery.

There is no need for the patient to fast prior preoperatively because serious complications are rare, sedation should be very light (if used at all) and the surgery will be performed under general anaesthesia at a later date if the local technique fails. The surgeon should be aware of any patient taking an α-adrenergic blocking agent (e.g. tamsulosin) for prostatic hyperplasia because these drugs are associated with the 'floppy iris syndrome', a major surgical challenge. The clinician performing the block should check that the axial length of the patient's eye has been measured because if it is 26 mm or greater there is an increased risk of globe perforation.

Monitoring and general care

Prior to the block the patient should empty the bladder, and then be positioned comfortably supine; the 'deck chair' position often suits the elderly, kyphotic population. Instrumental monitoring should include electrocardiography and pulse oximetry, and a sphygmomanometer cuff should be applied, but used with caution because it may disturb the patient. Intravenous access is mandatory for all sharp needle methods, and advisable when there is no dedicated anaesthetist in attendance or the patient is high risk, whatever the block technique.

Resuscitation equipment, drugs, and expertise should be immediately available.

Block techniques

As indicated already, there have been major changes in ophthalmic local anaesthetic techniques in the last 15–20 years. In 1996, general anaesthesia was used in only 24% of cataract procedures, with a 'sharp' needle (retro- or peribulbar) block being used in 83%, and a sub-Tenon's fascia block in 6.7%, of those receiving local anaesthesia (Eke & Thomson 1999). In contrast, an audit of 55,567 patients undergoing cataract extraction between 2001 and 2006 found that 20% of patients had a sharp needle block, 47% a sub-Tenon's fascia block, and 25% topical anaesthesia (El-Hindy et al. 2009). This change has been driven by evolving technology, surgical techniques, and, almost certainly, the medicolegal environment. Despite the widespread adoption of sub-Tenon's fascia block, the choice of technique for individual patients still depends on anaesthetic knowledge and experience, surgical preference, and patient factors. Not all patients are suitable for sub-Tenon's fascia block and the clinician needs to know how to use other methods.

All of the injection techniques should be performed after producing topical anaesthesia of the conjunctiva.

Retrobulbar block

The defining characteristic of retrobulbar (intraconal) block is the deep insertion of a sharp needle behind the globe and within the cone of the rectus muscles (Figure 20.5). Early proponents of the technique used 35–38-mm, 25-g needles, but these can reach the delicate structures at the rear of the orbit in a significant proportion of patients so 25-mm needles are now preferred (Katsev et al. 1989). Blunt needles have been used to increase tactile feedback and alert the clinician that the needle tip may be entering the tough fibrous wall of the sclera, but concerns that any subsequent damage could be worse prompted a return to fine, sharp needles (Grizzard et al. 1991).

Classically, the patient is asked to look upwards and inwards during needle insertion, but CT studies have shown that this rotates the optic nerve and ophthalmic artery into the path of the needle, so modern practice favours keeping the eye in the neutral position (Unsold et al. 1981). Similarly, the original needle insertion site was the junction of the lateral and middle thirds of the inferior orbital margin (Atkinson 1961), but this places the inferior

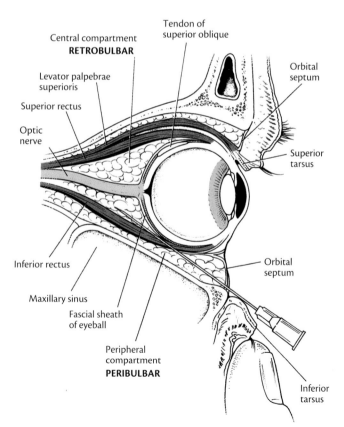

Figure 20.5 Needle position for retrobulbar block.

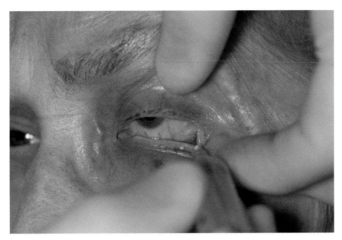

Figure 20.6 Needle insertion point for retrobulbar block.

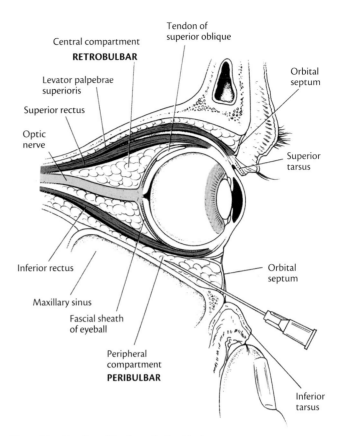

Figure 20.7 Needle position for peribulbar block.

oblique muscle in the needle path. However, if the needle is inserted as far laterally as is practicable (Figure 20.6), the path to the intraconal space is harmless, being through fat-filled tissues.

The needle may be inserted transcutaneously or transconjunctivally, but the latter is preferred because prior application of topical local anaesthetic in the conjunctival fornix minimizes discomfort, and it avoids needle insertion through another vascular layer. The needle is advanced straight back from the insertion site, with the bevel facing the globe, until the tip has passed the equator of the eye. At this point the needle is realigned, upwards and medially, to enter the muscular cone, but ensuring that it does not cross the mid-sagittal plane of the orbit. An aspiration test is performed to exclude vascular placement before 3–5 ml of local anaesthetic is injected slowly.

The onset of block is usually rapid and is assessed by noting the degree of akinesia; good analgesia cannot be assured if this does not develop. Retrobulbar injection does not block the facial nerve so the patient will still be able to squeeze the eye shut, a manoeuvre which can lead to serious complications during surgery. The facial nerve can be blocked using a variety of superficial injections along its course from the tragus to the lateral angle of the eye (Zahl 1990), but all are painful and each has its complications (Hamilton 1998).

Peribulbar block

Peribulbar (extraconal, parabulbar) block avoids the insertion of a sharp needle deep into the orbit (Figure 20.7). The needle (25 mm 25 g as described previously) is passed backwards, but no attempt is made to re-align it and place the tip within the muscle cone. Deposition of local anaesthetic at a greater distance from the target nerves requires use of a larger volume of solution and often more than one injection.

The landmarks and insertion site for the first injection are the same as for retrobulbar block, the needle being directed backwards in the inferotemporal quadrant until the tip lies beyond the equator of the eye at a depth of around 20 mm. An aspiration test is performed and 5 ml of local anaesthetic is injected. It is not unusual for there to be minimal akinesia in the medial aspect so a second injection may be needed, the same type of needle being used. With the eye in the neutral position, the needle is inserted at the most medial point of the medial canthus, and directed straight

backwards into the orbit (Figure 20.8). A slight resistance and subtle pop may be felt as the needle traverses the medial check ligament, but it should be inserted no more than 20 mm because it will be pointing directly at the optic canal and nerve. Again, an aspiration test is performed before 5 ml of local anaesthetic is injected. Some practitioners perform only the medial canthus injection. This can provide good anaesthesia although a larger volume, typically around 8 ml, is required and it may be more painful than an inferotemporal injection.

If complete akinesia does not develop a further injection may be performed, the site depending on the pattern of inadequacy of the

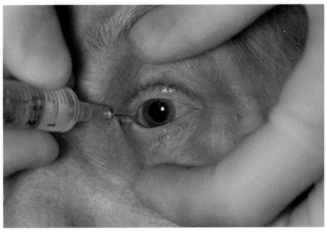

Figure 20.8 Needle insertion point for peribulbar block.

existing block. However, if a repeat injection is required, it is usually the inferotemporal injection which requires augmentation. The superonasal quadrant should be avoided because it contains structures (a rich network of blood vessels and both trochlea & superior oblique muscles) which are damaged easily.

Although local anaesthetic is placed outside the muscle cone, studies have shown that the local anaesthetic moves widely, spreading reliably into the cone (Ripart et al. 2001). The greater volume also pushes the solution anteriorly, filling the lids and blocking orbicularis oculi, thereby avoiding the need for a facial nerve block. Gentle pressure over a taped closed eye may be applied to help disperse the local anaesthetic and reduce the pressure in the eye before surgery.

Sub-Tenon's fascia block

Sub-Tenon's block has gained wide popularity because it does not involve the blind insertion of a sharp needle so that the feared complications of globe perforation, retrobulbar haemorrhage, and spread to the brainstem are almost completely avoided. However, there are disadvantages: the technique requires a degree of surgical dexterity and provision of a specific cannula.

As with the other blocks, the procedure begins with topical anaesthesia of the conjunctiva. This is followed by antiseptic drops (5% povidone iodine) before a speculum is inserted gently to keep the lids apart. The patient is asked to look upwards and outwards before a non-toothed forceps is used to grasp the conjunctiva 5–8 mm distal to the inferomedial limbus, the point where the conjunctiva is fused firmly with Tenon's fascia (Figure 20.9). A small nick is made in the conjunctiva and Tenon's fascia using round tipped spring scissors to reveal the space below. The conjunctival edge is held with the forceps to exert countertraction while the tip of a blunt cannula (connected to a loaded syringe) is passed gently down over the sclera and 15–20 mm into the space within the fascia (Figure 20.10).

If resistance is encountered, a little solution may be injected to 'hydrodissect' the tissue layers. If this is unsuccessful the cannula may be withdrawn and very gentle blunt dissection performed with round tipped scissors. The scissors should be used carefully to probe the space to find or form a passage for the cannula, but the jaws of the scissors should never be closed if they cannot be seen. With the tip of the cannula in the correct space a small volume

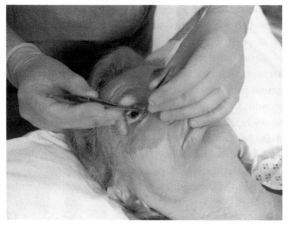

Figure 20.9 Site of conjunctival incision for sub-Tenon's fascia block.

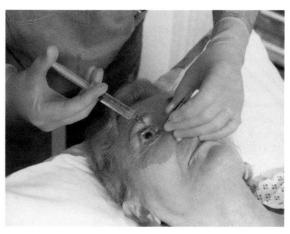

Figure 20.10 Cannula for sub-Tenon's fascia block partially inserted.

(3–6 ml) of local anaesthetic is injected. Within minutes a sensory block will have developed because the short ciliary nerves, which traverse the space, are bathed in local anaesthetic solution. Muscular akinesia takes longer, and often spares the lateral rectus and superior oblique muscles, but this should not represent a problem in simple cataract surgery.

There are few contraindications to sub-Tenon's fascia block, but previous placement of an encircling band during retinal detachment surgery obstructs access to the space so an alternative technique must be used. A pterygium, or other conjunctival lesion in the inferonasal quadrant, or previous medial rectus surgery also prevents access, but the inferotemporal quadrant can be used instead.

Systemic complications

Medical emergencies

Life-threatening events may be precipitated by the injection, or be a consequence of the physiological changes which can occur perioperatively (Rubin 1995). The patients undergoing ophthalmic surgery are often elderly with significant co-morbidity: 45% are hypertensive, 15% have had a myocardial infarct, and 15% are diabetic. On the day of surgery they are anxious, may omit their cardioprotective medication and then receive sympathomimetic dilating eye drops. They are required to lie almost flat under claustrophobic drapes and are then subjected to a potentially frightening surgical procedure. It is unsurprising that many have an increased heart rate and blood pressure, and that some decompensate to develop arrhythmias, heart failure, and cerebrovascular events. Despite this, such complications are relatively uncommon, 3.4 serious events being reported per 100,000 cataract extractions in 1996 (Eke & Thompson 1999), and none were related to any particular local anaesthetic technique.

Brainstem spread

Spread of local anaesthetic to the brainstem may be caused by inadvertent perforation of the dural cuff surrounding the optic nerve and injection of local anaesthetic into the CSF. It presents rapidly with confusion, cranial nerve palsies, coma, hypotension, bradycardia, and respiratory arrest. Treatment is supportive and requires skilled resuscitation. It is more easily caused by sharp needle techniques, estimations of the incidence with retrobulbar block being 0.3–0.8% (Hamilton 1992, Nichol et al. 1987), but it has been reported after sub-Tenon's fascia block (Ruschen et al. 2003).

Local anaesthetic toxicity

Systemic local anaesthetic toxicity may be due to an absolute over-dose of local anaesthetic or, more commonly, an intravascular injection of a normal dose of local anaesthetic. With the doses used for ophthalmic blocks intravenous injection is unlikely to have serious consequences, but if the same dose is injected at high pressure into an artery there may be retrograde spread to the brainstem provoking seizures, hypertension, arrhythmias, and coma. Treatment of systemic toxicity is considered in Chapter 8.

Local complications

Local complications can be sight threatening and the result of trauma from sharp needles or surgical dissection, or may be related to the constituents of the local anaesthetic solution.

Subconjunctival haemorrhage

Subconjunctival haemorrhage may occur with any technique, although it is more common with sub-Tenon's anaesthesia and in patients taking antiplatelet medication. It is essentially cosmetic and rarely presents a clinical problem.

Chemosis

Distension of the conjunctiva with local anaesthetic occurs most often with sub-Tenon's fascia block. It is rarely important except in glaucoma surgery where it may interfere with modelling of the scleral flap so some surgeons insist on sharp needle blocks in the belief that chemosis is less likely.

Retrobulbar haemorrhage

Retrobulbar haemorrhage may occur in about 1% of sharp needle blocks, although it has also been described after sub-Tenon's fascia block (Rahman & Ataullah 2004). It may present with pain, proptosis, immobility of the globe, subconjunctival haemorrhage, and extensive bruising around the eye, the sight of the eye being threatened if perfusion of the retina or optic nerve is compromised by arterial damage or increased orbital pressure. Successful management relies on early detection and surgical assessment of retinal perfusion, decompressive manoeuvres being required if this is inadequate. The risks of significant haemorrhage may be reduced by avoiding injections into the very vascular superonasal quadrant and in patients with coagulopathy.

Globe perforation

Estimates of the incidence of globe perforation vary widely, some reporting rates of less than 1 in over 10,000 blocks (Hamilton et al. 1988). However, in long eyes (axial length 26 mm or greater) rates of 1 in 140 have been calculated (Dukker et al. 1991). Increased axial length is significant because of the increasing prevalence of staphylomas, outward protrusions of the eye, often located posteriorly, and not obvious to the clinician performing the block. The staphyloma may be punctured by a needle which otherwise would have passed the eye safely. Other risk factors include uncooperative patients and inexperienced operators, but globe perforation has occurred in very experienced hands.

Globe perforation presents with pain, hypotony, loss of vision, and loss of a red reflex. It may be catastrophic because the needle detaches the retina and may provoke a rapid intraocular bleed. Treatment is rarely simple, and often requires further complex surgery. The prognosis can be good, but is more often poor. The risk may be reduced by measuring the length of the eye before the block, digital assessment of the space between the globe and the orbital margin, keeping the eye in the neutral position, and ensuring that the tip of the needle is not directed 'upwards and inwards' before it has passed the equator of the eye.

Optic nerve injury

The optic nerve may be damaged by direct needle trauma, intraneural injection of local anaesthetic and any interference with its blood supply.

Muscle injury

The delicate orbital muscles may be injured directly by the needle or by haemorrhage secondary to it, intramuscular injection of high concentrations of local anaesthetic (e.g. lidocaine 4%), elevation of orbital pressure compromising muscle perfusion, or by surgical manoeuvres. Inflammation of the damaged muscle may progress to fibrosis and contraction which can present as diplopia or strabismus. Sharp needle techniques are thought to have a higher incidence, but it has also been reported after sub-Tenon's fascia block (Jaycock et al. 2001). Hyaluronidase may have a protective effect by allowing more rapid dispersal of the local anaesthetic away from the muscle, but vasoconstrictors may worsen muscle injury.

Allergy

Allergy to local anaesthetics is extremely rare, but allergy to hyaluronidase has been reported (Agrawal et al. 2003). However, it tends to be relatively localized and systemic reactions or death have not been reported.

Key references

Report (2001) *Joint College Guidelines: Local Anaesthesia for Intraocular Surgery*. London: The Royal College of Anaesthetists and The Royal College of Ophthalmologists.

Stevens JD (1992) A new local anaesthetic technique for cataract extraction by one quadrant sub-Tenon's infiltration. *British Journal of Ophthalmology* 76: 670–4.

References

Agrawal A, McLure HA, Dabbs TR (2003) Allergic reaction to hyaluronidase after a peribulbar injection. *Anaesthesia* 58: 493–4.

Atkinson WS (1934) Local anaesthesia in ophthalmology. *Transactions of the American Ophthalmological Society* 32: 399–451.

Atkinson WS (1961) The development of ophthalmic anesthesia. *American Journal of Ophthalmology* 51: 1–14.

Davis DB, Mandel MR (1986) Posterior peribulbar anaesthesia: An alternative to retrobulbar anaesthesia. *Journal of Cataract and Refractive Surgery* 12: 182–4.

Dukker JS, Belmont JB, Benson WE, et al. (1991) Inadvertent globe perforation during retrobulbar and peribulbar anesthesia. Patient characteristics, surgical management, and visual outcome. *Ophthalmology* 98: 519–26.

Eke T, Thompson JR (1999) The National Survey of Local Anaesthesia for Ocular Surgery. I. Survey methodology and current practice. *Eye* 13: 189–95.

Eke T, Thompson JR (2007) Serious complications of local anaesthesia for cataract surgery: a 1 year national survey in the United Kingdom. *British Journal of Ophthalmology* 91: 470–5.

El-Hindy N, Johnston RL, Jaycock P, et al. (2009) The Cataract National Dataset Electronic Multi-centre Audit of 55,567 operations: anaesthetic techniques and complications. *Eye* 23: 50–5.

Grizzard WS, Kirk NM, Pavan PR, et al. (1991) Perforating ocular injuries caused by anesthesia personnel. *Ophthalmology* 98: 1011–16.

Hamilton RC (1992) Brain-stem anaesthesia as a complication of regional anaesthesia for ophthalmic surgery. *Canadian Journal of Ophthalmology* 27: 323–5.

Hamilton RC (1998) Complications of ophthalmic anesthesia. *Ophthalmological Clinics of North America* 11: 99–114.

Hamilton RC, Gimbel HV, Strunin L (1988) Regional anaesthesia for 12,000 cataract extraction and intraocular lens implantation procedures. *Canadian Journal of Anaesthesia* 35: 615–23.

Jaycock PD, Mather CM, Ferris JD, Kirkpatrick JN (2001) Rectus muscle trauma complicating sub-Tenon's local anaesthesia. *Eye* 15: 583–6.

Katsey DA, Drew RC, Rose BT (1989) An anatomic study of retrobulbar needle path length. *Ophthalmology* 96: 1221–4.

Knapp H (1884) On cocaine and its use in ophthalmic and general surgery. *Archives of Ophthalmology* 13: 402–48.

Nicoll JM, Acharya PA, Ahlen K, et al. (1987) Central nervous system complications after 6000 retrobulbar blocks. *Anesthesia & Analgesia* 66: 1298–302.

Rahman I, Ataullah S (2004) Retrobulbar haemorrhage after sub-Tenon's anesthesia. *Journal of Cataract & Refractive Surgery* 30: 2636–7.

Report (2001) *Joint College Guidelines: Local Anaesthesia for Intraocular Surgery*. London: The Royal College of Anaesthetists and The Royal College of Ophthalmologists.

Ripart J, Lefrant JY, de La Coussaye JE, et al. (2001) Peribulbar versus retrobulbar anesthesia for ophthalmic surgery: an anatomical comparison of extraconal and intraconal injections. *Anesthesiology* 94: 55–62.

Rubin AP (1995) Complications of local anaesthesia for ophthalmic surgery. *British Journal of Anaesthesia* 75: 93–6.

Ruschen H, Bremner FD, Carr C (2003) Complications after sub-Tenon's eye block. *Anesthesia & Analgesia* 96: 272–7.

Stevens JD (1992) A new local anaesthetic technique for cataract extraction by one quadrant sub-Tenon's infiltration. *British Journal of Ophthalmology* 76: 670–4.

Thomson I (1988) Addition of hyaluronidase to lignocaine with adrenaline for retrobulbar anaesthesia in the surgery of senile cataract. *British Journal of Ophthalmology* 72: 700–2.

Unsöld R, Stanley JA, Degroot J (1981) The CT-topography of retrobulbar anesthesia. Anatomic-clinical correlation of complications and suggestion of a modified technique. *Albrecht Von Graefes Archiv fur Klinische und Experimentelle Ophthalmologie* 217: 125–36.

Zahl K (1990) Blockade of the orbicularis oculi. In Zahl K, Meltzer MA (Eds) *Regional Anesthesia for intraocular surgery*, pp. 93–100. Philadelphia, PA: WB Saunders.

CHAPTER 21

Regional anaesthesia in obstetrics

Catriona Connolly and John McClure

Effective and safe regional anaesthesia in obstetrics requires a sound knowledge of the anatomy of the nervous system and reproductive tract, the physiology of pregnancy, and the pharmacology of local anaesthetic drugs. The anaesthetist learns to apply this knowledge through performing regional techniques under close senior supervision on the labour ward and in the operating theatre. The need to provide trainees with such supervised experience was the justification for introducing specialists in obstetric anaesthesia in the mid 20th century in the UK, largely through the efforts of the Faculty (now Royal College) of Anaesthetists and the Obstetric Anaesthetists Association.

It was James 'Young' Simpson (Simpson 1848) who originally proposed that 'local anaesthesia' might be used as an alternative to general anaesthesia, but this was not realized in obstetrics until 1900 when Kreis (1900) used spinal anaesthesia during operative vaginal delivery. Sacral epidural analgesia (with procaine) was first used during labour by Stoeckel (1909) who also warned of the risk of 'impairing the force of labour', but regional analgesia, especially lumbar epidural block, is now widely available, there being several reasons for its popularity.

The main alternative methods—parenteral and inhalational—have the potential to produce centrally mediated side effects in both mother (e.g. amnesia for the birth, confusion, disorientation, and nausea) and child. In the neonate, the effect can extend from mild neurobehavioural abnormalities, detectable only by sophisticated testing (Brockhurst et al. 2000), to severe respiratory depression with failure to initiate normal respiration at birth. Regional analgesia offers the possibility of maternal pain relief without clouding of consciousness or neonatal depression and has minimal effect on uterine blood flow or the fetus itself (Halpern et al. 1998). Further, low-dose combinations of local anaesthetic and opioid for epidural analgesia are now commonplace and associated with improved maternal satisfaction, a shorter second stage, and a lower incidence of instrumental delivery than earlier high dose local anaesthetic techniques (Cooper et al. 2010b, Hein et al. 2010, James et al. 1998). Additionally, bladder function is better preserved and allows a lower incidence of catheterization during labour (Wilson et al. 2009). Most elective and emergency operative deliveries are now performed under epidural or spinal anaesthesia, so reducing considerably the number of general anaesthetics required and contributing, almost certainly, to the decline in maternal deaths due to anaesthesia in the UK (Reports 1991–2008).

Thus pregnant women now have high expectations of safe, effective pain relief in labour, and regional anaesthesia for operative delivery if it is required. It is crucial that these expectations are realistic so written and verbal information should be available in both the antenatal setting (well before the pain of labour interferes with decision-making) and the labour ward for access in early labour. Patient information leaflets, in many languages, are available free-of-charge from the Obstetric Anaesthetists Association Website (www.oaa-anaes.ac.uk/content.asp?ContentID=185). Complete pain relief cannot be guaranteed so it is imperative that women understand that this is the case and that strategies are in place to deal with partial or complete failure of regional block.

Key principles

Innervation of the uterus and birth canal

The pain of uterine contractions is transmitted along visceral afferent Aδ and C fibres running through the sympathetic nerves and chain to the T_{10}–L_1 segments of the spinal cord (Figure 21.1). This pain is felt in the lower abdomen and back. Back pain may be very severe and extend into the sacral area if the fetal head persists in the occipitoposterior (OP) position and presses on the lumbosacral plexus and other structures in the pelvis. The pain of the second stage is caused by stretching of the birth canal and perineum. It is transmitted primarily through the (somatic) pudendal nerves to the S_2–S_4 segments cord, but the ilio-inguinal, genitofemoral (genital branches), and the posterior nerves of the thigh (perineal branches) may also be involved. This may explain, in part, the poor quality of analgesia obtained with pudendal nerve block.

Aorto-caval occlusion

The gravid uterus compresses the vena cava and aorta against the lumbar spine in all women at term, although not all will have symptoms of the 'supine hypotensive syndrome of pregnancy' (Holmes 1960). Venous return will depend on the adequacy of flow through the paravertebral and azygous veins, but there is, almost inevitably, some reduction in both cardiac output and uterine blood flow (Kerr et al. 1964, Lees et al. 1967). Lateral tilt may partially relieve the compression, but the full lateral position or manual uterine displacement may be required in some cases, particularly when the uterus is large (Kinsella et al. 1992). Arterial blood pressure may, to some extent, be maintained by compensatory vasoconstriction, but

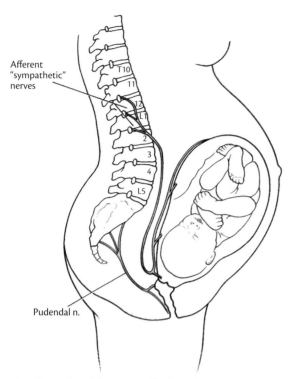

Afferent "sympathetic" nerves

Pudendal n.

Figure 21.1 Innervation of the uterus and birth canal.

regional anaesthesia will abolish this so hypotension should be anticipated and prevented by scrupulous attention to the woman's position and the maintenance of the circulation with vasopressors and intravenous fluid.

Epidural space

The anatomy and physiology of the epidural space are considered in Chapter 12. Recent work has questioned the existence of a negative pressure in the non-pregnant epidural space, earlier observations possibly reflecting indentation of the dura by needle or catheter (Aitkenhead et al. 1979). In late pregnancy, increases in intra-abdominal pressure and venous pressure (the latter by caval compression) both increase epidural pressure, as do the sitting position and the second stage of labour (Galbert & Marx 1974). It is therefore not surprising that Usubiaga and colleagues (1967) failed to demonstrate a negative epidural pressure in women undergoing Caesarean section. Venous distension and the humoral effects of progesterone reduce the compliance of the epidural space and are thought to cause the enhanced epidural drug spread seen in the pregnant woman (Datta et al. 1983, Fagraeus et al. 1983, Park 1988).

Ultrasound examination of the pregnant and non-pregnant epidural space showed that the soft-tissue 'channel' between the spinal processes, the skin–epidural distance and the epidural space are all narrower in pregnancy (Grau et al. 2001). The epidural space is also deformed by the tissue changes, and the ultrasonic 'visibility' of the ligamentum flavum, the dura mater, and the epidural space all decrease.

Management of hypotension

Hypotension induced by epidural or spinal anaesthesia can be prevented or treated with a vasopressor such as phenylephrine or

ephedrine (Ramanathan & Grant 1988, Ramanathan et al. 1984, Taylor & Tunstall 1991). Phenylephrine is the agent of choice during elective Caesarean section because it is associated with higher fetal pH than ephedrine (Prakash et al. 2010). It may be administered by continuous infusion or bolus dose, although the former has been found to produce better blood pressure control, and is associated with less nausea and vomiting than ephedrine (Cooper et al. 2002). In contrast though, a retrospective study of almost 400 women undergoing high-risk Caesarean section for fetal compromise, found that umbilical artery pH was similar whether ephedrine or phenylephrine was used to maintain maternal arterial pressure (Cooper et al. 2010a).

Fluid therapy

The technique of *preloading* (Ramanathan et al. 1983) with a fixed volume (500–1000 ml) of crystalloid solution *before* a central block is established is no longer common. Early work (Collins et al. 1978) demonstrated a significant decrease in the incidence of hypotension and fetal heart rate (FHR) abnormalities in a group of pre-loaded labouring women, but the epidurals were established using 10 ml bupivacaine 0.375%. More recent studies (Kinsella et al. 2000, Kubli et al. 2003) in women whose epidurals were established with bupivacaine 0.1% and fentanyl found that pre-loading had no influence on the incidence of hypotension or FHR abnormalities. *Co-loading* is the administration of intravenous fluid *while* the block is being administered, and a meta-analysis of eight studies comprising more than 500 women (Banerjee et al. 2010) found that there was no difference in maternal hypotension or neonatal outcome in comparison with pre-loading. Preloading risks overloading the circulation and should certainly be avoided in women with pre-eclampsia or cardiac disease with reduced left ventricular compliance. However, preloading should not be confused with, or regarded as a substitute for, the absolute requirement to maintain an adequate circulating volume. Hypovolaemia is very poorly tolerated in the presence of sympathetic block, and should be prevented or treated by volume replacement.

Peripheral techniques

Infiltration

Local anaesthetic infiltration is used widely by obstetricians and midwives before episiotomy or repair of a perineal tear. Lidocaine 1% is the agent of choice, but care must be taken with the total dose used in this very vascular area, the recommended maximum dose being 20 ml (200 mg) in a 70-kg adult. The addition of adrenaline 1:200,000 slows absorption and allows a larger dose of lidocaine (500 mg, 50 ml of 1%) to be given. Caesarean section has been performed under infiltration, mostly in countries where medical resources are limited.

Paracervical block

Paracervical block has largely disappeared from obstetric practice because of the risk of fetal bradycardia secondary to rapid uptake of local anaesthetic into the fetal circulation (Cibils 1976, Greiss et al. 1976), but it is still used for some gynaecological procedures. The visceral afferent fibres from the uterus are blocked by injecting 10 ml of lidocaine 1% on each side of the cervix below the mucosa of the lateral fornix. A guarded needle (Figure 21.2) is used and the injections should be made at '4' and '8 o'clock' to avoid the uterine

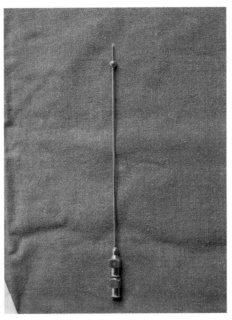
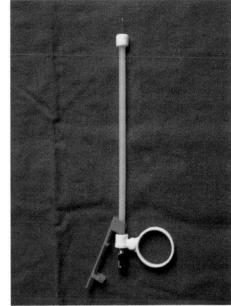

Figure 21.2 Kobak needle and disposable sheathed needle.

arteries and the fetal head. The duration of analgesia is limited (30–60 minutes) so the blocks may have to be repeated.

Pudendal nerve block

Bilateral pudendal nerve block may be used in the second stage of labour to reduce the discomfort of forceps delivery, but infiltration of the perineum and labia is also required to block the branches of the ilio-inguinal and genitofemoral nerves. The block is usually performed by the obstetrician, 5 minutes prior to delivery using lidocaine 1% and a transvaginal approach. This requires a guarded needle (Figure 21.2) to protect the vagina and the fetal head while the ischial spine is being located. The guide of the needle should be placed medial to the spine, at the point of attachment of the sacrospinous ligament. The needle is inserted through the vaginal wall and an initial dose of 5 ml of lidocaine 1% is injected. The needle is then advanced until a 'pop' indicates that it has penetrated the sacrospinous ligament and another 5 ml is injected. The procedure is repeated on the other side. A good block is not always guaranteed and a minimum of 5 minutes should be allowed for it to take effect (Hutchins 1980).

Transversus abdominal plane block

This relatively new block is described in Chapter 16. It has been used after Caesarean section (Issacs & Turner 2010), producing effective analgesia without opioid administration and allowing the mother to be ambulant 5 hours postoperatively.

Epidural block in labour

Caudal analgesia

Caudal block, performed through the sacral hiatus and described in Chapter 15, has been superseded by lumbar epidural techniques in obstetrics, but is of historical interest (Hingson & Edwards 1943. Stoeckel 1909).

Lumbar epidural analgesia

Ideally, an epidural catheter should be sited before the woman is distressed by severe pain to allow time for full patient assessment and informed consent to be obtained. Accurate catheter placement in an acutely distressed woman requires a degree of skill and dexterity that only comes with wide experience. The anaesthetist's task is easier, and safer for the woman, if she is cooperative and able to flex her spine in the sitting or lateral position. A skilled assistant is invaluable in supporting a distressed woman during epidural insertion, but occasionally a small dose (10–20 mcg) of intravenous fentanyl may be useful.

Ultrasound is becoming more widely used in regional techniques and, although pregnancy decreases the ultrasonic visibility of key structures (see 'Epidural space' section), Vallejo colleagues (2010) found that it decreased the epidural failure rate in first year trainees. It is anticipated that ultrasound will be of increasing use, particularly in placing epidurals in the obese women who are encountered more and more frequently on the labour ward.

Better mobility during labour, increasingly demanded by women, improves maternal satisfaction and enhances personal autonomy (Collis et al. 1995), and can be achieved by combining a low concentration of local anaesthetic with an opioid. However, increased mobility does not decrease the incidence of forceps or Caesarean delivery (Russell & Reynolds 1996).

Test doses

Various aspects of local anaesthetic test doses are described in Chapters 8, 11, and 14. The same principles apply when establishing a 'surgical' epidural for operative delivery so a formal test dose of a small volume of concentrated local anaesthetic (3–4 ml of lidocaine 2% or bupivacaine 0.5%) is recommended to exclude intrathecal or intravenous catheter placement. However, a formal test dose has become less necessary for an 'analgesic' epidural in labour with the introduction of low-dose techniques, the development of effective analgesia without motor block confirming accurate placement.

Intermittent injection technique

This technique has been in use since the 1970s. Typically, the epidural was established with a test dose of 4 ml lidocaine 2% followed by a loading dose of 6–8 ml bupivacaine 0.5%, and maintained by intermittent injections of bupivacaine 0.25–0.325% given 'on-demand'. This technique inevitably led to a degree of lower limb motor block and was associated with an increased risk of operative delivery. There was an element of 'patient-controlled analgesia' about the method, and it allowed for individual variability in analgesic requirements through labour, but severe pain could develop if the woman delayed her request or no one qualified to perform the injection was available.

Continuous infusion epidural analgesia (CIEA)

The introduction of accurate and reliable volumetric pumps, and concern about painful intervals, led to the development of CIEA. This was very popular in the 1980s because it reduced both the frequency of these intervals and the number of top-up injections required, but a fixed dose infusion does not allow for individual variability and causes an unacceptable degree of motor block in some women (Murphy et al. 1991, Thorburn & Moir 1981, Van Steenberge et al. 1987). Very low concentrations of bupivacaine (e.g. 0.08%) combined with fentanyl 2 mcg ml^{-1} reduce both the intensity of motor block and the number of supplementary injections required (Jones et al. 1989, Russell & Reynolds 1993).

Patient-controlled epidural analgesia (PCEA)

PCEA pumps can be programmed to give 'on demand' boluses (10–15 ml) of dilute local anaesthetic (e.g. bupivacaine 0.1%), usually with an opioid (e.g. fentanyl 2 mcg ml^{-1}). Each bolus is delivered at a rate of approximately 5 ml min^{-1}, and there is the further option of a low-volume background infusion, this approach providing the benefits of the earlier techniques, but avoiding their disadvantages. The hourly consumption can be limited to minimize drug toxicity, the low local anaesthetic dose reduces the risk of hypotension, and there is the additional bonus that the woman feels 'in control' (Gambling et al. 1988, Purdie et al. 1992). The low-dose drug combination allows greater mobility, improving both maternal satisfaction and the likelihood of spontaneous vaginal delivery (Murphy et al. 1991, Writer et al. 1998). As noted earlier a formal test dose is not required. With such low doses, lower limb motor block indicates that intrathecal injection has occurred, and lack of pain relief implies either venous injection or failure to place the catheter in the epidural space. However, a test dose should precede any subsequent administration of a larger dose of local anaesthetic.

Combined spinal–epidural analgesia (CSEA)

This technique was first described by Soresi (1937), and has since been adapted to provide good quality analgesia with minimal effect on motor power (Collis et al. 1994, Morgan 1995). As the name suggests, this technique comprises an initial intrathecal injection (usually of a small dose of local anaesthetic such as bupivacaine 2.5 mg and or a lipophilic opioid such as fentanyl 25 mcg) with the subsequent introduction of an epidural catheter for maintenance of analgesia. The intrathecal component provides rapid onset analgesia lasting approximately 1 hour and without loss of motor power, and the epidural catheter allows maintenance of analgesia thereafter using any of the techniques described earlier.

Three approaches have been described:

1. *Two needle, two interspace*: the first report of CSEA in obstetrics was by Brownridge (1981) who first placed an epidural catheter at the L$_1$–L$_2$ interspace, and then performed a spinal at L$_3$–L$_4$. Theoretically the spinal needle could cut the epidural catheter, but the risk is negligible with an atraumatic, pencil-point needle. If the spinal block is performed first, this approach can be particularly useful in women who are extremely distressed because it provides almost instant pain relief. Thus conditions for inserting the epidural needle and catheter are much improved, although there is some risk of trauma to anaesthetized tissue and nerves.

2. *Needle-through-needle, single interspace* (Carrie 1990): the now standard needle-through-needle technique (Figure 21.3) was popularized by Carrie and Donald (1991) and involves inserting a spinal needle through an epidural needle. There is a minimal risk of subsequently advancing the epidural catheter through the dural puncture hole (Robbins et al. 1995).

3. *'Double-barrel' needle* (Turner & Reifenberg 1995): This needle was designed to separate the dural puncture and epidural catheter placement sites, but is not in widespread use.

CSEA techniques have been the subject of a Cochrane review of 19 randomized controlled trials involving 2,500 women (Simmons 2007). This demonstrated a more rapid onset (approximately 10 minutes) of analgesia compared to standard low-dose epidural techniques. The high degree of mobility offered by this technique results in high maternal satisfaction (Collis et al. 1994, Price et al. 1998), but if women literally wish to walk about with such an epidural in place, it is recommended that they are supervised and assisted continuously by midwifery or clinical support staff because of the risk of falling.

Management of the second stage

If an epidural block is fully effective in the sacral segments, block of the afferent side of the bearing-down reflex will reduce its effectiveness. However, the actual ability to bear down should be unimpaired because the diaphragm and abdominal muscles produce this effort. There is limited evidence to assess the significance of a prolonged second stage (Report 2007), although there is an association between maternal morbidity and a second stage of longer than 2 hours

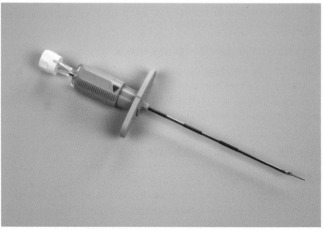

Figure 21.3 Needle-through-needle set for combined spinal epidural block.

(Cheng et al. 2004, Janni et al. 2002, Myles & Santolaya 2003, Saunders et al. 1992). Most obstetricians allow the fetal head to descend through the pelvis by uterine action before active 'pushing' is begun, considering it acceptable to let the second stage last longer than the notional 1 hour as long as maternal and fetal conditions are satisfactory and there is continued descent of the fetal head (Janni et al. 2002).

Analgesic drugs

Local anaesthetic drugs

The pharmacology of the local anaesthetic drugs is considered in Chapters 6–8.

Lidocaine

Lidocaine 1% (10 mg ml^{-1}) is most commonly used for local infiltration and peripheral blocks because of its rapid onset time. Epidural anaesthesia for Caesarean section requires 15–25 ml of lidocaine 2% (300–500 mg), a dose which may produce systemic toxicity so it is used with adrenaline 1:200,000 to reduce the speed of absorption and, hence, the plasma concentration. The same solution is still used in some centres if epidural analgesia is to be converted to a more intense anaesthetic block for Caesarean section or forceps delivery. Lidocaine is not suitable for continuous epidural analgesia in labour because it produces a high incidence of motor block.

Bupivacaine

Bupivacaine hydrochloride contains a racemic mixture of the S and R isomers of the butyl form of the pipecholylxylidine group of local anaesthetics. In equipotent doses it causes significantly less motor block than lidocaine, and is therefore a better agent for use during labour. Its onset is slower than lidocaine, but the duration of action is longer, although both variables depend on the dose given.

Levobupivacaine

The pure S isomer of bupivacaine is less cardiotoxic than the racemic mixture and is equipotent in terms of analgesia and motor block (Reynolds 1997). It is theoretically safer than racemic bupivacaine if a large dose is to be administered and it is less likely to produce life-threatening arrhythmias in the rare event of accidental intravenous administration (McLeod & Burke 2001).

Ropivacaine

Ropivacaine is the propyl form of the pipecholylxylidines and is produced as a single isomer (S). At equal doses it is less cardiotoxic than racemic bupivacaine, and it is available in 2-mg ml^{-1} and 7.5-mg ml^{-1} concentrations for use in obstetric epidural analgesia and anaesthesia (McClure 1996). Questions about its absolute potency raised by minimum local analgesic concentration studies (see next section) have perhaps limited its obstetric use, but it does produce greater sensory motor separation than equi-analgesic doses of bupivacaine (Zaric et al. 1996). The reduced intensity of motor block seen with ropivacaine increases maternal mobility and satisfaction, and the likelihood of a spontaneous vertex delivery (Writer et al. 1998), but perhaps these same ends can be achieved with lower concentrations of bupivacaine.

Chloroprocaine

Chloroprocaine 3% (20–25 ml) is a useful drug when rapid, profound epidural block is required. Onset is short (5–10 minutes), as is the duration of action (30–60 minutes) so additional injections of an alternative local anaesthetic may be required as the block regresses. An early preparation was associated with neurological toxicity (due to the bisulphite preservative) after accidental intrathecal injection. However, a new formulation with a higher pH appears to have reduced this risk, but subarachnoid administration is still contraindicated because of the risk of neurotoxicity (Gissen et al. 1984). Chloroprocaine is not available in the UK.

Minimum local analgesic concentration

The basis of this method of assessing local anaesthetics is discussed in Chapter 14. In obstetrics it has been used to provide numerical confirmation that greater concentrations of local anaesthetic are needed as labour progresses, and that the addition of an opioid to the solution reduces the local anaesthetic requirement (Capogna et al. 1998, Lyons et al. 1998, Polley et al. 1999).

Opioids

It quickly became apparent that morphine and other opioids, when used alone epidurally, were insufficient to provide satisfactory analgesia in labour (Heytens et al. 1987, Husemeyer et al. 1980), and mixtures of local anaesthetic and opioid have been in use since the early 1980s. Diamorphine (Lowson et al. 1995), meperidine (Perris & Malins 1981), fentanyl (Jones et al. 1989), and sufentanil (Russell & Reynolds 1993, Van Steenberge et al. 1987) are all used, usually with dilute bupivacaine. In the UK, the most commonly used agent is fentanyl, probably because it has featured most frequently in published studies.

α$_2$-adrenergic agonists

Clonidine is an α$_2$-adrenergic agonist and may be used in combination with epidural local anaesthetics and opioids (O'Meara & Gin 1993). Like opioids it decreases local anaesthetic requirements, but the combination is more likely to cause hypotension than a local anaesthetic with opoid (Dewandre et al. 2010). Thus clonidine is not used routinely in obstetric epidural analgesia, but 50–75 mcg may be given with an additional bolus dose of local anaesthetic (± opioid) when dealing with an inadequate or patchy block.

Indications for epidural block in labour

Pain relief

The primary indication for lumbar epidural analgesia in labour is the relief of pain, and for this it is unsurpassed. Barely 60% of women are satisfied with the pain relief afforded by carefully given parenteral and inhalational methods (Beazley et al. 1967); PCA with intravenous remifentanil is producing higher maternal satisfaction rates with little adverse neonatal effect, but maternal hypoxaemia may still occur (Blair et al. 2005). Most centres, which have established epidural services claim satisfactory analgesia in about 90% of cases. The pain from persisting OP position requires a greater spread of local anaesthetic within the epidural space to cover the sacral roots (Reynolds & O'Sullivan 1989).

Pre-eclampsia

The blood pressure of pre-eclamptic women is particularly sensitive to circulating catecholamines. Women with mild, untreated pre-eclampsia may show abrupt increases in blood pressure, particularly during uterine contractions. Those with more severe pre-eclampsia should already be established on antihypertensive drugs when they present in the labour ward, but the blood pressure may 'break through' this control during labour. Epidural analgesia is very effective in preventing the massive surges in blood pressure that occur with each contraction and should be established early in labour. However, lumbar epidural block alone will not control arterial blood pressure in severe pre-eclampsia and systemic antihypertensive therapy is required before an epidural block is performed.

The platelet count can fall precipitously in pre-eclampsia so a full blood count should be checked within 4 hours of inserting an epidural catheter. A platelet count $>100 \times 10^9 \, l^{-1}$ in that time frame is acceptable, but if it is lower, or has fallen rapidly, a full coagulation screen should be performed before the epidural is inserted (Valera et al. 2010). Such blood tests take time and it is realistic to expect at least an hour to elapse between sending the sample (marked urgent) to the laboratory and receiving the results. Therefore, these women should be seen as soon as possible on the labour ward so that options can be discussed and blood samples taken to avoid later delay in establishing an epidural. Constant communication with the midwifery and obstetric staff is essential to ensure that the anaesthetist is informed of new admissions to the labour ward. However, if there is a delay while test results are obtained, PCA with intravenous remifentanil is very useful in a distressed woman.

Multiple pregnancy

During vaginal delivery the second twin may be at risk from uterine inertia, cord compression or partial separation of the placenta, and modern obstetric opinion favours expediting delivery of the second twin. Oxytocin can be used to stimulate the flagging uterus, but if spontaneous delivery does not take place soon, forceps, an assisted breech delivery or Caesarean section may be required. An effective epidural allows the obstetrician to proceed immediately with the method of choice without the risks associated with general anaesthesia.

Diabetes mellitus

Diabetic mothers often have large babies, but may also have reduced placental function and their babies consequently have a high perinatal mortality rate. If elective Caesarean section is not planned, labour is usually induced at 37–38 weeks. Epidural analgesia is less likely to produce nausea, vomiting, and possible ketoacidosis than systemic analgesia.

Cardiovascular disease

Cardiac disease was the most common cause of maternal death in the 2006–08 Confidential Enquiry (Report 2011). It is impossible to generalize about heart disease because of the wide variety of congenital and acquired conditions that can be seen, and all patients, particularly those with fixed cardiac output conditions, should be discussed with a cardiologist during the antenatal period.

If a woman is to have a vaginal delivery, a carefully managed lumbar epidural best avoids most of the adverse factors of a painful labour, although the first dose of local anaesthetic should be small because hypotension is more likely to develop. The block allows labour to be augmented without maternal distress and, when extended to the sacral segments, it prevents uncontrolled bearing-down in the second stage and the Valsalva effect this can cause. Further, vasodilatation due to the epidural block helps to accommodate the increase in venous return which occurs in the third stage as caval occlusion is released and the uterus contracts after delivery. Slow administration

of intravenous oxytocin is a much safer alternative to ergometrine in the second stage in these women.

Obstetric anaesthetists are seeing an increasing number of women who have artificial heart valves. Their cardiac function is often extremely good, but they are usually receiving long-term anticoagulant therapy, often with low-molecular-weight heparin (LMWH). The anaesthetist should see these women in the antenatal period, when (in consultation with obstetrician, haematologist, and cardiologist) a plan should be made for the peripartum management of the anti-coagulation, and options for labour analgesia discussed. Pregnant women with ischaemic heart disease, and who may have had recent myocardial ischaemic events, are also being seen more frequently, and they and their antiplatelet drugs should be managed along similar lines.

The use of regional anaesthesia for Caesarean section in women with severe cardiac disease is contentious, and each case should be considered individually. Hypotension is much more likely with the high block required, particularly in fixed cardiac output conditions, and there may be sudden changes in haemodynamics. Many anaesthetists would consider general anaesthesia with full invasive cardiovascular monitoring the technique of choice.

Respiratory disease

Few women now come to the labour ward with severe disease of the lower respiratory tract, the most likely exceptions being those with asthma or an acute infection. They are likely to be very distressed during hyperventilation and Valsalva manoeuvres, so they find epidural analgesia very helpful. In recent years, more adult survivors of cystic fibrosis and those with heart–lung transplants have started to appear on labour wards. Detailed discussion of their management is beyond the scope of this book, but an obstetric anaesthetist should see them in the second trimester and a clear coordinated plan should be made for delivery.

For Caesarean section, mild respiratory disease has little effect on the choice between general and regional anaesthesia, but in more severe cases the choice depends largely on the degree of productive cough. Although some might advocate regional block, general anaesthesia avoids the distress of being unable to cough effectively when the abdominal muscles are relaxed due to central block and while the abdomen is open during surgery. However, epidural analgesia started at the end of surgery helps with effective postoperative coughing.

Contraindications to epidural block in labour

It is customary to classify certain conditions as 'absolute' or 'relative' contraindications to epidural anaesthesia in obstetrics. 'Absolute' contraindications include a bleeding diathesis (iatrogenic or due to disease), refusal by the woman to accept the technique, skin sepsis near the needle entry site and inadequate facilities for caring for the woman after the epidural has been performed. 'Relative' contraindications include conditions in which the risk–benefit ratio is less favourable than usual. Full explanation and discussion with the woman is essential.

Bleeding diathesis

This is most commonly caused by anticoagulant therapy, but may also be due to a platelet or coagulation factor deficiency (see Chapter 9). LMWH is used antenatally as prophylaxis against thromboembolic complications in high-risk groups, and each maternity unit should have a strategy for managing these women (Horlocker & Wedel 1998). The plan for managing the drugs during the peripartum period should be agreed with the woman and recorded in the case-notes antenatally.

Hypotension and hypovolaemia

The conditions which cause hypotension and hypovolaemia (e.g. haemorrhage, sepsis) must always be determined and treated before an epidural is performed.

Neurological disease

Multiple sclerosis is no longer considered to contraindicate epidural block in obstetrics although some neurologists still express anxiety about spinal anaesthesia (Bader et al. 1988, Confavreux et al. 1998). Evidence that central blocks cause acute demyelination is lacking and it seems unreasonable to refuse epidural analgesia to women with stable neurological disease if they might benefit. However, a full explanation should be given, existing neurological deficits documented, and informed consent obtained. Increasingly, the woman will have researched the literature in great detail beforehand.

Previous back trouble or spinal surgery

There is no reason why epidural anaesthesia per se should exacerbate previous problems. However, the removal of bony landmarks during previous spinal surgery, or subsequent skin scarring, may make identification of the epidural space difficult. Access to operation notes and radiographs may be helpful in such cases. After spinal surgery—especially some types of spinal fusion—adhesions may form in the epidural space, making the spread and effectiveness of the local anaesthetic unpredictable, and this possibility should be discussed fully beforehand. Daley and colleagues (1990) have shown that epidural block is almost as effective in women who have undergone lumbar spinal surgery as in those who have not. If the epidural block is inadequate or the epidural space cannot be found, a spinal may be successful.

Uterine scar

A uterine scar from a previous hysterotomy or Caesarean section may rupture during labour. The use of epidural block in this situation is controversial because any pain associated with uterine rupture may be concealed. However, pain is a relatively rare warning of scar rupture, and other clinical features, such as fetal distress and vaginal bleeding, are more common. All such women require meticulous maternal and fetal monitoring whether an epidural is used or not.

Fever

Mild pyrexia is common in labour and does not preclude the use of epidural analgesia, but it should not be used in the presence of high fever and systemic signs of sepsis.

Managing incomplete epidural analgesia in labour

A strategy should be in place for ensuring rapid assessment and correction of inadequate analgesia, starting with a check that the system delivering the solution is functioning properly without any leakage anywhere. Then the upper and lower levels of block should be defined, and any evidence of unilateral spread or a missed segment noted. An additional top-up injection of local anaesthetic and opioid can be given, and may include clonidine. The block should be reassessed after 15 minutes and, if it is still deficient, the catheter insertion site should be inspected (a number are pulled out inadvertently). If unilateral block persists, the catheter should be withdrawn 1–2 cm if possible, and another top-up injection given (either the same dose or a stronger solution), but if all these measures fail the catheter should be re-sited.

Immediate complications of epidural analgesia

Accidental dural puncture

Risk factors for accidental dural puncture include inexperienced clinician, morbidly obese parturient, technical difficulty, loss of resistance to air, and rotation of the needle after the epidural space has been located (Van de Velde et al. 2008). Most maternity units quote an incidence of less than 1% for this unfortunate complication, but the incidence of subsequent postdural puncture headache (PDPH) is over 50% (see 'Headache' section).

If dural puncture occurs one of two strategies of epidural management may be pursued:

1. The needle is withdrawn and the procedure repeated at an adjacent interspace. Particular care should be taken to identify whether the catheter has entered the subarachnoid space through the puncture hole created previously so a carefully observed test dose is essential. However, an extensive block may still occur, presumably due to local anaesthetic entering the cerebrospinal fluid (CSF) through the dural puncture.

2. Alternatively, the 'epidural' catheter is threaded into the subarachnoid space and analgesia provided by intermittent intrathecal injection. Only small doses of local anaesthetic (e.g. 2.5 mg bupivacaine, i.e. 1 ml of 0.25% solution), with or without opioid (e.g. 12.5–25 mcg fentanyl), are required, but the injections should be given by an anaesthetist. This technique provides effective analgesia without risking another dural puncture, but it does not decrease the likelihood of PDPH (Van de Velde et al. 2008).

Subsequent management of labour

Straining and pushing after accidental dural puncture might be thought to increase the risk of subsequent PDPH and there was a vogue for limiting the second stage or opting for elective forceps delivery, but this has largely been abandoned. A survey of UK maternity centres showed that 18% limited the length of the second stage, 11% avoided pushing and delivered using ventouse or forceps, and 69% allowed labour to continue without any intervention (Baraz & Collis 2005). However, there should be written guidance for management of labour if accidental dural puncture occurs.

Systemic toxicity

Systemic toxicity from excessive plasma concentrations of local anaesthetic is most commonly due to accidental intravascular injection (features, prevention, and management are considered in Chapter 8). The parturient is particularly sensitive to the cardiotoxic effects of the long-acting local anaesthetic drugs and prolonged skilled resuscitation may be required so every effort should be made to prevent such an event. A severe reaction will almost certainly require operative delivery under general anaesthesia, but if the episode was brief, treated quickly, and both woman and baby are stable the epidural may be re-sited. However, particular note should be made of the total dose of local anaesthetic administered.

Hypotension

The general aspects of hypotension during regional anaesthesia are considered fully in Chapter 11, and specific obstetric issues are discussed earlier in this chapter. The importance of reversing aortocaval compression with left lateral tilt, manual uterine displacement, or the full lateral position if necessary cannot be exaggerated. Early use of a vasoconstrictor (e.g. intravenous boluses of ephedrine 3–6 mg or phenylephrine 20–40 mcg) is recommended in addition to intravenous Hartmann's solution. Oxygen should be administered, particularly if there is fetal bradycardia.

Total spinal

This is a life-threatening emergency requiring prompt recognition and treatment to avoid permanent sequelae. Immediate treatment should comprise left lateral tilt, administration of oxygen, assisted ventilation with a tight fitting face-mask, and intravenous administration of a vasopressor, possibly even 1:10,000 adrenaline, to maintain blood pressure. Bradycardia, if present, should be treated with intravenous atropine, and subsequent circulatory support provided by increments of ephedrine or phenylephrine, or an infusion of adrenaline 1:100000 (10 mcg ml^{-1}). The trachea should be intubated if the woman is unconscious and, if the circulation is maintained, she should be transferred rapidly to theatre for immediate Caesarean section. Consideration should be given to administering an intravenous induction agent to ensure unconsciousness, and inhalational anaesthesia, along with intense respiratory and circulatory support, continued until the effects of the spinal anaesthetic begin to wear off.

If there is no cardiac output, the situation is even more urgent and the baby should be delivered by immediate Caesarean section on the labour ward within 4 minutes of the onset of cardiac arrest to improve the chances of successful maternal resuscitation (Howell et al. 2007) and decrease the risk of neonatal hypoxic brain injury or death.

Urinary retention

Bladder sensation is impaired during epidural analgesia, particularly in the presence of opioid analgesia. The possibility of urinary retention should be considered regularly during labour to avoid significant bladder distension with possible long-term effects on maternal bladder control.

Later complications of epidural block

Headache

PDPH will occur in over 50% of pregnant women who suffer accidental dural puncture with a Tuohy needle. It usually becomes apparent on mobilization after delivery, but may develop during labour (Van de Velde et al. 2008). The clinical features and basic aspects of management are considered in Chapter 13, but conservative measures often need supplementation with an epidural blood

patch in this group. A severe headache, worse when the woman is sitting or standing and relieved by lying down, is particularly distressing because it interferes with her attempts to feed and care for her new baby.

Epidural blood patch

A Cochrane systematic review of epidural blood patching concluded that 'too few patients have been included in randomized trials to allow a reliable assessment of the potential benefits and harms of the technique' (Boonmak & Boonmak 2010). However, the success rate for curing the headache is 70–98% if the patch is performed more than 24 hours after the onset of symptoms (Crawford 1980). If the first blood patch is unsuccessful, a repeat patch has the same chance of success. This, combined with the low incidence of complications, has established blood patching as the definitive treatment for PDPH, although it is contraindicated if the women is pyrexial or there is other evidence of bacteraemia.

The procedure should be performed under strict aseptic conditions in the theatre or anaesthetic room by an experienced anaesthetist assisted, if possible, by a trainee anaesthetist who can both learn and take the blood sample. The lateral position is preferred for obvious reasons and an epidural needle is inserted in the usual way, preferably at the same level as the dural puncture occurred. A venous blood sample is then obtained from the antecubital fossa under equally strict aseptic conditions, 20 ml for the patch plus sufficient for sending to the laboratory for culture. The blood is then injected slowly into the epidural space, either until the woman complains of any discomfort, or until all 20 ml have been used. The woman should lie flat for 30 minutes, after which she should mobilize gradually with help. Previous blood patch treatment does not affect the success of subsequent epidural block and is certainly not a contraindication to one (Abouleish et al. 1975).

If the epidural needle insertion was very difficult (leading to anxiety about ease of repetition) and a catheter is still in place, an alternative is to infuse saline at 60 ml h^{-1} for 24 hours, this being successful in 70% of women (Crawford 1972), although mobility is severely restricted.

Backache

Retrospective surveys have found an association between epidural analgesia in labour and postpartum backache (MacArthur et al. 1990, 1992, MacLeod et al. 1995, Russell et al. 1993), but the association was not confirmed in prospective cohort studies (MacArthur et al. 1997, Russell & Reynolds 1998). Women who have backache during pregnancy are more likely to have long-term backache, the sensory block produced by the epidural possibly allowing them to adopt postures during labour that would otherwise cause pain. In those who do not have backache during pregnancy poor posture during the second stage of labour, with acute flexion of the hips and spine in the presence of motor and sensory block, may lead to symptoms subsequently although they are generally short-lived. During pregnancy advice should be given to all women about taking care with posture during labour.

Neurological deficit

All women who have received central nerve block in labour require routine anaesthetic follow-up. All residual neurological symptoms require full assessment, but care must be taken to identify whether the nerve injury has an obstetric cause (Scott & Hibbard 1990).

Neurological deficit due to a block must be identified early and monitored regularly until full recovery occurs, with any delay in the expected rate of recovery prompting urgent referral for specialist neurological assessment.

Regional anaesthesia for Caesarean section

Infiltration anaesthesia

Caesarean section can be performed under local infiltration, but a large volume (at least 100 ml) of local anaesthetic is required so a dilute solution (lidocaine 0.5% with adrenaline 1:200,000) must be used, and many would advocate doubling the volume (and halving the concentration) by dilution with an equal volume of normal saline. However, in the developed world few obstetricians, and even fewer anaesthetists, have seen or administered infiltration anaesthesia for Caesarean section, although its use in the developing world may be life-saving. Absolute requirements are a gentle surgical technique and careful infiltration using a 25-g spinal needle of all relevant structures (midline skin, subcutaneous tissue, anteior, lateral, and posterior rectus sheath, and the peritoneum) as surgery progresses (Ranney & Stanage 1975). A Pfannenstiel incision is not appropriate because of the greater surgical dissection required.

Central neural block

Because an extensive block, with significant sympathetic nerve block, is needed for Caesarean section it is vital that aortocaval compression is avoided so a solid or inflatable wedge (Carrie 1982) must be placed under the right flank to ensure uterine displacement.

An extensive block is required (T_6–S_5), but it is also essential that it is both complete and intense. The *extent* of spread is generally easy to define by touch, light pinprick, or application of cold, but the *intensity* of block is more difficult to assess. However, some indication may be given by observing the degree of motor block and the response to a vigorous pinch of the skin of the lower abdomen. Visceral sensation is never completely abolished because the peritoneum is innervated by the vagus nerves, which remain unblocked, and mothers should be warned that pressure and tugging sensations may be felt. Exteriorization of the uterus after delivery should be avoided, particularly if epidural anaesthesia is used, but on occasion exteriorization is necessary to control haemorrhage. It is useful to warn the woman in advance that she may suffer transient abdominal pressure and nausea, feelings which usually resolve quickly after the uterus is returned gently to the abdomen.

Epidural anaesthesia

Epidural anaesthesia may be used for Caesarean section in one of two situations: establishment of a new block if one of slow onset for an elective procedure is indicated; or augmentation of an analgesic block in labour if operative delivery is required. Lidocaine and all of the long-acting local anaesthetics are appropriate, but the most widely used are lidocaine 2% (with adrenaline 1:200,000) and levobupivacaine 0.5% (Howell et al. 1990). The risk of systemic toxicity dictates an incremental approach, a suitable regimen consisting of a 4-ml test dose followed by three or four further aliquots (at 1-minute intervals) to a total of 20 ml, with an opioid such as fentanyl (75 mcg) (Noble et al. 1991) or diamorphine 3 mg often added to the final increment.

Some anaesthetists vary the woman's position with each increment to ensure even spread, but it is doubtful if this is necessary (Norris & Dewan 1987). If 20 ml does not seem to produce adequate anaesthesia, one or two further aliquots of 5 ml may be given cautiously, or spinal anaesthesia should be administered. The volume of local anaesthetic injected intrathecally should be half of the usual dose to avoid extensive CSF spread because the previous epidural injection will have reduced the compliance of the spinal canal.

When starting an epidural *de novo*, a minimum of 30 minutes should be allowed before the start of surgery in a conscious patient, but a shorter period may suffice if overt epidural block has developed during labour. However, current practice is to provide less intense block during labour so plenty of time should still be allowed for the development of a block adequate for surgery. A significant number of 'analgesic' epidurals are converted for Caesarean section in the event of fetal distress or failure to progress (or for forceps delivery or manual removal of placenta). The same solutions are used as for a new epidural, but the volume should be reduced according to the extent and intensity of the existing block. Epidural opioid given prior to surgery will improve the quality of analgesia during operative delivery, but it may also be administered after surgery to provide postoperative pain relief.

Spinal anaesthesia

Spinal anaesthesia usually produces a more intense block (especially in the sacral segments) of faster onset than an epidural. Hyperbaric bupivacaine 0.5%, the most commonly used agent, may be injected in the sitting or lateral position, but the patient should then be placed in the supine 'wedged' position. A volume of 2.0–2.5 ml should ensure spread to the midthoracic region, but some prefer a slightly larger dose (2.5–3.0 ml) to increase the density of block, using pillows under the head and upper thorax to prevent excessive spread. A third alternative is to use 2.5–3.0 ml of plain bupivacaine 0.5%, although its spread is more variable and the upper extent of the block less predictable (Carrie & O'Sullivan 1984). A small dose of opioid (e.g. diamorphine 300 mcg in saline) may be added to improve both intraoperative and postoperative analgesia provided an appropriate level of care and monitoring is available after surgery.

Its speed of onset may allow spinal anaesthesia to be used for emergency Caesarean section provided that fetal distress is not profound, but the decision requires full discussion of the degree of urgency with the obstetrician. Spinal anaesthesia may be used in severe eclampsia if the platelet count is adequate (see 'Pre-eclampsia' section) (Hood & Curry 1999, Sharwood-Smith et al. 1999), but treatment with magnesium increases the risk of hypotension. Magnesium can be antagonized by calcium, but the hypotension usually responds to cautious treatment with a vasopressor (James 1998).

Spinal anaesthesia is also useful for 'trial' of forceps delivery. This does not, itself, require an extensive block, but one of the described techniques should be used because immediate Caesarean section may be necessary if the trial fails.

Combined spinal–epidural anaesthesia (CSEA)

This combines the rapid onset of dense block provided by a spinal with the flexibility to extend the spread and duration of block by supplementation through an epidural catheter, the three techniques being described earlier. The intrathecal dose can be smaller than is used for spinal anaesthesia alone because it is supplemented, and eventually superseded, by epidural drug administration. This reduces the incidence of hypotension, but the risk of intrathecal catheter placement should always be considered and cautious epidural increments of local anaesthetic given (Robbins et al. 1995).

Immediate complications

Hypotension

Hypotension may be sudden in onset, particularly with spinal anaesthesia, and may cause severe nausea and vomiting in the mother. Careful positioning, with adequate lateral tilt to prevent aortocaval compression and elevation of the head and shoulders on pillows to restrict local anaesthetic spread, can reduce the risk. Both vasoconstrictors and intravenous fluids are used to try and prevent hypotension, but a Cochrane review of various prophylactic measures found that, while they can reduce the incidence of hypotension, none eliminates the need to treat maternal hypotension during the procedure (Cyna et al. 2002).

Respiratory distress or depression

A potential disadvantage of extensive central block in a woman at term is the possibility of respiratory embarrassment. A block to T_1 paralyses the intercostal muscles, but leaves the diaphragm (C_3–C_5) unaffected and preserves adequate inspiratory reserve, but in the recumbent woman at term the gravid uterus may impede diaphragmatic excursion. In any patient, the abdominal muscles are paralysed and this reduces the ability to cough effectively, potentially causing respiratory distress or embarrassment (Gamil 1989). In practice these effects only cause problems in women with significant respiratory disease or copious sputum production.

Inadequate block

If an epidural block is found to be inadequate before surgery, and time is available, it should be managed as previously described, ultimately with recourse to spinal or general anaesthesia depending on the urgency of the situation. An inadequate spinal anaesthetic may be repeated, but cautiously (see Chapter 13) and with full appreciation of the degree of urgency and the time available before delivery must be assured.

If the block is found to be inadequate during surgery, the strategy followed should be that agreed with the woman *before* surgery starts. Depending on the degree and nature of the discomfort, and the stage of surgery, local anaesthetic infiltration by the obstetrician, a further epidural top-up (both require regard to the total dose used) and small intravenous doses of opioid may each be tried. However, discomfort that is poorly tolerated should result in an immediate alert to the surgeon to stop operating, after which general anaesthesia is induced. There is no place for benzodiazepines unless the core problem is maternal, anxiety although the risk of anterograde amnesia of unpredictable duration clouding her first memories of the baby should be explained before a benzodiazepine is given.

Pruritus

Pruritus after neuraxial opioids has been reported in 70% of pregnant and recently delivered women (Bonnet 2008). The symptoms are difficult to control, but naloxone, naltrexone, nalbuphine, ondansetron, and droperidol are all effective in preventing the condition (Kjellberg & Tramer 2001), although nalbuphine (2–3 mg) may be used for treatment without reversing analgesia (Somrat et al. 1999).

Urinary retention

As noted under the complications of epidural analgesia, bladder sensation is impaired by central neural block, but the bladder should be catheterized before Caesarean section whatever the form of anaesthesia.

Later complications

Headache

PDPH after accidental dural puncture is considered earlier in this chapter (see 'Accidental dural puncture' section), and is also relatively common after spinal anaesthesia in pregnant women. The incidence is related to spinal needle size and is 3–10% in this population, even with 26-g needles, and although even smaller gauge needles have been produced (Carrie & Collins 1991) they are more difficult to use (Flaatten et al. 1989, Dahl et al. 1990). Atraumatic or 'pencil-point' tip needles (24 and 27 g) are now in common use and have reduced the incidence of PDPH to less than 2% (Carrie & Donald 1991, Cesarini et al. 1990, Reid & Thorburn 1991). Postpartum headache may have other causes, and each should be considered before the diagnosis of PDPH is made (Klein & Loder 2010), but it is reasonable to treat a posturally related and persistent headache with an epidural blood patch if conservative measures (Chapter 13) are unsuccessful. All women who have had central neural block should be followed-up the day after delivery and should be made aware of the small risk of headache developing days, or even weeks, after dural puncture and of the need to report it if troublesome.

Neurological deficit

As with epidural block for labour analgesia, routine anaesthetic follow-up after central nerve block for Caesarean section or other peripartum procedures should including identification, and appropriate management, of any neurological sequelae.

The obese parturient

Obesity is an increasing problem, recent UK data indicating that in 2009 5% of pregnant women had a body mass index (BMI) ≥35 kg m², and that in 2% it was ≥40 kg m², the defining figure for morbid obesity (Report 2010). Obesity is an independent risk factor for adverse obstetric outcome, and is associated with a significantly increased Caesarean delivery rate (Weiss et al. 2004). It increases the risks of both general and regional anaesthesia (Saravanakumar et al. 2006), and is associated with technical difficulties and reduced efficacy with epidural analgesia. The Caesarean section rate of women receiving epidural analgesia during labour shows a marked positive correlation with BMI (Dresner et al. 2006).

The Centre for Maternal and Child Enquiries recommends (Report 2010) that:

◆ All pregnant women with a booking BMI ≥40 should have an antenatal consultation with a senior experienced obstetric anaesthetist;

◆ A similarly qualified clinician should be available for the care of all women with a BMI > 40 during labour; and that

◆ Careful consideration should be given to the timing of an epidural, particularly for women with a BMI ≥40. Some units advocate its early institution.

- Appropriately sized general equipment (e.g. delivery beds, operating tables, blood pressure cuffs, etc) will be required during labour or operative delivery.
- Longer than standard epidural and atraumatic spinal needles must be available.

Identification of the midline is somewhat easier with the woman in the sitting position, the skin being indented by its attachment to the spinous processes, and she may herself be able to confirm from the sense of pressure that the needle has been inserted in the midline. Ultrasound scanning can be very helpful in such situations and its increasing availability should help greatly.

Many clinicians insert a longer than usual length of catheter into the epidural space of obese subjects to reduce the risk displacement because of the greater mobility of the subcutaneous tissues. Standard introducers for spinal needles may not be long enough, and an epidural needle is a useful substitute. However, care should be taken that the spinal needle does protrude too far from the epidural guide needle's tip, especially if a formal CSE technique is being used using longer epidural and spinal needles than are available in standard kits. CSE may be the technique of choice, particularly if operative delivery might be prolonged. Increased adipose tissue and venous engorgement in the epidural space reduce the compliance of the vertebral canal in the morbidly obese and lower doses of local anaesthetic are needed.

Key reference

Report (2010) *Saving Mothers' Lives: reviewing maternal deaths to make motherhood safer: 2006–08. The Eighth Report on Confidential Enquiries into Maternal Deaths in the United Kingdom.* London: Centre for Maternal and Child Enquiries. Also available in *British Journal of Obstetrics & Gynaecology* 2011; 118 (Suppl 1):1–203.

On-line resource

http://www.oaa-anaes.ac.uk/ Obstetric Anaesthetists Association website.

References

Abouleish E, Wadhwa RK, de la Vega S, et al. (1975) Regional analgesia following epidural blood patch. *Anesthesia & Analgesia* 54: 634–6.

Aitkenhead AR, Hothersall AP Gilmour DG, Ledingham IMcA (1979) Dural dimpling in the dog. *Anaesthesia* 34: 14–19.

Bader AM, Hunt CO, Datta S, et al. (1988) Anesthesia for the obstetric patient with multiple sclerosis. *Journal of Clinical Anesthesia* 1: 21–4.

Banerjee A, Stocche RM, Angle P, Halpern SH (2010) Preload or coload for spinal anesthesia for elective Cesarean delivery: a meta-analysis. *Canadian Journal of Anaesthesia* 57: 24–31.

Baraz R, Collis R (2005) The management of accidental dural puncture during labour epidural analgesia: a survey of UK practice. *Anaesthesia* 60: 673–9.

Beazley JM, Leaver EP, Morewood JH, Bircumshaw J (1967) Relief of pain in labour *Lancet* 13: 1033–5.

Bezov D, Ashina S, Lipton R (2010) Post-dural puncture headache: part II—prevention, management, and prognosis. *Headache* 50: 1482–98.

Blair JM, Dobson GT, Hill DA, et al. (2005) Patient controlled analgesia for labour: a comparison of remifentanil with pethidine. *Anaesthesia* 60: 22–7.

Bonnet MP, Marret E, Josserand J, Mercier FJ (2008) Effect of prophylactic 5-HT3 receptor antagonists on pruritus induced by neuraxial opioids: a quantitative systematic review. *British Journal of Anaesthesia* 101: 311–19.

Brockhurst NJ, Littleford JA, Halpern SH (2000) The neurologic and adaptive capacity score. A systematic review of its use in obstetric anesthesia research. *Anesthesiology* 92: 237–46.

Brownridge P (1981) Epidural and subarachnoid analgesia for elective Caesarean section. *Anaesthesia* 36: 70.

Capogna D, Celleno D, Lyons G, et al. (1998) Minimum local analgesic concentration of extradural bupivacaine increases with the progression of labour. *British Journal of Anaesthesia* 80: 11–13.

Carrie LES (1982) An inflatable obstetric anaesthetic 'wedge'. *Anaesthesia* 37: 745–7.

Carrie LES (1990) Extradural, spinal and combined block for obstetric surgical anaesthesia. *British Journal of Anaesthesia* 65: 225–33.

Carrie LES, Collins PD (1991) 29-gauge spinal needles. *British Journal of Anaesthesia* 66: 145–6.

Carrie LES, Donald F (1991) A 26-gauge pencil-point needle for combined-epidural anaesthesia for Caesarean section. *Anaesthesia* 46: 230–1.

Carrie LES, O'Sullivan GM (1984) Subarachnoid bupivacaine 0.5% for Caesarean section. *European Journal of Anaesthesia* 1: 275–83.

Cesarini M, Torrielli R, Lahaye F, et al. (1990) Sprotte needle for intrathecal anaesthesia for Caesarean section: incidence of postdural puncture headache. *Anaesthesia* 45: 656–8.

Cheng Y, Hopkins L, Caughey A (2004) How long is too long: Does a prolonged second stage of labor in nulliparous women affect maternal an neonatal outcomes? *American Journal of Obstetrics and Gynecology* 191: 933–8.

Cibils LA (1976) Response of human uterine arteries to local anesthetics. *American Journal of Obstetrics and Gynecology* 126: 202–10.

Collins KM, Bevan DR, Beard RW (1978) Fluid loading to reduce abnormalities of fetal heart rate and maternal hypotension during epidural analgesia in labour. *British Medical Journal* 2: 1460–1.

Collis RE, Baxandall ML, Srikantharajah ID, et al. (1994) Combined spinal epidural (CSE) analgesia; technique, management, and outcome in 300 mothers. *International Journal of Obstetric Anaesthesia* 3: 75–81.

Collis RE, Davies DWL, Aveling W (1995) Randomised comparison of combined spinal–epidural and standard epidural analgesia in labour. *Lancet* 345: 1413–16.

Confavreux C, Hutchinson M, Hours MM, et al. (1998) Rate of pregnancy-related relapse in multiple sclerosis. Pregnancy in Multiple Sclerosis Group. *New England Journal of Medicine* 339: 285–91.

Cooper D, Carpenter M, Mowbray P, et al. (2002) Fetal and maternal effects of phenylephrine and ephedrine during spinal anaesthesia for Caesarean delivery. *Anesthesiology* 97: 1582–90.

Cooper D, Sharma S, Orakkan P, Gurung S (2010a) Retrospective study of association between choice of vasopressor given during spinal anaesthesia for high-risk Caesarean delivery and fetal pH. *Anesthesia & Analgesia* 110: 154–8.

Cooper GM, MacArthur C, Wilson MJ, et al. (2010b) Satisfaction, control and pain relief: short- and long-term assessments in a randomised controlled trial of low-dose and traditional epidurals and a non-epidural comparison group. *International Journal of Obstetetric Anaesthesia* 19: 31–7.

Crawford JS (1972) The prevention of headache consequent upon dural puncture. *British Journal of Anaesthesia* 44: 598–600.

Crawford JS (1980) Experience with epidural blood patch. *Anaesthesia* 35: 513–15.

Cyna AM, Andrew M, Emmett RS, et al. (2002) Techniques for preventing hypotension during spinal anaesthesia for Caesarean Section. *Cochrane Database Systematic Reviews* 3: CD002251.

Dahl JB, Schultz P, Anker-Moller E (1990) Spinal anaesthesia in young patients using a 29-gauge needle: technical considerations and an evaluation of postoperative complaints compared with general anaesthesia. *British Journal of Anaesthesia* 64: 178–82.

Daley MD, Rolbin SH, Hew EM, et al. (1990) Epidural anesthesia for obstetrics after spinal surgery. *Regional Anesthesia* 15: 280–4.

Datta S, Lambert DH, Gregus J (1983) Differential sensitivities of mammalian nerve fibers during pregnancy. *Anesthesia & Analgesia* 62: 1070–2.

Dewandre PY, Decurninge V, Bonhomme V, et al. (2010) Side effects of the addition of clonidine 75µg or sufentanil 5µg to 0.2% ropivacaine for labour epidural analgesia. *International Journal of Obstetric Anaesthesia* 19: 149–54.

Dresner M, Brocklesby J, Bamber J (2006) Audit of the influence of body mass index on the performance of epidural analgesia in labour and the subsequent mode of delivery. *BJOG: An International Journal of Obstetrics and Gynaecology* 113: 1178–81.

Fagraeus L, Urban BJ, Bromage PR (1983) Spread of epidural analgesia in early pregnancy. *Anesthesiology* 58: 184–7.

Flaatten H, Rodt SA, Vamnes J, et al. (1989) Postdural puncture headache. A comparison between 26- and 29-gauge needles in young patients. *Anaesthesia* 44: 147–9.

Galbert MW, Marx GF (1974) Extradural pressures in the parturient patient. *Anesthesiology* 40: 449–502.

Gambling DR, McMorland GH, Yu P, Lazlo G (1988) A comparison of patient-controlled epidural analgesia and intermittent 'top-ups' during labour. *Anesthesia & Analgesia* 35: 249–54.

Gamil M (1989) Serial peak expiratory flow rates in mothers during Caesarean section under extradural anaesthesia. *British Journal of Anaesthesia* 62: 415–18.

Gissen AJ, Datta S, Lambert D (1984) The chloroprocaine controversy. II. Is chloroprocaine neurotoxic? *Regional Anesthesia* 9: 135–45.

Grau T, Leipold RW, Horter J, et al. (2001) The lumbar epidural space in pregnancy: visualization by ultrasonography. *British Journal of Anaesthesia* 86: 798–804.

Greiss FC, Still JG, Anderson SG (1976) Effects of local anesthetic agents on the uterine vasculature and myometrium. *American Journal of Obstetrics and Gynecology* 124: 889–98.

Halpern SH, Leighton BL, Ohnsson A, et al. (1998) Effect of epidural vs parenteral opioid analgesia on the progress of labor: a meta-analysis. *Journal of the American Medical Association* 280: 2105–10.

Hein A, Rösblad P, Norman M, et al. (2010) Addition of low-dose morphine to intrathecal bupivacaine/sufentanil labour analgesia: A randomised controlled study. *International Journal of Obstetric Anaesthesia* 19: 384–9.

Heytens L, Cammu H, Camu F (1987) Extradural analgesia during labour using alfentanil. *British Journal of Anaesthesia* 59: 331–7.

Hingson RA, Edwards WB (1943) Continuous caudal analgesia. An analysis of the first ten thousand confinements thus managed with the report of the authors' first thousand cases. *Journal of the American Medical Association* 123: 538–46.

Holmes F (1960) Incidence of the supine hypotensive syndrome in late pregnancy. A clinical study in 500 subjects. *Journal of Obstetrics and Gynaecology* 67: 274–5.

Hood DD, Curry R (1999) Spinal versus epidural anesthesia for cesarean section in severely pre-eclamptic patients; a retrospective survey. *Anesthesiology* 90: 1276–82.

Horlocker TT, Wedel DJ (1998) Spinal and epidural blockade and perioperative low molecular weight heparin: Smooth sailing on the Titanic. *Anesthesia & Analgesia* 86: 1153–6.

Howell C, Grady K, Cox C (2007) *Managing Obstetric Emergencies and Trauma—The MOET Course Manual*, 2nd edn. London: RCOG Press.

Howell P, Davies W, Wrigley M, et al. (1990) Comparison of four local extradural anaesthetic solutions for elective Caesarean section. *British Journal of Anaesthesia* 65: 648–53.

Husemeyer RP, O'Connor MC, Davenport HT (1980) Failure of epidural morphine to relieve pain in labour. *Anaesthesia* 35: 161–3.

Hutchins CJ (1980) Spinal analgesia for instrumental delivery. A comparison with pudendal nerve block. *Anaesthesia* 35: 376–7.

Issacs R, Turner M (2010) 'Itching to do a TAP block?' *International Journal of Obstetric Anaesthesia* 19: 468–9.

James MFM (1998) Magnesium in obstetric anaesthesia. *International Journal of Obstetric Anaesthesia* 7: 115–23.

James KS, McGrady E, Quasim I, Patrick A (1998) Comparison of epidural bolus administration of 0.25% bupivacaine and 0.1% bupivacaine with 0.0002% fentanyl for analgesia during labour. *British Journal of Anaesthesia* 81: 507–10.

Janni W, Schiessl B, Peschers U, et al. (2002) The prognostic impact of a prolonged second stage of labor on maternal and fetal outcome. *Acta Obstetricia Gynecologica Scandinavica* 81: 214–21.

Jones G, Paul DL, Elton RA, McClure JH (1989) Comparison of bupivacaine and bupivacaine with fentanyl in continuous extradural analgesia during labour. *British Journal of Anaesthesia* 63: 254–9.

Kerr MG, Scott DB, Samuel E (1964) Studies of the inferior vena cava in late pregnancy. *British Medical Journal* 1: 532–3.

Kinsella SM, Whitwam JG, Spencer JA (1992) Reducing aortocaval compression: how much is enough? *British Medical Journal* 305: 539–40.

Kinsella S M, Pirlet M, Mills M S, et al. (2000. Randomised study of fluid preload before epidural analgesia during labour. *British Journal of Anaesthesia* 85: 311–13.

Kjellberg F, Tramèr MR (2001) Pharmacological control of opioid-induced pruritus: a quantitative systematic review of randomized trials. *European Journal of Anaesthesiology* 18: 346–57.

Klein AM, Loder E (2010) Postpartum headache. *International Journal of Obstetric Anaesthesia* 19: 422–30.

Kreis O (1900) Uber Medullarnarkose bei Gebarenden. *Zentralblatt Fur Gynaekologie* 24: 724.

Kubli M, Shennan A, Seed PT, O'Sullivan G (2003) A randomised controlled trial of fluid pre-loading before low dose epidural analgesia for labour. *International Journal of Obstetric Anaesthesia* 12: 256–60.

Lees MM, Scott DB, Kerr MG, Taylor SH (1967) The circulatory effects of recumbent postural change in late pregnancy. *Clinical Science* 32: 453–65.

Lowson SM, Eggers KA, Warwick JP, et al. (1995) Epidural infusions of bupivacaine and diamorphine in labour *Anaesthesia* 50: 420–2.

Lyons G, Columb M, Wilson RC, Johnson RV (1998) Epidural pain relief in labour: potencies of levobupivacaine and racemic bupivacaine. *British Journal of Anaesthesia* 81: 899–901.

MacArthur AJ, MacArthur C, Weeks SK (1997) Is epidural anesthesia in labor associated with chronic low back pain? A prospective cohort study. *Anesthesia & Analgesia* 85: 1066–70.

MacArthur C, Lewis M, Knox EG, Crawford JS (1990) Epidural anaesthesia and long term backache after childbirth. *British Medical Journal* 301: 9–12.

MacArthur C, Lewis M, Knox EG (1992) Investigation of long-term problems after obstetric epidural anaesthesia. *British Medical Journal* 304: 1279–82.

McClure JH (1996) Ropivacaine. *British Journal of Anaesthesia* 76: 300–7.

McLeod GA, Burke D (2001) Levobupivacaine. *Anaesthesia* 56: 331–41.

MacLeod J, Macintyre C, McClure JH, Whitfield A (1995) Backache and epidural analgesia. A retrospective survey of mothers 1 year after childbirth. *International Journal of Obstetric Anaesthesia* 4: 21–5.

Morgan BM (1995) 'Walking' epidurals in labour. *Anaesthesia* 50: 839–40.

Murphy JD, Henderson K, Bowden MI, et al. (1991) Bupivacaine versus bupivacaine plus fentanyl for epidural analgesia: effect on maternal satisfaction. *British Medical Journal* 302: 564–7.

Myles T, Santolaya J (2003) Maternal and neonatal outcomes in patients with a prolonged second stage of labor. *Obstetrics and Gynecology* 102: 52–8.

Noble DW, Morrison LM, Brockway MS, McClure JH (1991) Epinephrine, fentanyl or epinephrine and fentanyl as adjuncts to bupivacaine for extradural anaesthesia in elective Caesarean section. *British Journal of Anaesthesia* 66: 645–50.

Norris MC, Dewan DM (1987) Effect of gravity on the spread of extradural anaesthesia for Caesarean section. *British Journal of Anaesthesia* 59: 338–41.

O'Meara ME, Gin T (1993) Comparison of 0.125% bupivacaine with 0.125% bupivacaine and clonidine as extradural analgesia in the first stage of labour. *British Journal of Anaesthesia* 71: 651–6.

Park WY (1988) Factors influencing the distribution of local anaesthetics in the epidural space. *Regional Anesthesia* 13: 49–57.

Perris BW, Malins AF (1981) Pain relief in labour using epidural pethidine and epinephrine. *Anaesthesia* 36: 631–3.

Polley LS, Columb MO, Naughton NN, et al. (1999) Relative analgesic potencies of ropivacaine and bupivacaine for epidural analgesia in labor. *Anesthesiology* 90: 944–50.

Prakash S, Pramanik V, Chellani H, et al. (2010) Maternal and neonatal effects of bolus administration of ephedrine and phenylephrine during spinal anaesthesia for caesarean delivery: a randomised study. *International Journal of Obstetric Anaesthesia* 19: 24–30.

Price C, Lafreniere L, Brosnan C, Findley I (1998) Regional analgesia in early active labour: combined spinal–epidural vs. epidural. *Anaesthesia* 53: 951–5.

Purdie J, Reid J, Thorburn J, Asbury AJ (1992) Continuous extradural analgesia: Comparison of midwife top-ups, continuous infusions and patient controlled administration. *British Journal of Anaesthesia* 68: 580–4.

Ramanathan S, Friedman S, Moss P, et al. (1984) Phenylephrine for the treatment of maternal hypotension due to epidural anesthesia. *Anesthesia & Analgesia* 63: 262.

Ramanathan S, Grant GJ (1988) Vasopressor therapy for hypotension due to epidural anesthesia Caesarean section. *Acta Anaesthesiologica Scandinavica* 32: 559–65.

Ramanathan S, Masih A, Rock I, et al. (1983) Maternal and fetal effects of prophylactic hydration with crystalloids or colloids before epidural anesthesia. *Anesthesia & Analgesia* 62: 673–8.

Ranney B, Stanage WF (1975) Advantages of local anesthesia for Cesarean section. *Obstetrics and Gynecology* 45: 163–7.

Reid JA, Thorburn J (1991) Headache after spinal anaesthesia. *British Journal of Anaesthesia* 67: 674–77.

Report (2007) *Intrapartum care of healthy women and their babies during childbirth*. London: Nice Clinical Guideline, 55 (available at http://www.nice.org.uk/CG055)

Report (2010) *Maternal obesity in the UK: Findings from a national project*. London: Centre for Maternal and Child Enquiries.

Reports (1991–2011) *Confidential Enquiries into Maternal Deaths in the United Kingdom, 1985–87 (1991); 1988–90 (1994); 1991–93 (1996); 1994–96 (1998); 1997–1999 (2001); 2000–2002 (2004); 2003–2005 (2007); 2006–2008 (2011)*. London: HMSO & TSO.

Reynolds F (1997) Does the left hand know what the right hand is doing? An appraisal of single enantiomer local anaesthetics. *International Journal of Obstetric Anaesthesia* 6: 257–69.

Reynolds F, O'Sullivan G (1989) Epidural fentanyl and perineal pain in labour. *Anaesthesia* 44: 341–4.

Robbins PM, Fernando R, Lim GH (1995) Accidental intrathecal insertion of an extradural catheter during combined spinal–extradural anaesthesia for Caesarean section. *British Journal of Anaesthesia* 75: 355–7.

Russell R, Reynolds F (1993) Epidural infusions for nulliparous women in labour. A randomised double-blind comparison of fentanyl/bupivacaine and sufentanil/bupivacaine. *Anaesthesia* 48: 856–61.

Russell R, Reynolds F (1996) Epidural infusion of low-dose bupivacaine and opioid in labour. Does reducing motor block increase the spontaneous delivery rate? *Anaesthesia* 51: 266–73.

Russell R, Reynolds F (1998) Epidural analgesia and chronic backache. *Anesthesia and Analgesia* 87: 747–8.

Russell R, Groves P, Taub N, et al. (1993) Assessing long-term backache after childbirth. *British Medical Journal* 306: 1299–303.

Saravanakumar K, Rao SG, Cooper GM (2006) Obesity and obstetric anaesthesia. *Anaesthesia* 61: 36–48.

Saunders N, Paterson C, Wadsworth J (1992) Neonatal and maternal morbidity in relation to the length of the second stage of labour. *British Journal of Obstetrics and Gynaecology* 99: 381–5.

Scott DB, Hibbard BM (1990) Serious non-fatal complications associated with extradural block in obstetric practice. *British Journal of Anaesthesia* 64: 537–41.

Sharwood-Smith G, Clark V, Watson E (1999) Regional anaesthesia for Caesarean section in severe pre-eclampsia: spinal anaesthesia is the preferred choice. *International Journal of Obstetric Anaesthesia* 8: 85–9.

Simmons SW, Cyna AM, Dennis AT, Hughes D (2007) Combined spinal-epidural versus epidural analgesia in labour. *Cochrane Database of Systemic Reviews* 18: CD003401.

Simpson JY (1848) Local anaesthesia, notes on its production by chloroform etc. in the lower animals and in man. *Lancet* ii: 39–42.

Somrat C, Oranuch K, Ketchada U, et al. (1999) Optimal dose of nalbuphine for intrathecal-morphine induced pruritus after Caesarean section. *Journal of Obstetric and Gynaecological Research* 25: 209–13.

Soresi AL (1937) Episubdural anesthesia. *Anesthesia and Analgesia* 16: 306–10.

Stoeckel W (1909) Uber sakrale Anaesthesie. *Zentralblatt Fur Gynaekologie* 33: 1.

Boonmak P, Boonmak S (2010) Epidural blood patching for preventing and treating post-dural puncture headache. *Cochrane Database of Systemic Reviews* 1: CD001791.

Taylor JC, Tunstall ME (1991) Dosage of phenylephrine in spinal anaesthesia for Caesarean section. *Anaesthesia* 46: 314–16.

Thorburn J, Moir DD (1981) Extradural analgesia: the influence of volume and concentration of bupivacaine on the mode of delivery, analgesic efficacy and motor block. *British Journal of Anaesthesia* 53: 933–9.

Turner MA, Reifenberg NA (1995) Combined spinal–epidural anaesthesia. The single space double-barrel technique. *International Journal of Obstetric Anaesthesia* 4: 158–60.

Usubiaga JE, Wikinski JA, Usubiaga LE (1967) Epidural pressure and its relation to spread of anaesthetic solutions in the epidural space. *Anesthesia & Analgesia* 46: 440–6.

Valera MC, Parant O, Vayssiere C, et al. (2010) Physiologic and pathologic changes of platelets in pregnancy *Platelets* 21: 587–95.

Vallejo MC, Phelps AL, Singh S, et al. (2010) Ultrasound decreases the failed labour epidural rate in resident trainees *International Journal of Obstetric Anaesthesia* 19: 4373–8.

Van de Velde M, Schepers R, Berends N, et al. (2008) Ten years of experience with accidental dural puncture and post-dural puncture headache in a tertiary obstetric anaesthesia department. *International Journal of Obstetric Anaesthesia* 17: 329–35.

Van Steenberge A, Debroux HC, Noorduin H (1987) Extradural bupivacaine with sufentanil for vaginal delivery. *British Journal of Anaesthesia* 59: 1518–22.

Weiss JL, Malone FD, Emig D, et al. (2004) Obesity, obstetric complications and cesarean delivery rate—a population-based screening study. *America Journal of Obstetrics and Gynecology* 190: 1091–7.

Wilson MJ, Macarthur C, Shennan A (2009) Urinary catheterization in labour with high-dose vs mobile epidural analgesia: a randomized controlled trial. *British Journal of Anaesthesia* 102: 97–103.

Writer WDR, Stienstra R, Eddleston JM, et al. (1998) Neonatal outcome and mode of delivery after epidural analgesia for labour with ropivacaine and bupivacaine: a prospective meta-analysis. *British Journal of Anaesthesia* 81: 713–17.

Zaric D, Nydahl P, Philipson I, et al. (1996) The effect of continuous lumbar epidural infusion of ropivacaine (0.1%, 0.2% and 0.3%) and 0.24% bupivacaine on sensory and motor blockade in volunteers—a double-blind study. *Regional Anesthesia* 21: 14–25.

CHAPTER 22

Regional anaesthesia in children

Steve Roberts

Regional anaesthesia is now firmly placed at the heart of paediatric anaesthesia. However, it differs from adult practice in that it is almost always performed in combination with general anaesthesia. Indeed, as a general rule, it would be neither safe nor possible to attempt regional blocks in the awake child. This is because a child cannot be guaranteed to remain still and calm; and paraesthesiae and peripheral nerve stimulation are techniques that would be difficult for young children to understand or accept. The possible exceptions to this are teenagers undergoing relatively minor surgery or premature infants undergoing hernia repair.

Neurobiology of pain

In outline, the pain pathway is much the same in children as in adults (Chapter 2). However, there are important functional differences (Fitzgerald & Walker 2009).

- The receptive fields of individual neurones may be much larger, implying less accurate pain localization in the immature nervous system;

- Activity in non-nociceptive fibres (Aδ) can, in the neonate, activate neurones in dorsal horn laminae which are predominantly nociceptive in the adult;

- Descending inhibitory pathways are less well developed, allowing unmodulated nociceptive input to the spinal cord;

- There may be differences in the proportion of subclasses of opioid receptors in neonates, and this may contribute to their reduced ability to modulate nociceptive transmission.

These factors suggest that younger patients may experience more pain than adults. In addition, it is very likely that later response to pain in children can be affected adversely by previous inadequate control of pain, for example, during and after circumcision (Taddio et al. 1997). All of this information argues strongly for the use of regional anaesthesia, whenever possible, in the anaesthetic management of children.

Injury results in repetitive C-fibre activation which, through spinal cord N-methyl-D-aspartate (NMDA) and neurokinin receptors, gives rise to the development of secondary hyperalgesia, increasing the patient's perception of pain. Regional anaesthesia will reduce this C-fibre activity, thereby inhibiting the development of hyperalgesia.

Local anaesthetic pharmacology

In general terms, the principles of local anaesthetic pharmacology outlined in Chapters 6–8 apply as much to children as adults. However, several reports of toxicity (Ludot et al. 2008), especially in association with continuous infusion (Larsson et al. 1994), indicate that children, particularly neonates and infants, need separate consideration. Bupivacaine is widely used, but increasingly it is being superseded by the newer enantiomers levobupivacaine and ropivacaine.

Pharmacokinetics

There has been limited study of local anaesthetic pharmacokinetics in children, particularly in infants and with regard to the newer agents, but the available information does indicate key differences in comparison to the adult state.

Absorption is dependent on the same factors as in adults, but can be faster in certain circumstances. This has been clearly documented after intercostal block where a combination of increased vascularity, greater cardiac index, and a greater surface area from which to absorb (due to the greater volume injected in relation to patient size) allows greater uptake of drug (Rothstein et al. 1986). The choice of drug also makes a difference, ropivacaine, having less vasodilator action, has a longer T_{max} than bupivacaine after caudal injection (Karmakar et al. 2002).

Distribution of local anaesthetics in children is influenced markedly by age-related changes in body fluid compartments. Water is 80% of body water in the premature, 75% in term neonates, 65% in infants, and only decreases to the adult 60% in older children, intracellular fluid increasing from 20% of body weight in the premature to 30% in adults. In addition, the concentrations of α-1-acid-glycoprotein and albumin, the main proteins which bind local anaesthetics, are lower in young infants (Booker et al. 1996). The influence of such differences is complex, but the overall effect is that, at steady state, the volume of distribution is higher in infants than in adults (Weston & Bourchier 1995). Despite surgery stimulating a potentially protective rise in α-1-acid-glycoprotein there is a substantial risk of toxicity with infusions lasting longer than the recommended 48 hours (Larsson et al. 1997).

Metabolism of local anaesthetic drugs is by the same routes as in adults, but what information there is suggests that the capacity of the liver to deal with these drugs is limited in neonates compared to older children. Lidocaine and bupivacaine are metabolized predominantly by cytochrome CYP3A4, ropivacaine by CYP1A2 and levobupivacaine by both. The CYP3A4 system matures within the first 9 months of life, but CYP1A2 not until ages 5–8 years.

The elimination half-lives of the local anaesthetics are longer in neonates and infants than in adults. This is true of bupivacaine, even though its clearance is relatively greater, because its volume of distribution is also much larger (Weston & Bourchier 1995).

Risk of toxicity

The risk of toxicity after a local anaesthetic injection is dependent upon many factors (Chapters 7 and 8), no matter what the age of the patient, but some specific points need to be considered, especially in the very young. Most obviously, there is the problem of adjusting the dose used to the size of the patient, even without allowing for the impact of certain physiological differences. Rate of rise of plasma concentration is proportional to cardiac output which is higher (relatively) in neonates, and this effect will be increased by the slower metabolism noted above. The immaturity of the blood–brain barrier may be relevant, although the practice of performing blocks *after* the administration of general anaesthesia will obscure the early features of systemic toxicity.

There is no doubt that plasma concentrations are influenced by the age of the recipient, plasma concentrations of local anaesthetics associated with the risk of toxicity being reported after ilio-inguinal and caudal block in infants, despite apparently conservative doses (Luz et al. 1998). Technique may also prove important, higher plasma concentrations of ropivacaine being found with ultrasound when it was compared with a landmark method for ilioinguinal block (Weintraud et al. 2009). It was postulated that the landmark technique, being less accurate, often results in local anaesthetic being deposited intramuscularly where the surface area for absorption is low. However, with ultrasound the injection would be placed precisely in the correct fascial plane where there is a greater surface area for absorption. The implication is that lower doses should be used for fascial blocks with ultrasound.

Although the actual plasma concentration is not the only factor in the generation of toxicity, the general principle is that conservative doses should be used in young patients. Bearing that in mind, 'single-shot' injections are generally safe, but cumulation remains a significant hazard in neonates and infants receiving continuous infusions (Cheung et al. 1997). Levobupivacaine and ropivacaine have wider safety margins and should be preferred to bupivacaine for infusion.

Treatment of toxicity

Systemic toxicity from local anaesthetic drugs results in progressive depression of central nervous and cardiovascular systems with readily recognizable symptoms and signs. However, the prior administration of general anaesthesia to most children means that there will be no obvious warning features, and that cardiac arrhythmias or cardiovascular collapse may be the first manifestation. Extrasystoles, broadening of the QRS complex, ventricular tachycardia and fibrillation may all occur, especially with the longer acting agents.

If toxicity does occur the anaesthetist should stop any injection or infusion, ensure oxygenation, lung ventilation, and venous access, seek further assistance, and follow basic life support guidelines. Seizures are treated with small doses of benzodiazepine,

thiopental, or propofol. The cardiovascular system should be monitored constantly and standard protocols followed if the patient develops arrhythmias or cardiac arrest. Arrhythmias may be refractory, and resuscitation may be prolonged, but lipid emulsion (see Chapter 8) has been used with equally dramatic effect in these situations in children as in adults (Ludot et al. 2008).

Prevention of toxicity

Prevention is preferable to treatment, and the introduction of ultrasound may have a major effect by minimizing total doses and identifying intravascular injection. Further, the newer local anaesthetics should be used where possible. However, even with these developments, it remains vital that the basic principles of safe use are followed (Table 22.1), slow careful injection with repeated aspiration being the hallmark of good practice. The value of a test dose is reduced by the concurrent administration of general anaesthesia, which also reduces the sensitivity of adrenaline as a marker of intravenous injection. In neonates local anaesthetic infusions should be limited to 48 hours due to the increased risk of toxicity.

Local anaesthetic doses in children

Making recommendations about 'safe' doses in children is difficult. Adult recommendations are based on the results of clinical studies, but these are relatively rare in children, particularly across the whole paediatric population age range from neonate to teenager. Age, body weight, and height have all been used as a basis for dosage, but weight has generally been adopted as the standard (Table 22.2). However, the uncritical application of 'ml kg^{-1}' regimens has potential pitfalls which are considered in Chapters 7 and 8.

Peripheral techniques

Topical application

Two topical local anaesthetic preparations are available to facilitate venepuncture and cannulation, their use making these procedures much less traumatic for child and anaesthetist alike.

The eutectic mixture of local anaesthetics (EMLA) is an oil-in-water emulsion of equal amounts of the base forms of lidocaine and prilocaine. In this formulation these agents can penetrate the skin and produce cutaneous analgesia, but taking at least an hour to be fully effective, and with a duration of action limited to 30–60 minutes. EMLA has also been used for neonatal circumcision, skin grafting and the insertion of grommets through the eardrum in older children.

Amethocaine is more lipid soluble, and Ametop (a 4% gel) is more rapid in onset (30–40 minutes) (Jain 2000), has a duration of up to 3 hours and may further facilitate venepuncture by its

Table 22.1 Basic recommendations for the safe conduct of local anaesthetic injections in children

1. Aspirate prior to each injection
2. Evaluate the effect of a test dose of 0.5–1.0 ml containing adrenaline
3. Inject slowly over a period of approximately 90 seconds
4. Repeat aspirations should be performed during the course of the injection
5. Stop the injection if any abnormal signs or symptoms occur

Table 22.2 Dose ranges of local anaesthetic agents (bupivacaine, levobupivacaine, and ropivacaine) for various common blocks. The upper limits quoted should not be exceeded. When performed with ultrasound these volumes can be significantly reduced—see text for details

Block name	Local anaesthetic 0.25%	Block	Operations
Axillary/infraclavicular	0.4–0.6 ml kg^{-1}	Brachial plexus	Arm and hand surgery
Supraclavicular	0.4–0.6 ml kg^{-1}	Brachial plexus	Arm and hand surgery
Interscalene	0.4–0.6 ml kg^{-1}	Brachial plexus	Shoulder surgery
Femoral	0.4–0.6 ml kg^{-1}	Femoral	Femoral fracture Surgery to femur
Fascia iliaca compartment	0.8 ml kg^{-1}	Femoral Obturator Lateral cutaneous	Femoral fracture Surgery to femur
Sciatic	0.5 ml kg^{-1}	Sciatic	Lower limb*
Popliteal	0.5 ml kg^{-1}	Sciatic	Below the knee surgery**
Inguinal	0.4–0.6 ml kg^{-1}	Ilio-inguinal Iliohypogastric	Inguinal hernia Orchidopexy
Rectus sheath	0.2–0.4 ml kg^{-1} per side	T_9–T_{11}	Pyloroplasty Umbilical hernia
Penile	0.2 ml kg^{-1} per side	Dorsal penile	Circumcision Meatoplasty
Intercostal	Max 0.8 ml kg^{-1} with 1: 200 000 adrenaline	Intercostal 1–6	Thoracotomy
		Intercostal 6–12	Abdominal surgery
Paravertebral	0.3–0.5 ml kg^{-1}	T_7–T_9	Thoracotomy Abdominal surgery

*Combined with femoral.
**Combined with saphenous nerve block

vasodilator properties (EMLA is a vasoconstrictor). Both preparations can cause some local oedema, and Ametop a degree of erythema.

Peripheral nerve blocks

Peripheral blocks (Table 22.2) are the mainstay of analgesic management for paediatric ambulatory surgery, being suitable for peripheral and body surface procedures. They also avoid the problems of central block. Lower limb plexus and compartment techniques provide good unilateral analgesia, but maintain sensory and motor function in the other leg, and without disturbing urinary control.

However, special care is needed because the child under general anaesthesia cannot report needle trauma to the nerve or intravascular injection. Standard landmark approaches have long been supported by peripheral nerve stimulation, but in recent years ultrasound has contributed further to nerve identification and needle guidance (Marhofer et al. 2006, Roberts 2006) (Table 22.3). Generally, the quality of ultrasound imaging is superior in children because the structures are more superficial, this allowing higher frequency probes to be used with consequent better image resolution although some nerves (e.g. lateral cutaneous nerve of the thigh) are too small to be identified in the youngest patients. Children weighing less than 15 kg require a probe with a small

'footprint'. For all ages a 22-g short-bevelled needle is appropriate, because this improves 'feel' as it is advanced through the tissues, while a short extension catheter between the syringe and needle prevents dislodgment of the needle during injection.

Where prolonged analgesia is required thought should be given to the insertion of a catheter using stimulation or ultrasound to confirm its position. The catheter should be inserted using a strict aseptic technique, and 'tunnelled' to diminish the chance of

Table 22.3 Advantages of ultrasound guided nerve blocks in children

No ionizing radiation
Portability (laptop sized machines)
Visualization of the nerve and adjacent structures e.g. vessels, pleura, kidney
Visualize the spread of local anaesthetic (avoid intravascular or intraneural injection)
Increased efficacy (faster onset, longer duration, and increased success rates)
Decreased incidence of complications
Allows lower volumes of local anaesthetic to be used
Can be performed in presence of muscle relaxants
Can be performed in patients with neuropathy

dislodgement. Tissue adhesive can be applied to the skin puncture site to aid fixation and reduce local anaesthetic leakage which can lead to the dressing lifting off the skin. As confidence with nerve catheter techniques has grown their use after discharge home has been described (Dadure et al. 2005, Ilfeld et al. 2004), this aided by the development of disposable elastometric pumps (Dadure et al. 2003). Infusion (0.1–0.3 ml kg^{-1} h^{-1}) of levobupivacaine 0.125%, can be continued for as long as necessary (but limited to 48 hours in neonates).

The actual techniques are much the same as in adults, but some points require particular mention.

Brachial plexus block

Traditionally, only the axillary route of brachial plexus block has been used in children due to the risk of pneumothorax with other techniques; supraclavicular and infraclavicular approaches are being used now (De Jose Maria et al. 2008, Marhofer et al. 2004), but not interscalene because shoulder surgery is uncommon in children (Van Geffen et al. 2006). Ultrasound and nerve stimulation may be used to facilitate each of the techniques (Marhofer et al. 2006, Tobias 2001), but in children with severe musculoskeletal problems (e.g. club arm) ultrasound is superior because it is difficult to elicit a motor response if joints are fused and muscles absent, hypoplastic or fibrosed (Ponde & Diwan 2009). When a catheter is used the infraclavicular approach may provide the most reliable fixation.

Lower limb blocks

Blocks of the lumbar plexus (Kirchmair et al. 2004), femoral nerve (Oberndorfer et al. 2007), fascia iliaca compartment, lateral cutaneous nerve of thigh, and sciatic nerve (Oberndorfer et al. 2007, Schwemmer et al. 2004) can all be performed in children (Tobias 2003). However, they are specialized techniques and caudal epidural injection is probably more reliable in less experienced hands. As with the upper limb blocks, and for identical reasons, ultrasound is superior to peripheral nerve stimulation in children with cerebral palsy although it can hinder ultrasound imaging. For example, the sciatic nerve can be obscured by fibrosed muscle (homogenous hyperechoic appearance) and, at the popliteal level, the 'see-saw' sign (Schafhalter-Zoppoth et al. 2004) is absent if the limb is fixed.

Ilio-inguinal–iliohypogastric block

This block is used for inguinal hernia repair, orchidopexy, hydrocele, and varicocele surgery. The needle is inserted medial to the anterior superior iliac spine (ASIS), 2.5 mm along a line from the ASIS to the umbilicus, and advanced perpendicular to the skin until a single loss of resistance is felt when the local anaesthetic (0.4–0.6 ml kg) is injected. In experienced hands, ultrasound has facilitated significant reduction in the volume injected (to 0.075 ml kg^{-1}) without diminishing the success rate (96%) (Willschke et al. 2006), something which will hopefully decrease the risk of systemic toxicity in infants. There is a 10% incidence of femoral block (Lipp et al. 2004), and reports of intraperitoneal injection causing visceral damage with the landmark technique have appeared, but the wider use of ultrasound will, hopefully, also decrease the risk of these complications (Weintraud et al. 2008).

A second injection may be made immediately lateral to the pubic tubercle to block the medial end of the incision.

Rectus sheath block

This technique, placing local anaesthetic between the rectus muscle and its posterior sheath so that it spreads both cephalad and caudad, is indicated for umbilical hernia repair, pyloromyotomy, and simple duodenal atresia repair. With the landmark technique the needle is inserted level with the umbilicus, at the lateral margin of the rectus muscle and at an angle of 60° to the skin aiming in a lateral to medial direction. An initial 'pop' is felt as the needle passes through the anterior sheath, and then the 'scratch' sensation of contact with the posterior sheath is sought. After aspiration 0.2–0.4 ml kg^{-1} of local anaesthetic is injected, and the process repeated on the other side. With ultrasound the volume of local anaesthetic can be decreased to 0.1 ml kg^{-1} per side (Willschke et al. 2006).

Transversus abdominis plane block

This is a relatively new block which is indicated for abdominal surgery when an epidural is too invasive or contraindicated, although there are debates about extent of spread and efficacy (Chapter 16). It may be used unilaterally for open appendectomy, inguinal surgery, and iliac crest graft harvesting (Fredrickson 2009), or bilaterally for laparoscopic surgery or laparotomy. The aim is to place local anaesthetic between the transversus abdominis and internal oblique muscles, the anterior rami of T_7–L_1 running in the fascial plane between them to supply the anterior abdominal wall.

A standard regional block needle is used: 40 mm for a neonate or infant, 50 mm for a child, and 100 mm for a teenager. The patient lies supine and the ultrasound probe is placed in the transverse plane over the mid axillary line, half way between the costal margin and the iliac crest except for inguinal surgery when it is placed just above the iliac crest. Using an 'in-plane' technique the needle is inserted, the fascial plane identified and 0.5 ml kg^{-1} of local anaesthetic injected.

Penile block

The main indication for this block is circumcision; it is unsuitable for proximal hypospadias repair. The penis is drawn downwards, the pubic symphysis identified and the skin marked on either side, 0.5–1.0 cm from the midline at the root of the penis (note that the penile vessels lie in the midline). From these points, the needle is directed medially and caudally, inferior to the pubic ramus, until there is a characteristic 'give' as Scarpa's fascia is pierced. This will be at a depth of 0.5–3.0 cm, although it is *independent* of the age or size of the patient. Local anaesthetic *without vasoconstrictor* must be used, and ropivacaine should also be avoided (Burke et al. 2000). There should be no resistance to injection. The block has been shown to be as effective as caudal analgesia, but with a lower incidence of urinary retention (Metzelder et al. 2010) and no lower limb motor block.

Intercostal block

Percutaneous intercostal block is technically easy to perform, but is associated with a significant risk of pneumothorax, especially in children less than 10 years old, and the failure rate may be as high as 25%. The technique may be used for the placement of chest drains and for inpatients with fractured ribs, and should be performed in the mid-axillary line, where the inner intercostal muscles separate the nerve from the parietal pleura, so that the likelihood of pneumothorax is reduced. Only experienced practitioners should perform this block.

A safer and more reliable technique is to place an epidural catheter adjacent to the intercostal neurovascular bundle, under direct vision, at the time of operation. This is especially useful after surgery for the harvesting of costal cartilage. A loading dose of bupivacaine 0.25% (0.5 ml kg^{-1}) is followed by an infusion of levobupivacaine 0.125%.

Paravertebral block

This technique is useful for chest surgery, and it has also been shown to be as effective as epidural block for renal surgery in children (Lonnquist & Olsson, 1994). When compared to ilio-inguinal nerve block for inguinal hernia repair it was found to provide significantly improved and prolonged analgesia (Naja et al. 2006). It has the advantage that there is no risk of spinal cord trauma, but pneumothorax and spinal anaesthesia are possible complications. Diffusion of local anaesthetic to the epidural space occurs in up to 70% of cases and this may be an important site of action.

With the patient prone or lateral, the thoracic spines at the level to be blocked are marked, and a line parallel to the spines, is drawn on the side to be blocked, at a distance from the spines equal to the space between them (1–2 cm) (Figure 22.1). A short-bevelled or Tuohy needle of appropriate size is inserted on this line at a point level with the inferior border of the upper spinous process, and advanced until there is loss of resistance to injection of saline.

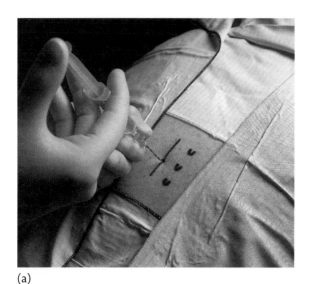

(a)

(b)

Figure 22.1 (a) Needle insertion for paravertebral block in a child. (b) Location of paravertebral space by loss of resistance to liquid.

The endpoint is not as well defined as with an epidural loss of resistance, and catheter insertion tends to be harder, but the depth of insertion may be estimated from the formula 0.48 × weight (kg) + 18.7 mm. Peripheral nerve stimulation has been used for locating the paravertebral space (Naja et al. 2005), and ultrasound may prove useful though evidence is presently lacking. Alternatively, the catheter can be placed under direct vision by the surgeon at thoracotomy.

Eng and Sabanathan (1992) infused 0.5% bupivacaine at a rate of 0.2 ml kg^{-1} h^{-1} for up to 5 days in children aged 7–16 years who had undergone thoracotomy, and obtained excellent analgesia. However, this dose rate (equivalent to 1 mg kg^{-1} h^{-1}) would result in significant accumulation and toxicity if used in neonates or infants, and potentially toxic plasma concentrations have been reported in infants who received only half that dose for up to 48 hours (Karmakar et al. 1996), so a further reduction in dosage is clearly necessary in this age group. Plasma concentrations remained within safe limits in neonates and infants when bupivacaine 0.125% with adrenaline 1: 400,000 was infused at 0.25 mg kg^{-1} h^{-1}, (0.2ml kg^{-1} h^{-1}), but the analgesia was less effective, up to 18% of patients needing opioid supplements (Cheung et al. 1997). Nevertheless, it is better to accept the need for supplementation than to risk local anaesthetic toxicity.

Central techniques

Caudal epidural block has been widely used in paediatric practice for many years, but only since the late 1980s have the lumbar and thoracic epidural techniques gained in popularity. However, all specialized UK paediatric centres now use continuous epidural analgesia routinely, even in neonates and infants (Llewellyn & Moriarty 2007). These central blocks provide excellent pain control—and this is their main advantage—but they may, in addition, reduce the stress response to surgery, facilitate early extubation, and improve postoperative respiratory function. The latter may be of value in high-risk neonates and infants undergoing major surgery.

Caudal block

Equipment

A 22-g, 50-mm cannula allows easy injection from a 10- or 20-ml syringe and is long enough to reach the sacrococcygeal ligament in all but the most obese child. The 24-g, 30-mm needle is more suitable for neonates and small infants.

Technique

The child is turned into the left lateral position (for the right-handed anaesthetist). Accurate location of the sacral cornua is essential for success, and it is important to realize that these bony protuberances, which represent the unfused laminae of the fifth sacral segment, appear to be more cephalad than in the adult. They are palpated best by moving the left thumb up and down across the base of the sacrum (Figure 22.2) and can be thought of as forming the base of an isosceles triangle whose apex points cephalad. The apex is formed by the fusion of the sacral bones in the midline and the area of the triangle is filled by the sacrococcygeal ligament (Figure 22.3).

When the cornua have been identified, the thumb is moved cephalad so that it lies over the apex of the triangle and the cannula is inserted immediately caudad to the thumb at an angle of about 20° (Park 2006) (Figure 22.4). After passing through the skin and

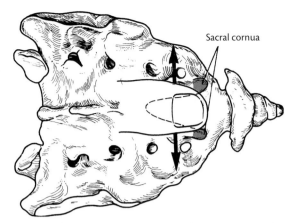

Figure 22.2 Identification of sacral cornua using sideways movement of the thumb.

subcutaneous fat the cannula meets the resistance of the sacrococcygeal ligament, and there is a distinct loss of resistance as it is penetrated. The cannula should be inserted close to the apex of the triangle because the sacral cavity is comparatively deep at that point and it is easier to appreciate that the cavity has been entered. The cannula may then be advanced gently up the sacral canal, but this should not be done if a needle is used because it increases the risk of venous puncture.

If blood appears at the hub, the cannula should be withdrawn until the flow ceases, and the lumen cleared with saline. Aspiration may then produce blood-stained saline, but as long as frank blood does not appear, local anaesthetic may be injected. If a needle is used, aspiration tests for blood sometimes give false negative results because the vessel wall is sucked onto the needle bevel. This risk can be minimized by the prior injection of 1 ml of solution to distend the vein, followed by gentle aspiration. The appearance of blood is not an indication for abandoning the block as long as the needle or cannula can be repositioned satisfactorily.

The dose regimen for paediatric caudal anaesthesia is well established (Table 22.4), but the advent of ultrasound allows the spread of local anaesthetic to be monitored in real time (Raghavan & Arnold 2007). Levobupivacaine, ropivacaine, and bupivacaine all provide effective analgesia (Locatelli et al. 2005) and have similar onset times. Levobupivacaine and ropivacaine provide approximately 1 hour less analgesia than bupivacaine, but also

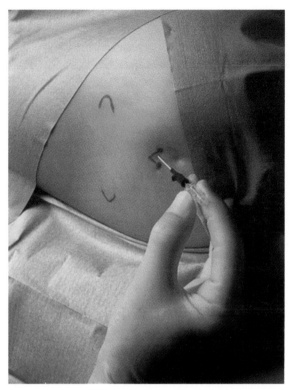

Figure 22.4 Cannula insertion for caudal block in a child.

cause less motor block in the first 3 postoperative hours. The use of additives for caudal block is considered later.

As well as being highly effective, the technique has a good safety record, the incidence of complications being very low (0.07% Giaufre et al. 1996). However, the seriousness of these complications has led to the development of techniques to identify correct needle placement, the most promising being electrostimulation (Tsui et al. 1999) and ultrasound (Roberts 2005). The latter has greater potential (Figure 22.5) allowing identification of the dural sac, observation of a test bolus of saline to discount intravascular placement, and monitoring of local anaesthetic spread. Ultrasound can also be used for screening patients with stigmata of spinal dysraphism.

In children the straighter spinal column and less dense packing of the epidural space by fat and fibrous tissue allows catheters to be threaded up to the thoracic region from the sacral hiatus. This provides thoracic segmental analgesia, yet avoids the hazards associated

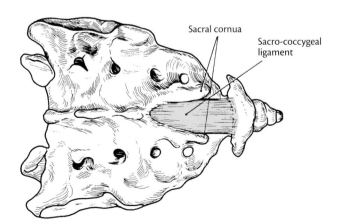

Figure 22.3 Sacrococcygeal ligament.

Table 22.4 Paediatric caudal dosages for 0.25% levobupivacaine, ropivacaine, and bupivacaine

	Loading dose (ml kg^{-1})	Infusion dose (ml kg^{-1} h^{-1})
Neonates		
Low (L$_5$–S$_5$)	0.3–0.5	0.16–0.2
High (T$_{12}$–S$_5$)	1.0*	0.16–0.2
Infants and children		
Low (L$_5$–S$_5$)	0.3–0.5	0.32–0.4
High (T$_{12}$–S$_5$)	1.0	0.32–0.4

*When administering large volumes to neonates the use of 0.125% is as effective and safer.

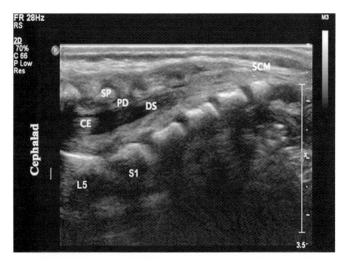

Figure 22.5 Longitudinal paramedian ultrasound scan of an infant sacrum using a linear 5–12-MHZ transducer (CE = cauda equina, DS = termination of dural sac, PD = posterior dura, SP = spinous process, SCM = sacrococcygeal membrane, L5, S1 = fifth lumbar and first sacral vertebral bodies).

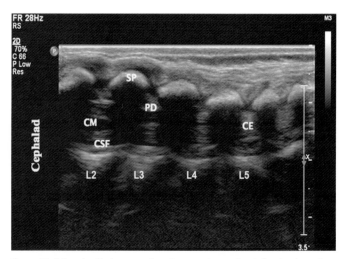

Figure 22.6 Longitudinal paramedian ultrasound scan of an infant lumbar spine using a linear 5–12-MHZ transducer (CE = cauda equina, CM = conus medullaris, CSF = cerebrospinal fluid, L = lumbar vertebral bodies, PD = posterior dura, SP = spinous process).

with introducing a needle at the thoracic level (Bosenberg et al. 1988). Until recently it has been difficult to assess the level of the catheter tip, but several novel methods have been described, including ultrasound (Chawathe et al. 2003, Roberts 2005), electrostimulation and electrocardiographic methods (Tsui et al. 1998, 2002). The caudal route is close to the perineum, and there are concerns regarding infection, but while colonization rates are higher there does not seem to be an increased infection rate (McNeely et al. 1997); tunnelling reduces the incidence of colonization (Bubeck et al. 2004).

Epidural block

The epidural space may be approached by the lumbar or thoracic routes in children and is popular for a wide range of surgery.

Identifying the epidural space

The technique for identification of the epidural space has been the subject of much debate in the literature, following reports of complications associated with the use of air for loss of resistance. Serious sequelae, including fatalities possibly secondary to venous air embolism, have been reported in children (Flandin-Blety & Barrier 1995) and a review of adult practice identified wide-ranging complications (pneumocephalus, spinal cord and nerve root compression, subcutaneous emphysema, venous air embolism, incomplete analgesia, and paraesthesia) after the use of air (Saberski et al. 1997). However, in many of the cases cited there were basic failures of technique which, if avoided, could have prevented the complications described.

Nevertheless, air does present potential hazards in children not seen in adults. It is easier to inject relatively large volumes rapidly, and the incidence of venous air embolism is known to be associated with both the volume injected and the rate of injection. Moreover, intracardiac communications with variable right-to-left shunt (the foramen ovale is patent in 50% of children up to 5 years of age) allow air to cross into the arterial circulation. The low venous epidural pressure makes detection of inadvertent venous cannulation difficult, so air can enter the circulation readily, even when the injection pressure is low. The only disadvantage of saline is that it can make dural puncture harder to detect, but

well-described methods exist for confirmation in cases of doubt. Provided that standard techniques are followed carefully, and repeated attempts to identify the epidural space are avoided, the incidence of complications related to venous air embolism is low, but avoiding air injection altogether will minimize the risk of accidents.

The prevention of inadvertent dural puncture requires not only a sensitive method for detecting loss of resistance, but also a careful technique because the epidural space in neonates and infants may be as little as 5 mm from the skin. However, ultrasound can aid location of the epidural space, prepuncture scans being used to measure its depth (Marhofer et al. 2005) and identify clinically important structures (e.g. the conus medullaris) (Figure 22.6).

Equipment

Packs specially designed for paediatric use are commercially available (Portex, UK). The 18-g and 19-g, Huber tip, Tuohy needles are 50 mm long and have graduations at 5-mm intervals. The '18-g' catheter has the standard three helically placed eyes, this design having a much lower incidence of kinking and occlusion is now used in all ages (Figure 22.7).

Technique

As noted previously, ultrasound can be used to identify the depth of the epidural space, but where it is not yet available an estimate can be obtained using one of several formulae. At the lumbar level a simple guide is to allow 1 mm kg^{-1} (Bosenberg & Gouws 1995), but formulae for the thoracic spine are more complex (Masir 2006): depth of epidural space (cm) = 1.95 + (0.045 × weight in kg), *or* 2.15 + (0.01 × age in months). However, caution must prevail because there is little margin for error given that the average distance from dura to spinal cord is 4.3 mm in those aged 2–10 years. Both paramedian and midline approaches are possible, but the latter, used with cephalad angulation, is preferred for both lumbar and thoracic approaches, the landmarks and technique being the same as for the adult (Chapter 14). At present there is limited evidence for the use of ultrasound-*guided* placement in children

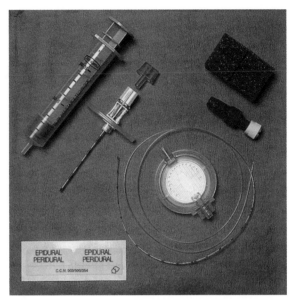

Figure 22.7 Half-length 18-g Tuohy needle and 21-g catheter for paediatric epidural analgesia.

(Tsui & Pillay 2010), even though their small size and lower degree of ossification make them more suitable subjects.

Catheters should be sited as close as possible to the dermatomes to be blocked in order to ensure effective anaesthesia. Consideration should be given to subcutaneous tunnelling because this may prevent accidental dislodgement and, in the longer term, protect against bacterial colonization, but there should be an immediate check that the catheter has not kinked.

Dosage regimens

After confirming catheter position a bolus is administered and the infusion is started in theatre (Table 22.5) because this allows the drug delivery system to be assessed and simplifies fluid management. In neonates a plain bolus and infusion of 0.125% ropivacaine or bupivacaine is used, this being just as effective as higher concentrations due to the lack of myelination and the small diameter of the nerves. The low concentration decreases the risk of local anaesthetic toxicity, but the infusion should be stopped after 48 hours for reasons noted earlier. In young infants, even doses as low as

Table 22.5 Dose ranges of local anaesthetic (levobupivacaine, ropivacaine, and bupivacaine) for epidural use

	Loading dose: 0.25% plain (ml kg^{-1})	Infusion dose: 0.125% plain (ml kg^{-1} h^{-1})
Neonates		
Lumbar	0.5–0.75	0.16–0.2
Thoracic	0.5	0.16–0.2
Infants and children		
Lumbar	0.5–0.75	0.32–0.4
Thoracic	0.5	0.32–0.4

NB: infants and children are best managed with a mixture of local anaesthetic and opioid or clonidine. Preservative-free morphine (10 mcg ml^{-1}) should be added to the infusate. The morphine infusion rate should not exceed 5 mcg kg^{-1} h^{-1}.

bupivacaine 0.25% at 0.38 mg kg^{-1} h^{-1} (0.15 ml kg^{-1} h^{-1}), may result in significant accumulation after as little as 32 hours (Peutrell et al. 1997). Additives are not recommended in neonates because they increase the risk of apnoeic episodes.

In older children a lower concentration of local anaesthetic causes fewer complications (e.g. hypotension), but an additive is necessary for effective analgesia (see next section). A comparison of bupivacaine, levobupivacaine, and ropivacaine (all at 0.125%) found no difference in quality of analgesia, but less motor block with the newer agents (De Negri et al. 2004). The use of patient-controlled epidural analgesia in children of 7 years and older has been shown to be as effective as continuous infusion, but with lower local anaesthetic requirements (Antok et al. 2003).

Epidural additives

The aim of adding other analgesic drugs to solutions of epidural local anaesthetic is to provide effective, balanced analgesia with minimal side effects by using lower rates of administration than is needed with a single drug. Multiple epidural drug combinations are recommended (except in infants), with simple systemic analgesics having an important role also. Many drugs have been administered epidurally in children (e.g. midazolam, neostigmine, ketorolac), but the practice is irresponsible given the lack of safety data and the availability of the well-known and effective additives described here.

Epidural opioids

Adding an opioid to an epidural infusion can enhance the quality of analgesia, but achieving this with lipophilic opioids (e.g. fentanyl) requires that the catheter tip lies adjacent to the dermatomes to be blocked or it will not be effective segmentally. In contrast, hydrophilic opioids such as morphine enter the cerebrospinal fluid (CSF) so catheter position is less critical. In situations where it is difficult to be certain of catheter position, preservative-free morphine may be the logical choice. Morphine, diamorphine, and fentanyl are well established for epidural use in children, and recently sufentanil has been shown to provide superior analgesia to fentanyl, but unfortunately has a higher incidence of pruritus (Cho et al. 2008). However, not all opioids are effective as epidural supplements, tramadol, for example, having little effect when given with bupivacaine for hypospadias repair (Prosser et al. 1997).

The disadvantage of epidural opioids is the increase in side effects such as urinary retention, pruritus, nausea, vomiting, and respiratory depression. The incidence, especially of urinary retention, is increased in older children, but routine urinary catheterization is not generally required. The impact of side effects can be minimized by restricting the opioid dose, ensuring adequate postoperative fluids and using naloxone early for pruritus and retention (0.5 mcg kg^{-1} repeated at 10-minute intervals to a maximum of 2 mcg kg^{-1}). For these reasons opioids should not be used in single-shot caudals for day-case surgery or in neonates and infants.

The incidence of respiratory depression in patients receiving epidural opioids is less than 1% when management is by a pain control team, although sedation and slight reduction in respiratory rate are more common (6.5%) (Lloyd-Thomas & Howard 1994). Infusion analgesia probably has a more predictable effect on respiration than large intermittent bolus doses (Bozkurt et al. 1997). During epidural opioid infusions in children the dose should not exceed morphine 5 mcg kg^{-1} h^{-1} or fentanyl at 0.4 mcg kg^{-1} h^{-1} (Berde 1994).

Clonidine

Clonidine, an α_2-adrenergic agent, is not a suitable additive in neonates because of the risk of apnoea.

There is close correlation between the lumbar CSF concentration of clonidine and the degree of analgesia. When combined with other analgesics, 1–2 mcg kg^{-1} of clonidine effectively doubles the duration of analgesia after caudal local anaesthetic injection (Cook et al. 1995, Jamali et al. 1994). For lumbar or thoracic administration 2 mcg kg^{-1} should be given with the initial local anaesthetic bolus and sufficient should be added to the infusion to provide a dose rate of 0.08–0.12 mg kg^{-1} h^{-1} (De Negri et al. 2001). There may be a synergistic effect between clonidine and opioids, but some centres prefer clonidine to opioid additives because of the side effects of the latter, the mild sedation produced by clonidine often being beneficial in the early postoperative period.

Ketamine

Ketamine, an NMDA receptor antagonist, should not be used in children less than a year old because the central nervous system is at an early stage of development. Only the preservative-free preparation should be used in the epidural space.

Caudal administration of ketamine 0.5 mg kg^{-1} with bupivacaine 0.25% increased the duration of analgesia (time to first treatment request) from a median of 3.2 to 12.5 hours (Cook et al. 1995). Increasing the dose to 1 mg kg^{-1} further prolonged the analgesia (16.5 hours), but at the expense of behavioural side effects (Semple et al. 1996). There is no clinical evidence of such side effects when less than 0.5 mg kg^{-1} is employed. The enantiomer, S-ketamine, has recently been shown to be effective (Locatelli et al. 2008), has the advantage of being preservative free and has a synergistic effect with clonidine (Hager et al. 2002).

Ketamine cannot be recommended for epidural infusion in any form.

Complications

For a comprehensive review of epidural complications and their incidence in children the UK National Paediatric Epidural Audit provides informative reading (Llewellyn & Moriarty 2007). There were five serious incidents in 10,633 epidurals, but only one child had a persistent problem at 1 year. That audit, and one by Strafford et al. (1995), have shown that the incidence of infection is very low, but that epidural abscess should remain a cause for concern.

The possibility that *compartment syndrome* may be masked by an epidural block has been a long-standing concern in orthopaedic surgery. However, it should not be considered a contraindication to epidural anaesthesia. Indeed it may aid diagnosis by providing good pain relief through which the pain of compartment syndrome breaks through (Dunwoody et al. 1997), the increased requirement for analgesia having been shown to precede other clinical symptoms (Bae et al. 2001). In high-risk cases only low concentration local anaesthetic should be used for both bolus and infusion, pressure monitoring should be used (monitor the anterior compartment) and, most importantly, the orthopaedic and nursing staff must have a high index of suspicion.

Nurses must be aware that sensory block increases the risk of *compression neuropraxia* and *pressure sores*, and frequent turning should be part of the nursing care of all patients with epidural blocks.

Unlike the situation in adults, haemodynamic stability is the norm during the onset of an epidural block in children up to the age of 8 years, and left ventricular function, as assessed by M-mode echocardiography, is unaffected. However, mild decreases in mean blood pressure and heart rate may be seen.

Dural puncture is rare in experienced hands, but postdural puncture headache may require treatment with a dural blood patch if it does occur. In children, persistent CSF leakage may present with atypical symptoms such as orthostatic nausea and dizziness.

Spinal block

Spinal anaesthesia has gained in popularity for infants of less than 44 weeks postconceptual age—a group known to be at risk of postoperative apnoea after general anaesthesia. The incidence of this complication may be reduced by the use of spinal anaesthesia, though apnoea can still occur. The success rate of spinal anaesthesia in these patients is variable, with some authors reporting a need for supplementation (general anaesthesia or sedation) in up to 45% (Webster et al. 1991). However, if supplementation is given, the advantage of the spinal is lost because the risk of apnoea becomes the same as with a full general anaesthetic. A recent Cochrane Database review (Craven et al. 2003) found no evidence that spinal anaesthesia was beneficial in this patient group, but the technique will continue to be popular with enthusiasts. However, others will consider the high failure rate, lack of evidence, and the alternative of a caudal supplemented desflurane general anaesthetic preferable. Spinal anaesthesia has also been used in older children, but surgery awake is generally poorly tolerated in this population (Kokki et al. 1998).

Spinal anaesthesia has the advantage of producing low plasma concentrations of local anaesthetic, with consequent minimal risk of systemic toxicity (Beauvoir et al. 1996), but use in infants is limited to surgery lasting less than 60 minutes because of its short duration of action. This is secondary to a larger volume of CSF (4 ml kg^{-1} compared to 2 ml kg^{-1} in adults, with 50% of it spinal compared to 25% in adults) and a proportionately higher blood flow aiding rapid absorption of the local anaesthetic.

Technique

Given the quick onset (1–2 minutes) and a limited duration of spinal anaesthesia in the premature infant; the surgical team should be scrubbed and ready. Skin at the intended puncture site (L$_4$–L$_5$ or L$_5$–S$_1$ because the conus terminates at L$_3$ in this age group) should be anaesthetized either topically or by local infiltration, and insertion of the appropriate size of paediatric lumbar puncture needle may be facilitated by making a small incision in the skin. The block can be performed with the infant in the lateral, prone, or sitting position, but the latter has the advantages that it is easier to identify the midline and that CSF pressure is higher so that backflow is better. Kokki et al. (1998) found that hyperbaric bupivacaine (0.5% in 8% glucose) at a dose of 0.3–0.5 mg kg^{-1} (0.06–0.1 ml kg^{-1}) produced more successful blocks than the same dose of the glucose-free solution, but tetracaine 1% at 0.8 mg kg^{-1} (0.08 ml kg^{-1}) is probably better than either because of its longer duration of action. More recently, the newer agents levobupivacaine and ropivacaine have been used (Kokki et al. 2004, 2005).

A successful block at the L$_1$ level is identified by the loss of hip flexion. The infant's legs should not be raised (e.g. to place the diathermy plate) because this can cause a high block. To minimize discomfort and disturbance, monitoring devices and intravenous access can be placed on the lower limbs. A pacifier coated in 10% dextrose may also help calm the infant.

Key references

Tsui BC, Pillay JJ (2010) Evidence-based medicine: Assessment of ultrasound imaging for regional anesthesia in infants, children and adolescents. *Regional Anesthesia and Pain Medicine* 35: 47–54.

Willscke H, Marhofer P, Machata AM, et al. (2010) Current trends in paediatric regional anaesthesia, *Anaesthesia* 65 (supplement 1): 97–104.

On-line resources

http://www.nysora.com/regional_anesthesia/neuraxial_techniques/3010-caudal_anesthesia.html

http://www.usgraweb.hk/en/Start.html Open video tab to access caudal videos

References

Antok E, Bordet F, Duflo F, et al. (2003) Patient-controlled epidural analgesia versus continuous epidural infusion with ropivacaine for postoperative analgesia in children. *Anesthesia & Analgesia* 97: 1608–11.

Aynsley-Green A, Lloyd-Thomas AR, Ward-Platt MP (1995) Paediatric pain. In Aynsley-Green A, Ward-Platt MP, Lloyd-Thomas AR (Eds) *Clinical paediatrics: stress and pain in infancy and childhood*, 3 edn, pp. ix–xi. London: Ballière.

Bae DS, Kadiyala RK, Waters PM (2001) Acute compartment syndrome in children: contemporary diagnosis, treatment, and outcome. *Journal of Pediatric Orthopaedics* 21: 680–8.

Beauvoir C, Rochette A, Desch G, D'Athis F (1996) Spinal anaesthesia in newborns: total and free bupivacaine plasma concentration. *Paediatric Anaesthesia* 6: 195–9.

Berde C (1994) Epidural analgesia in children. *Canadian Journal of Anaesthesia* 41: 555–60.

Booker PD, Taylor C, Saba G (1996) Perioperative changes in α-1-acid-glycoprotein concentrations in infants undergoing major surgery. *British Journal of Anaesthesia* 76: 365–8.

Bosenberg AT, Gouws E (1995) Skin-epidural distance in children. *Anaesthesia* 50: 895–7.

Bosenberg AT, Bland BAR, Schulte-Steinberg O, Downing JW (1988) Thoracic epidural anesthesia via caudal route in infants. *Anesthesiology* 69: 265–9.

Bozkurt P, Kaya G, Yeker Y (1997) Single-injection lumbar epidural morphine for postoperative analgesia in children. *Regional Anesthesia* 22: 212–17.

Bubeck J, Boos K, Krause H, et al. (2004) Subcutaneous tunneling of caudal catheters reduces the rate of bacterial colonization to that of lumbar epidural catheters. *Anesthesia & Analgesia* 9: 689–93.

Burke D, Joypaul V, Thomson MF (2000) Circumcision supplemented by dorsal penile nerve block with 0.75% ropivacaine: A complication. *Regional Anesthesia & Pain Medicine* 25: 424–7.

Chalkiadis GA, Anderson BJ, Tay M, et al. (2005) Pharmacokinetics of levobupivacaine after caudal epidural administration in infants less than 3 months of age. *British Journal of* Anaesthesia 95: 524–9.

Chawathe MS, Jones RM, Gildersleve CD (2003) Detection of epidural catheters with ultrasound in children. *Paediatric Anaesthesia* 13: 681–4.

Cheung SLW, Booker PD, Franks R, Pozzi M (1997) Serum concentrations of bupivacaine during prolonged continuous paravertebral infusion in young infants. *British Journal of Anaesthesia* 79: 9–13.

Cho JE, Kim JY, Kim JE, et al. (2008) Epidural sufentanil provides better analgesia from 24 h after surgery compared with epidural fentanyl in children *Acta Anaesthesiologica Scandinavia* 52: 1360–3.

Cook B, Grubb DJ, Aldridge LA, Doyle E (1995) Comparison of the effects of adrenaline, clonidine and ketamine on the duration of caudal analgesia produced by bupivacaine in children. *British Journal of Anaesthesia* 75: 698–701.

Craven PD, Badawi N, Henderson-Smart DJ, O'Brien M (2003) Regional (spinal, epidural, caudal) versus general anaesthesia in preterm infants undergoing inguinal herniorrhaphy in early infancy. *Cochrane Database of Systemic Reviews* 3: CD003669.

Dadure C, Pirat P, Raux O, et al. (2003) Perioperative continuous peripheral nerve blocks with disposable infusion pumps in children: a prospective descriptive study. *Anesthesia & Analgesia* 97: 687–90.

Dadure C, Motais F, Ricard C, et al. (2005) Continuous peripheral nerve blocks at home for treatment of recurrent complex regional pain syndrome I in children. *Anesthesiology* 102: 387–91.

De Jose Maria B, Banus E, Egea MN (2008) Ultrasound-guided supraclavicular vs. infraclavicular brachial plexus blocks in children. *Paediatric Anaesthesia* 18: 838–44.

De Negri P, Ivani G, Tirri T, et al. (2004) A comparison of epidural bupivacaine, levobupivacaine, and ropivacaine on postoperative analgesia and motor blockade. *Anesthesia & Analgesia* 99: 45–8.

De Negri P, Ivani G, Visconti C (2001) The dose-response relationship for clonidine added to a postoperative continuous epidural infusion of ropivacaine in children. *Anesthesia & Analgesia* 93: 71–6.

Dunwoody JM, Reichert CC, Brown KL (1997) Compartment syndrome associated with bupivacaine and fentanyl epidural. *Journal of Pediatric Orthopedics* 17: 285–8.

Eng J, Sabanathan S (1992) Continuous paravertebral block for post-thoracotomy analgesia in children. *Journal of Pediatric Surgery* 27: 556–7.

Fitzgerald M, Walker S M (2009) Infant pain management: a developmental neurobiological approach. *Nature Clinical Practice Neurology* 5: 35–50.

Flandin-Blety C, Barrier G (1995) Accidents following extradural analgesia in children. The results of a retrospective study. *Paediatric Anaesthesia* 5: 41–6.

Fredrickson MJ (2009) Ultrasound (US) guided transversus abdominis plane (TAP) block for paediatric inguinal hernia surgery – a pilot study. *Pediatric Anaesthesia* 5: 556–7.

Giaufre E, Dalens B, Gombert A (1996) Epidemiology and morbidity of regional anesthesia in children: a one-year prospective survey of the French-Language Society of Paediatric Anesthesiologists. *Anesthesia and Analgesia* 83: 904–12.

Hager H, Marhofer P, Sitzwohl C, et al. (2002) Caudal clonidine prolongs analgesia from caudal (S)-ketamine in children. *Anesthesia & Analgesia* 94: 1169–72.

Ilfeld BM, Smith DW, Enneking FK (2004) Continuous regional analgesia following ambulatory pediatric orthopedic surgery. *American Journal Orthopedics* 33: 405–8

Jain A, Rutter N (2000) Topical amethocaine gel in the newborn infant: how soon does it work and how long does it last? *Archives of Diseases of Childhood* 83: 211–14.

Jamali S, Monin S, Begon C, et al. (1994) Clonidine in pediatric caudal anesthesia. *Anesthesia & Analgesia* 78: 663–6.

Jennings E, Fitzgerald M (1996) C-fos can be induced in the neonatal rat spinal cord by both noxious and innocuous stimulation. *Pain* 68: 301–6.

Karmakar MK, Booker PD, Franks R, Pozzi M (1996) Continuous extrapleural paravertebral infusion of bupivacaine for post-thoracotomy analgesia in young infants. *British Journal of Anaesthesia* 76: 811–15.

Karmakar MK, Aun CST, Wong EL, et al. (2002) Ropivacaine undergoes slower systemic absorption from the caudal epidural space in children than bupivacaine. *Anesthesia & Analgesia* 94: 259–65.

Kirchmair L, Enna B, Mitterschiffthaler G, et al. (2004) Lumbar plexus in children. A sonographic study and its relevance to pediatric regional anesthesia. *Anesthesiology* 101: 445–50.

Kokki H, Tuovinen K, Hendolin H (1998) Spinal anaesthesia for paediatric day-case surgery: a double blind, randomized, parallel group, prospective comparison of isobaric and hyperbaric bupivacaine. *British Journal of Anaesthesia* 81: 502–6.

Kokki H, Ylönen P, Heikkinen M, Reinikainen M (2004) Levobupivacaine for pediatric spinal anesthesia. *Anesthesia & Analgesia* 98: 64–7.

Kokki H, Ylönen P, Laisalmi M, et al. (2005) Isobaric ropivacaine 5 mg/mL for spinal anesthesia in children. *Anesthesia & Analgesia* 100: 66–70.

Larsson BA, Olsson GL, Lonnqvist PA (1994) Plasma concentrations of bupivacaine in young infants after continuous epidural infusion. *Paediatric Anaesthesia* 4: 159–62.

Larsson BA, Lonnqvist PA, Olsson GL (1995) Plasma concentrations of bupivacaine in neonates after continuous epidural infusion. *Anesthesia & Analgesia* 84: 501–5.

Lawson RA, Smart NG, Gudgeon AC, Morton NS (1995) Evaluation of an amethocaine gel preparation for percutaneous analgesia before venous cannulation in children. *British Journal of Anaesthesia* 75: 282–5.

Lipp AK, Woodcock J, Hensman B, Wilkinson K (2004) Leg weakness is a complication of ilio-inguinal nerve block in children. *British Journal of Anaesthesia* 92: 273–4.

Llewellyn N, Moriarty A (2007) The National Pediatric Epidural Audit. *Pediatric Anesthesia* 17: 520–33.

Lloyd-Thomas AR, Howard RF (1994) A pain service for children. *Paediatric Anaesthesia* 4: 3–15.

Locatelli BG, Ingelmo P, Sonzogni V, et al. (2005) Randomized, double-blind, phase III, controlled trial comparing levobupivacaine 0.25%, ropivacaine 0.25% and bupivacaine 0.25% by the caudal route in children. *British Journal of Anaesthesia* 94: 366–71.

Locatelli BG, Frawley G, Spotti A, et al. (2008) Analgesic effectiveness of caudal levobupivacaine and ketamine. *British Journal of Anaesthesia* 100: 701–6.

Lonnquist PA, Olsson GL (1994) Paravertebral versus epidural block in children. Effects on postoperative morphine requirements after renal surgery. *Acta Anaesthesiologica Scandinavica* 38: 346–9.

Ludot H, Tharin JY, Belouadah M, et al. (2008) Successful resuscitation after ropivacaine and lidocaine-induced ventricular arrhythmia following posterior lumbar plexus block in a child. *Anesthesia & Analgesia* 106: 1572–4.

Luz G, Wieser CH, Innerhofer P, et al. (1998) Free and total bupivacaine plasma concentrations after continuous epidural anaesthesia in infants and children. *Paediatric Anaesthesia* 8: 473–78.

Marhofer P, Frickey N (2006) Ultrasonographic guidance in pediatric regional anesthesia Part 1: Theoretical background. *Paediatric Anaesthesia* 16: 1008–18.

Marhofer P, Greher M, Sitzwohl C, Kapral S (2004) Ultrasonographic guidance for infraclavicular plexus anaesthesia in children. *Anaesthesia* 59: 642–6.

Marhofer P, Bosenberg A, Willschke H (2005) Pilot study of neuraxial imaging by ultrasound in infants and children. *Paediatric Anaesthesia* 15: 671–67.

Masir F, Driessen JJ, Thies KC, et al. (2006) Depth of the thoracic epidural space in children. *Acta Anaesthesiologica Belgica* 57: 271–5.

McNeely JK, Trentadue NC, Rusy LM, et al. (1997) Culture of bacteria from lumbar and caudal epidural catheters used for postoperative analgesia in children. *Regional Anesthesia and Pain Medicine* 22(5): 428–31.

Metzelder ML, Kuebler JF, Glueer S, et al. (2010) Penile block is associated with less urinary retention than caudal anesthesia in distal hypospadia repair in children. *World Journal of Urology* 28: 87–91.

Naja ZM, Raf M, El Rajab M, et al. (2005) Nerve stimulator-guided paravertebral blockade combined with sevoflurane sedation versus general anaesthesia with systemic analgesia for postherniorrhaphy pain relief in children: a prospective randomized trial. *Anesthesiology* 103: 600–5.

Naja ZM, Raf M, El Rajab M, et al. (2006) A comparison of nerve stimulator guided paravertebral block and ilio-inguinal nerve block for analgesia after inguinal herniorrhaphy in children. *Anaesthesia* 61: 1064–8.

Newman PJ, Bushnell TG, Radford P (1996) The effect of needle size and type in paediatric caudal analgesia. *Paediatric Anaesthesia* 6: 459–61.

Oberndorfer U, Marhofer P, Bösenberg A, et al. (2007) Ultrasonographic guidance for sciatic and femoral nerve blocks in children. *British Journal Anaesthesia* 98: 797–801.

Park JH, Koo BN, Kim JY, et al. (2006) Determination of the optimal angle for needle insertion during caudal block in children using ultrasound imaging. *Anaesthesia* 61: 946–9.

Peutrell JM, Holder K, Gregory M (1997) Plasma bupivacaine concentrations associated with continuous extradural infusions in babies. *British Journal of Anaesthesia* 78: 160–2.

Ponde VC, Diwan S (2009) Does ultrasound guidance improve the success rate of infraclavicular brachial plexus block when compared with nerve stimulation in children with radial club hands? *Anesthesia & Analgesia* 108: 1967–70.

Prosser DP, Davis A, Booker PD, Murray A (1997) Caudal tramadol for postoperative analgesia in paediatric hypospadias surgery. *British Journal of Anaesthesia* 79: 293–6.

Raghavan K, Arnold R (2007) Spread of local anaesthetic solution in epidural space visualisation with ultrasound in single shot caudals. *Pediatric Anaesthesia* 17: 608–9.

Roberts S (2006) Ultrasonographic guidance in pediatric regional anesthesia. Part 2: techniques. *Paediatric Anaesthesia* 16: 1112–24.

Roberts SA, Galvez I (2005) Ultrasound assessment of caudal catheter position in infants. *Paediatric Anaesthesia* 15: 429–32.

Roberts SA, Guruswamy V, Galvez I (2005) Caudal injectate can be reliably imaged using portable ultrasound: a preliminary study. *Paediatric Anaesthesia* 15: 948–52.

Rothstein P, Arthur G, Feldman HS, et al. (1986) Bupivacaine for intercostal nerve blocks in children: Blood concentrations and pharmacokinetics. *Anesthesia & Analgesia* 65: 625–32.

Saberski LR, Kondamuri S, Osinubi OYO (1997) Identification of the epidural space: is loss of resistance to air a safe technique? *Regional Anesthesia* 22: 3–15.

Schafhalter-Zoppoth I, Younger SJ, Collins AB, Gray AT (2004) The 'seesaw' sign: improved sonographic identification of the sciatic nerve. *Anesthesiology* 101: 808–9.

Schwemmer U, Markus CK, Greim CA, et al. (2004 Sonographic imaging of the sciatic nerve and its division in the popliteal fossa in children. *Pediatric Anaesthesia* 14: 1005–8.

Semple D, Findlow D, Aldridge LM, Doyle E (1996) The optimal dose of ketamine for caudal epidural blockade in children. *Anaesthesia* 51: 1170–2.

Semsroth M, Plattnew O, Horcher E (1996) Effective pain relief with continuous intrapleural bupivacaine after thoracotomy in infants and children. *Paediatric Anaesthesia* 6: 303–10.

Stayer SA, Pasquariello CA, Schwartz RE, et al. (1995) The safety of continuous pleural lignocaine after thoracotomy in children and adolescents. *Paediatric Anaesthesia* 5: 307–10.

Strafford MA, Wilder RT, Berde CB (1995) The risk of infection from epidural analgesia in children: a review of 1620 cases. *Anesthesia & Analgesia* 80: 234–8.

Taddio A, Katz J, Illersich AL, Curran G (1997) Effect of neonatal circumcision in pain response during subsequent routine vaccination. *Lancet* 349: 599–603.

Thong WY, Pahel V, Khalil S (2000) Inadvertent administration of intravenous ropivacaine in a child. *Paediatric Anaesthesia* 10: 563–4.

Tobias JD (2001) Brachial plexus anaesthesia in children. *Paediatric Anaesthesia* 11: 265–75.

Tobias JD (2003) Regional anaesthesia of the lower extremity in children. *Paediatric Anaesthesia* 13: 152–63.

Tsui BC, Pillay JJ (2010) Evidence-based medicine: assessment of ultrasound imaging for regional anesthesia in infants, children, and adolescents. *Regional Anesthesia and Pain Medicine* 35(Suppl 2): S47–54.

Tsui BC, Gupta S, Finucane B (1998) Confirmation of epidural catheter placement using nerve stimulation. *Canadian Journal of Anaesthesia* 45: 640–4.

Tsui BCH, Tarkkila P, Gupta S, Kearney R (1999) Confirmation of caudal needle using nerve stimulation. *Anesthesiology* 91: 374–8.

Tsui BC, Seal R, Koller J (2002) Thoracic epidural catheter placement via the caudal approach in infants by using electrocardiographic guidance. *Anesthesia & Analgesia* 95: 326–30.

Van Geffen GJ, Luc T, Gielen M (2006) Ultrasound-guided interscalene brachial plexus block in a child with femur fibula ulna syndrome. *Paediatric anaesthesia* 16: 330–2.

Wall PD (1988) The prevention of postoperative pain. *Pain* 33: 289–90.

Webster AC, McKishnie JD, Kenyon CF, et al. (1991) Spinal anaesthesia for inguinal hernia repair in high-risk neonates. *Canadian Journal of Anaesthesia* 38: 281–6.

Weinberg GL, Ripper R, Feinstein DL, Hoffman W (2003) Lipid emulsion infusion rescues dogs from bupivacaine-induced cardiac toxicity. *Regional Anesthesia and Pain Medicine* 28: 198–202.

Weinberg GL (2008) Lipid infusion therapy: translation to clinical practice. *Anesthesia and Analgesia* 106: 1340–2.

Weintraud, M, Marhofer P, Bösenberg A, et al. (2008) Ilioinguinal/iliohypogastric blocks in children: Where do we administer the local anesthetic without direct visualization? *Anesthesia & Analgesia* 106: 89–93.

Weintraud M, Lundblad M, Kettner SC, et al. (2009) Ultrasound versus landmark-based technique for ilioinguinal-iliohypogastric nerve blockade in children: The implications on plasma levels of ropivacaine. *Anesthesia & Analgesia* 5: 1488–92.

Weston PJ, Bourchier D (1995) The pharmacokinetics of bupivacaine following interpleural nerve block in infants of very low birthweight. *Paediatric Anaesthesia* 5: 219–22.

Willschke H, Bösenberg A, Marhofer P, et al. (2006) Ultrasonography-guided rectus sheath block in paediatric anaesthesia—a new approach to an old technique. *British Journal of Anaesthesia* 97: 244–9.

Willschke H, Bosenberg A, Marhofer P, et al. (2006) Ultrasonographic guided ilioinguinal/iliohypogastric nerve block in pediatric anesthesia – what is the optimal volume? *Anesthesia & Analgesia* 102: 1680–4.

CHAPTER 23

Pain and autonomic nerve blocks

Mick Serpell and Andreas Goebel

The sympathetic nervous system was, for a long time, the target for pain relieving techniques, but they are now used much less frequently than in the past because the mechanisms of pain are better understood. The role of the sympathetic nervous system in the generation and maintenance of pain may have been overemphasized previously (Schott 1998) so the rational for sympathetic block in chronic pain management is being re-evaluated. Systemic medication, stimulation techniques, physical therapy, and psychological techniques are all used much more widely than previously. When it is used, sympathetic block can be produced in one of three ways:

1. Direct injections of the sympathetic chain or related ganglia using local anaesthetic or neurolytic solutions;

2. Venous injection, with the circulation excluded by tourniquet, of drugs which deplete adrenergic transmitters—intravenous regional sympathetic block (IVRSB); and

3. Systemic administration (by intravenous infusion) of α-adrenergic antagonist drugs.

The analgesic effect of most nerve block techniques (e.g. an epidural in labour or coeliac plexus for cancer pain) is a result of the interruption of transmission in *afferent* nociceptive fibres, but the effects of sympathetic nerve block can be more complex. The sympathetic nervous system is directly involved in the pathophysiology of some painful states ('sympathetically maintained pain'), and the analgesic action is due primarily to block of sympathetic *efferent* activity. There may also be disruption of reflex control systems so that peripheral or central sensory processing is altered. Finally, peripheral vasodilatation can relieve pain due to ischaemia.

General principles

Indications for sympathetic block

Peripheral vascular disease

Sympathetic blocks may be used for the following:

1. *Acute vascular disorders*: post-traumatic vasospasm; acute arterial or venous occlusion; cold injury; inadvertent intra-arterial injection of drugs (e.g. thiopental or contaminated drugs of abuse);

2. *Chronic vasospastic conditions*: Raynaud's syndrome; acrocyanosis; livedo reticularis; sequelae of spinal cord injury or disease (e.g. polio);

3. *Chronic obliterative arterial diseases*: thromboangiitis obliterans (Buerger's disease); atherosclerosis;

4. *Perioperative purposes*: microvascular surgery; arteriovenous fistula formation for dialysis.

In spite of this long list, there are no controlled trials of sympathetic block in peripheral vascular disease, much of the evidence being anecdotal (Gordon et al. 1994). For example, lumbar sympathectomy with phenol produced long-lasting (24–120 months) pain relief and healing of ulcers in 59% of 373 patients, the best responses occurring in diabetics with rest pain (not claudication) and non-diabetics with digital gangrene or ulcers (Mashiah et al. 1995). The traditional view is that sympathectomy increases skin, but not muscle blood flow, although Gleim and colleagues (1995) reported immediate improvement in painless walking distance, the benefit lasting for 6–9 months during which time the patient may develop collateral circulation. Such results are comparable to surgical sympathectomy, but with reduced morbidity and mortality. If amputation is necessary, a preoperative block may aid in defining the limits of tissue viability and also facilitate healing of the stump.

Visceral pain

Nociceptive fibres from the viscera accompany sympathetic nerves, their block interrupting these pathways, and also viscero-visceral reflexes so that ischaemia and spasm are relieved. Situations in which blocks may be considered are as follows:

1. *Abdominal cancer*. Neurolytic coeliac plexus block produces partial to complete pain relief lasting for the remainder of life in about 70–90% of patients with pain arising from carcinoma of the pancreas, stomach, gall bladder, or liver (Brown et al. 1987, Eisenberg et al. 1995). Mercadante (1993) showed that coeliac plexus block was equally effective, but with fewer side effects, as systemic analgesia in a series of 20 patients. The pain of other abdominal malignancies and rectal tenesmus due to pelvic carcinoma may also be helped (Bristow & Foster 1988). Neurolytic superior hypogastric plexus blocks have been used for chronic pelvic pain related to cancer (Plancarte et al. 1990a, de Leon-Casasola et al. 1993, 2008). Block of the ganglion impar at the inferior end of the sacrum has been used for perineal pain.

2. *Chronic non-malignant abdominal pain*. Sympathectomy for chronic pancreatitis is not as effective as for cancer pain

(Gress et al. 2001). Unilateral block of the coeliac plexus at the L_1 level is sometimes helpful in the loin-pain haematuria syndrome. It has been claimed that some chronic perineal pain syndromes respond to bilateral lumbar sympathetic block, and superior hypogastric block has been used for chronic non-malignant pelvic pain syndromes.

3. *Acute abdominal pain.* There may be some benefit in the pain of pancreatitis and ureteric colic, but this is usually managed with systemic analgesics.

4. *Cardiac pain.* The pain of acute myocardial infarction, and intractable angina, is eased by upper thoracic sympathetic or stellate ganglion block. Stellate ganglion block is used for intractable angina before and even after cardiac by-pass surgery (Chester et al. 2000). Endoscopic transthoracic sympathectomy was found to be beneficial in an uncontrolled trial involving 24 patients with severe angina (Wettervik et al. 1995).

5. *Perioperative purposes.* Anaesthesia for upper abdominal surgery may be achieved using a combination of coeliac plexus and intercostal nerve blocks or wound infiltration. However, Hamid and colleagues (1992) found that the technique provided only partial attenuation of postoperative pain and the neuroendocrine response because total afferent block was not produced.

Hyperhidrosis

Sympathetic blocks produce anhidrosis and patients with hyperhidrosis may be referred for sympathectomy although the patient should have a thorough trial of conservative treatment first because side effects such as Horner's syndrome are common after neurolytic procedures. Endoscopic transthoracic sympathectomy of the upper limb is a safe and effective alternative to open cervical sympathectomy in the management of hyperhidrosis, as well as in vasospastic conditions and sympathetically maintained pain (Byrne et al. 1990).

Neuropathic pain

The aetiology of neuropathic pain (Chapter 2) may be metabolic, ischaemic, hereditary, compressive, traumatic, toxic, infectious, or immune mediated (Woolf & Mannion 1999). Typically, there are sensory deficits, abnormal sensations (e.g. paraesthesiae), and pain which may be maintained by sympathetic efferent activity or by circulating catecholamines. After partial nerve injury, both injured and uninjured axons become sensitive to circulating catecholamines and to noradrenaline released from postganglionic sympathetic terminals (Woolf & Mannion 1999). The cell bodies of sensory neurones in the dorsal root ganglion also come under the closer influence of sympathetic axons after nerve injury, so that sympathetic activity may be capable of initiating or maintaining activity in sensory fibres (McLachlan et al. 1993). The use of sympathectomy for neuropathic pain is based on very weak evidence, most of the literature describing retrospective case series with very small sample sizes and no control groups. There is usually inadequate assessment of the response (including pain reduction), the duration of response is typically not reported, and the possible complications are often ignored (Mailis-Gagnon & Furlan 2008).

Acute herpes zoster: sympathetic block is claimed to reduce pain and promote healing during the acute phase, but the incidence of post-herpetic neuralgia is not reduced (Ali 1995, Hogan 1993).

Sympathetic blocks are unproven in established postherpetic neuralgia (Wu et al. 2000).

Carcinomatous neuropathy: invasion by carcinoma, particularly of the brachial or lumbar plexus, and carcinoma of head and neck may produce a neuropathic pain which is partially responsive to sympathetic block.

Complex regional pain syndrome: complex regional pain syndrome (CRPS) is a condition characterized by unrelenting pain, disturbances of sensory, motor, and autonomic function, and with trophic changes affecting skin, hair, and bone. Older terms for the condition ('reflex sympathetic dystrophy', 'shoulder-hand syndrome', 'Sudeck's atrophy', or 'causalgia') are now outdated, and diagnosis is based on the complaint of disproportionate pain, exclusion of other pathology, and the presence of a range of symptoms and signs related to disordered neurological function (Table 23.1). These criteria have yet to be adopted by the International Association for the Study of Pain, but the use of earlier definitions is discouraged.

Although 90% of cases occur after limb injury, the rest being 'spontaneous' (Veldman et al. 1993), the cause of CRPS is unknown. Many pathophysiological abnormalities have been identified or proposed, but it is unclear whether they are primary or secondary in nature:

1. Aberrant sympathetic nervous system activation (Wasner et al. 1999), although the concentration of noradrenaline in venous blood draining the limb is *decreased* (Drummond et al. 1991);

2. Increased release of peptides from nerve endings (Birklein et al. 2001) although the mechanism of action is unclear;

3. Primary microcirculatory problems (Groeneweg et al. 2008);

4. Changes in the cortical representation (the homunculus) of the affected limb, successful treatment leading to its normalization (Maihofner et al. 2004);

5. The fluid from skin blisters on affected limbs contains high concentrations of pro-inflammatory markers indicating an inflammatory process (Huygen et al. 2002), but there is no correlation between concentration and severity of symptoms, and steroids, while beneficial in some early states, are unlikely to be effective in the established condition (Munts et al. 2009);

Table 23.1 Budapest criteria for CRPS derived from Harden and colleagues (2007). ***Essential components***: continuing disproportionate pain with no other diagnosis possible. ***Other clinical features***: there should be at least one symptom in each of three of the following categories, and one sign in at least two of them*

Category	Symptoms/signs
Sensory	Allodynia/hyperalgesia
Vasomotor	Changes (or asymmetry) in skin temperature or colour
Sudomotor/oedema	Changes (or asymmetry) in sweating/oedema
Motor/trophic	Decreased range of movement
	Weakness/tremor/dystonia
	Trophic changes in hair, skin or nails

*If the essential requirements are met, but fewer symptoms/signs are present a diagnosis of 'CRPS-NOS' (not otherwise specified) may be made.

6. An autoimmune mechanism is supported by some patients having antibodies which bind to peripheral nerve (Goebel et al. 2005, Kohr et al. 2009), and others responding to immunoglobulin therapy (Goebel et al. 2010); and

7. Central sensitization at least sustains the condition, low-dose ketamine producing temporary pain relief (Sigtermans et al. 2009).

With precise aetiology so uncertain, it is not surprising that treatment is both non-specific and difficult. Somatic nerve blocks which are anatomically appropriate for the distribution of the pain can be used for its relief, especially to facilitate physiotherapy (Charlton 1990). Sympathetic blocks can produce good pain relief in over 50% of patients initially, but there are no known prognostic factors to indicate who will respond, and the proportion decreases with time. However, 10% of otherwise refractory patients still respond after 12 years (Schattschneider et al. 2006, Torebjork et al. 1995).

What is less clear is whether sympathetic blocks have any therapeutic effect, although some patient subgroups may benefit (Carroll et al. 2009, Meier et al. 2009, Price et al. 1998). Local anaesthetics do not produce long-lasting relief, and a series of blocks is unlikely to prolong the effect (Rodriguez et al. 2006). There is no evidence to indicate that neurodestructive procedures are any better than placebo, a comparative study of radiofrequency ablation and phenol injection of the sympathetic chain showing no difference between them other than an incidence of chronic neuralgia with phenol (Manjunath et al. 2008). A recent, high-quality, albeit small study did show promising results from the injection of botulinum toxin (Carroll et al. 2009). Other forms of sympathetic block, primarily IVRSB, have been tried, but the results of formal studies have been mixed at best.

Reference to a text on pain medicine (e.g. Binder & Barron 2009) is recommended for more detailed consideration of this condition.

Other indications

In addition to the indications discussed already, other suggested uses for sympathetic block include stellate ganglion block for Bell's palsy, quinine toxicity, retinal artery occlusion, tinnitus, and certain types of acute hearing loss.

Contraindications to sympathetic block

In general, the conditions which raise concerns about performing sympathetic blocks are as for other techniques, but a few specific points should be made:

Abnormalities of coagulation: many of the target nerves are deeply placed and close to major blood vessels. A large haematoma may result if there is any disorder of coagulation.

Hypovolaemia: splanchnic, coeliac, and bilateral lumbar sympathetic blocks produce extensive vasodilation so precautions should be taken to avoid hypotension.

Anatomical abnormality: spinal scoliosis or tissue distortion by tumour may make the block more difficult to perform and so reduce the success rate. Anomalous vessels (e.g. those feeding tumours) increase the risk of accidental needle puncture and haematoma.

Local neoplasm: needles should not be inserted through neoplastic tissue because there is a risk of spread to deeper structures, but there are circumstances when this is unavoidable.

Inadequate facilities: full facilities for resuscitation and radiographic control must be available.

Clinical application of sympathetic blocks

Sympathetic blocks should only be used as part of a comprehensive multidisciplinary approach utilizing all the other components of holistic care, and a modern Pain Clinic should also provide drug therapy, physical therapy, stimulation techniques (e.g. transcutaneous electrical nerve stimulation (TENS), acupuncture), and psychological approaches. However, there are circumstances (e.g. lumbar sympathectomy for a patient under the care of a vascular surgeons; coeliac plexus block for a patient with carcinoma of the pancreas) in which the role of the anaesthetist is to perform the sympathetic block only while the other aspects of management are coordinated by another doctor, but the anaesthetist should still work as a part of the team.

Diagnostic blocks can be used to differentiate between somatic and visceral pain, to identify a sympathetic component, to assess whether blood flow increases, or if sweating decreases. If an attempt is being made to define the sympathetic contribution to any particular pain syndrome the diagnostic block must be a pure sympathetic block without any accompanying somatic block. This can only be achieved by precise interruption of the sympathetic chain and neither epidural injection nor IVRSB with local anaesthetic or guanethidine are selective enough because they also block somatic sensory components. Objective signs of sympathetic block must be identified using changes in skin temperature (assessed by touch, surface thermometer, or thermal-sensitive strips with a liquid crystal display) or conductivity, or tests of sweat production with ninhydrin, cobalt blue, or starch iodine. When sympathetic supply to a limb has been blocked, the veins visibly dilate and the increased blood flow in skin (laser-Doppler) and deeper veins (venous plethysmography) can be measured (Breivik & Cousins 2009).

False positive results may be due to spread of solution to adjacent somatic nerves or into the epidural space, systemic effects of absorbed local anaesthetic, or the placebo response. False negative results may follow an incomplete or inappropriate block, and inadequate assessment before or after the block. Confounding factors are the difficulty of achieving complete sympathetic block (Malmqvist et al. 1987), the possibility of both sympathetic and somatic contributions to the patient's pain, the lack of correlation between the durations of sympathetic block and pain relief, and the variability of responses on different occasions. Some patients demonstrate unexpected or unusual responses, such as contralateral or delayed blocks, and some pain is made worse (Purcell-Jones & Justins 1988).

Intravenous phentolamine (an α-adrenergic blocking drug) has been suggested as a test of sympathetic involvement in chronic pain, and as a predictor of the outcome of sympathetic block (Arner 1991, Raja et al. 1991), but there are uncertainties about its sensitivity, specificity, and reliability.

A *prognostic block* can be used to demonstrate to the patient the effect on pain, blood flow, or sweating, but there may be poor correlation between its result and the outcome of any subsequent surgical or neuroablative procedure. Local anaesthetic injection may produce greater block of nerve function than a neurolytic technique because larger volumes tend to be used. If neuroablation is to be based upon the results of prognostic blocks, more than one should be performed and a consistent response demonstrated. Sometimes the prognostic block will produce an increase in pain or an increase in limb temperature, which the patient finds uncomfortable and unacceptable.

Therapeutic blocks using local anaesthetic drugs result in temporary block, whilst neurolytic agents (alcohol or phenol) destroy the sympathetic chain and result in a more persistent effect. Surgical ablation can be performed by open removal or electrocoagulation of the sympathetic chain, or minimally invasive procedures using stereotactic thermal, laser interruption, or percutaneous radiofrequency lesioning. Neurolytic blocks are indicated primarily for painful abdominal cancer and peripheral vascular disease, and should be used with great caution and reluctance in all other conditions. There are no clear guidelines on the indications for different techniques, and the optimal frequency and duration of treatment have not been established.

Essential requirements for sympathetic block

1. The performance of sympathetic blocks requires a full understanding of the relevant anatomy and the pathophysiology of the underlying condition.

2. Informed consent must be obtained before the block is performed so that the patient has a full understanding of the potential benefits and side effects.

3. Resuscitation equipment must be immediately available.

4. Secure venous access is essential for all patients, and facilities for the treatment of hypotension must be available. A pre-load of intravenous crystalloid solution is usually given before bilateral blocks (splanchnic, coeliac, lumbar sympathetic, superior hypogastric).

5. Patients may experience discomfort when the blocks are being performed and some practitioners employ sedation with drugs such as midazolam and alfentanil in addition to infiltration with local anaesthetic. General anaesthesia is rarely necessary, and it has been argued that nerve damage will not be recognized in a patient who is unable to speak or respond.

6. Constant monitoring should include pulse oximetry and regular measurement of blood pressure. Oxygen desaturation may occur during sedation, especially in the prone patient.

7. Radiological control in the form of an image intensifier, ultrasound, or computed tomography (CT) scanner is mandatory for splanchnic, coeliac, lumbar sympathetic, and superior hypogastric blocks. Whenever possible a permanent print should be made and filed in the patient's notes, especially for any neurolytic procedure. The image intensifier allows a faster, safer procedure, overcomes the problem of variable anatomical landmarks, allows precise needle placement, demonstrates the spread of injected solution, and reveals inadvertent intravascular injection even when aspiration tests have been negative. With accurate needle placement small volumes of neurolytic solution can be used, thereby minimizing the risk of complications.

8. An aseptic technique is essential.

Neurolytic solutions for sympathetic blocks

A number of different solutions will destroy nerves, but phenol and alcohol are used most commonly for neurolytic sympathetic blocks.

Phenol destroys all nerve fibre types by protein denaturation. It is not selective and will destroy both motor and sensory nerves although the fibres can regenerate so the blocks should not be regarded as permanent. The strongest aqueous solution is 6%, but higher concentrations can be obtained using an oily base such as X-ray contrast medium and this is recommended. Contact with somatic nerves may cause neuritis. Toxic reactions may occur if a dose of 600 mg is exceeded in a 70-kg man.

Alcohol has a similar non-selective destructive effect on nerves, but it produces a very high incidence of neuritis and is usually reserved for coeliac plexus block where the large injection volumes preclude the safe use of phenol.

Sympathetic block techniques

Stellate ganglion block

Anatomy

The stellate ganglion is formed by the fusion of the inferior cervical and first thoracic sympathetic ganglia. It is present in only 80% of the population, so a more correct term would be either lower cervical or upper thoracic sympathetic block (cervicothoracic sympathetic trunk block (Elias 2000)). It lies anterior to the prevertebral fascia, the transverse process of the seventh cervical and first thoracic vertebrae, and the neck of the first rib (Figure 23.1). It may be covered in its lower parts by the dome of the pleura, and lies posterior to the carotid sheath.

Technique

A number of approaches to the stellate ganglion have been described, but the simplest and most satisfactory is the anterior paratracheal. With the patient in the supine position, the head is extended and a point is marked level with, and 2 cm lateral to, the cricoid cartilage (at C_6). Pressure is applied with two fingers in the groove between the trachea and the carotid sheath (Figure 23.2). In a very thin patient it may be possible to feel the transverse process of C_6. A 23-g, 30-mm needle is inserted directly backwards to pass between the trachea and the carotid sheath until it strikes the transverse process of C_6, some 2.5–3 cm from the skin. The needle should then be withdrawn 2–3 mm so that the tip lies anterior to

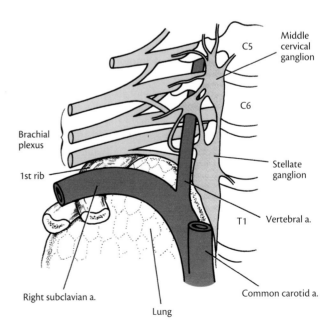

Figure 23.1 Anatomy of the stellate ganglion. Note that, at the level of injection (C6), the vertebral artery is a posterior relation.

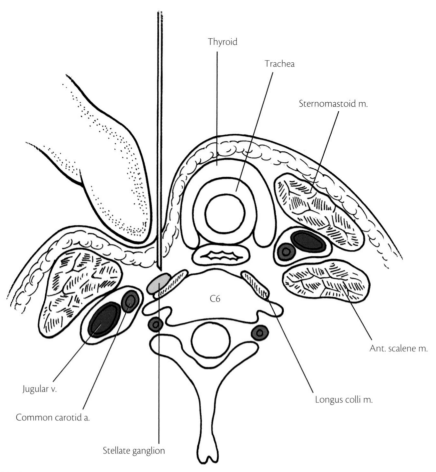

Figure 23.2 Stellate ganglion block.

the prevertebral fascia and the longus colli muscle. The needle is fixed in this position with one hand, whilst an aspiration test is performed. A small portion (1–2 ml) of the local anaesthetic should be injected and, if there are no adverse effects, the remainder is injected slowly, with repeated aspiration tests. The use of a short catheter between needle and syringe allows an assistant to perform the injection while the needle is kept 'immobile'. The patient should be instructed to open the mouth slightly and not to talk or swallow during the injection, but to raise a hand as a signal to stop if the injection is painful. If the needle is in the correct fascial plane, there should be slight resistance to injection, but no swelling should be apparent. To produce full sympathetic block of the upper limb the solution must extend to the T_3 ganglion and volumes larger than 10 ml may be necessary. Although it is often done, there may be little advantage in sitting the patient to aid spread to the thoracic ganglia (Hardy & Wells 1987, Hogan et al. 1992).

Other approaches: lateral and posterior approaches have a much higher incidence of complications, including epidural and intrathecal injection, and should only be used when the anterior approach is difficult because of anatomical distortion. Ultrasound-guided techniques are being used increasingly and are claimed to reduce complications (Narouze et al. 2007).

Choice of solution

Lidocaine 1% is suitable for a diagnostic block, but bupivacaine 0.25% or 0.5% is preferred for other indications; 10 ml should produce sympathetic block of the head, as evidenced by the development of a Horner's syndrome. However, this does not guarantee sympathetic block of the arm, this requiring spread to T_2 & T_3, an injection volume of 15 ml, and confirmation of effect by demonstrating an increase in skin temperature of at least 2°C. Continuous infusion has been described using the technique described previously to insert an epidural catheter, and infusion of bupivacaine 0.25% at up to 8 ml h^{-1} to maintain sympathetic block in the arm (Owen-Falkenberg & Olsen 1992).

Only 1 ml of solution should be used for diagnostic or prognostic blocks to better predict the response to destruction by radiofrequency ablation or phenol. Using a larger volume can confuse the outcome and prognosis of the block because it may also affect somatic and visceral afferent nerves.

Neurolytic stellate ganglion block is potentially very hazardous and should be performed only by an experienced practitioner. If the technique is used only a very small volume (less than 1 ml) containing radio-opaque medium should be injected under X-ray control to ensure that surrounding structures are not damaged (Racz & Holubec 1989). A technique for producing radiofrequency lesions has been described (Geurts & Stolker 1993), but transthoracic endoscopic techniques are safer and more predictable.

Complications

Systemic toxicity: the stellate ganglion is closely related to several major blood vessels, particularly the vertebral artery. Intra-arterial injection of even a minute dose of local anaesthetic will produce immediate signs of central toxicity (convulsions) because the drug is delivered directly to the brain.

Vaso-vagal reactions: these are readily triggered from the neck and should be distinguished from local anaesthetic toxicity. The patient becomes anxious, pale, sweaty, and nauseated, with bradycardia and hypotension. Withdrawal of the needle and elevation of the legs is usually sufficient treatment.

Horner's syndrome: unilateral miosis, ptosis, enophthalmos, and anhidrosis are inevitable results of successful stellate ganglion block, and the patient must be warned of this beforehand. Vasodilatation of the conjunctiva and tympanic membrane, and unilateral nasal congestion demonstrated by a 'stuffy' nose (Guttmann's sign) may also occur. No special treatment is required, although the miosis may be reversed with 10% phenylephrine drops.

Other nerve block: if the injection is in the wrong tissue plane, the local anaesthetic may affect the roots of the brachial plexus. No treatment is required, but the block may lead to diagnostic and prognostic confusion. Phrenic nerve block will occur if the solution is injected too far anteriorly, and only causes problems in those with severe respiratory disease who are dependent on diaphragmatic function. Spinal or epidural injection will cause significant problems and may occur if the needle passes between the transverse processes of the adjacent vertebrae. Local anaesthetic solution may also spread to the recurrent laryngeal nerve and cause hoarseness, and also to the contralateral ganglion and cause bilateral Horner's syndrome (Wallace & Milholland 1993). The patient should be warned of these possible complications.

Tissue damage: the dome of the pleura rises above the first rib and is closely related to the ganglion so there is a risk of pneumothorax if the needle is inserted caudally. The oesophagus may also be damaged by a misplaced needle, and intercostal neuralgia, presenting as severe chest wall pain, has been described after stellate ganglion block (McCallum & Glynn 1986).

Bilateral stellate blocks should never be performed because of the risk of pneumothorax, phrenic nerve block and recurrent laryngeal nerve palsy.

Thoracic sympathetic block

The upper thoracic sympathetic ganglia lie on the heads of the ribs covered by pleura, and the interconnecting chain is just anterior to the somatic nerves. The lower two or three ganglia are on the sides of the vertebral bodies, but the close relationship between somatic nerves and sympathetic chain for most of its thoracic course means that injections are likely to spread to affect both. The risk of other complications (e.g. pneumothorax, subarachnoid injection, somatic nerve needle injury) is also high. Thus when thoracic sympathetic ablation is indicated (e.g. for hyperhidrosis) an endoscopic surgical procedure is used (Byrne et al. 1990, Gordon & Collin 1994) and the reader is referred elsewhere for a description of the block technique (Breivik & Cousins 2009).

An alternative for producing unilateral sympathetic block of the arm is interpleural injection (see Chapter 16), Reiestad and colleagues (1989) describing daily injections of 3 ml bupivacaine 0.5% with adrenaline through an indwelling catheter. Finally, a thoracic epidural infusion can be used to produce sympathetic as well as somatic block.

Splanchnic nerve block

Anatomy

The greater, lesser, and least splanchnic nerves sweep forward across the side of the body of T_{12} to pierce the diaphragm and form the coeliac plexus (Figure 23.3). The pleura, lying lateral to the nerves, is attached posteriorly to the vertebral bodies and creates a well-defined compartment (Boas 1983).

Technique

With the patient prone, and under image intensifier control, the lateral end of the transverse process of L_1 is identified. The needle is inserted just lateral to this, and directed to pass beneath the twelfth rib on to the side of the body of T_{12}. The needle is manoeuvred, in the lateral view, until the tip is just posterior to the anterior edge of the T_{12} vertebra. Injection of contrast should show that the spread is limited antero-inferiorly by the crus of the diaphragm, and posteriorly by the attachment of the pleura to the vertebrae.

Choice of solution

Up to 15 ml of either bupivacaine 0.5% or phenol 6% can be injected using constant radiographic monitoring. Volumes as small as 3 ml have been used.

Complications

A *pneumothorax* may be produced if the needle is not kept close to the side of the body of T_{12}, and both intrathecal and epidural injection may occur.

Coeliac plexus block

Anatomy

The coeliac plexus, the largest of the prevertebral plexuses, is formed by the union of the greater (T_5–T_{10}), lesser (T_{10}–T_{11}) and least (T_{12}) splanchnic nerves with the coeliac branch of the right vagus so contains both sympathetic and parasympathetic fibres.

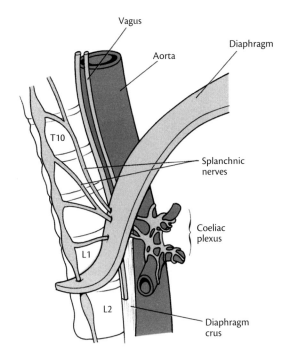

Figure 23.3 Position of the splanchnic nerves and coeliac plexus. Note that the latter lies more anterior than the sympathetic chain.

There are usually two semilunar-shaped ganglia lying in the retro-peritoneal tissue at the T_{12}–L_1 level (Figure 23.4) between the suprarenal glands, posterior to the stomach, pancreas, and the left renal vein, anterior to the crura of the diaphragm, and mainly ante-rolateral to the aorta. The kidneys are in close relationship. The ganglia surround the origin of the coeliac and superior mesenteric arteries and bilateral spread of the solution is necessary to ensure complete block.

In the classic retrocrural technique, first described by Kappis in 1919, two needles are positioned posterior to the crura of the diaphragm, but this may only block the splanchnic nerves. The needle must penetrate the diaphragm and lie 1–2 cm anterior to the vertebral body to be certain of reaching the whole of the plexus. This is easier on the right side, but the needle is likely to encounter the aorta on the left. A combined approach has been described involving a right transcrural injection and a left retrocrural injec-tion (Brown & Moore 1988).

Technique

With the patient prone the spinous process and transverse proc-esses of the first lumbar vertebra are identified using the image intensifier, and a point is marked 6–7 cm lateral to the spine making sure that it is inferior to the transverse processes and the twelfth rib (Figure 23.5). The skin and deeper tissues are infiltrated with local anaesthetic before a 15-cm, 20-g needle is inserted at the marked point and directed towards the side of the body of L_1 (Figure 23.6). The needle is likely to damage the kidney if the inser-tion point is more than 7.5 cm lateral to the spine (Moore et al. 1981). The needle is advanced slightly cephalad and at about 60° to the coronal plane.

Once contact has been made with the vertebral body the needle is guided anteriorly, monitored in the lateral view. The needle tip should be kept close to the vertebral body until it lies at the anterior edge of the body. A second needle is inserted on the opposite side. The coeliac plexus lies more anterior than the sympathetic chain so

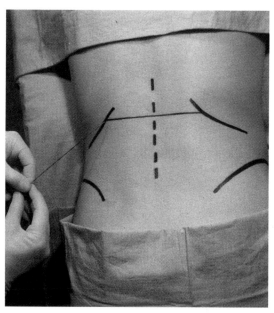

Figure 23.5 Landmarks and needle alignment (supine patient viewed from above) for coeliac plexus block. The posterior spines of T_{11}–L_4 have been marked.

the right needle should be advanced to lie about 1–2 cm anterior to the vertebral body, the left a little less because of the presence of the aorta. An anteroposterior X-ray view at this stage should show the needle points situated medial to the lateral edge of the L_1 vertebra and clearly anterior to the vertebral body (Figure 23.7). Injection of contrast solution should demonstrate spread in the longitudinal axis without any lateral or posterior extension. Careful aspiration tests should precede the injection, which should be very easy; resistance suggests that the needle tip lies in the wrong place. A small volume of local anaesthetic should be injected before the alcohol because the latter can produce consid-erable discomfort.

A single-needle, transaortic approach has been described by Ischia and colleagues (1983). The needle is inserted on the left side and positioned to ensure that its point is in the middle of the coe-liac plexus. In a modified version of this technique, the needle is inserted as for the standard approach and advanced until a charac-teristic 'click' and aspiration of blood confirm that the tip is in the

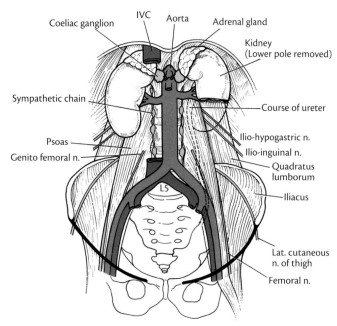

Figure 23.4 Posterior abdominal wall to show the position and relations of the coeliac plexus and lumbar sympathetic chain.

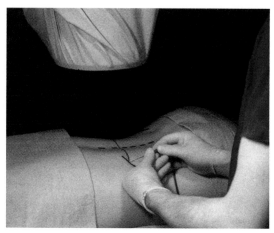

Figure 23.6 Needle inserted for coeliac plexus block.

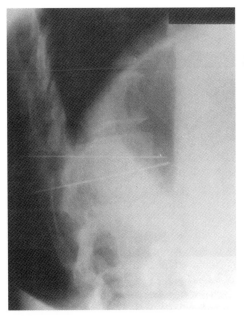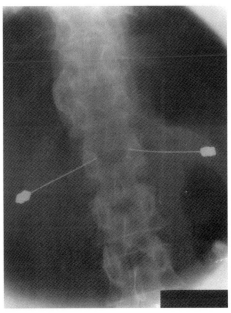

Figure 23.7 Correct needle positions for bilateral coeliac plexus block. Note that the needle tip is clearly anterior to the body of the vertebra.

aorta. The needle is then advanced through the anterior aortic wall. The point must lie in an area of very low resistance to injection, and not in the wall of the aorta. This technique is only recommended if difficulties are encountered when the standard approach is used for a neurolytic plexus block in a patient with cancer.

It is claimed that the use of CT scanning (Figure 23.8) improves the safety and effectiveness of coeliac plexus block (Brown & Moore 1988, Filshie et al. 1983), and a CT-guided, single-needle transaortic approach requiring only 12 ml of neurolytic solution has been described (Lieberman & Waldman 1990). The advantages of percutaneous ultrasonic guidance for both lumbar sympathetic and coeliac plexus block have also been outlined (Kirvela et al. 1992), but the best imaging modality has yet to be determined (Rathmell et al. 2000). Finally, an endoscopic technique has been described (Michaels 2007).

The procedure can be performed in the lateral position if the patient is unable to lie prone, and the single-needle, ultrasound-guided, anterior approach is also an option for such patients. It is claimed that this technique reduces the risk of neurological complications because the needle is never near the spinal cord or spinal arteries (Montero-Matamala et al. 1989).

Choice of solution

Diagnostic and therapeutic local anaesthetic injections may be performed with up to 20 ml of plain bupivacaine 0.25% on each side. Depot preparations of steroid can be added for chronic pancreatitis, although the value of this remains unproven (Kennedy 1983). For a neurolytic block, up to 20 ml of alcohol 50% is injected on each side. Absolute alcohol can be diluted with bupivacaine 0.25%. Repeated aspiration tests must be performed and the dispersion of the contrast solution observed. Brown and Moore (1988) advocate the injection of larger volumes because they claim that standard ones result frequently in incomplete neurolysis and inadequate pain relief. Phenol can be used in smaller volumes of 5–10 ml per side.

Complications

Hypotension is an almost inevitable consequence, and it can persist for many days after a neurolytic block, so coeliac plexus block is contraindicated in hypovolaemic patients. *Diarrhoea* is also a common complication.

Paraplegia has been reported. The needles or neurolytic solution may cause damage to, or spasm of, the spinal blood vessels, particularly the artery of Adamkiewicz, the largest artery supplying the lumbar spinal cord (Davies 1993). Other *neurological sequelae* may follow spread of neurolytic solution to the lumbar somatic nerves, and inadvertent epidural or intrathecal injection may cause paraplegia.

Either the needle or the neurolytic solution may damage other adjacent structures such as the aorta, the coeliac and superior mesenteric arteries, the pleura, the thoracic duct, or the kidneys.

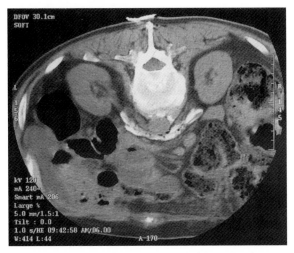

Figure 23.8 CT scan though abdomen at the level of the coeliac plexus. Note the dye lying in the plane *anterior* to the diaphragm.

Finally, *failure of ejaculation* is a significant risk so neurolytic blocks must be avoided in young males or any man unwilling to accept the risk of this side-effect.

Davies (1993) reviewed 2730 neurolytic coeliac plexus blocks and estimated that major complications (paraplegia with or without loss of sphincter function) happened once every 683 blocks. A meta-analysis by Eisenberg and colleagues (1995) reported local pain in 96%, diarrhoea in 44%, hypotension in 38%, and major neurological complications such as weakness or paraesthesia in 1% of patients.

After neurolysis, new pain syndromes may develop. *Post-sympathectomy neuralgia* is a poorly understood condition occurring in up to 20% of patients and explained as a complex neuropathic, central reafferentation and deafferentation syndrome (Nelson & Stacey 2006). Additional features, such as compensatory hyperhidrosis and gustatory sweating, may appear (Mailis-Gagnon & Furlan 2008).

Lumbar sympathetic block

Anatomy

The lumbar sympathetic trunk is situated in the retroperitoneal connective tissue anterior to the vertebral bodies and the medial margin of psoas muscle (Figures 23.4 and 23.9). The aorta and the inferior vena cava are anterior relations, the genitofemoral nerve lies laterally on psoas, and the kidney and ureter are posterolateral in position. All the sympathetic fibres pass through or synapse at the L_2 ganglion, so in theory a block at the upper level of L_3 should abolish all the sympathetic supply to the lower limb, but opinions differ over the number of levels which need to be injected to produce optimal lower limb sympathectomy. Boas (1983) reviewed 500 patients and was unable to demonstrate any difference between single (L_2 or L_3), double (L_2 & L_3, or L_3 & L_4) or triple level injections (L_2, L_3 & L_4), although Walsh and colleagues (1984), reporting over 400 cases, claimed that the latter produced the best results. Umeda and colleagues (1987) studied 19 cadavers and concluded that the optimal site was level with either the lower third of the L_2 vertebral body or the upper third of L_3. A single level injection is safer and faster to perform, and the spread of solution can be observed with the image intensifier. If it is insufficient, the injection can be repeated at an adjacent level.

Usually, four pairs of lumbar arteries arise from the aorta and wind around the upper four lumbar vertebral bodies, deep to the sympathetic trunks and under the tendinous arches which give origin to psoas. The arteries are often accompanied by lumbar veins which may form plexiform networks, and all of these vessels are vulnerable to needle penetration.

Technique

The injection can be performed with the patient prone or lateral, but both patient and the various landmarks are more stable in the prone position, and bilateral blocks can be performed more easily. Thus, the lateral position is reserved for the patient who cannot lie prone. The essence of the prone approach is the same for splanchnic, lumbar sympathetic, superior hypogastric, and coeliac plexus injections although the needle lies more anterior for the latter.

The needle can be inserted at any lumbar level, but lower limb blocks (e.g. for peripheral vascular disease) usually target L_3/L_4, and injection at L_1 is indicated for renal pain. Mandl (1947) described the classical approach, which depended upon needle contact with the transverse process to gauge depth. A more lateral approach, designed to avoid the transverse process, was described by Reid and colleagues (1970) and can be used with an image intensifier so that the needle misses this obstacle.

Prone position: the spinous process of L_3 is identified with the image intensifier and a point marked 7–10 cm lateral to it, midway between the transverse processes of L_3 and L_4. It is essential that the transverse process does not obstruct the passage of the needle, otherwise correct placement will be difficult or even impossible. The skin and deeper tissues are infiltrated with local anaesthetic before a 15-cm, 20-g needle is inserted at the point marked and directed towards the side of the body of L_3 (Figure 23.10). The needle should be at approximately 60° to the coronal plane, and some practitioners find it helpful to rotate the image intensifier to 60° as well, so that the needle is inserted along the direction of the X-ray view.

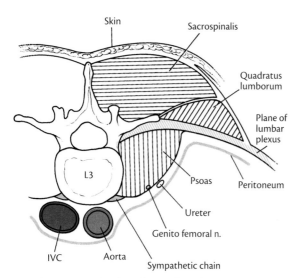

Figure 23.9 Transverse section through L3 to show the position and relations of the lumbar sympathetic chain.

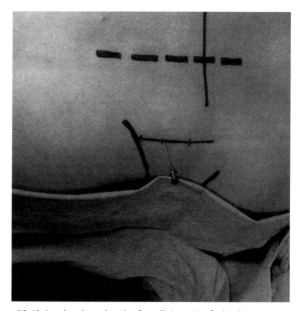

Figure 23.10 Landmarks and angle of needle insertion for lumbar sympathectomy at the level of L3.

Once contact is made with the vertebral body, the needle is manoeuvred anteriorly, monitored in the lateral view. The needle tip should remain close to the vertebra and its final position should be level with the anterior edge of the vertebral body (Figure 23.11). A characteristic 'click' is often felt as the needle passes through the psoas fascia. An anteroposterior X-ray at this stage should show that the needle tip lies midway between the lateral edge of the vertebral body and the spinous process.

Injection of contrast solution should demonstrate linear spread in the longitudinal axis alone without any lateral or posterior extension (Figure 23.11). Injection into psoas muscle produces a characteristic pattern which radiates inferolaterally away from the vertebral body. Occasionally, the contrast medium will be 'whisked' away in a small vessel, even though aspiration tests were negative. If the pattern of spread from the initial level of injection is satisfactory, then all the solution should be injected at that level. If the spread is not entirely satisfactory it may be possible to use a small volume at that level and to repeat the procedure at vertebral levels above or below. The same needle can usually be partially withdrawn, then redirected on to the adjacent vertebra. If difficulty is encountered, a second needle should be inserted at the appropriate level.

For an injection at L_1 the insertion point should not be more than 7.5 cm lateral to the spinous process in order to avoid penetration of the kidney. Insertion should be at the level of the L_1–L_2 interspace with the needle directed slightly cephalad to reach the side of the body of L_1.

Lateral position: very little modification in technique is needed for the lateral position. The major problem is positioning the patient so that the X-rays are truly anteroposterior and lateral.

Continuous block: a catheter can be inserted into the prevertebral area and a continuous sympathetic block maintained by an infusion of local anaesthetic (Betcher et al. 1953). Some authors recommend a prognostic block for up to 5 days as a prerequisite to neurolytic block (Breivik et al. 1997). Such an infusion may be indicated in young patients when there is doubt about the long-term effect of a chemical sympathectomy. CT-guided single-needle

techniques have been described, and some authors claim that they offer advantages (Dondelinger & Kurdziel 1984, Redman et al. 1986).

Choice of solution

A diagnostic block requires a small volume to be placed precisely: 2–5 ml of bupivacaine 0.5% at each level should suffice. For therapeutic injections of local anaesthetic 5–10 ml bupivacaine 0.5% may be given at a single level. Aqueous phenol 6%, or a stronger, dissolved in X-ray contrast medium is used for neurolysis, 2–5 ml usually being satisfactory, although recommendations range from 1–10 ml (Boas 1983, Walsh et al. 1984). The needle should be flushed with local anaesthetic before withdrawal to avoid leaving a track of phenol through the more superficial tissues. Radiofrequency lumbar sympathectomy has been described (Rocco 1995) and Botox A (75 units in 10 ml of bupivacaine) has also been used (Carroll et al. 2009).

Complications

Major complications such as inadvertent injection of phenol into the vertebral canal, the peritoneal cavity, or a blood vessel should not occur with a correct technique performed under radiographic control. Similarly, damage to the kidney, renal pelvis, ureter, and intervertebral discs by the needle or neurolytic solution should also be avoidable. Injury to blood vessels in the posterior abdominal wall is not uncommon, but a significant retroperitoneal haematoma is unlikely in a patient with normal coagulation. However, phenol damage to blood vessels may explain some otherwise unaccountable neurological complications (Clarke 1984).

Mild backache is common and is likely to be more severe if neurolytic solution is deposited inadvertently in the posterior abdominal wall. Destruction of sympathetic fibres may cause a characteristic cramp-like or burning pain and dysaesthesia in the anterior thigh—so-called '*sympathalgia*' (Boas 1983, Kramis et al. 1996)—which may also follow surgical sympathectomy (Tracy & Cockett 1957). *Neuropathic pain* may be caused by spread of phenol to the genitofemoral nerve where it lies on psoas. Occasionally, other somatic nerves may be damaged by the needle or by injected

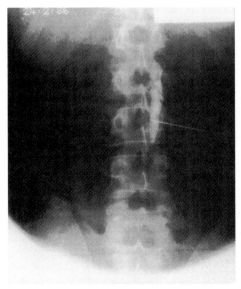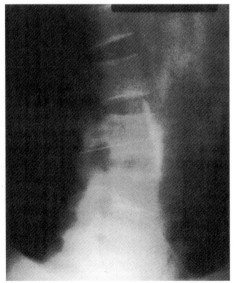

Figure 23.11 Films taken after completion of injection for lumbar sympathectomy. Note how the dye has spread longitudinally from the single injection point.

phenol. Treatment of both sympathalgia and neuritis may include amitriptyline or the gabapentinoids and TENS, but these are not always immediately effective and the patient will need to be reassured that remission should occur over a period of several weeks.

The vasodilatation produced by sympathectomy may result in *hypotension*, especially in the elderly or after bilateral blocks. Blood pressure should be monitored for at least 2 hours after the procedure and the patient supervised during mobilization in case there is postural hypotension. Hypotension usually responds quickly to elevation of the legs so vasopressors or intravenous fluids are required rarely. *Intravascular 'steal'* may occur after sympathectomy in arteriosclerotic patients and result in diversion of blood from compromised distal vessels into the more proximal or less diseased circulation.

Failure of ejaculation is a real risk after bilateral block and this risk must be explained to male patients (Baxter & O'Kafo 1984).

Superior hypogastric plexus block

Anatomy

The superior hypogastric plexus, which innervates pelvic viscera, is situated retroperitoneally in front of the lower third of the fifth lumbar vertebra and the upper third of the first sacral segment.

Technique

The method was described by both Plancarte and colleagues (1990a) and de Leon-Casasola and colleagues (1993). The L_4/L_5 interspace is identified and bilateral needle entry points are marked 5–7 cm lateral to the midline at that level. Using the same general principles as for a lumbar sympathectomy, the two needles are inserted to lie anterolateral to the L_5/S_1 interspace. If blood is aspirated, the recommendation is to advance the needle so that aspiration ceases (de Leon-Casasola et al. 1993). Injected contrast solution should remain anterior to the L_5/S_1 interspace. For a diagnostic block 8–10 ml bupivacaine 0.25% is injected through each needle, and for a neurolytic block 8 ml aqueous phenol on each side.

Waldman and colleagues (1991) described a modified technique using a single needle with CT guidance. An anterior, ultrasound-guided approach is advocated for patients who have difficulty in lying prone because it is a bedside procedure, is less time-consuming, and avoids the radiation exposure involved with a CT-guided anterior approach (Mishra et al. 2008).

Ganglion impar

Two techniques have been described for presacral block of the ganglion impar for intractable perineal pain associated with cancer. The injection may be performed with a bent needle inserted just anterior to the tip of the coccyx and then directed to the front of the sacrococcygeal junction under X-ray guidance (Plancarte et al. 1990b). After a test dose of local anaesthetic, 4–10 ml phenol 6% or 10% can be injected. Alternatively, in a paracoccygeal approach said to be easier, the needle is inserted alongside the coccyx and guided through three discrete steps with a rotating or corkscrew trajectory (Foye & Patel 2009).

Intravenous regional sympathetic blocks

IVRSB, a development of intravenous regional anaesthesia (IVRA), is a simple and relatively inexpensive technique which involves the injection of a drug into an exsanguinated limb isolated from the circulation by a tourniquet. Guanethidine (Hannington-Kiff 1974), the drug most frequently used in the UK, blocks re-uptake of noradrenaline and depletes stores in the postganglionic nerve terminals. Complete repletion takes up to 10 days, but the effect of the block may last much longer. Other drugs which have been used include ketanserin, bretylium, reserpine, labetalol, ketorolac, hydralazine, methyldopa, clonidine, and droperidol. However, the evidence base for IVRSB is weak, and systematic reviews find little objective support for its use (Forouzanfar 2002, Goebel et al 2012).

Technique

The technique is essentially the same as for IVRA, but sedation may be necessary before the tourniquet is inflated and exsanguination performed by elevation rather than compression if the limb is particularly sensitive. Drug injection (see 'Complications' section) may cause burning pain, possibly related to the release of catecholamines by guanethidine. Most practitioners keep the tourniquet inflated for 15–20 minutes, and reactive hyperaemia may follow its release. Blood pressure should be monitored carefully, prolonged hypotension requiring active treatment (Sharpe et al. 1987).

It is not possible to give firm guidelines on the optimal frequency or the total number of blocks if a series is planned, but an interval of 1 week between blocks is usual. There seems to be little point continuing beyond 3–4 blocks if no benefit develops, although some disagree, but if there is only short-term pain relief, it should be used for physiotherapy and exercise.

Choice of solution

Guanethidine 10–20 mg in up to 40 ml of preservative-free prilocaine or lidocaine 0.5% is used for an arm, and 20–30 mg in up to 50 ml for a leg. Bretylium (1–1.5 mg kg^{-1}) is used outside the UK instead of guanethidine.

Complications

Prolonged hypotension, *bradycardia*, and *dizziness* may be very troublesome (Jadad et al. 1995). *Pain on injection* may occur despite the use of prilocaine or lidocaine. Onset may be immediate or it may develop while the tourniquet is inflated. Occasionally, the presenting condition is exacerbated and the patient returns the next day with a painful, red, swollen hand or foot. In this case the block should not be repeated.

Key references

Binder A, Baron R (2009) Complex regional pain syndrome, including applications of neural blockade. In Cousins MJ, Carr DB, Horlocker TT, Bridenbaugh PO (Eds) *Neural blockade*, 4th edn, pp. 1154–68. Philadelphia, PA: Wolters Kluwer, Lippincott-Williams & Wilkins.

Breivik H, Cousins MJ (2009) Sympathetic neural blockade of upper and lower extremity. In Cousins MJ, Carr DB, Horlocker TT, Bridenbaugh PO (Eds) *Neural blockade*, 4th edn, pp. 848–85. Philadelphia, PA: Wolters Kluwer, Lippincott-Williams & Wilkins.

Forouzanfar T, Koke AJ, van KM, et al. (2002) Treatment of complex regional pain syndrome type I. *European Journal of Pain* 6: 105–22.

Harden RN, Bruehl S, Stanton-Hicks M, et al. (2007) Proposed new diagnostic criteria for complex regional pain syndrome. *Pain Medicine* 8: 326–31.

On-line resource

http://pdver.atcomputing.nl/english.html Evidence Based Guidelines CRPS type 1.

References

Ali NMK (1995) Does sympathetic ganglionic block prevent postherpetic neuralgia? *Regional Analgesia* 20: 227–33.

Arner S (1991) Intravenous phentolamine test: diagnostic and prognostic use in reflex sympathetic dystrophy. *Pain* 46: 17–22.

Baxter AD, O'Kafo BA (1984) Ejaculatory failure after chemical sympathectomy. *Anesthesia & Analgesia* 63: 770–1.

Betcher AM, Bean G, Casten DF (1953) Continuous procaine block of paravertebral sympathetic ganglions: observations on one hundred patients. *Journal of the American Medical Association* 151: 288–92.

Binder A, Baron R (2009) Complex regional pain syndrome, including applications of neural blockade. In Cousins MJ, Carr DB, Horlocker TT, Bridenbaugh PO (Eds) *Neural blockade*, 4th edn, pp. 1154–68. Philadelphia, PA: Wolters Kluwer, Lippincott-Williams & Wilkins.

Birklein F, Schmelz M, Schifter S, et al. (2001) The important role of neuropeptides in complex regional pain syndrome. *Neurology* 57: 2179–84.

Blanchard J, Ramamurthy S, Walsh N, et al. (1990) Intravenous regional sympatholysis: a double blind comparison of guanethidine, reserpine, and normal saline. *Journal of Pain and Symptom Management* 5: 357–61.

Boas RA (1983) The sympathetic nervous system and pain. In Swerdlow M (Ed) *Relief of intractable pain*, pp. 215–37. Amsterdam: Elsevier.

Boas RA (1998) Sympathetic nerve blocks: in search of a role. *Regional Anesthesia and Pain Medicine* 23: 292–305.

Breivik H (1997) Chronic pain and the sympathetic nervous system. *Acta Anaesthesiologica Scandinavica Supplementum* 110: 131–4.

Breivik H, Cousins MJ (2009) Sympathetic neural blockade of upper and lower extremity. In Cousins MJ, Carr DB, Horlocker TT, Bridenbaugh PO (Eds) *Neural blockade*, 4th edn, pp. 848–85. Philadelphia, PA: Wolters Kluwer, Lippincott-Williams & Wilkins.

Bristow A, Foster JMG (1988) Lumbar sympathectomy in the management of rectal tenesmoid pain. *Annals of the Royal College of Surgeons of England* 70: 38–9.

Brown DL, Moore DC (1988) The use of neurolytic celiac plexus block for pancreatic cancer: anatomy and technique. *Journal of Pain and Symptom Management* 3: 206–9.

Brown DL, Bulley CK, Quiel EL (1987) Neurolytic celiac plexus block for pancreatic cancer pain. *Anesthesia and Analgesia* 66: 869–73.

Byrne J, Walsh TN, Hederman WP (1990) Endoscopic transthoracic electrocautery of the sympathetic chain for palmar and axillary hyperhidrosis. *British Journal of Surgery* 77: 1040–9.

Cacchio A, De BE, Necozione S, et al. (2009) Mirror therapy for chronic complex regional pain syndrome type 1 and stroke. *New England Journal of Medicine* 361: 634–6.

Carroll I, Clark JD, Mackey S (2009) Sympathetic block with botulinum toxin to treat complex regional pain syndrome. *Annals of Neurology* 65: 348–51.

Casale R, Glynn C, Buonocore M (1992) The role of ischaemia in the analgesia which follows Bier's block technique. *Pain* 50: 169–75.

Charlton JE (1990) Reflex sympathetic dystrophy: non-invasive methods of treatment. In Stanton-Hicks M, Janig W, Boas RA (Eds) *Reflex sympathetic dystrophy*, pp. 151–164. Boston, MA: Kluwer.

Chester M, Hammond C, Leach A (2000) Long-term benefits of stellate ganglion block in severe chronic refractory angina. *Pain* 87: 103–5.

Clarke IMC (1984) Nerve blocks. *Clinics in Oncology* 3: 181–193.

Cossins L, Okell RW, Cameron H, et al. (submitted) Treatment of complex regional pain syndrome in adults: A systematic review of randomised controlled trials published June 2000 until April 2010.

Davies DD (1993) Incidence of major complications of neurolytic coeliac plexus block. *Journal of the Royal Society of Medicine* 86: 264–6.

de Leon-Casasola OA, Kent E, Lema MJ (1993) Neurolytic superior hypogastric plexus block for chronic pelvic pain associated with cancer. *Pain* 54: 145–51.

de Leon-Casasola OA (2008) Neurolysis of the sympathetic axis for cancer pain management. In Benzon HT (Ed) *Raj's Practical Management of Pain*, 4th edn, pp. 683–8. Philadelphia, PA: Mosby Elsevier.

Dondelinger R, Kurdziel JC (1984) Percutaneous phenol neurolysis of the lumbar sympathetic chain with computed tomography control. *Annals of Radiology* 27: 376–9.

Drummond PD, Finch PM, Smythe GA (1991) Reflex sympathetic dystrophy: the significance of differing plasma catecholamine concentrations in affected and unaffected limbs. *Brain* 114: 2025–36.

Eisenberg E, Carr DB, Chalmers TC (1995) Neurolytic celiac plexus block for treatment of cancer pain: a meta-analysis. *Anesthesia & Analgesia* 80: 290–5.

Elias M (2000) Cervical sympathetic and stellate ganglion blocks. *Pain Physician* 3: 294–304.

Filshie J, Golding S, Robbie DS (1983) Unilateral computerised tomography guided coeliac plexus block: a technique for pain relief. *Anaesthesia* 38: 498–503.

Forouzanfar T, Koke AJ, van KM, et al. (2002) Treatment of complex regional pain syndrome type I. *European Journal of Pain* 6: 105–22.

Foye PM, Patel SI (2009) Paracoccygeal corkscrew approach to ganglion impar injections for tailbone pain. *Pain Practice* 9: 317–21.

Geurts JWM, Stolker RJ (1993) Percutaneous radiofrequency lesion of the stellate ganglion in the treatment of pain in upper extremity reflex sympathetic dystrophy. *The Pain Clinic* 6: 17–25.

Gleim M, Maier C, Melchert U (1995) Lumbar neurolytic sympathetic blockades provide immediate and long-lasting improvement of painless walking distance and muscle metabolism in patients with severe peripheral vascular disease. *Journal of Pain and Symptom Management* 10: 98–104.

Goebel A, Vogel H, Caneris O, et al. (2005) Immune responses to Campylobacter and serum autoantibodies in patients with complex regional pain syndrome. *Journal of Neuroimmunology* 162: 184–9.

Goebel A, Baranowski AP, Maurer K, et al. (2010) Intravenous immunoglobulin treatment of complex regional pain syndrome: A randomized trial. *Annals of Internal Medicine* 152: 152–8.

Goebel A, Barker CH, Turner-Stokes L, et al. (2012) Complex regional pain syndrome in adults: UK guidelines for diagnosis, referral and management in primary and secondary care. London: RCP

Gordon A, Collin J (1994) Thoracoscopic sympathectomy. *European Journal of Vascular Surgery* 8: 247–8.

Gordon A, Zechmeister K, Collin J (1994) The role of sympathectomy in current surgical practice. *European Journal of Vascular Surgery* 8: 129–37.

Gress F, Schmitt C, Sherman S, et al. (2001) Endoscopic ultrasound-guided celiac plexus block for managing abdominal pain associated with chronic pancreatitis: a prospective single center experience. *American Journal of Gastroenterology* 96: 409–16.

Groeneweg G, Huygen FJ, Niehof SP, et al. (2008) Effect of tadalafil on blood flow, pain, and function in chronic cold complex regional pain syndrome: a randomized controlled trial. *BMC Musculoskeletal Disorders* 9: 143.

Hamid SK, Scott NB, Sutcliffe NP, et al. (1992) Continuous coeliac plexus blockade plus intermittent wound infiltration with bupivacaine following upper abdominal surgery: a double-blind randomised study. *Acta Anaesthesiologica Scandinavica* 36: 534–9.

Hannington-Kiff JG (1974) Intravenous regional sympathetic block with guanethidine. *Lancet* i: 1019–20.

Harden RN, Bruehl S, Stanton-Hicks M, et al. (2007) Proposed new diagnostic criteria for complex regional pain syndrome. *Pain Medicine* 8: 326–31.

Hardy PAJ, Wells JCD (1987) Stellate ganglion blockade with bupivacaine: effect of volume on extent of sympathetic blockade. *British Journal of Anaesthesia* 59: 933P–934P.

Hogan QH (1993) The sympathetic nervous system in post-herpetic pain. *Regional Anesthesia* 18: 271–3.

Hogan QH, Erickson SJ, Haddox JD, Abram SE (1992) The spread of solutions during stellate ganglion block. *Regional Anesthesia* 17: 78–83.

Huygen FJ, De Bruijn AG, De Bruin MT, et al. (2002) Evidence for local inflammation in complex regional pain syndrome type 1. *Mediators of Inflammation* 11: 47–51.

Ischia S, Luzzani A, Ischia A, Faggion S (1983) A new approach to the neurolytic celiac plexus block: the transaortic technique. *Pain* 16: 333–41.

Jadad AR, Carroll D, Glynn CJ, et al. (1995) Intravenous regional sympathetic blockade for pain relief in reflex sympathetic dystrophy: a systematic review and a randomized, double-blind crossover study. *Journal of Pain Symptom Management* 10: 13–20.

Kennedy SF (1983) Celiac plexus steroids for acute pancreatitis. *Regional Anesthesia* 8: 39–40.

Kirvela O, Svedstrom E, Lundblom N (1992) Ultrasonic guidance of lumbar sympathetic and coeliac plexus block. A new technique. *Regional Anesthesia* 17: 43–6.

Kohr D, Tschernatsch M, Schmitz K, et al. (2009) Autoantibodies in complex regional pain syndrome bind to a differentiation-dependent neuronal surface autoantigen. *Pain* 143: 246–51.

Kramis RC, Roberts WJ, Gillette RG (1996) Post-sympathectomy neuralgia: hypothesis on peripheral and central mechanisms. *Pain* 64: 1–9.

Lieberman R, Waldman SD (1990) Celiac plexus neurolysis with the modified transaortic approach. *Radiology* 175: 274–6.

Mailis-Gagnon A, Furlan AD (2008) Sympathectomy for neuropathic pain. The Cochrane Database of Systematic Reviews. *The Cochrane Library, The Cochrane Collaboration, 2008* Vol 2. Updated Oct 14. Issue 1. Art. No.: CD002918. DOI: 10.1002/14651858.CD002918.

Maihofner C, Handwerker HO, Neundorfer B, et al. (2004) Cortical reorganization during recovery from complex regional pain syndrome. *Neurology* 63: 693–701.

Malmqvist L-A, Bengtsson M, Bjornsson G, et al. (1987) Sympathetic activity and haemodynamic variables during spinal analgesia in man. *Acta Anaesthesiologica Scandinavica* 31: 467–73.

Mandl F (1947) *Paravertebral Block*. London: Heinemann.

Manjunath PS, Jayalakshmi TS, Dureja GP, et al. (2008) Management of lower limb complex regional pain syndrome type 1: an evaluation of percutaneous radiofrequency thermal lumbar sympathectomy versus phenol lumbar sympathetic neurolysis—a pilot study. *Anesthesia & Analgesia* 106: 647–9.

Manriquez RG, Pallares V (1978) Continuous brachial plexus block for prolonged sympathectomy and control of pain. *Anesthesia & Analgesia* 57: 128–30.

Mashiah A, Soroker D, Pasik S, Mashiah T (1995) Phenol lumbar sympathetic block in diabetic lower limb ischemia. *European Journal of Cardiovascular Prevention & Rehabilitation* 467–70.

McCabe CS, Haigh RC, Ring EF, et al. (2003) A controlled pilot study of the utility of mirror visual feedback in the treatment of complex regional pain syndrome (type 1). *Rheumatology (Oxford)* 42: 97–101.

McCallum MID, Glynn CJ (1986) Intercostal neuralgia following stellate ganglion block. *Anaesthesia* 41: 850–2.

McLachlan EM, Janig W, Devor M, Michaelis M (1993) Peripheral nerve injury triggers noradrenergic sprouting within dorsal root ganglia. *Nature* 363: 543–6.

Meier PM, Zurakowski D, Berde CB, et al. (2009) Lumbar sympathetic blockade in children with complex regional pain syndromes: a double blind placebo-controlled crossover trial. *Anesthesiology* 111: 372–80.

Mercadante S (1993) Celiac plexus block versus analgesics in pancreatic cancer pain. *Pain* 52: 182–92.

Merskey H, Bogduk N (Eds) (1994) Classification of chronic pain, 2nd edn, pp. 40–3. Seattle, WA: IASP Press.

Michaels AJ, Draganov PV (2007) Endoscopic ultrasonography guided celiac plexus neurolysis and celiac plexus block in the management of pain due to pancreatic cancer and chronic pancreatitis. *World Journal of Gastroenterology* 13: 3575–80.

Mishra S, Bhatnagar S, Gupta D, Thulkar S (2008) Anterior ultrasound-guided superior hypogastric plexus neurolysis in pelvic cancer pain. *Anaesthesia and Intensive Care* 36: 732–5.

Montero-Matamala AM, Lopez FV, Sanchez JLA, Bach LD (1989) Percutaneous anterior approach to the coeliac plexus using ultrasound. *British Journal of Anaesthesia* 62: 637–40.

Moore DC, Bash WH, Burnett LL (1981) Celiac plexus block: a roentgenographic, anatomic study of technique and spread of solution in patients and corpses. *Anesthesia & Analgesia* 60: 369–79.

Munts AG, van der Plas AA, Ferrari MD, et al. (2009) Efficacy and safety of a single intrathecal methylprednisolone bolus in chronic complex regional pain syndrome. *European Journal of Pain* 14: 523–8.

Narouze S, Vydyanathan A, Patel N (2007) Ultrasound-guided stellate ganglion block successfully prevented esophageal puncture. *Pain Physician* 10: 747–52.

Nelson DV, Stacey BR (2006) Interventional therapies in the management of complex regional pain syndrome. *Clinical Journal of Pain* 22: 438–42.

Nikolajsen L, Jensen TS (2001) Phantom limb pain. *British Journal of Anaesthesia* 87: 107–16.

Owen-Falkenberg A, Olsen KS (1992) Continuous stellate ganglion blockade for reflex sympathetic dystrophy. *Anesthesia & Analgesia* 75: 1041–2.

Plancarte R, Amescua C, Patt RB, Aldrete JA (1990a) Superior hypogastric plexus block for pelvic cancer pain. *Anesthesiology* 73: 236–9.

Plancarte R, Amescua C, Patt RB, et al. (1990b) Presacral blockade of the ganglion of Walther (ganglion impar). *Anesthesiology* 73: A751.

Price DD, Long S, Wilsey B, et al. (1998) Analysis of peak magnitude and duration of analgesia produced by local anesthetics injected into sympathetic ganglia of complex regional pain syndrome patients. *Clinical Journal of Pain* 14: 216–26.

Purcell-Jones G, Justins DM (1988) Delayed contralateral sympathetic blockade following chemical sympathectomy – a case history. *Pain* 34: 61–4.

Racz GB, Holubec JT (1989) Stellate ganglion neurolysis. In Racz GB (Ed) *Techniques of neurolysis*, pp. 133–44. Boston, MA: Kluwer.

Raja SN, Treede R-D, Davis KD, Campbell JN (1991) Systemic alpha-adrenergic blockade with phentolamine: a diagnostic test for sympathetically maintained pain. *Anesthesiology* 74: 691–8.

Rathmell JP, Gallant JM, Brown DL (2000) Computed tomography and the anatomy of celiac plexus block. *Regional Anesthesia and Pain Management* 25: 411–16.

Redman DRO, Robinson PN, Al-Kutoubi MA (1986) Computerized tomography guided lumbar sympathectomy. *Anaesthesia* 41: 39–41.

Reid W, Watt JK, Gray TG (1970) Phenol injection of the sympathetic chain. *British Journal of Surgery* 57: 45–50.

Reiestad F, McIlvaine WB, Kvalheim L, et al. (1989) Interpleural analgesia in treatment of upper extremity reflex sympathetic dystrophy. *Anesthesia & Analgesia* 69: 671–3.

Rocco AG (1995) Radiofrequency lumbar sympatholysis. The evolution of a technique for managing sympathetically maintained pain. *Regional Anesthesia* 20: 3–12.

Rodriguez RF, Bravo LE, Tovar MA, et al. (2006) Study of the analgesic efficacy of stellate ganglion blockade in the management of the complex regional pain syndrome in patients with pain mediated by sympathetic nervous system: preliminary study. *Revista de la Sociedad Espanola del Dolor* 4: 230–7.

Schattschneider J, Binder A, Siebrecht D, et al. (2006) Complex regional pain syndromes: the influence of cutaneous and deep somatic sympathetic innervation on pain. *Clinical Journal of Pain* 22: 240–4.

Schott GD (1998) Interrupting the sympathetic outflow in causalgia and reflex sympathetic dystrophy. *British Medical Journal* 316: 792–3.

Schutzer SF, Gossling HR, Connecticut F (1984) The treatment of reflex sympathetic dystrophy syndrome. *Journal of Bone and Joint Surgery* 66A: 625–9.

Serpell M (2008) The role of the sympathetic nervous system and pain. *Anaesthesia & Intensive Care Medicine* 9: 75–8.

Sharpe E, Milaszkiewicz R, Carli F (1987) A case of prolonged hypotension following intravenous guanethidine block. *Anaesthesia* 42: 1081–4.

Sigtermans MJ, Van Hilten JJ, Bauer MC, et al. (2009) Ketamine produces effective and long-term pain relief in patients with complex regional pain syndrome type 1. *Pain* 145: 304–11.

Straube S, Derry S, Moore RA, McQuay HJ (2010) Cervico-thoracic or lumbar sympathectomy for neuropathic pain and complex regional pain syndrome. *Cochrane Database of Systematic Reviews* 7: CD002918. DOI: 10.1002/14651858.CD002918.pub2.

Taskaynatan MA, Ozgul A, Tan AK, et al. (2004) Bier block with methylprednisolone and lidocaine in CRPS type I: a randomized, double-blinded, placebo-controlled study. *Regional Anesthesia & Pain Medicine* 29: 408–12.

Torebjork E, Wahren L, Wallin G, et al. (1995) Noradrenaline-evoked pain in neuralgia. *Pain* 63: 11–20.

Tracy GD, Cockett FB (1957) Pain in the lower limb after sympathectomy. *Lancet* i: 12–14.

Umeda S, Arai T, Hatano Y (1987) Cadaver anatomic analysis of the best site for chemical lumbar sympathectomy. *Anesthesia & Analgesia* 66: 643–6.

Veldman PH, Reynen HM, Arntz IE, et al. (1993) Signs and symptoms of reflex sympathetic dystrophy: prospective study of 829 patients. *Lancet* 342: 1012–16.

Verdugo RJ, Ochoa JL (1994) 'Sympathetically maintained pain.' I. Phentolamine block questions the concept. *Neurology* 44: 1003–10.

Waldman SD, Wilson WL, Kreps RD (1991) Superior hypogastric block using a single needle and computed tomography guidance: description of a modified technique. *Regional Anesthesia* 16: 286–7.

Walker SM, Cousins MJ (1997) Complex regional pain syndromes: including 'reflex sympathetic dystrophy' and 'causalgia'. *Anaesthesia and Intensive Care* 25: 113–25.

Wallace MS, Milholland VS (1993) Contralateral spread of local anesthetic with stellate ganglion block. *Regional Anesthesia*; 18: 55–9.

Walsh JA, Glynn CJ, Cousins MJ, Basedow RW (1984) Blood flow, sympathetic activity and pain relief following lumbar sympathetic blockade or surgical sympathectomy. *Anaesthesia and Intensive Care* 13: 18–24.

Wasner G, Heckmann K, Maier C, et al. (1999) Vascular abnormalities in acute reflex sympathetic dystrophy (CRPS I): complete inhibition of sympathetic nerve activity with recovery. *Archives of Neurology* 56: 613–20.

Wettervik C, Claes G, Drott C, et al. (1995) Endoscopic transthoracic sympathectomy for severe angina. *Lancet* 345: 97–8.

Woolf CJ, Mannion RJ (1999) Neuropathic pain: aetiology, symptoms, mechanisms and management. *Lancet* 353: 1959–64.

Wu CL, Marsh RH, Dworkin RH (2000) The role of sympathetic nerve blocks in herpes zoster and postherpetic neuralgia. *Pain* 87: 121–9.

CHAPTER 24

Regional anaesthesia for day-care surgery

Stuart Grant

Local anaesthesia should be used on as many day patients as possible;
alone, with sedation or with general anaesthesia. It maintains the best balance
between effectiveness and side effects for postoperative analgesia.
If it can be used, use it.

(Rudkin 1997)

The continued growth of day surgery has led to more invasive, more prolonged, and increasingly painful procedures being performed (McGrath et al. 2004). With such large numbers of patients undergoing routine surgery the working practices of day units must be geared to proper selection of suitable patients, efficient management of operating time, and the rapid restoration of the patients to 'street fitness' so that they can be discharged home with the minimum of postoperative morbidity. In well-run units, the unplanned admission of patients to an in-patient bed after surgery should be no more than 2–3% of total activity, and many units manage a lower incidence than this.

A number of factors predict unanticipated admission after day-care surgery, but the common reasons include pain, excessive drowsiness, and postoperative nausea & vomiting (PONV) (Chung & Mezei 1999, Fortier et al. 1998). The ability to discharge patients home and avoid subsequent readmission relies greatly on the appropriate use of regional anaesthesia to minimize these sequelae, either directly or by reducing general anaesthetic and opioid requirements (Chan et al. 2001).

General considerations

Role of regional anaesthesia

Regional anaesthesia is employed increasingly as the main technique because it improves the efficiency of a day surgery unit, decreases unplanned admission rates, and reduces costs (Dexter & Tinker 1995) An unplanned overnight stay in an acute hospital bed can double the cost of a surgical procedure.

Pain control

Ineffectual pain control is often the primary reason for delayed discharge and, because surgeons are performing increasingly complex surgery on a day-stay basis, effective pain management becomes both more important and more difficult to achieve. Regional anaesthesia can provide a quality and intensity of analgesia, especially in the early postoperative period, which is unsurpassed by any other

regimen (Report 1990). Not only is the analgesia of regional anaesthesia superior to that attainable with opioids, but it is also free from their side effects—PONV, sedation, and dysphoria.

Nausea and vomiting

PONV is very common, having an incidence of up to 30% after general anaesthesia (Le et al. 2010), and being strongly related to opioid administration (Roberts et al. 2005); like pain, it is often a major factor in delayed discharge after day surgery (Fortier et al. 1998). Regional anaesthesia is associated with significantly less risk of PONV (McCartney et al. 2004), provided that side effects such as hypotension and bradycardia are avoided, and that the surgical technique is modified to avoid stimulation outside the area of the block. Such stimulation is an important cause of morbidity in procedures such as inguinal hernia repair where traction on the spermatic cord can produce visceral pain resulting in nausea and hypotension despite a fully functional inguinal field block.

Sedation and dysphoria

Whether regional anaesthesia is used as the sole technique, with minimal intravenous sedation or in combination with light general anaesthesia, patients often recover more quickly than with general anaesthesia alone. Opioid requirements are reduced, and there is less sedation, so the patients spend less time in the postanaesthetic recovery area, require nursing care for a shorter period and can mobilize and cooperate with the physiotherapist at an earlier stage (McCartney et al. 2004).

Nursing workload

The demands on nursing time in the early recovery phase after surgery are reduced, allowing staff to concentrate on ensuring that the patients' analgesic and other requirements are properly met.

Discharge time

The combination of decreased pain, minimal PONV, and less post-operative sedation allows for earlier tolerance of both oral intake and mobilization. Significant reductions in the time to discharge have been demonstrated after a variety of procedures (Liu et al. 2005).

Patient preparation

There are no set rules for determining the most appropriate regional technique for a particular surgical procedure and, similarly, the choice of supplement (none, sedation, or light general anaesthesia) is a matter for the particular team involved. However, both patient and surgical team must be consulted carefully about the benefits and risks of the intended approach. Patients have often had many months to build a relationship with their surgeon and therefore surgical support for regional techniques is very influential. With prior supportive discussion from surgical and nursing staff the subsequent consultation with the anaesthetist is usually much more straightforward. Many day-care surgery units have nurse-managed preoperative assessment clinics and, subject to agreed guidelines, suitable regional anaesthetic techniques can also be discussed with the patient at this stage.

Careful discussion of the risks and benefits of regional anaesthesia and, more importantly, written documentation of that discussion are important (Brull et al. 2007, 2008). Careful explanations should be provided of strategies for dealing with failure of the regional anaesthetic, and also of the common side effects. For example, before interscalene brachial plexus block the symptoms of phrenic nerve and recurrent laryngeal nerve palsy are described; before spinal anaesthesia both the risk of postdural puncture headache and its management are outlined, and the possibility of delayed micturition mentioned.

In most circumstances, fasting guidelines should be identical to those for general anaesthesia in the event of the need to convert from regional to general. Inadequate local anaesthesia, an uncooperative patient, surgical complications, and other unforeseen factors may necessitate this so the stomach should be empty preoperatively. Additionally, it is important to discuss the necessity for a patient chaperone to be available during the journey home *and* over the night after surgery (Ip & Chung 2009).

Patients are more amenable to remaining awake during surgery if the prevailing atmosphere within the unit is geared towards the routine use of regional anaesthesia. Explanation and reassurance can begin during the admission process with emphasis on the positive benefits of early recovery, fewer side effects, and that first cup of tea or coffee. Nevertheless, reassurance about appropriate levels of sedation during both block performance and surgery may also be needed to convince most patients that a regional technique is the correct choice.

The patient is entitled to a degree of privacy and dignity while the block is performed, and both warmth and comfortable support for the head and other pressure areas is appreciated. Conversation between members of staff should be limited to matters relating to the patient and the operation. Patients like to be informed about the progress of surgery, and some may need to be distracted with quiet, gentle conversation, but incessant talking soon becomes irritating and does nothing to promote a relaxed atmosphere. With the increasing use of video technology, many patients enjoy the chance to watch the operation, while the surgeon can describe relevant aspects as the operation proceeds.

The planned utilization of the nerve block will guide the dose and concentration of the local anaesthetic to be used. If the block is to be combined with a general anaesthetic the concentration of the local anaesthetic can be reduced appropriately to avoid unnecessary motor paralysis. By reducing the concentration, but maintaining the volume of local anaesthetic injected the total dose is decreased, yet the duration of analgesia is broadly similar (Mulroy et al. 2001). The use of additives to the local anaesthetic solution to prolong analgesia without extensive block is an attractive concept for day surgery, but adrenaline has little impact on the duration of the long-acting drugs and clonidine has limited applicability because of its side effects—bradycardia, hypotension, and sedation (Popping et al. 2009). Similarly, opioids produce little improvement in analgesia compared to long-acting local anaesthetics used alone (Gormley et al. 1996), and their side effects may delay discharge.

Consideration should also be given to the precise point of nerve block, the aim being to minimize the extent of both numbness and muscle weakness. More distal locations (e.g. the wrist rather than the axilla) may provide the analgesia needed, but limit the risk of injury to anaesthetized tissues after discharge and allow maximum use of the limb. It may even be more appropriate to ask the surgeon to administer the required local anaesthetic through the incision, or even to avoid a block altogether if it will interfere with a particular patient's function.

The precise social circumstances need to be assessed particularly carefully when blocks are used in day-stay surgery. Unless high-quality supervision by a responsible adult can be assured absolutely, continuous peripheral block techniques should not be used, and the risks of even single-shot blocks may outweigh the benefits. However, once all factors have been considered patients may be sent home safely with an 'anaesthetized' upper or lower extremity after day surgery (Klein et al. 2002).

Appropriate written information, packs of oral analgesic drugs for patients to take home, and efficient back-up facilities in the event of postoperative complications must be provided to ensure that the full benefits of regional anaesthesia are realized and complications avoided.

Use of regional anaesthesia by surgeons

Although anaesthetists perform the majority of formal local anaesthetic techniques, some of the simpler blocks are suitable for use by surgeons, either as the sole anaesthetic technique or as a supplement to general anaesthesia (Table 24.1). However, all but the most minor techniques carry the risk of systemic toxicity from overdose or inadvertent intravascular injection, so surgeons must be properly trained in the safe use of local anaesthetic drugs and in the recognition and treatment of systemic toxicity if they use these

Table 24.1 Local techniques suitable for use by surgeons

Local Technique	Examples of use
Topical drops, gels and cream	Eye surgery; urology
Wound irrigation; wound edge infiltration	Skin incisions; superficial surgery
Infiltration and field blocks	Breast biopsy/surgery; inguinal hernia
Intra-articular injection	Arthroscopy of knee, elbow, and ankle
Discrete nerve block under direct vision	Spermatic cord; carpel tunnel
Intraorbital blocks	Cataract surgery
Intravenous regional	Forearm (and foot) surgery

techniques without an anaesthetist present. Full resuscitation facilities and patient monitoring equipment must be immediately available, and formal arrangements for an anaesthetist to attend if necessary should be in place.

Regional techniques for day-care surgery

The demands on day-care anaesthesia are increasing as new surgical techniques allow more major cases to be undertaken. Not only the complexity, but also the duration, of surgery is increasing, and it is now considered reasonable to undertake major gynaecological, orthopaedic, and general surgical procedures in this way (White 2000). However, effective and skilfully applied methods of pain management are required if these patients are to recover rapidly and be discharged safely. As a result all possible regional techniques, from the most central (including spinal anaesthesia) to the very peripheral, are now used for this form of surgery although some modification, as noted earlier, may be necessary to restrict the duration and, particularly, the extent of the block to minimize interference with postoperative mobility and safety. For minor surgery, a long-lasting peripheral nerve block can provide all the analgesia necessary, but after more major surgery a balanced multimodal regimen will be required.

Upper limb blocks (Chapter 17)

Intravenous regional anaesthesia

This technique may be considered for minor surgery distal to the elbow if a tourniquet is to be used. It is easy and quick to perform, and ensures rapid return of function. Its main drawback is the lack of residual analgesia, but this can be overcome with a supplementary peripheral block or local infiltration of the wound site by the surgeon prior to tourniquet deflation.

Brachial plexus block

Brachial plexus block is particularly suited to day surgery for upper limb procedures, with supraclavicular, infraclavicular, and axillary techniques all having been used (Gebhard 2005, Neal et al. 2009). However, anxiety about the risk of pneumothorax occurring after discharge has made practitioners reluctant to use the supraclavicular approach for day surgery although the introduction of ultrasound has led to a resurgence in it's popularity. Unfortunately, pneumothorax can still occur, even in the most expert of hands (Bhatia et al. 2010), so it remains a method of doubtful suitability for day surgery.

Shoulder surgery can be particularly painful, and interscalene block can provide significant analgesic benefit (Hadzic et al. 2005), having been used as both anaesthetic technique and analgesic adjunct with either a single injection or catheter technique (Ciccone et al. 2008, Le et al. 2008, Liu et al. 2009, Mariano et al. 2009). With ultrasound guidance lower volumes of local anaesthetic can be used without reducing the effectiveness or duration of block (Renes et al. 2009, Riazi et al. 2008), and this may also reduce the duration of phrenic nerve block.

For more distal surgery careful consideration needs to be given to the location of the incision and the need for a surgical tourniquet in choosing which brachial plexus technique to use, remembering that their likely distributions of block vary considerably (Chapter 17). Surgery can be performed under brachial plexus block with a drug of short duration (or under general anaesthesia),

while a more discrete peripheral nerve block with a long-acting drug is used to provide postoperative analgesia once the surgical anaesthetic has receded.

Distal nerve block for shoulder surgery

Suprascapular nerve block, at the suprascapular notch, can be performed as an isolated technique for shoulder surgery with the advantage of providing partial analgesia without the risk of phrenic palsy. A comparison of this block with both intra-articular local anaesthetic and interscalene block for shoulder arthroscopy found that the latter provided the best quality analgesia, but that suprascapular block is a viable alternative when interscalene injection is contraindicated by respiratory concerns (Singelyn et al. 2004). It should also be noted that due to problems with glenohumeral chondrolysis it is no longer recommended to use intra-articular local anaesthetic techniques for pain after shoulder surgery (Webb & Ghosh 2009). Price (2008) has described a promising technique combining suprascapular and axillary nerve blocks for shoulder surgery.

Lower limb blocks (Chapter 18)

Femoral nerve and fascia iliaca blocks

Both of these techniques can be extremely valuable for the more extensive knee procedures, but careful assessment of the patient's need to walk after discharge is necessary. If the surgery is extensive, and marked postoperative pain is anticipated, a perineural catheter can be placed and the patient discharged home with a continuous infusion provided that proper instruction is provided about potential motor weakness and care with mobilization (Klein et al. 2001, Williams et al. 2003, 2006). If the surgery is not anticipated to be overly painful, a catheter is not indicated or a long-acting nerve block is not deemed appropriate then a medium duration amide such as lidocaine can be used for surgical anaesthesia.

Popliteal nerve block

Foot and ankle surgery produce extreme pain, and its control can be difficult using opioids alone. Popliteal nerve block for day-care surgery usually causes no more disability than the operation itself because most patients have a cast or dressing at least halfway up the calf and they are invariably instructed not to weight bear by the surgeon (Capdevila et al. 2006, di Benedetto et al. 2002, Ilfeld et al. 2002). A single injection technique can last between 14 and 18 hours, but if extended analgesia is required because of particularly painful surgery a catheter technique can be used (Ilfeld et al. 2002).

Saphenous nerve block

A single injection saphenous block can complement a popliteal block for surgery on the medial side of the leg and ankle. The saphenous is a purely sensory nerve, and previous block techniques did not have high success rates, particularly in obese patients, but ultrasound imaging has greatly improved matters (Horn et al. 2009, Redborg et al. 2009).

Ankle block

Ankle block is useful for distal foot surgery because it does not produce the motor block which limits the use of more proximal techniques (Redborg et al. 2009), and thus it preserves the ability to walk unimpeded postoperatively. For most procedures it is only necessary to block the tibial, saphenous, deep and superficial peroneal nerves because the sural nerve territory is rarely involved.

Intra-articular injection for knee surgery

Intra-articular injections of local anaesthetic are often combined with general anaesthesia, but with appropriate local anaesthetic injection at port sites the technique can be used as a regional-only method (Boden et al. 1994).

Blocks in the trunk (Chapter 16)

Blocks of the thoracic nerves have their primary use as adjuncts to general anaesthesia to minimize opioid requirements and subsequent PONV, although thoracic paravertebral block has been used as the sole anaesthetic for breast surgery (Coveney et al. 1998, Pusch et al. 1999, Weltz et al. 1995).

The more distal forms of thoracic nerve (e.g. rectus sheath and transversus abdominis plane) block are also very useful for specific procedures in the day-care setting although they can rarely be used alone because visceral innervation is unaffected. The traditional technique for inguinal hernia repair is block of the ilio-inguinal and iliohypogastric nerves (combined with local infiltration in the awake patient), but an alternative is to use the transversus abdominis plane block. This more proximal injection has two advantages: it blocks the lateral branches of the intercostal nerves, and local anaesthetic solution does not distort the surgical field. The standard technique can be used for a range of lower abdominal surgery, and there is a subcostal version which can be used for the upper abdominal wall (Hebbard 2008).

Central neuraxial block

At one time central blocks were thought to be contraindicated in the day-care setting, but modern evidence supports their carefully controlled use (Liu et al. 2005). However, they have limitations, particularly longer times to ambulation and micturition than general anaesthesia. In addition, the more recent increase in popularity of peripheral nerve blocks has reduced the frequency of use of central techniques. Despite this, they remain very important for selected day-care surgical populations and for patients with contraindications to other techniques.

Caudal block (see Chapters 15 and 22)

Caudal nerve blocks have been used for many years in paediatric day-care practice, and the technique is very useful for lower limb and urogenital procedures. Lower limb weakness and a delay in return of bladder function can prolong time to discharge (Brenner et al. 2010, Menzies et al. 2009, Yao et al. 2009).

Spinal and epidural block

Spinal anaesthesia is quickly performed, has low cost, allows rapid turnover between patients, and provides predictable anaesthesia (Mulroy & Salinas 2005, Nair et al. 2009, Sell et al. 2008). Recovery is reliable, but can be delayed occasionally by slow return of bladder or bowel function. The complications need to be considered carefully prior to use, postdural puncture headache occurring more frequently in day-care patients (up to 2%) than in-patients, although the incidence is less with very fine (27-g) Whitacre needles (Shaikh et al. 2003). Transient neurological symptoms (see Chapter 13) are common after day-care procedures performed in the lithotomy position, but the incidence can be minimized by using local anaesthetics other than lidocaine (Zaric & Pace 2009). Epidural or combined spinal epidural techniques have also been used successfully for day surgery in selected cases (Urmey et al. 1995).

Discharge criteria

Patients who have had day-care surgery under spinal anaesthesia need to meet specific criteria prior to discharge from the day-care unit (see British Association of Day Surgery link in 'On-line resources'). Before allowing ambulation it is important to demonstrate that motor, sensory and sympathetic blocks have regressed. Normal perianal sensation (S_4–S_5), plantar flexion of the foot, and proprioception of the great toe indicate return of normal function (Marshall & Chung 1999).

Urinary retention may complicate an otherwise uneventful recovery from spinal anaesthesia. Risk factors include bupivacaine dose greater than 7 mg, age older than 70 years, history of voiding difficulty, and having hernia, rectal, or urological surgery. Patients unable to void may be catheterized and then asked to return to the day surgical unit the following day for trial without catheter. However, Mulroy and colleagues (2002) have demonstrated that patients can be discharged safely provided that the spinal has regressed and bladder ultrasound has shown that the residual volume is less than 400 ml. If patients are to be discharged prior to voiding they should be instructed to return to the hospital if they have not passed urine within 8 hours of discharge.

Nerve catheter techniques for day surgery

Certain orthopaedic procedures, particularly of the shoulder joint, are suitable for day-care management except that they are followed by severe and prolonged postoperative pain, although this is readily managed with continuous nerve block. Careful selection of both patient and method will allow such catheter techniques to be used safely and successfully after day surgery, some centres having over a decade of experience with this approach (Grant et al. 2001, Klein et al. 2001). The introduction of disposable, pressurized systems for infusing local anaesthetic solutions was an important advance in facilitating the use of these techniques.

The principles of patient assessment, selection of surgical and anaesthetic techniques, and requirements for postoperative care are as outlined already for the use of any regional technique, but with additional emphasis and careful planning at every stage. Of particular importance is the role of the chaperone who must not only be present throughout the period of infusion, but also understand the infusion system, be able to undertake certain manoeuvres (e.g. catheter removal), and recognize the features of complications (e.g. of local anaesthetic toxicity). Extensive written documentation (Table 24.2) should support both patient and chaperone, with photographs or diagrams of the system in use being very helpful. It is clear that continuous techniques can only be used after day surgery when a very high standard of domestic support is available.

The aim of the infusion in these circumstances is *not* to produce total pain relief through nerve block alone because that will result in extensive numbness, significant muscle weakness, systemic local anaesthetic toxicity, or all three. Dilute solutions, at relatively low volume infusion rates, are used such that good pain relief is attained by supplementation with oral analgesics. All involved must recognize that this is the aim, and the patient information document should outline how pain is to be controlled during and after the infusion. Clearly, there must be ready access to an anaesthetist (with knowledge and experience of these techniques) for advice throughout the duration of the infusion although the need for consultation will be minimized by making sure that the patient documentation anticipates all possible anxieties and concerns.

Table 24.2 Sample patient instructions for peripheral nerve catheter care at home

General considerations for caring for a blocked body part
Protect your arm/leg. The blocked extremity may be numb, weak, and difficult for your brain to locate.
Avoid placing hot or cold items on a numb limb. You could cause heat or cold damage to the skin if you are unable to feel the temperature.
Carefully pad your limb. Normally, we continually adjust the position of our bodies because this helps prevent sores and other injuries.
Be careful not to bang or bump the numb body part. This may result in unrecognized injuries and worsen pain when the block wears off.
Elevate the limb. This will help decrease swelling, which will help increase comfort when the block wears off.
You may regain some movement or feeling or experience some breakthrough pain when the initial strong numbing medicine wears off. This is normal.
It is normal to have some leaking at the catheter site.
If the catheter becomes disconnected or if you notice large amounts of drainage, call the on-call anaesthetist at the number provided.

Taking care of your peripheral nerve catheter
Avoid pulling or tugging on the catheter.
Do not shower or get the dressing wet. This could loosen the dressing and dislodge the catheter.
Keep the catheter site dry while sponge bathing.
Avoid pinching or kinking the catheter and tubing.
If the site around the catheter becomes red, painful, or swollen, contact your anaesthetist. These could be signs of infection. You should close the clamp on your catheter and call the on-call anaesthetist at the number provided.

What should I call about?
If you develop any of the following symptoms, you should close the clamp on your catheter and call the on-call anaesthetist at the number provided immediately:
Numb lips
Metallic taste in the mouth
Ringing in the ears
Dizziness
Increased anxiety
Shortness of breath
Sudden unexpected sleepiness
Seizures
Tremors, shakes, twitching
If you are having severe pain in a previously numbed arm/leg and are unable to move your fingers or toes or the fingers/toes are not pink, close the clamp on the catheter and call the surgeon or on-call anaesthetist immediately.

Taking care of your blocked body part
Arm and shoulder blocks:
Ensure that your entire arm is supported, including the wrist. Do not let the wrist dangle over the end of the sling.
Pad and cushion the elbow and wrist.
Leg, knee, and foot blocks:
Do NOT bear any weight on the numb limb until you completely recover the feeling and strength after the block wears off.
Always have assistance getting up and moving about.
Pad the knee, ankle, and heel.

Postoperative care

Normal recovery room discharge criteria should be met, and the ability to walk safely (using crutches or a walking frame if needed) must be checked by the nursing or physiotherapy staff prior to hospital discharge (Muraskin et al. 2007, Williams et al. 2007a) unless the patient is in a wheelchair. The ability to void urine is not essential for discharge after every day-care procedure, but is necessary with urological, gynaecological, and hernia surgery. However, a risk factor for patient injury after day-care surgery is the short trip to the toilet, patients often feeling that such a short 'hop', literally in some cases, can be made without mechanical or human support. Careful explanation is necessary to emphasize that some kind of support will be needed for even the shortest trip. Similar warnings are required for a patient who is discharged in a wheelchair.

Explicit instructions about care of an 'anaesthetized' limb need to be given before discharge. Both heat and cold can cause injury so instructions on the safe use of ice packs and heat pads are vital

for patient safety. There should be a full discussion of postoperative care instructions with both patient *and* chaperone, with these discussions supported by the issue of written instructions (Table 24.2). Time spent before discharge covering the details of common patient worries can greatly reduce the number of subsequent telephone calls to the unit (or other healthcare providers) for advice. The use of co-analgesic drugs along with a nerve block is a common area of questioning, and the provision of a detailed patient information leaflet covering this is invaluable.

A detailed education about what to do when the nerve block wears off is important. Provision should be made for adequate rescue analgesia to be given to the patient before discharge, or a prescription issued to allow the drugs to be collected by the chaperone on the way home (Williams et al. 2007b). The nerve block is only one part of the analgesic regimen, with oral analgesics providing the 'balance' of pain control; opioids, paracetamol, and non-steroidal anti-inflammatory drugs, alone or in combination, are used as appropriate for patient and procedure. Patients should be instructed to start this medication as soon as they feel the block start to regress, or before going to bed, rather than waiting for pain to develop.

Overview

In conclusion, increasingly complex and painful surgical procedures are being performed on a day-care basis, but poor pain control and PONV are common reasons for delayed discharge or in-patient admission. Regional anaesthesia provides a very important component of pain control which, in combination with other techniques of pain relief, allows the successful performance of surgical procedures otherwise impossible with general anaesthesia alone. The use of continuous peripheral nerve blocks at home has further improved pain control, but careful patient selection is essential.

Further reading

Steele S (Ed) (2004) *Ambulatory Anesthesia and Perioperative Analgesia.* New York: McGraw Hill.

Twersky RS, Philip BK (Eds) (2008) *Handbook of Ambulatory Anesthesia,* 2nd edn. New York: Springer.

On-line resources

http://www.ncbi.nlm.nih.gov/pmc/articles/PMC2745079/?tool=pubmed— Regional Anesthesia At Home

http://www.anesthesia-analgesia.org/content/101/6/1663.long—Peripheral Nerve Block Techniques For Ambulatory Surgery

http://www.daysurgeryuk.net/bads/joomla/files/Handbooks/ SpinalAnaesthesia.pdf—British Association of Day Surgery

References

Bhatia A, Lai J, Chan VW, Brull R (2010) Case report: pneumothorax as a complication of the ultrasound-guided supraclavicular approach for brachial plexus block. *Anesthesia & Analgesia* 111: 817–19.

Boden BP, Fassler S, Cooper S, et al. (1994) Analgesic effect of intraarticular morphine, bupivacaine, and morphine/bupivacaine after arthroscopic knee surgery. *Arthroscopy* 10: 104–7.

Brenner L, Kettner SC, Marhofer P, et al. (2010) Caudal anaesthesia under sedation: a prospective analysis of 512 infants and children. *British Journal of Anaesthesia* 104: 751–5.

Brull R, McCartney CJ, Chan VW, El-Beheiry H (2007) Neurological complications after regional anesthesia: contemporary estimates of risk. *Anesthesia & Analgesia* 104: 965–74.

Brull R, McCartney CJ, Chan VW, et al. (2007) Disclosure of risks associated with regional anesthesia: a survey of academic regional anesthesiologists. *Regional Anesthesia and Pain Medicine* 32: 7–11.

Brull R, Wijayatilake DS, Perles A, et al. (2008) Practice patterns related to block selection, nerve localization and risk disclosure: a survey of the American Society of Regional Anesthesia and Pain Medicine. *Regional Anesthesia and Pain Medicine* 33: 395–403.

Capdevila X, Dadure C, Bringuier S, et al. (2006) Effect of patient-controlled perineural analgesia on rehabilitation and pain after ambulatory orthopedic surgery: a multicenter randomized trial. *Anesthesiology* 105: 566–73.

Chan VW, Peng PW, Kaszas Z, et al. (2001) A comparative study of general anesthesia, intravenous regional anesthesia, and axillary block for outpatient hand surgery: clinical outcome and cost analysis. *Anesthesia & Analgesia* 93: 1181–4.

Chung F, Mezei G (1999) Factors contributing to a prolonged stay after ambulatory surgery. *Anesthesia & Analgesia* 89: 1352–9.

Ciccone WJ, Busey TD, Weinstein DM, et al. (2008) Assessment of pain relief provided by interscalene regional block and infusion pump after arthroscopic shoulder surgery. *Arthroscopy* 24: 14–19.

Coveney E, Weltz CR, Greengrass R, et al. (1998) Use of paravertebral block anesthesia in the surgical management of breast cancer: experience in 156 cases. *Annals of Surgery* 227: 496–501.

Dexter F, Tinker JH (1995) Analysis of strategies to decrease postanesthesia care costs. *Anesthesiology* 82: 94–101.

di Benedetto P, Casati A, Bertini L, et al. (2002) Postoperative analgesia with continuous sciatic nerve block after foot surgery: a prospective, randomized comparison between the popliteal and subgluteal approaches. *Anesthesia & Analgesia* 94: 996–1000.

Fortier J, Chung F, Su J (1998) Unanticipated admission after ambulatory surgery—a prospective study. *Canadian Journal of Anaesthesia* 45: 612–19.

Gebhard RE (2005) Outpatient regional anesthesia for upper extremity surgery. *International Anesthesiology Clinics* 43: 177–83.

Gormley WP, Murray JM, Fee JP, Bower S (1996) Effect of the addition of alfentanil to lignocaine during axillary brachial plexus anaesthesia. *British Journal of Anaesthesia* 76: 802–5.

Grant SA, Nielsen KC, Greeengrass RA, et al. (2001) Continuous peripheral nerve block for ambulatory surgery. *Regional Anesthesia and Pain Medicine* 26: 209–14.

Hadzic A, Williams BA, Karaca PE, et al. (2005) For outpatient rotator cuff surgery, nerve block anesthesia provides superior same-day recovery over general anesthesia. *Anesthesiology* 102: 1001–7.

Hebbard P (2008) Subcostal transversus abdominis plane block under ultrasound guidance. *Anesthesia & Analgesia* 106: 674–5; author reply 675.

Horn JL, Pitsch T, Salinas F, Benninger B (2009) Anatomic basis to the ultrasound-guided approach for saphenous nerve blockade. *Regional Anesthesia and Pain Medicine* 34: 486–9.

Ilfeld BM, Morey TE, Enneking FK (2002) Continuous popliteal sciatic nerve block for postoperative pain control at home: a randomized, double-blinded, placebo-controlled study. *Anesthesiology* 97: 959–65.

Ip HY, Chung F (2009) Escort accompanying discharge after ambulatory surgery: a necessity or a luxury? *Current Opinion in Anaesthesiology* 22: 748–54.

Klein SM, Greengrass RA, Grant SA, et al. (2001) Ambulatory surgery for multi-ligament knee reconstruction with continuous dual catheter peripheral nerve blockade. *Canadian Journal of Anaesthesia* 48: 375–8.

Klein SM, Nielsen KC, Greengrass RA, et al. (2002) Ambulatory discharge after long-acting peripheral nerve blockade: 2382 blocks with ropivacaine. *Anesthesia & Analgesia* 94: 65–70.

Le LT, Loland VJ, Mariano ER, et al. (2008) Effects of local anesthetic concentration and dose on continuous interscalene nerve blocks: a dual-center, randomized, observer-masked, controlled study. *Regional Anesthesia and Pain Medicine* 33: 518–25.

Le TP, Gan TJ (2010) Update on the management of postoperative nausea and vomiting and postdischarge nausea and vomiting in ambulatory surgery. *Anesthesiology Clinics* 28: 225–49.

Liu SS, Strodtbeck WM, Richman JM, Wu CL (2005) A comparison of regional versus general anesthesia for ambulatory anesthesia: a meta-analysis of randomized controlled trials. *Anesthesia & Analgesia* 101: 1634–42.

Liu SS, Zayas VM, Gordon MA, et al. (2009) A prospective, randomized, controlled trial comparing ultrasound versus nerve stimulator guidance for interscalene block for ambulatory shoulder surgery for postoperative neurological symptoms. *Anesthesia & Analgesia* 109: 265–71.

Mariano ER, Afra R, Loland VJ, et al. (2009) Continuous interscalene brachial plexus block via an ultrasound-guided posterior approach: a randomized, triple-masked, placebo-controlled study. *Anesthesia & Analgesia* 108: 1688–94.

Marshall SI, Chung F (1999) Discharge criteria and complications after ambulatory surgery. *Anesthesia & Analgesia* 88; 508–17.

McCartney CJ, Brull R, Chan VW, et al. (2004) Early but no long-term benefit of regional compared with general anesthesia for ambulatory hand surgery. *Anesthesiology* 101: 461–7.

McGrath B, Elgendy H, Chung F, et al. (2004) Thirty percent of patients have moderate to severe pain 24 hr after ambulatory surgery: a survey of 5,703 patients. *Canadian Journal of Anaesthesia* 51: 886–91.

Menzies R, Congreve K, Herodes V, et al. (2009) A survey of pediatric caudal extradural anesthesia practice. *Paediatric Anaesthesia* 19: 829–36.

Mulroy MF, Salinas FV (2005) Neuraxial techniques for ambulatory anesthesia. *International Anesthesiology Clinics* 43: 129–41.

Mulroy MF, Larkin KL, Batra MS, et al. (2001) Femoral nerve block with 0.25% or 0.5% bupivacaine improves postoperative analgesia following outpatient arthroscopic anterior cruciate ligament repair. *Regional Anesthesia and Pain Medicine* 26: 24–9.

Mulroy MF, Salinas FV, Larkin KL, Polissar NL (2002) Ambulatory surgery patients may be discharged before voiding after short-acting spinal and epidural analgesia. *Anesthesiology* 97: 315–19.

Muraskin SI, Conrad B, Zheng N, et al. (2007) Falls associated with lower-extremity-nerve blocks: a pilot investigation of mechanisms. *Regional Anesthesia and Pain Medicine* 32: 67–72.

Nair GS, Abrishami A, Lermitte J, Chung F (2009) Systematic review of spinal anaesthesia using bupivacaine for ambulatory knee arthroscopy. *British Journal of Anaesthesia* 10: 307–15.

Neal JM, Gerancher JC, Hebl JR, et al. (2009) Upper extremity regional anesthesia: essentials of our current understanding, 2008. *Regional Anesthesia and Pain Medicine* 34: 134–70.

Pöpping DM, Elia N, Marret E, et al. (2009) Clonidine as an adjuvant to local anesthetics for peripheral nerve and plexus blocks: a meta-analysis of randomized trials. *Anesthesiology* 111: 406–15.

Price DJ (2008) Axillary (circumflex) nerve block used in association with suprascapular nerve block for the control of pain following total shoulder joint replacement. *Regional Anesthesia and Pain Medicine* 33: 280–1.

Pusch F, Freitag H, Weinstabl C, et al. (1999) Single-injection paravertebral block compared to general anaesthesia in breast surgery. *Acta Anaesthesiologica Scandinavica* 43: 770–4.

Redborg KE, Antonakakis JG, Beach ML, et al. (2009) Ultrasound improves the success rate of a tibial nerve block at the ankle. *Regional Anesthesia and Pain Medicine* 34: 256–60.

Renes SH, Rettig HC, Gielen MJ, et al. (2009) Ultrasound-guided low-dose interscalene brachial plexus block reduces the incidence of hemidiaphragmatic paresis. *Regional Anesthesia and Pain Medicine* 34: 498–502.

Report (1990) *Report of the working party on pain after surgery*. London: The Royal College of Surgeons of England and the College of Anaesthetists, p 20.

Riazi S, Carmichael N, Awad I, et al. (2008) Effect of local anaesthetic volume (20 vs 5 ml) on the efficacy and respiratory consequences of ultrasound-guided interscalene brachial plexus block. *British Journal of Anaesthesia* 101: 549–56.

Roberts GW, Bekker TB, Carlsen HH, et al. (2005) Postoperative nausea and vomiting are strongly influenced by postoperative opioid use in a dose-related manner. *Anesthesia & Analgesia* 101: 1343–8.

Rudkin GE (1997) Pain management in the adult day surgery patient. In Millar JM, Rudkin GE, Hitchcock M (Eds) *Practical anaesthesia and analgesia for day surgery*, pp. 89–105. Oxford: Bios Scientific Publishers.

Sell A, Tein T, Pitakänen M (2008) Spinal 2-chloroprocaine: effective dose for ambulatory surgery. *Acta Anaesthesiologica Scandinavica* 52: 695–9.

Shaikh S, Chung F, Imarengiaye C, et al. (2003) Pain, nausea, vomiting and ocular complications delay discharge following ambulatory microdiscectomy. *Canadian Journal of Anaesthesia* 50: 514–18.

Singelyn FJ, Lhotel L, Fabre B (2004) Pain relief after arthroscopic shoulder surgery: a comparison of intraarticular analgesia, suprascapular nerve block, and interscalene brachial plexus block. *Anesthesia & Analgesia* 99: 589–92.

Urmey WF, Stanton J, Peterson M, Sharrock NE (1995) Combined spinal-epidural anesthesia for outpatient surgery. Dose-response characteristics of intrathecal isobaric lidocaine using a 27-gauge Whitacre spinal needle. *Anesthesiology* 83: 528–34.

Webb ST, Ghosh S (2009) Intra-articular bupivacaine: potentially chondrotoxic? *British Journal of Anaesthesia* 102: 439–41.

Weltz CR, Greengrass RA, Lyerly HK (1995) Ambulatory surgical management of breast carcinoma using paravertebral block. *Annals of Surgery* 222: 19–26.

White PF (2000) Ambulatory anesthesia advances into the new millenium. *Anesthesia & Analgesia* 90: 1234–35.

Williams BA, Kentor ML, Vogt MT, et al. (2003) Femoral-sciatic nerve blocks for complex outpatient knee surgery are associated with less postoperative pain before same-day discharge: a review of 1,200 consecutive cases from the period 1996–1999. *Anesthesiology* 98: 1206–13.

Williams BA, Kentor ML, Vogt MT, et al. (2006) Reduction of verbal pain scores after anterior cruciate ligament reconstruction with 2-day continuous femoral nerve block: a randomized clinical trial. *Anesthesiology* 104: 315–27.

Williams BA, Kentor ML, Bottegal MT, et al. (2007a) The incidence of falls at home in patients with perineural femoral catheters: a retrospective summary of a randomized clinical trial. *Anesthesia & Analgesia* 104: 1002.

Williams BA, Bottegal MT, Francis KA, et al. (2007b) Rebound pain scores as a function of femoral nerve block duration after anterior cruciate ligament reconstruction: retrospective analysis of a prospective, randomized clinical trial. *Regional Anesthesia & Pain Medicine* 32: 186–92.

Yao YS, Qian B, Chen BZ, et al. (2009) The optimum concentration of levobupivacaine for intra-operative caudal analgesia in children undergoing inguinal hernia repair at equal volumes of injectate. *Anaesthesia* 64: 23–6.

Zaric D, Pace NL (2009) Transient neurologic symptoms (TNS) following spinal anaesthesia with lidocaine versus other local anaesthetics. *Cochrane Database of Systematic Reviews* 2: CD003006.

CHAPTER 25

Regional anaesthesia in the elderly

Bernadette Veering

The elderly population, particularly those aged 85 and over, continues to increase rapidly in every developed country, leading to a progressive growth in the number of surgical interventions in this age group. Knowledge of age-related changes in anatomy and physiology is important for the selection of an optimal anaesthetic regimen, and regional techniques are chosen frequently in such patients, especially during orthopaedic, genitourinary, gynaecological, cataract, and hernia surgery. However, their use raises some general points which, while not exclusive to the elderly, apply particularly to them.

General considerations

Preservation of consciousness

Advantages

Properly performed regional anaesthesia leaves consciousness unimpaired and minimizes the disorientation and confusion (see later in chapter) which may follow a general anaesthetic. It also allows the patient to act as his or her own monitor and communicate with attendant staff. Thus, a diabetic patient can recognize and report the symptoms of hypoglycaemia, and distress during transurethral resection of the prostate can give early warning that bladder irrigation fluid has entered the circulation. Although some elderly patients are apprehensive about being conscious during surgery, the majority are remarkably phlegmatic about it, and they often appreciate that the presence of intercurrent disease, which is so common in this age group, may increase the risk of general anaesthesia.

Disadvantages

The elderly find it very difficult to lie still on a hard operating table for a long time, and considerable discomfort may develop in those parts of the body not affected by the block. Joints stiffen and bony prominences, being less well covered, are at risk of skin breakdown. Special care should be given to these pressure areas if a regional block has rendered them insensitive or immobile. In addition, deafness, or the mental slowing which accompanies old age, impairs the communication which is so essential during the performance of the block and throughout surgery.

Anatomical changes

Distortion, such as curvature or rotation of the spine, can make central blocks difficult to perform. Intervertebral spaces may be narrowed, ligaments may be calcified, and osteophytes are often present. Limitation of abduction at the shoulder joint may make the axillary approach to the brachial plexus difficult or impossible. At the cellular level, one-third of myelinated fibres have disappeared from peripheral nerves by the age of 90.

Physiological changes

Changes in body composition, hepatic blood flow, and hepatic mass that occur with normal ageing may have an impact on the rate and extent of the systemic absorption, distribution, metabolism, and excretion of local anaesthetics (Sadean & Glass 2003). The increase in body fat with age may result in greater volumes of distribution of lipophilic local anaesthetics. Hepatic blood flow declines with age, so there is decreased clearance of local anaesthetics with a high hepatic extraction ratio such as lidocaine and mepivacaine. There is also a gradual decline in hepatic mass, and consequently, the clearance of local anaesthetics with relatively low hepatic extraction ratios (which are mostly dependent upon metabolizing hepatic enzyme activity) may also decrease with age.

This chapter focuses on the issues relating to the impact of age on the pharmacodynamics and pharmacokinetics of central neural block and peripheral blocks.

Central neural block

Factors which modify central neural block

Changes in anatomy, physiology, and pharmacokinetics may directly or indirectly alter certain aspects of central neural block in elderly patients. Decline in the neuronal population within the spinal cord and in peripheral nerves, deterioration of myelin sheaths and connective tissue barriers, a decrease in the size of nerve fibres, and slowing of conduction velocity, especially in motor nerves, contribute to altered nerve block characteristics after epidural and subarachnoid administration of local anaesthetics (Bromage 1978, Ferrer-Brechner 1986). These factors are accelerated by arteriosclerosis (Bromage 1978). Furthermore, changes occur in the lumbar and thoracic spine; for example, elderly patients often have a dorsal kyphosis and a tendency to flex the hips and knees because of osteoarthritis and cartilage calcification, and the intervertebral foramina are narrowed by sclerosis and calcification. Degenerative disc and joint changes result in distortion and compression of the epidural space; the dura becomes more permeable to local anaesthetics because of a significant increase in the size of the arachnoid villi, and there is an associated reduction in volume and an increase in the specific gravity of cerebrospinal fluid (CSF) (May et al. 1990). All these factors contribute to an increased sensitivity to local anaesthetics.

Advantages of central neural block

Epidural or spinal anaesthesia has advantages compared with general anaesthesia for surgical procedures performed commonly in the elderly. Intraoperative blood loss is reduced in patients undergoing hip replacement surgery, probably due to a reduction in central venous pressure (Macfarlane et al. 2009, Parker et al. 2004). Several studies have shown that when regional anaesthesia is employed, there is a significantly lower incidence of thromboembolic events, and this is associated with lower morbidity and mortality due, probably, to a combination of increased blood flow to the lower extremities, favourable changes in coagulation and fibrinolysis, and inhibition of platelet aggregation (Parker et al. 2004). Catley and colleagues (1985) demonstrated that when regional anaesthesia (either epidural or intercostal nerve block) is used for postoperative pain control, it has a greater margin of safety in terms of respiratory side effects than the continuous intravenous administration of morphine.

Continuous epidural catheter techniques provide safe and excellent postoperative analgesia in elderly patients. In addition, epidural and spinal anaesthesia are associated with a reduction in postoperative negative nitrogen balance and an amelioration of endocrine stress responses to surgery, particularly in operations on the lower abdomen and lower extremities (Kehlet 1989). Data suggest that the cortisol response is increased in elderly patients, whereas other responses may be similar to those of younger patients (Hakanson et al. 1984).

Clinical aspects of epidural anaesthesia

Age influences the spread of local anaesthetic in the epidural space with most investigators finding a slight increase in the extent of analgesic spread with age after administration of a fixed volume of a local anaesthetic agent (Figure 25.1) (Simon et al. 2002, 2004, 2006, Veering et al. 1987, 1992). More specifically, Hirabayashi & Shimizu (1993) found that age was associated with a higher upper level of analgesia after the thoracic epidural administration of a fixed dose.

Increased epidural compliance and decreased epidural resistance (considered to be due to degeneration of fatty tissue within the epidural space), increased residual epidural pressure, and progressive sclerotic closure of the intervertebral foramina with advancing age may all contribute to enhanced spread in the elderly (Bromage 1978, Tsui et al. 2004). The onset time to maximal caudal spread has been reported to decrease with age (Veering et al. 1987, 1992), so surgery in areas innervated by these segments can be started sooner in older than in younger patients. In addition, a more rapid onset and enhanced intensity of motor block have been demonstrated.

Adrenaline can be used as a test for accidental intravascular injection (Tsui et al. 2004), but elderly patients may have a reduced responsiveness to a given dose because the beta-receptor affinity for adrenergic agonists is diminished.

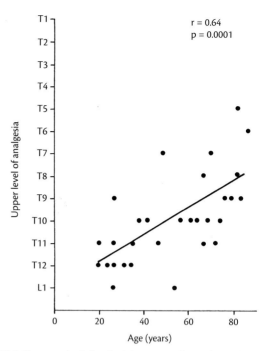

Figure 25.1 The upper level of analgesia increases with age after epidural administration of bupivacaine. (Reproduced with permission from Veering BT, Burm AGL, Van Kleef JW et al, Epidural anaesthesia with bupivacaine: effects of age on neural blockade and pharmacokinetics, *Anesthesia & Analgesia*, 66, 7, pp. 589–94, Wolters Kluwer. Copyright *International Anesthesia Research Society* 1987.)

Lumbar epidural anaesthesia with lidocaine stimulates the ventilatory response to hypercapnoea to the same degree as in young patients (Sakura et al. 1995) and does not affect the resting ventilation parameters such as minute ventilation and tidal volume. It therefore appears to be a safe technique in elderly patients.

Clinical aspects of spinal anaesthesia

Spinal anaesthesia permits the use of small doses of local anaesthetic agents with minimal risk of systemic toxicity. Other advantages of spinal anaesthesia over epidural anaesthesia are a visible indication of successful needle placement, rapid onset, and profound analgesia. Studies on possible correlations between age and onset, duration, and spread of analgesia following subarachnoid administration of a local anaesthetic are confusing because of the variation in the types and doses of local anaesthetic agents used, and the differences in the baricity of the injected solutions (Tsui et al. 2004).

With hyperbaric solutions both the level of analgesia and the onset of motor block increase with age. Injection of hyperbaric bupivacaine at the $L_4–L_5$ instead of the $L_3–L_4$ interspace does not influence the final height of block (Veering et al. 1996). A gradual degeneration of the central and peripheral nervous system, changes in the anatomical configuration of the lumbar and thoracic spine, and, possibly, a reduction of the volume of the CSF may all contribute to the increased spread of analgesia with a hyperbaric solution.

Glucose-free (plain) bupivacaine is slightly hypobaric at body temperature, but the effect of age on the maximal height of analgesia is marginal The complete, profound, long-lasting motor block and the increased duration of analgesia with glucose-free bupivacaine in elderly patients provide satisfactory conditions for orthopaedic procedures in the lower limbs. Glucose-free and hyperbaric bupivacaine solutions result in increased duration of analgesia at the T_{12} dermatome, and this gives more time for operations in the lower abdominal or inguinal region.

Epidural and spinal analgesia with opioids

Intrathecal and epidural opioids are administered in order to prolong postoperative analgesia, and older patients show an increased responsiveness to them (Sadean & Glass 2004). A reduction in the requirements of epidural morphine in older patients has been reported and is thought to be due to relatively high concentrations of morphine in the CSF (Figure 25.2) (Ready et al 1991).

The rationale for combining local anaesthetics with adjuvant drugs is to use lower doses of each agent, and to preserve analgesia with fewer side effects. A reduced dose of hyperbaric bupivacaine (7.5 mg) in combination with sufentanil, or a 'mini-dose' of plain bupivacaine (4 mg) in combination with fentanyl (20 mcg), provided reliable spinal anaesthesia for the repair of hip fracture in aged patients, with few events of hypotension and little need for vasopressor support of blood pressure (Ben-David et al. 2000).

Spinal anaesthesia with bupivacaine in combination with fentanyl decreases pain intensity in the immediate postoperative period and does not alter the mental state of geriatric patients receiving pre- and intraoperative benzodiazepines for sedation (Fernandez-Galinski et al. 1996), but 25 mcg of spinal fentanyl does induce oxygen desaturation and pruritus. On the other hand, in unpremedicated elderly patients, spinal anaesthesia with bupivacaine and 25 mcg fentanyl does not decrease oxygen saturation (Varrassi et al. 1992). Caution should be used when intraspinal opioids are administered to elderly patients and extra vigilance is required to detect unpredictable sedation or respiratory depression.

Pharmacokinetic aspects

Plasma concentrations of local anaesthetics are of clinical importance with respect to their systemic toxicity. These concentrations are dependent upon vascular uptake (absorption) from the extravascular injection site and systemic disposition (distribution

into the bloodstream and elimination from the body). Knowledge of the absorption rate is important, as this affects the duration of the nerve block.

Most data on the effect of age on the pharmacokinetics of lidocaine are available after intravenous administration (Simon & Veering 2010, Tsui et al. 2004). The plasma elimination half-life of lidocaine is prolonged in the elderly, a change secondary to either an increase in the apparent volume of distribution or a decrease in the clearance. The greater percentage of body fat contributes to the greater volume of distribution. After a single epidural dose of lidocaine, the peak plasma concentrations are unaffected by age, but the terminal half-life is prolonged and the clearance is decreased. This may lead to increased accumulation of lidocaine with continuous epidural infusions, or with intermittent bolus doses. In elderly patients the free lidocaine concentration increased during thoracic epidural anaesthesia, so caution should be exercised to avoid such accumulation (Fukada et al. 2003).

In order to evaluate the pharmacokinetics of bupivacaine in the elderly, a stable isotope method has been used (Burm et al 1988). After epidural administration, bupivacaine, levobupivacaine, and ropivacaine show a biphasic absorption profile: a rapid initial phase followed by a much slower phase (Burm 1989, Simon & Veering 2010, Tsui et al. 2004). The initial fast absorption rate is a reflection of the high initial concentration gradient and the vascularity of the epidural space. The slower second absorption phase is believed to be due to slow uptake of local anaesthetics sequestered in the epidural fat.

The systemic absorption of bupivacaine after subarachnoid administration is also biphasic. The initial absorption is much slower than after epidural administration because the subarachnoid space is less well perfused than the epidural space. However, the mean absorption of bupivacaine after subarachnoid administration is shorter in elderly patients because of a faster late absorption rate. In view of this, a shorter duration of spinal anaesthesia might be expected in older patients, but this has not been demonstrated.

The results of absorption studies confirm that elderly patients are more sensitive to both epidural bupivacaine, levobupivacaine, and ropivacaine and subarachnoid bupivacaine. This is more likely to be due to changes in pharmacodynamics than to impairment of vascular absorption. The consequences of reduced clearance of bupivacaine will be most apparent during continuous block when it is probable that plasma concentrations will rise to higher levels, with consequent reduction in the safety margin. Infusion rates and bolus doses may therefore need to be adjusted. This should not necessarily affect the quality of block because of the increased sensitivity to bupivacaine in older patients. Prolonged epidural infusion of racemic bupivacaine in an elderly population showed that unbound plasma concentrations did not increase over time (Veering et al. 2002). Changes in the concentration of free drug are buffered by the high volume of distribution (Simon & Veering 2010).

Because bupivacaine and ropivacaine exhibit a relatively low hepatic extraction ratio, the observed age-related decline in clearance is more likely to be due to a change in the drug-metabolizing hepatic enzyme activity or serum protein binding than to an alteration in liver blood flow. However, age has not been shown to affect the protein binding of bupivacaine, so the decline in clearance is best explained by a decrease in hepatic enzyme activity. Whether this is due to decreased activity of the hepatic enzymes per se or to a reduction in the size of the liver remains to be clarified.

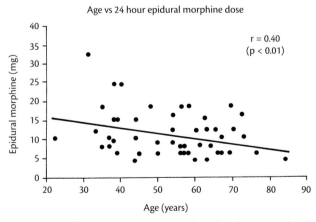

Age vs 24 hour epidural morphine dose

$r = 0.40$
$(p < 0.01)$

Epidural morphine (mg) / Age (years)

Figure 25.2 The effective 24-hour epidural morphine dose decreases with age after abdominal hysterectomy. (Reproduced with permission from Ready LB, Chadwick HS, Ross B, Age predicts effective epidural morphine dose after abdominal hysterectomy, *Anaesthesia & Analgesia*, 66, 12, pp. 1215–18, Wolters Kluwer. Copyright *International Anesthesia Research* Society 1987.)

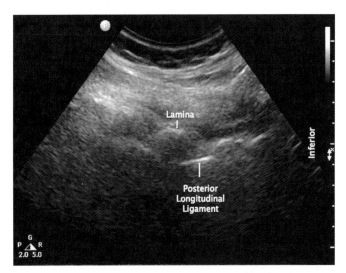

Figure 25.3 Paramedian lumbar sonogram in a 70-year-old female with a significant scoliosis. Compare with Figure 14.4 and note that the laminae, dura, and posterior longitudinal ligaments are readily apparent in the 'young' subject, but the view is far less well defined in the 'elderly' patient.

Olofsen and colleagues (2008) developed a pharmacokinetic/pharmacodynamic model for epidural anaesthesia which may help to explain a part of the variability by introducing to the model covariates such as age, different sites of injection, different local anaesthetics, and variations in dosage. However, this model should be validated for different clinical situations (Simon & Veering 2010).

Disadvantages of central neural block

Technical difficulty

The techniques of spinal and epidural anaesthesia are more difficult in the elderly because of the anatomical changes already described, so there is always a chance of failure. Unfortunately, these anatomical changes also impair the view of the vertebral canal which can be obtained with ultrasound (Figure 25.3).

Postdural puncture headache

This is the most common complication of spinal anaesthesia. Although it is largely related to the size of the needle, the incidence decreases with age, possibly because decreased elasticity of the tissues allows less stretching of the dura mater, so that less CSF leaks from the subarachnoid space (Gielen 1989).

Hypotension

Untreated hypotension, secondary to sympathetic nerve block, leading to relative hypovolaemia and decreased venous return, can be very detrimental to the elderly patient, especially those with limited cardiac reserve. Ageing is associated with a reduction in the baroreceptor mediated heart rate response to hypotension, so elderly patients may not produce the same increase in sympathetic activity as young ones (Priebe 2000). Carpenter and colleagues (1992) found that high levels of sensory block and increasing age appeared to be the two main risk factors for the development of hypotension. Decreased cardiac reserve, structural changes in the arterioles, and changes in the autonomic nervous system with increasing age may play a role. Transthoracic electrical bioimpedance studies of subarachnoid block in elderly patients (53–96 years) revealed that systolic blood pressure decreased by 25% as early as

6–9 minutes after the block (Critchley et al. 1994). Cardiac output was unaffected because a decrease in stroke index in the more severe cases of hypotension was compensated for by an increase in heart rate. The higher the block, the more aggressive was the treatment required.

Opinions on managing hypotension in elderly patients during central nerve block range from the administration of moderate volumes of intravenous fluid to the use of vasopressors. Administration of ephedrine prophylactically with a fluid preload, usually about 7 ml kg^{-1}, has been recommended (Critchley 1996). It should be emphasized, however, that rapid preloading constitutes a potential risk in older patients with limited cardiac reserve, and hypotension commonly follows spinal anaesthesia in normovolaemic elderly patients undergoing elective procedures, irrespective of whether or not any fluid is given (Buggy et al. 1997). Since the potential for exaggerated cardiovascular changes during a subarachnoid block is directly related to the height of the block, one of the most effective methods of preventing hypotension is to avoid a high sensory block. Unfortunately, injection at the L_4/L_5 interspace offers no advantage in this respect compared with injection at L_3/L_4 (Veering et al 1996).

The incidence and severity of hypotension can be reduced by injecting local anaesthetic solutions incrementally. There is some control over the level of block and the slower onset allows time for auto-compensation. Continuous spinal (CSA), continuous epidural, and the combined technique can all be used to minimize hypotension, not only while the block is being established, but throughout the course of the anaesthetic. Miville and colleagues (2006) found that small, titrated doses of hyperbaric bupivacaine, injected using CSA, produced better haemodynamic stability in elderly patients than single-dose spinal anaesthesia. When haemodynamic stability is critically important a catheter technique may be optimum in the elderly.

Confusion

Prompt and complete postoperative recovery of mental function to the preoperative state is particularly important in elderly patients if mental faculties are already compromised by age-related disease or drug therapy. Elderly surgical, particularly orthopaedic (Silverstein et al 2007), patients are prone to non-specific symptoms of central nervous system dysfunction such as confusion, delirium, transient fluctuations of consciousness and mood, and severe disruption of sleep in the first week after surgery. In most cases, recovery of cognitive function is prompt and complete within 1 week. The cause is probably multifactorial (Silverstein et al. 2007), but sensitivity to benzodiazepines and anticholinergic drugs is increased, and even the relatively sparing use of intravenous sedation may delay the recovery of mental function which usually occurs after regional anaesthesia. Prolongation of an altered mental state for more than a week after surgery is most common in patients with a previous history of psychiatric disturbance, particularly clinical depression. Choice of anaesthesia technique (general or regional) has not been found to be significant (Rasmussen 2006).

Hypothermia

Hypothermia (a decrease in core temperature) is common in patients undergoing surgery under central nerve block. Elderly patients are at particular risk because low core temperature may not trigger protective vasomotor reflexes, so their responses may be delayed or less efficient than in younger subjects (Sessler 2008). The impaired autonomic response may explain why elderly patients have a lower threshold for shivering during spinal anaesthesia. This is a potentially serious problem because the elderly have a higher incidence of ischaemic heart disease and may not be able to tolerate the increased oxygen demands associated with shivering. Body temperature is reduced more by general anaesthesia than epidural block when the operating theatre temperature is cold, but there is little difference when the environment is relatively warm. The time required for postoperative rewarming also appears to increase directly with advancing age.

Peripheral nerve block

Peripheral blocks are used frequently in elderly patients especially as supplementary analgesic techniques for upper limb trauma, hip and knee surgery, but more studies need to be performed to establish their characteristics in this group. However, both sensory and motor effects have been shown to last approximately 2.5 times longer in elderly than younger patients after both brachial plexus block with ropivacaine (Paqueron et al 2002) and sciatic nerve block with mepivacaine (Hanks et al. 2006). Femoral nerve (3-in-1) block was found to provide prolonged pain relief without local anaesthetic toxicity in elderly patients (Snoeck et al. 2003).

Regional versus general anaesthesia

The issues surrounding the choice between regional and general anaesthesia are considered at length in Chapters 3 and 5. Many of the studies, and thus the subsequent meta-analyses (e.g. Rodgers et al. 2000, which have addressed this question include elderly patients, but few have focused on this age group, those which have raising the same issues (e.g. Ballantyne 2004) as are considered in the earlier chapters. A few examples will illustrate the point:

- Several studies showed that regional anaesthesia decreased the incidence of postoperative arterial graft occlusion in elderly patients (Christopherson et al. 1993, Rosenfeld et al. 1993, Tuman et al. 1991), but this specific benefit may no longer apply because new antithrombotic drugs have been developed.

- Norris and colleagues (2001) performed a randomization of 168 elderly patients undergoing major aortic surgery to one of four groups, each receiving a different combination of intraoperative anaesthetic and postoperative care regimens. Postoperative outcome was uninfluenced by these variations, superficially suggesting that the standard of perioperative care is more important that than the specific anaesthetic of analgesic regimen. This may be an important issue, but the numbers of patients involved were small compared to those now considered to be valid for such studies.

- Hip fracture is common in the elderly, and regional anaesthesia was once thought to reduce long-term mortality, but the current view is that there is *insufficient evidence from randomized trials* to support this view (Parker & Griffith 2004). Modern data confirm that it can reduce postoperative pain, morphine consumption, and nausea and vomiting compared with systemic analgesia (Macfarlane 2009), but length of stay is not reduced and rehabilitation after total hip arthroplasty does not appear to be facilitated.

- A meta-analysis showed that thoracic epidural analgesia was superior to the lumbar route in reducing postoperative myocardial infarction (Beattie et al. 2001), suggesting that wider use of thoracic block is warranted in elderly, high-risk patients.

Age-related disease, as opposed to old age per se, is primarily responsible for the progressive increase in morbidity and mortality of elderly surgical patients. Factors other than the choice of anaesthesia may be crucial for long-term survival.

Overview

Elderly patients are more sensitive to local anaesthetic agents. Central techniques produce greater degrees of sensory and motor block, and the risk of hypotension due to sympathetic block is greater also. What little evidence there is suggests that the effects of this greater sensitivity are seen after peripheral nerve block as well. However, this group is also very sensitive to the side effects of other analgesic drugs, especially the opioids, so regional techniques have much to offer, especially given the greater incidence of intercurrent disease. Distorted anatomy increases the technical challenge of block placement in many patients, and particular care is needed to avoid injury to joints and skin, so the use of regional techniques in this age group requires particular skill and experience.

Key references

Sadean MR, Glass PS (2003) Pharmacokinetics in the elderly. *Bailliere's Best Practice & Research in Clinical Anaesthesiology* 17: 191–205.

Tsui BC, Wagner A, Finucane B (2004) Regional anaesthesia in the elderly: a clinical guide. *Drugs and Aging* 21: 895–910.

On-line resources

http://www.aaa-online.org.uk Age Anaesthesia Association.

http://www.sagahq.org/ Society for the Advancement of Geriatric Anesthesia.

References

Ballantyne JC (2004) Does epidural analgesia improve surgical outcome? *British Journal of Anaesthesia* 92: 4–6.

Beattie W, Badner N, Choi P (2001) Epidural analgesia reduced postoperative myocardial infarction: a meta-analysis. *Anesthesia & Analgesia* 93: 853–8.

Ben-David B, Frankel R, Arzumonov T, et al. (2000) Minidose bupivacaine-fentanylspinal anesthesia for surgical repair of hip fracture in the aged. *Anesthesiology* 92: 6–10.

Bromage PR (1978) *Epidural analgesia*. Philadelphia, PA: WB Saunders.

Buggy D, Higgins P, Moran C, et al. (1997) Prevention of spinal anesthesia-induced hypotension in the elderly: comparison between preanesthetic administration of crystalloids, colloids and no prehydration. *Anesthesia & Analgesia* 84: 106–10.

Burm AGL (1989) Clinical pharmacokinetics of epidural and spinal anaesthesia. *Clinical Pharmacokinetics* 16: 283–311.

Burm AG, Van Kleef JW, Vermeulen NP, et al. (1988) Pharmacokinetics of lidocaine and bupivacaine following subarachnoid administration in surgical patients: simultaneous investigation of absorption and disposition kinetics using stable isotopes. *Anesthesiology* 69: 584–92.

Catley DM, Thornton C, Jordan C, et al. (1985) Pronounced, episodic oxygen desaturation with ventilatory pattern and analgesic regimen. *Anesthesiology* 63: 20–8.

Carpenter RL, Caplan RA, Brown DL, et al. (1992) Incidence and risk factors for side effects of spinal anesthesia. *Anesthesiology* 76: 906–12.

Christopherson R, Beattie C, Meinert CL, et al. (1993) Perioperative Ischemia Randomized Anaesthesia Trial Study Group: Perioperative morbidity in patients randomized to epidural or general anaesthesia for lower extremity vascular surgery. *Anesthesiology* 79: 422–34.

Critchley LAH (1996) Hypotension, subarachnoid block and the elderly patient. *Anaesthesia* 51: 1139–43.

Critchley LH, Stuart JC, Short TG, Gin T (1994) Haemodynamic effects of subarachnoid block in elderly patients. *British Journal of Anaesthesia* 73: 464–70.

Fernandez-Galinski D, Rué M, Moral V, et al. (1996) Spinal anaesthesia with bupivacaine and fentanyl in geriatric patients. *Anesthesia & Analgesia* 83: 537–41.

Ferrer-Brechner T (1986) Spinal and epidural anaesthesia in the elderly. *Seminars in Anesthesiology* V: 54–61.

Fukuda T, Kakiuchi Y, Miyabe M, et al. (2003) Free lidocaine concentrations during continuous epidural anesthesia in geriatric patients. *Regional Anesthesia and Pain Medicine* 28: 215–20.

Gielen M (1989) Postdural headache (PDPH). *A review. Regional Anesthesia* 14: 101–1

Hakanson E, Rutberg H, Jorfeldt L, Wiklund L (1984) Endocrine and metabolic responses after standardized moderate surgical trauma: Influence of age and sex. *Clinical Physiology* 4: 461–73.

Hanks RK, Pietrobon R, Steele SM, et al. (2006) The effect of age on sciatic nerve block duration. *Anesthesia & Analgesia* 102: 588–92.

Hirabayashi Y, Shimizu R (1993) Effect of age on extradural dose requirement in thoracic extradural anaesthesia. *British Journal of Anaesthesia* 71: 445–6.

Kehlet H (1989) Surgical stress: the role of pain and analgesia. *British Journal of Anaesthesia* 63: 189–95.

Macfarlane AJ, Prasad GA, Chan VW, Brull R (2009) Does regional anaesthesia improve outcome after total hip arthroplasty? A systematic review. *British Journal of Anaesthesia* 103: 335–45.

May C, Kaye JA, Atack JR, et al. (1990) Cerebrospinal fluid production is reduced in healthy aging. *Neurology* 40: 500–3.

Minville V, Fourcade O, Grousset D, et al. (2006) Spinal anesthesia using single injection small-dose bupivacaine versus continuous catheter injection techniques for surgical repair of hip fracture in elderly patients. *Anesthesia & Analgesia* 102: 1559–63.

Norris EJ, Beattie C, Perler BA, et al. (2001) Double-masked randomized trial comparing alternate combinations of intraoperative anesthesia and postoperative analgesia in abdominal aortic surgery. *Anesthesiology* 95: 1054–67.

Olofsen E, Burm AGL, Simon M, et al. (2008) Population pharmacokinetic-pharmacodynamic modeling of epidural anesthesia. *Anesthesiology* 109: 664–74.

Paqueron X, Boccara G, Bendahou M, et al. (2002) Brachial plexus nerve block exhibits prolonged duration in the elderly. *Anesthesiology* 97: 1245–9.

Parker M J, Handoll HH, Griffiths R (2004) Anaesthesia for hip fracture surgery in adults. *Cochrane Database of Systemic Reviews* 4: CD000521.

Priebe HJ (2000) The aged cardiovascular risk patient. *British Journal of Anaesthesia* 85: 763–78.

Rasmussen LS (2006) Postoperative cognitive dysfunction: incidence and prevention. *Baillieres Best Practice & Research in Clinical Anaesthesiology* 20: 315–30.

Ready LB, Chadwick HS, Ross B (1987) Age predicts effective epidural morphine dose after abdominal hysterectomy. *Anesthesia & Analgesia* 66: 1215–18.

Ready LB, Loper KA, Nessley M, Wild L (1991) Postoperative epidural morphine is safe on surgical wards. *Anesthesiology* 75: 452–6.

Rodgers A, Walker N, Schug S, et al. (2000) Reduction of postoperative mortality and morbidity with epidural or spinal anaesthesia: results from overview of randomised trials. *British Medical* Journal 321: 1493.

Rosenfeld BA, Beattie C, Christopherson R, et al. (1993) Perioperative Ischemia Randomized Anaesthesia Trial Study Group: The effects of different anesthetic regimen on fibrinolysis and the development of postoperative arterial thrombosis. *Anesthesiology* 79: 435–43.

Sadean MR, Glass PS (2003) Pharmacokinetics in the elderly. *Bailliere's Best Practice & Research in Clinical Anaesthesiology.* 17: 191–205.

Sakura S, Saito Y, Kosaka Y (1995) The effects of epidural anesthesia on ventilatory response to hypercapnia and hypoxia in elderly patients. *Anesthesia & Analgesia* 82: 306–11.

Sessler DI (2008) Temperature monitoring and perioperative thermoregulation. *Anesthesiology* 109: 318–38.

Silverstein JH, Timberger M, Reich DL, et al. (2007) Central nervous system dysfunction after noncardiac surgery and anesthesia in the elderly. *Anesthesiology* 106: 622–8.

Snoeck MM, Vree TB, Gielen MJ, Lagertweit AJ (2003) Steady state bupivacaine plasma concentrations and safety of a femoral '3-in-1' nerve block with bupivacaine in patients over 80 years of age. *International Journal of Clinical Pharmacology and Therapeutics* 41: 107–13.

Simon MJ, Veering BT (2010) Factors affecting the pharmacokinetics and neural block characteristics after epidural administration of local anaesthetics. *European Journal of Pain (Supplement)* 4: 209–18.

Simon MJ, Veering BT, Stienstra R, et al. (2002) The effects of age on neural blockade and hemodynamic changes after epidural anesthesia with ropivacaine. *Anesthesia & Analgesia* 94: 1325–30.

Simon MJ, Veering BT, Stienstra R, et al. (2004) Effect of age on the clinical profile and systemic absorption and disposition of levobupivacaine after epidural administration. *British Journal of Anaesthesia* 93: 512–20.

Simon MJG, Veering BT, Burm AGL, et al. (2006) The effect of age on the systemic absorption and disposition of ropivacaine following epidural anesthesia. *Anesthesia & Analgesia* 101: 276–82.

Tsui BC, Wagner A, Finucane B (2004) Regional anaesthesia in the elderly: a clinical guide. *Drugs and Aging* 21: 895–910.

Tuman KJ, McCarthy RJ, Marck RJ, et al. (1991) Effects of epidural anaesthesia and analgesia on coagulation and outcome after major vascular surgery. *Anesthesia & Analgesia* 73: 696–70.

Varrassi G, Celleno D, Capogna G, et al. (1992) Ventilatory effects of subarachnoid fentanyl in the elderly. *Anaesthesia* 47: 558–62.

Vassilieff N, Rosencher N, Sessler DI, Conseiller C (1995) Shivering threshold during spinal anaesthesia is reduced in elderly patients. *Anesthesiology* 83: 1162–6.

Veering BT, Burm AGL, Van Kleef JW, et al. (1987) Epidural anaesthesia with bupivacaine: effects of age on neural blockade and pharmacokinetics. *Anesthesia & Analgesia* 66: 589–94.

Veering BT, Burm AGL, Vletter AA, et al. (1992) The effect of age on the systemic absorption and systemic disposition of bupivacaine after epidural administration. *Clinical Pharmacokinetics* 22: 75–84.

Veering BT, Ter Riet PM, Burm AGL, et al. (1996) Spinal anaesthesia with hyperbaric 0.5% bupivacaine in elderly patients: effect of the site of injection on the spread of analgesia. *British Journal of Anaesthesia* 77: 1–4.

Veering BT, Burm AGL, Feyen HM, et al. (2002) Pharmacokinetics of bupivacaine during postoperative epidural infusion; enantioselectivity and role of protein binding. *Anesthesiology* 96: 1062–9.

Index